Chronic Wound Care:
The Essentials

A Clinical Source Book for
Healthcare Professionals

Edited by
Diane L. Krasner, PhD, RN, FAAN

With more than 50 contributors

Chronic Wound Care:
The Essentials

A Clinical Source Book for
Healthcare Professionals

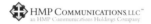
HMP COMMUNICATIONS, LLC™
an HMP Communications Holdings Company

President: **Bill Norton**
Executive Vice President: **Peter Norris**
Vice President/Group Publisher: **Jeremy Bowden**
Special Projects Editor: **Amanda Wright**
Creative Director: **Vic Geanopulos**
Senior Production Manager: **Andrea Steiger**
Production/Circulation Director: **Kathy Murphy**

Copyright ® 2014
HMP Communications, LLC
83 General Warren Blvd., Suite 100
Malvern, PA 19355

ISBN 978-1-893446-09-0

DEDICATION

To people with chronic wounds
and their caregivers,
their wound care team
and the entire interprofessional team:
May we all strive to improve
chronic wound care
by sharing & caring!

ACKNOWLEDGEMENT

To the CWCE contributors:
Thank you for sharing your expertise and for
your commitment to chronic wound care.

To the staff at HMP Communications:
Thank you for your ongoing support of the
Chronic Wound Care series.

To my mentor, Dr. George Rodeheaver:
Your guidance and support for almost thirty years
are appreciated beyond words.

To my husband, David A. Welber,
Your love and friendship make every day special!

TABLE OF CONTENTS

TABLE OF CONTENTS

Afsaneh Alavi, MD, FRCPC (Derm)
Department of Medicine (Dermatology)
Women's College Hospital
University of Toronto, Toronto
Ontario, Canada

David G. Armstrong, DPM, PhD, MD
University of Arizona Department of Surgery
Professor of Surgery, Director, Southern Arizona
Limb Salvage Alliance (SALSA)
Tucson, Arizona

Richard Barry, BBA, CHT-A
Vice President of Safety and Technical
Healogics
Jacksonville, Florida

Jennifer A. Berry, FNP-BC
Barnes-Jewish Hospital
Saint Louis, Missouri

Nicholas J. Bevilacqua, DPM, FACFAS
North Jersey Orthopaedic Specialists, P.A.
Teaneck, New Jersey

Shirley Blanchard, PhD, ABDA, OTR/L, FAOTA
Associate Professor of Occupational Therapy
School of Pharmacy and Health Professions
Creighton University
Omaha, Nebraska

Barbara J. Braden, PhD, RN, FAAN
Dean Emerita
Graduate School and University College
Creighton University
Omaha, Nebraska

A.C. Browne, MB, MICGP
General Practitioner
Department of General Practice,
Mercers Medical Centre
Royal College of Surgeons of Ireland
Dublin, Ireland

Sarah M.E. Cockbill, PhD, LL.M, B.Pharm, M.Pharm, DAgVetPharm, MIPharmM, FCPP, FRPharmS
Honorary Lecturer
Cardiff School of Pharmacy & Pharmaceutical
Sciences, Cardiff University, Cardiff
Wales, UK

Gregory A. Compton, MD, CMD
OpenDelta Consulting, LLC
Johns Island, South Carolina

Patricia Coutts, RN
Wound Care and Clinical Trials Coordinator
Toronto Regional Wound Healing Clinic
Mississauga, Ontario, Canada

Linda Cowan, PhD, ARNP, FNP-BC, CWS
Research Health Scientist, Center of Innovation for
Disability and Rehabilitation Research (CIDRR8),
North Florida/South Georgia Veterans Health
System
Adjunct Associate Professor at the University of
Florida College of Nursing
Gainesville, FL

Sue Currence, BSN, RN, CWON
University of Maryland, St. Joseph Medical Center
Towson, Maryland

Jean M. de Leon, MD
Professor, Department of Physical Medicine and
Rehabilitation
University of Texas Southwestern
Dallas, Texas

Morty Eisenberg, MD, MScCH, CCFP, FCFP
Hospitalist Division Head and Wound Consultant,
Sunnybrook Health Sciences Centre
St. John's Rehab Hospital, Toronto
Assistant Professor, Department of Family and
Community Medicine and Dalla Lana School of Public
Health, Faculty of Medicine, University of Toronto
Ontario, Canada

CONTRIBUTORS

Cynthia Ann Fleck, RN, BSN, MBA, APN/CNS, ET/WOCN, CWS, CFCN, DNC
Cynthia Fleck & Associates, LLC
St. Louis, Missouri

Robert G. Frykberg, DPM, MPH
Chief, Podiatry, Carl T. Hayden VA Medical Center
Phoenix, Arizona

Harriet W. Hopf, MD
Professor and Vice Chair, Department of
Anesthesiology, Associate Dean for Academic Affairs
University of Utah School of Medicine
Salt Lake City, Utah

Dean P. Kane, MD, FACS
Johns Hopkins Hospital
The Center for Cosmetic Surgery and MediSpa
Baltimore, Maryland

David Keast, BSc (Hon), MSc, DipEd, MD, CCFP, FCFP
Centre Director, Aging, Rehabilitation and Geriatric
Care Research Centre, Lawson Health Research
Institute, St. Joseph's Parkwood Hospital
London, Ontario, Canada

John P. Kirby, MD, MS, FCCWS, FACS
Medical Director, Surgical & Wound Care Clinic,
Barnes-Jewish Hospital, Assistant Professor of
Surgery, Section of Acute & Critical Care Surgery,
Department of Surgery, Washington University in St.
Louis School of Medicine
Saint Louis, Missouri

Diane L. Krasner, PhD, RN, CWCN, CWS, MAPWCA, FAAN
Wound & Skin Care Consultant, Adjunct Faculty,
Nursing & Allied Health, Harrisburg Area,
Community College – York Campus, Instructor,
Achieve Test Prep – York Campus, APPRISE (PA
SHIP) Counselor, York County Area Agency of Aging
York, Pennsylvania

Stephan J. Landis, MD, FRCPC
Department of Hospital Medicine, and Ambulatory
Wound Clinic, Guelph General Hospital
Guelph, Ontario, Canada
Dermatology Day Care and Wound Clinic
Women's College Hospital
Toronto, Ontario, Canada

James B. Lutz, MS, CCRA
Lutz Consulting, LLC, Medical Writing Services
Buellton, CA

Heather McConnell, RN, BScN, MA (Ed)
Associate Director, International Affairs and Best
Practice Guidelines Centre, Registered Nurses'
Association of Ontario
Ontario, Canada

Jeffery A. Niezgoda, MD, FACHM, MAPWCA, CHWS
President, The American College of Hyperbaric
Medicine, President and Chief Medical Officer,
WebCME.net, Medical Director AZH Centers,
Medical Director, Sheehan Care Plan Centers,
Consultant in Wound Care & Hyperbaric Medicine
Milwaukee, Wisconsin

Linda Norton, BScOT, OT Reg (ONT), MScCH
National Educator, Shoppers Home Health Care
Director, Interprofessional Team, Canadian
Association of Wound Care Institute
Toronto, Ontario

Heather L. Orsted, RN, BN, ET, MSc
Principal, eQuadra Solutions Inc.
Abbotsford, BC, Canada

Priscilla Phillips, PhD
Department of Oral Biology
University of Florida
Gainesville, Florida

Mary Ellen Posthauer, RDN, CD, LD
Consulting Dietitian, Past Director/President
National Pressure Ulcer Advisory Panel

Patricia Price, BA (Hons), PhD, AFBPsS, CPsychol, FHEA
Department of Wound Healing
School of Medicine, Cardiff University
Cardiff, United Kingdom

Catherine R. Ratliff, PhD, APRN-BC, CWOCN, CFCN
University of Virginia Health System
Charlottesville, Virginia

George T. Rodeheaver, PhD
Professor and Director
Plastic Surgery Research
University of Virginia Medical Center
Charlottesville, Virginia

Siobhan Ryan, MD, FRCPC
Assistant Professor
Division of Dermatology
Department of Medicine
University of Toronto
Toronto, Ontario, Canada

Pamela Scarborough, PT, DPT, MS, CDE, CWS, CEEAA
Director of Public Policy and Education
American Medical Technologies
Irvine, California

Jos M.G.A. Schols, MD, PhD
Professor of Old Age Medicine
Department of Family Medicine and Department of Health Services Research
Caphri - School for Public Health and Primary Care,
Maastricht University
Maastricht, The Netherlands

Gregory Schultz, PhD
UF Research Foundation Professor
Department of Obstetrics and Gynecology
Institute for Wound Research
University of Florida
Gainesville, Florida

R. Gary Sibbald, BSc, MD, MEd, FRCPC (Med), FRCPC (Derm), MACP, FAAD, MAPWCA
Professor of Medicine and Public Health
University of Toronto, Director
International Interprofessional Wound Care Course
(IIWCC- University of Toronto, Stellenbosch
University, New York University, Abu Dhabi) and
Masters of Science in Community Health
(Prevention and Wound Care)
Dalla Lana Faculty of Public Health, Past President,
World Union of Wound Healing Societies

Adrianne P. S. Smith, MD
President and CEO
APS Medical Consultants
San Antonio, Texas

Stephen Sprigle, PhD, PT
Professor, Applied Physiology, Bioengineering &
Industrial Design
Georgia Institute of Technology
Atlanta, Georgia

Linda A. Stamm[†], APRN-BC, CWS (deceased)
Formerly at Barnes- Jewish Hospital at Washington
University, School of Medicine
Saint Louis, Missouri

Joyce Stechmiller, PhD, ACNP-BC, FAAN
Department Chair
Department of Adults and Elderly
Associate Professor of Nursing
College of Nursing, University of Florida
Gainesville, Florida

CONTRIBUTORS

Nancy A. Stotts, RN, EdD, FAAN
Professor Emeritus
University of California, San Francisco
San Francisco, California

Terence D. Turner, OBE, FRPharmS, MPharm
University of Wales College of Medicine
Cardiff, United Kingdom

Lia van Rijswijk, MSN, RN, CWCN
Instructor, Holy Family University School of Nursing
and Allied Health Professions
Philadelphia, Pennsylvania
Clinical Editor *Ostomy Wound Management*, HMP
Communications
Malvern, Pennsylvania

**Robert A. Warriner, III‡, MD, FCCP, FACWS,
FAPWCA (deceased)**
Former Chief Medical Officer, Healogics
Jacksonville, Florida

Dot Weir, RN, CWON, CWS
Osceola Regional Medical Center
Kissimmee, Florida

**James R. Wilcox, RN, BSN, ACHRN, CWCN,
CFCN, CWS, WCC, DAPWCA, FCCWS**
Immediate Past President, Baromedical Nurses
Association, Director of Research & Quality for
Medical Affairs, Healogics
Jacksonville, FL

Deidre D. Wipke-Tevis, RN, PhD
Associate Professor & PhD Program Director
Sinclair School of Nursing
University of Missouri-Columbia,
Columbia, Missouri

Kathy Whittington, RN, MS, CWCN
Clinical Support Manager
Span-America
Greenville, South Carolina

Laurel A. Wiersema-Bryant, APRN, BC, CWS
Barnes-Jewish Hospital at Washington University,
School of Medicine
Saint Louis, Missouri

Kevin Y. Woo, PhD, RN, FAPWCA
Assistant Professor, School of Nursing
Queen's University
Kingston, Ontario, Canada

Stephanie C. Wu, DPM, MS
Biomechanics, Dr. William M. Scholl College of
Podiatric Medicine
Associate Professor, Center for Stem Cell and
Regenerative Medicine
Rosalind Franklin University of Medicine and Science
North Chicago, Illinois

With the aging of the baby boomers and impending epidemics of diabetes, Alzheimer's disease, and other chronic illnesses, there has never been a more urgent need for knowledgeable chronic wound care providers. **Chronic Wound Care: The Essentials (CWCE)** does just that: it presents **the essentials** of chronic wound care that all wound team members need to know—from nurse aides to physicians. Unfortunately, the education that healthcare practitioners of all levels receive contains very little emphasis on the details of wound care. Practitioners interested in wound care usually have to educate themselves. This new book in HMP Communications' **Chronic Wound Care series** will be an invaluable resource for clinicians. Administrators, industry members, insurers, legal professionals, healthcare students, and others with an interest in wound care will also find **CWCE** to be an **essential** reference.

In this time of technological advancement, education is a continuous lifelong process. Even those practitioners and researchers who have dedicated their careers to wound care have difficulty keeping pace with the rapidly expanding information on the subject. This wealth of new information is manageable only if there is a well-organized, basic foundation upon which to correctly add and interpret the importance of these new bricks of information. Without the basic foundation, the dedicated practitioner is buried in a random pile of facts and figures.

Since 1990, nurse specialist Diane Krasner has been recruiting interprofessional wound care experts to share their expertise and insights in the **Chronic Wound Care series** (1990-2012, Editions 1-5). **CWCE** contains 23 of the most **essential** chapters from recent editions of the **Chronic Wound Care series** plus two new chapters. Over fifty leaders in the field of wound care share their clinical experiences, research results, expertise, and current opinions. Each of these chapters is an **essential** brick for building the foundation of knowledge required of each wound care practitioner. Whether you are a beginning practitioner or an experienced professional, this book will educate or re-educate you on the optimal ways to care for patients with chronic wounds.

George T. Rodeheaver, PhD
Director, Plastic Surgery Research Lab
University of Virginia School of Medicine
Charlottesville, Virginia

Whether you are new to healthcare, a seasoned healthcare professional with a new focus, need to update yourself on wound care, or are an interested professional (eg, administrator, industry member, insurer, or legal professional), chronic wound care is a hard topic to grasp. The goal of **Chronic Wound Care: The Essentials (CWCE)** is to provide you with **essential** information on the topic in one easy-to-use reference.

I gleaned need-to-know information from the last two editions of **Chronic Wound Care: A Clinical Source Book for Healthcare Professionals** (CWC4 2007; CWC5 2012) to form this book. Two new chapters were added and several others were updated. The result is a resource that covers all of the fundamental aspects of chronic wound care. I encourage you to start your journey by reading Chapter 1, a new overview chapter by Dr. Gregory Compton and me. Then select chapters by specific topic based on your professional needs. Be sure to review the objectives and Take-Home Messages For Practice in each chapter and if you are preparing for a certification exam, each chapter has several self-assessment questions at the end.

Fifty-three contributors—national and international thought-leaders in wound care—share their experience and expertise with you in the 25 chapters of **CWCE**. I hope that you will incorporate this information into your practice and share it with others.

**If you have knowledge,
Let others light their candles by it.**

-Sarah Margaret Fuller

Diane L. Krasner
PhD, RN, CWCN, CWS, MAPWCA, FAAN
Wound & Skin Care Consultant
York, Pennsylvania

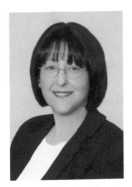

Diane L. Krasner, PhD, RN, CWCN, CWS, MAPWCA, FAAN

Dr. Diane L. Krasner is a board certified wound specialist with experience in wound, ostomy & incontinence care across the continuum of care. She is a Fellow of the American Academy of Nursing and a Master of the American Professional Wound Care Association. Dr. Krasner is a wound & skin care consultant and part-time nursing instructor in York, PA. She is a volunteer at the York County Area Agency on Aging.

Krasner graduated from The Johns Hopkins University with a B.A. and M.A. in Ancient Near Eastern History and Egyptology. She went on to receive her BSN, MS and PhD from the University of Maryland School of Nursing and a M.S. in Adult and Continuing Education from Johns Hopkins School of Continuing Studies. Dr. Krasner was a Johnson & Johnson Medical Post Doctoral Fellow at the Center for Nursing Research at Johns Hopkins University School of Nursing.

Dr. Krasner served as the lead co-editor of five editions of *Chronic Wound Care: A Clinical Source Book for Healthcare Professionals* (1991–2012, HMP Communications, Malvern, PA). She is the sole editor of the new text *Chronic Wound Care: The Essentials* (2014, HMP Communications, Malvern, PA). She has served on numerous editorial boards and currently is on the editorial boards of *The Journal of Legal Nurse Consulting, Ostomy Wound Management, Long-Term Living, The International Journal of Wound Care, World Wide Wounds, WoundSource,* and *WOUNDS*. Since 1992, Dr. Krasner has served on the Board of Directors and as an officer of several national wound care organizations.

Dr. Krasner's research interests include wound pain, palliative wound care and legal issues related to wound care. She has numerous publications in the wound care literature and lectures nationally and internationally on wound & skin care.

CHAPTER 1

Chronic Wound Care: An Overview

Diane L. Krasner, PhD, RN, CWCN, CWS, MAPWCA, FAAN
Gregory A. Compton, MD, CMD

Objectives

The reader will be challenged to:
- Describe the phenomenon of chronic wounds with its growing importance for patients, caregivers, healthcare providers, systems, and society
- Appraise the challenges of caring for people with chronic wounds
- Identify 7 skills and 5 principles for chronic wound care

What is a Chronic Wound?

Most people are familiar with acute wounds (eg, abrasions, minor burns, incontinence-associated dermatitis, lacerations, skin tears) that go on to heal without complications following the normal healing trajectory. Individuals with chronic wounds—wounds that do not heal in the normal manner—often learn about the phenomenon for the first time when confronted with one of the major categories of chronic wounds: vascular (eg, arterial, venous, or mixed ulcers); pressure ulcers; neuropathic ulcers (eg, diabetic foot wounds); or non-healing/palliative wounds. PLATES 1-6, page 342, illustrate common types of chronic wounds.

A widely used, formal definition of a chronic wound was published by the Wound Healing Society group in 1994. They define chronic wounds as wounds that "fail to progress through a normal, orderly, and timely sequence of repair or wounds that pass through the repair process without restoring anatomic and functional results."[1] In 2009 the European Pressure Ulcer Advisory Panel (EPUAP) and the National Pressure Ulcer Advisory Panel (NPUAP) in the US, published a clinical practice guideline entitled, *Pressure Ulcer Prevention & Treatment*, that defined a chronic wound as "a wound that does not proceed through the normal stages of healing but becomes stuck in one phase."[2] Other definitions include a time component, such as a wound that fails to heal in 3 months.[3] *The goals and plans of care for chronic wound patients are different than those for acute wound patients. The underlying pathology that causes the healing process to stall*

Krasner DL, Compton GA. Chronic Wound Care: An Overview. In: Krasner DL, ed. Chronic Wound Care: The Essentials. Malvern, Pa: HMP Communications, 2014:1–6.

must be addressed. The care of chronic wounds is much more challenging than the management of acute wounds.

One of the most common and challenging chronic wound types is the pressure ulcer (older terms are decubitus ulcer and bedsore).[4] In 2009 the National Pressure Ulcer Advisory Panel (NPUAP) in the US collaborated with the European Pressure Ulcer Advisory Panel (EPUAP) to develop and publish a clinical practice guideline entitled *Pressure Ulcer Prevention & Treatment.* In this document a pressure ulcer is defined as a "localized injury to the skin and/or underlying tissue, usually over a bony prominence, as a result of pressure or pressure in combination with shear. A number of contributing or confounding factors are also associated with pressure ulcers; the significance of these factors has yet to be elucidated."[2] The pressure ulcer is a common geriatric syndrome that healthcare providers need to address in older, frail populations.[4]

When healing stalls, an acute wound can become a chronic wound and should be reassessed and documented as such. For example, an acute surgical incision that dehisces secondary to wound infection becomes a chronic wound. Another common example is a lower leg traumatic abrasion that becomes a chronic venous ulcer in the person with chronic venous insufficiency. A chronic wound can become an acute wound. For example, a chronic pressure ulcer after surgical myocutaneous flap repair becomes an acute surgical wound. *It is important that such changes in wound status are recognized and correctly documented along with other assessment parameters and treatment information in the medical record as mandated by payers, especially on government data base assessments such as the MDS and OASIS[5,6]* (see Chapter 4 for more information on assessment and documentation).

Why are Chronic Wounds an Important Issue for Patients, Caregivers, the Healthcare System, and Society?

The toll that chronic wounds take on patients, caregivers, the healthcare system, and society is staggering. From the patient and caregiver perspective, chronic wounds may significantly impact quality of life, activities of daily living, and productivity. For certain individuals, they may also be a source of anxiety, depression, pain, and suffering[7] (see Chapters 9 and 10 for a more detailed discussion).

Chronic wounds are currently estimated to affect over 7.5 million people in the United States. These numbers are projected to rise due to our aging population with chronic conditions and the increase in the number of people with diabetes.[8,9] The drain on our healthcare system both in terms of dollars and human resources is extraordinary due to the intensity of care that chronic wound patients require. The financial burden to the US healthcare system alone has been estimated at $20 billion annually.[10]

Chronic wounds of the lower extremity [vascular (eg, arterial, venous, or mixed ulcers); pressure ulcers; neuropathic ulcers (eg, diabetic foot ulcers)] are the most prevalent chronic wounds. Chronic venous insufficiency (CVI) is the most common underlying cause and an estimated 600,000 new ulcers develop annually.[11] Current projections are that 25% of the elderly will experience chronic limb ulceration by the year 2050.[3]

Among people with diabetes, almost 10% develop chronic wounds of the lower extremity with 84% of non-healing ulcers resulting in amputation. The 3-year survival rate following amputation is 50%.[12]

The incidence of chronic wounds in people with dementia, end-stage chronic illness, and at end-of-life is significant and often requires different management approaches.[13] See Chapter 23, *Skin Changes At Life's End* (SCALE), for a detailed discussion.

Should Chronic Wounds be Considered a Quality Indicator?

The notion that chronic wounds should be linked to quality of care actually goes all the way back in written history to Florence Nightingale. In *Notes on Nursing,*[14] originally published in 1859, Ms. Nightingale wrote:

If a patient is cold, if a patient is feverish, if a patient is faint, if he is sick after taking food, if he has a bedsore, it is generally the fault not of the disease, but of the nursing.

Today the majority of wound care professionals appreciate how the interplay of multiple chronic medical conditions and other risk factors converge and create high risk for chronic wounds and impaired wound healing in vulnerable populations. There is a minority viewpoint that pressure ulcers are largely preventable and a result of substandard care.[15]

In the past decade, regulatory agencies, payers, and quality organizations have used pressure ulcer prevalence and incidence as a quality measure. In acute care settings in the United States, facilities are no longer paid for pressure ulcers that develop during a hospital admission.[16] In long-term care, pressure ulcer rates and care are scrutinized by surveyors from state departments of health as well as federal surveyors. Long-term care facilities may receive citations or monetary fines for avoidable pressure ulcers under F Tag 314. It would not be surprising that the facility acquired rates of other types of chronic wounds will be monitored with equal vigilance in the future by regulatory agencies, payers, and quality organizations. Wound care professionals should measure their own facility's chronic wound prevalence and incidence rates and benchmark these rates against national rates if they are not yet doing so.

Are Chronic Wounds a Marker for End-of-Life?

Most chronic wounds reach closure when underlying factors are addressed, but a subset of chronic wounds are non-healable and the best practice is palliative. These wounds and related skin findings that occur at the end of life have been labeled with terms including: the Kennedy Terminal Ulcer,[17] skin failure,[18] and most recently, Skin Changes At Life's End (SCALE).[19]

The first modern historical observation of a pressure ulcer linked to a dying patient was made by Jean-Martin Charcot (1825-1893).[20,21] In a French medical textbook written in 1877, Charcot described a specific type of ulcer that is butterfly in shape and occurring over the sacrum. Patients that developed the ulcers usually died shortly thereafter, so he termed the ulcer **Decubitus Ominosus.** However, Charcot attributed the ulcers to being neuropathic rather than pressure in origin. Charcot's writings of *Decubitus Ominosus* were all but forgotten in the medical literature until recently with renewed interest in skin organ compromise.[20]

Another historical example of chronic wounds

as a marker for end of life comes from the writings of Dr. Alois Alzheimer in Germany. He was on call in 1901 when a 51-year-old woman, Frau August D, was admitted to his asylum for the insane in Frankfort. Dr. Alzheimer followed this patient, studied her symptoms, and presented her case to his colleagues as what came to be known as Alzheimer's disease. When Frau Auguste D died on April 8, 1906, her medical record listed the cause of death as "septicemia due to decubitus."[22] Alzheimer noted, "at the end, she was confined to bed in a fetal position, was incontinent and in spite of all the care and attention given to her, she suffered from decubitus." Here we have the first identified patient with Alzheimer's disease having developed immobility and two pressure ulcers with end-stage Alzheimer's. In our modern times, end-stage Alzheimer's has become an all-too-frequent scenario with multiple complications including SCALE.

Contemporary discussions of the Kennedy Terminal Ulcer, skin failure, and Skin Changes At Life's End (SCALE) add to our understanding of chronic wounds as markers for the end of life. Both quantitative and qualitative research is urgently needed to expand our understanding of this phenomenon and to explicate an evidence base for practice.

The Challenge of Chronic Wound Care

Because chronic wounds do not heal in the usual, predictable manner, they present challenges for patients, caregivers, wound team members, healthcare team members, and health systems. Typical interventions often do not produce easy resolution to healing. Members of the interprofessional wound team must identify specific pathologic host and wound conditions and address them to the extent practicable. Even with the best care some chronic wounds will not heal. *Every wound is unique and every patient is unique. This is a process that requires knowledge, skill, experience, and tenacity. It requires a commitment to care that is person/patient-centered, meets the standard of care, and is as evidence-informed as possible.*[23]

Non-healing wounds can be the result of many conditions or a combination of systemic and local factors[24] such as:

- Chronic disease states (eg, diabetes, renal, or liver disease)
- Immune dysfunction (eg, cancer, HIV)
- Compromised perfusion (eg, arterial or venous insufficiency)
- Infection (eg, local, deep, systemic)
- Drug therapy (eg, anticoagulants, steroids)
- Nutritional issues (eg, obesity, malnutrition)
- Life style issues (eg, smoking, non-adherence)
- Access to care issues (eg, no insurance coverage for optimal treatment modalities)

See Chapter 7, *Cofactors in Impaired Wound Healing*, for additional information.

In the United States, patients with chronic wounds typically are frequent users of the healthcare system and its resources. They experience hospital re-admissions and often require additional care in alternative settings (wound clinics, home care, or long-term care). Holistic care with wound care provided by an interprofessional wound care team is the ideal (see Chapter 2).

Wound care providers must strive to provide care that meets the standard of care and incorporates evidence-informed practice for all patients with chronic wounds. Providing access for people with chronic wounds to the comprehensive care and support that they require will be the most pressing wound care-related challenge in the next decade.

With all of these challenges, here are **7 SKILLS** that should be developed for success in the field of chronic wound care:

1. Respect for patients and caregivers
2. Respect for patient preferences
3. Tenacity
4. Perseverance
5. Creativity
6. Compassion
7. Sharing & Caring

Lifelong learning is a hallmark of every profession. All healthcare professionals need to keep abreast of advances and new discoveries in wound care and incorporate them into patient care.

The wound care offered to each individual must reflect his or her overall goals and plan of care. Chapter 2 discusses three distinct wound care pathways: 1) aggressive, 2) maintenance, and 3) non-healable or palliative. Using patient-centered care approaches, the wound care team should plan the pathway that optimizes the patient's outcome and improves his or her quality of life. This challenge requires excellent assessment skills, open communication, and commitment on the part of the entire healthcare team. For people with non-healing/palliative wounds, expert palliative wound care can help to prevent wound deterioration, infection, and provide comfort.[19]

In conclusion, we challenge you to commit to:

FIVE Chronic Wound Care PRINCIPLES

1. Focus on prevention
2. Use gentle techniques
3. Provide timely interventions that meet or exceed the standard of care
4. Be respectful of patient preferences
5. Maintain a holistic perspective

Take-Home Messages for Practice

- Because chronic wounds do not heal in the usual, predictable manner, they present challenges for patients, caregivers, wound care team members, healthcare providers, and health systems.
- Wound care providers must strive to deliver services for patients with chronic wounds across the continuum of care that meet the standard of care and incorporate evidence-informed practice.
- Commit to 7 skills and 5 chronic wound care principles to be successful in the field of chronic wound care.

Multiple Choice Questions

1. A patient who develops a chronic wound six weeks prior to dying is likely exhibiting which of the following phenomena?
   A. A quality of care issue
   B. SCALE
   C. Acute wound becoming chronic
   D. Chronic wound becoming acute

2. Which of the following is NOT a skill that enhances a chronic wound care practitioner's success?
   A. Adherence to the evidence-base for wound care at all times
   B. Respect for patient preferences
   C. Compassion
   D. Sharing & Caring

Answers: 1 – B, 3 – A

References

1. Lazarus G, Cooper D, Knighton D, et al. Definitions and guidelines for assessment of wounds and evaluation of healing. *Archives of Dermatology*. 1994;130:489-493.

2. National Pressure Ulcer Advisory Panel and European Pressure Ulcer Advisory Panel. Prevention and treatment of pressure ulcers: clinical practice guideline. Washington, DC: National Pressure Ulcer Advisory Panel, 2009.

3. Mustoe TA, O'Shaughnessy K, Kloeters O. Chronic wound pathogenesis and current treatment strategies: a unifying hypothesis. *Plast Reconstr Surg*. 2006;117(7 Suppl):35s-41s.

4. Thomas DR, Compton G, eds. *Pressure Ulcers in the Aging Population: A Guide for Clinicians*. Aging Medicine Series. New York, NY: Humana Press – Springer; 2014.

5. Bryant RA, Nix DP, eds. *Acute and Chronic Wounds: Current Management Concepts*. 4th ed. St. Louis, MO: Mosby Elsevier; 2012.

6. Brown P, ed. *Quick Reference Guide to Wound Care: Palliative, Home and Clinical Practices*. 4th ed. Burlington, MA: Jones & Bartlett Learning; 2013.

7. Reddy M, Cottrill R. *Healing Wounds, Healthy Skin: A Practical Guide for Patients with Chronic Wounds*. New Haven, CT: Yale University Press; 2011.

8. Greer N, Foman N, Dorruan J, et al. *Advanced Wound Care Therapies for Non-Healing Diabetic, Venous and Arterial Ulcers: A Systematic Review*. VA-ESP Project #09-009; 2012.

9. Sen CK, Gordillo GM, Roy S, et al. Human skin wounds: a major and snowballing threat to public health and the economy. *Wound Repair Regen*. 2009;17(6);763-771.

10. Brem H, Maggi J, Nierman D, et al. High cost of stage IV pressure ulcers. *Am J Surg*. 2010;200:473-477.

11. Evidence-Based Clinical Practice Guideline: Chronic Wounds of the Lower Extremity. American Society of Plastic Surgeons, Arlington Heights, IL, 2007.

12. Harrington C, Zagan M, Corea J, et al. A cost analysis of diabetic lower-extremity ulcers. *Diabetes Care*. 2000;23:1333.

13. Collier KS, Protus BM, Bohn CL, Kimbrel JM. *Wound Care At End of Life: A Guide for Hospice Professionals*. Montgomery, AL: HospiScript Services, A Catamaran Company; 2013.

14. Nightingale F. *Notes on Nursing: What It Is and What It Is Not*. Commemorative Edition. Philadelphia, PA: Lippincott; 1992.

15. Olshansky K. Only you can prevent pressure ulcers. *Long-term Living*. 2002. www.ltlmagazine.com. Accessed December 20, 2013.

16. Meddings JA, Reichert H, Hofer T, McMahon LF. Hospital Report Cards for Hospital-Acquired Pressure Ulcers: How Good are the Grades? *Ann Intern Med*. 2013;159:505-513.

17. Kennedy KL. The prevalence of pressure ulcers in an intermediate care facility. *Decubitus*. 1989;2(2):44-45.

18. Langemo DK, Brown G. Skin fails too: acute, chronic, and end-stage skin failure. *Adv Skin Wound Care*. 2006;19(4):206-211.

19. Sibbald RG, Krasner DL, Lutz JB, et al. The SCALE Expert Panel: Skin Changes At Life's End. Final Consensus Document. October 1, 2009.

20. Levine JM. Historical perspective on pressure ulcers: the decubitus ominosus of Jean-Martin Charcot. *J Am Geriatr Soc*. 2005;53(7):1248-1251.

21. Charcot JM. *Lectures on the Diseases of the Nervous System*. Translated by G. Sigerson. London: The New Sydenham Society; 1877.

22. Shenk D. I Have Lost Myself. In: *The Forgetting: Alzheimer's: Portrait of an Epidemic*. Anchor; 2003.

23. Sackett DL, Straus SE, Richardson WS, Rosenberg W, Haynes RB. *Evidence-based Medicine: How to Practice and Teach EBM*. 2nd ed. Edinburgh, Scotland: Churchill Livingstone; 2000.

24. Woo KY, Krasner DL, Sibbald RG. Palliative Wound Care and Treatment at End of Life. In: Thomas DR, Compton G, eds. *Pressure Ulcers in the Aging Population: A Guide for Clinicians*. Aging Medicine Series. New York, NY: Humana Press – Springer; 2014.

CHAPTER 2

International Interprofessional Wound Caring

Diane L. Krasner, PhD, RN, CWCN, CWS, MAPWCA, FAAN;

George T. Rodeheaver, PhD;

R. Gary Sibbald, BSc, MD, MEd, FRCPC (Med, Derm), MACP, FAAD, MAPWCA;

Kevin Y. Woo, PhD, RN, FAPWCA

Objectives

The reader will be challenged to:

- Conceptualize the dimensions of the International Interprofessional Wound Caring Model 2012©
- Analyze his or her own practice by comparing and contrasting it to the International Interprofessional Wound Caring Model 2012
- Commit to completing a personal scorecard and construct a personal learning portfolio
- Relate the needs of his or her practice and the needs of the person with wounds to his or her social responsibility for care at community, national, and international levels.

Introduction

A person with a chronic wound often suffers from a myriad of biopsychosocial problems, such as physical disability, pain, social needs, and mental anguish. Addressing these multiple issues properly requires skilled help from knowledgeable wound care professionals; however, wound care expertise and knowledge of the evidence base for practice alone usually are not enough to heal a chronic wound and improve the life of the person with that wound.

In this chapter, the editors of *Chronic Wound Care: A Clinical Source Book for Healthcare Professionals* present the International Interprofessional Wound Caring Model 2012© (Figure 1 and Plate 7 on page 343). Our goals for you are to think about your own work environment and to reflect on whether your environment enables you to practice interprofessional wound care. We challenge you to analyze how your current practice model compares and contrasts with ours. Then ask yourself and other members of your team if you can improve your interprofessional wound caring practice model. Additionally, we challenge you to complete your own personal scorecard and to construct your personal learning portfolio for your continuous professional development and lifelong learning.

We conceptualize *person*, *patient*, and *circle of care* will be utilized in the following manner. When the term *person* is used, this refers to an autonomous individual with no specific healthcare relationship for diagnosis and treatment. When the term *patient* is used, the healthcare provider-

Krasner DL, Rodeheaver GT, Sibbald R.G, Woo KY. International interprofessional wound caring. In: Krasner DL, ed. *Chronic Wound Care: The Essentials.* Malvern, PA: HMP Communications; 2014:7–16.

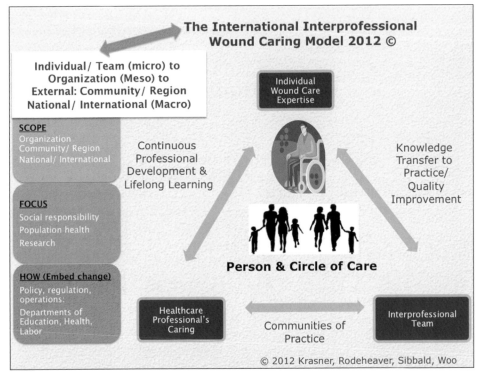

Figure 1. The International Interprofessional Wound Caring Model 2012. © 2012 Krasner, Rodeheaver, Sibbald, Woo.

patient relationship is implied, including the legal obligation to care. To facilitate expression of all those involved in a person's biopsychosocial environment, we use the expression, *the person's circle of care*. This is not used as a legal term in this textbook as outlined elsewhere. It is utilized as a social term that includes all of the stakeholders in the patient's health and well-being. The circle includes, but is not limited to, the patient, a legal guardian or responsible party, a spouse or significant other, interested friends or family members, caregivers, and any other individual(s) who may have active involvement or interest in the patient's care and well-being.

A person with a wound and his or her circle of care need the wound care expert's professional knowledge and skill, but they also require the expertise of other members of the interprofessional team, including generalist physicians and nurses, physical therapists, dietitians, pharmacists, social workers, discharge planners, and so on. The mix of professionals that one patient needs will dif-

fer from another patient's through individualized patient-centered care.

Each individual healthcare professional's caring behavior is an essential dimension of our model. We sincerely believe that without this commitment to the call to care by all members of the team, wound care cannot be optimized. The human touch — reaching out to the person with a wound and his or her circle of care — builds the trust and the confidence that heals wounds, people, and lives.

Person, Circle of Care, and Population

The first dimension that is central to the model is that of the person with a wound and his or her circle of care. Several key factors often contribute to the development of chronic wounds. People with chronic wounds are often older — the average age is 70 years for venous leg ulcer sufferers and 60 years for people with diabetic neuropathic foot ulcers. These individuals frequently have coexisting medical conditions that can impair healing. Oral drugs prescribed for patients' medical needs often interfere with the wound healing process. Chronic wound patients often experience pain that has not been adequately addressed by their healthcare team. Several international pain surveys have demonstrated that pain is the third to fifth most important component of care for healthcare providers and may be the first priority for patients.[1] This disconnect emphasizes the need to address individualized patient-centered concerns as part of any chronic wound treatment plan.

Chronic wounds usually interfere with a person's quality of life and activities of daily living. Imagine the social isolation that a person with a leg ulcer feels when he or she cannot eat with the rest of the family because the odor from the wound is offensive. The person with a diabetic neurotrophic foot ulcer can lay awake for hours because of burning and shooting neuropathic pain in both feet at night. The chronic pain, suffering, and diminished quality of life often lead to depression. Depression is particularly common in persons with diabetes due to multiple complications, including neuropathy as well as ischemia, infection, and deformity. Individuals suffering from chronic wounds often have decreased capacity for activities of daily living. They often lack the physical stamina for employment, leading to a high number of absentee days, or even can be trapped into long-term disability. Frequent dressing changes may interfere with employment opportunities, and the cost of supplies may not be covered by the healthcare system. Affected individuals often are unable to walk long distances or stand for any prolonged period of time. They may have difficulty sleeping and even maintaining an adequate level of self-care. We must address all of these patient-centered concerns.

Historically, patients often are given instructions on how to treat a wound with minimal discussion to explain the cause(s) or address patient-centered concerns. The patient may not comprehend the pathophysiology of the wound and the importance of his or her cooperation (and his or her family's and caregiver's cooperation) to promote wound healing. This is typical of the concept of *compliance*, which is the act or process of obeying an order or command. This is very provider-centered care — not patient-centered care. Recent literature has emphasized

the concept of *adherence* or the ability of a patient to follow through on a treatment or regime.[2] The emphasis shifts away from provider-centered care and refocuses on the patient's perspective. To increase the collaborative network even further, the term *coherence* refers to frank discussion between the healthcare professional and the person with a wound, allowing both points of view to be considered and a negotiated treatment plan that incorporates both perspectives to be developed.

We must work toward collaboration to include persons with chronic wounds and their circle of care. We must acknowledge the fact that every person who has a social network of caregivers, family, friends, and concerned acquaintances is likely to have far better outcomes than those individuals who are socially isolated.[3]

Wound Care Expertise

Wound care expertise consists of evidence-based wound care knowledge of the skills and expert knowing gained from clinical experience and of the attitudes and values that we bring to practice as individuals. Healthcare providers can acquire knowledge of the evidence base for wound care by reading or by attending formalized courses, conferences, and seminars. Novice healthcare professionals transition to expert practitioners with time and experience as described by Benner[4] and others. As healthcare providers, we need to treat the whole patient and not just the hole in the patient (Figure 2). Our knowledge base should include expertise about the cause(s) of common chronic wounds, such as venous leg ulcers, pressure ulcers, diabetic neurotrophic foot ulcers, and nonhealing surgical wounds. We also need to know about uncommon chronic wounds, palliative wounds, and deteriorating wounds. This knowledge needs to be complemented with the ability to assess and treat pain, other patient-centered concerns, and local wound care expertise.

Traditional wound care has often been delivered with saline wet-to-dry gauze dressings. Removal of these dressings can cause local bleeding and pain, and the procedure is nursing time-intensive. Since the classic work of Winter[5] in 1962, several advantages for moist wounds have been identified and include a faster healing rate with occlusion and enhanced re-epithelization with removal of eschar. To translate this into everyday practice,

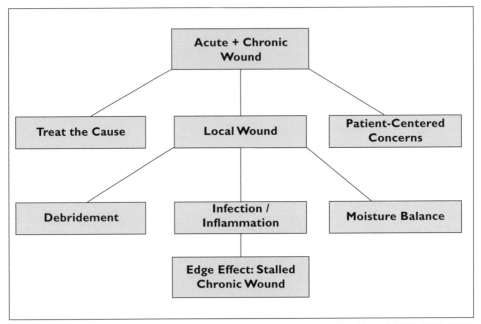

Figure 2. Wound bed preparation paradigm for holistic patient care. Sibbald et al. 2000, 2003, 2006, 2007, WHO 2010, 2011.

several newer, moist, interactive wound dressings have been added to our therapeutic toolkit.

Local wound care expertise goes well beyond the selection of the appropriate dressing to look at criteria to benchmark healing and when to use advanced products, including growth factors, skin substitutes, complementary therapies, and other procedures, such as skin grafting. We often teach the principles of local wound care with the mnemonic: **DIM** before **DIME** for adequate Debridement, Infection and Inflammation control, and Moisture balance before the Edge effect, signaling stalled healing and the need for active local therapy. The optimal wound care practices outlined in the preparing the wound bed algorithm are essential before advanced and often expensive therapies are considered.[6-8] If a wound with the ability to heal is not 30% smaller at Week 4, despite optimal local wound care, it is unlikely to heal by Week 12, and advanced therapies should be considered.[9] Clinicians are reminded that if a wound is unlikely to heal (eg, due to inadequate vasculature or coexisting illness), advanced therapies are seldom indicated and their chance of success is minimal (nonhealable wound). In addition,

a maintenance wound does not heal at the expected rate because the patient may refuse to wear the compression that is required to correct venous disease or because the healthcare system does not provide plantar pressure redistribution for a person with a neurotrophic foot ulcer and the patient cannot afford the treatment.

There is a need to link our new knowledge and research findings in wound care to the improved outcomes of patients with wounds worldwide. This process involves the inclusion of evidence from 3 different perspectives:[10]

- *Efficacy* — it works in idealized patients
- *Efficiency* — it works in usual patients
- *Effectiveness* — it has benefit at a reasonable cost.

The current organization of the evidence base for wound care may not encompass all 3 perspectives. One of the pitfalls of randomized controlled trials (RCTs) in wound research is the strict subject selection, eliminating most "usual" patients, and the disadvantage when attempting to extrapolate the RCT results to the real world of clinical practice for patients who would not meet the entry criteria of the study. Efficacy studies compare strictly controlled patients without confounding variables to a placebo. These conceptual studies are necessary for proof of concept. These studies need to be complemented with RCTs comparing the new treatment to usual practices or evidence-informed practice in a clinic that includes usual current treatment for all patients assessed with wounds that have the ability to heal. This treatment must be cost neutral or cost saving for the practice to be translated into day-to-day care by obtaining reimbursement within a healthcare system (effectiveness). There is a need to build economic models to test the feasibility of integrating a new treatment that may be expensive but have cost savings or may be cost neutral to the healthcare system.

Sackett et al[11] emphasized the importance of combining clinical expertise and the best available external evidence, expert knowledge, and patient preference. Without clinical expertise, practice risks becoming tyrannized by evidence — even excellent external evidence may be inappropriate for an individual patient. Without current best evidence, clinical practice rapidly will be out of date, to the detriment of patients. This combination of the scientific evidence base with expert opinion contextualized to local practice is referred to as *evidence-informed practice*. We also must remember the central needs of the patient and the consultation with patients to determine their preferences for treatment. The person's experiences with illness and the experiences of his or her circle of care are often forgotten in the rush for RCTs and other levels of evidence.

To translate the evidence-based paradigm, we can develop a clinical practice guideline. However, all guidelines are not created equal. The methodological quality of a guideline can be assessed through the Appraisal of Guidelines for Research & Evaluation (AGREE II) Instrument (www.agreetrust.org). This instrument examines 6 domains: scope and purpose, stakeholders, rigor, clarity, applicability, and editorial independence. Through this process, we can identify high-quality guidelines and recommendations for translation into practice without continually creating new guidelines or reinventing the wheel.

The Interprofessional Team

Professionals involved in wound care come from diverse professional backgrounds. Each professional brings unique expertise, adding strength to the team. Team collaboration helps fill knowledge gaps, broadens perspectives, and optimizes patient care delivery.

Teams are not created overnight. Individuals in a multiprofessional network need to respect each other's expertise and work toward improving patient outcomes. The next step is to form an interprofessional team with group care plans and sharing of situational learning from experience. In some cases, this may even evolve to a transprofessional team. Advanced practice team members can often perform the functions of more than one team member when required. Highly functioning teams have a flattened structural framework with shared care of patients and do not exemplify the pyramidal structure of a dominant leader and followers that have little to do with key patient care decisions.

Each of us as individuals requires a network of other individuals with complementary expertise in wound care. Let us conceptualize our team for this chapter. George Rodeheaver, PhD, as the basic scientist, brings us new perspectives, treatments, or diagnostic procedures from the laboratory or clinical investigations for consideration. Diane Krasner, RN, as a nurse and allied healthcare professional, focuses on prevention, local treatment, and allied healthcare issues across the continuum of care. Gary Sibbald, MD, as the physician key opinion leader, evaluates innovative treatments or procedures and trials them before identifying the strengths and weaknesses as well as the advantages and disadvantages for patient care before translating a new modality into everyday clinical practice. Kevin Woo, RN, as a nurse researcher and educator, shares his passion for knowledge generation, synthesis, and translation. These 4 distinct professional perspectives broaden our base and strengthen our team.

By practicing as a team, healthcare professionals are able to balance the amount of responsibility and the workload, particularly in challenging cases. It is imperative that all team members share their knowledge and experience in order to provide better care. Tuckman[12] has defined 4 stages to team development: forming, storming, norming, and performing. Several aspects are more likely to be found in successful teams, including clear communication, flexibility, adaptability, openness, shared leadership, and mutual respect.

Healthcare Professional's Caring

Wound care experts must realize that working in a silo even with individual caring cannot offer the person and his or her circle of care optimal treatment. Many individuals who have become healthcare professionals do so because they truly want to help others. The journey to successful healthcare professional status requires a formalized training program that often supplies the basics of nursing, medicine, podiatry, physical therapy, occupational therapy, and other healthcare professional disciplines. It is important to complement professional knowledge with skills to work within a healthcare system. Professionals in health disciplines need to develop communication, collaboration, and management skills. A caring healthcare professional must have a patient-centered approach. This can be exemplified by the Keller and Carroll model[13] to patient communication:

- Engage
- Empathize
- Educate
- Enlist.

For each patient, we should know something about him or her other than the reason for the visit (*engagement*). This information may include hobbies, important family events, or milestones in his or her life. We need to be good listeners, and we need to *empathize* with patients' pain and suffering and not dismiss their concerns with trivial sympathetic comments. Establishing patients' perspectives on their disease processes allows healthcare professionals to *educate* individuals from current beliefs to a negotiated treatment plan, taking patients' wishes into account and having a consensus on the next steps. We then need to *enlist* the patient to be an active participant and take personal responsibility for the diagnostic and treatment process.

As individuals, healthcare professionals need to be in tune with their own belief systems and have a balance with attention to their physical, spiritual, psychological, and social needs. Professionalism refers to the behavior of a professional to uphold ethical and interpersonal values. Healthcare professionals are expected to demonstrate respect for others and uphold appropriate boundaries between themselves, coworkers, and patients.

We should create a comfortable work environment with compassion for others and commitment to improving illness and promoting wellness. There is a need to be a health advocate and to promote a healthy living style and wellness by setting a good example. Other ways to advocate for health include developing new and better healthcare systems with universal access, treating illness early, educating the general public, and supporting wellness.

Continuous Professional Development and Lifelong Learning

Continuous professional development (CPD) refers to lifelong learning that is learner- and workplace-centered. This is also referred to as situational learning because it is determined by practice and problems with patient care. Continuous professional development relates to day-to-day activities. The outcomes from CPD are more likely to change behavior and improve patient care outcomes than an accredited classroom event or traditional continuing education programs.

Single educational events without secondary enabling or reinforcing strategies to bring the information back to the workplace are often unsuccessful in changing practice. Enablers, reference guides, and toolkits are examples of products that can be utilized to change practice. An enabler or quick reference guide is a 20-second to 2-minute reading time summary of relevant strategies for bedside or patient care. An educational toolkit is designed for the implementation of best clinical practices and may consist of educational materials, measuring guides, monofilaments, and other useful aids to clinical practice. Mentorship after an educational event or small learning groups and educational outreach visits (during which an expert may translate the information learned in the formalized setting for the workplace) can also facilitate the integration of new knowledge into practice.

As healthcare professionals, we also must commit to lifelong learning through experience. We learn from the literature, but we also must learn from our experiences and dialogues with colleagues. The first step is to create a network of individuals with whom we can consult when we do not have an answer to a clinical question. We may need to involve a preceptor to learn a skill or task that is important to our job or clinical activities. Preceptorships are often time-limited and driven by specific goals and objectives. Beyond preceptorships, we also may need a mentor. A mentor is an individual who, in a nonjudgmental, comfortable manner, can provide guidance for job-related, personal, and other decisions to achieve life goals and balance as well as to advance a career and promote wound care expertise. Some mentorship relationships have a time-limited spectrum, while others can evolve into a co-mentorship relationship. A younger mentee may be a computer "native" and can teach a computer "immigrant" mentor tricks of the new technologies. At the same time, the senior mentor can continue to add contextual knowledge from lifelong experience, solving difficult situational clinical problems for the younger mentee.

We often learn from relaying case studies or case series and then discussing diagnoses and management. Another dimension to a case history is storytelling. In storytelling, the emotional and situational components of the history and the sequence of events are related with a personal analysis or honesty that may not be contextualized in the formal case history dominated by facts in the sequential history, physical, investigation, and treatment process. Storytelling and the personal anecdote remain critically important methods — even with the current trend of evidence-informed healthcare.

Knowledge Transfer into Practice

Knowledge transfer into practice refers to the link between scientific evidence and the need to change clinical practice. This is a conceptual framework of moving new knowledge from the laboratory bench to the literature/classroom and ultimately to the bedside in order to improve patient care outcomes. This concept requires the transfer of knowledge from efficacy or proof-of-concept RCTs in idealized patients to the trial of the same principles in usual everyday wound care clinics in order to demonstrate that the integration of the concept improves patient care outcomes.

Wikipedia, the Internet's free encyclopedia, describes 3 related concepts in the health sciences: knowledge utilization, research utilization, and implementation. These concepts describe the process of bringing a new idea, practice, or technology into consistent and appropriate use in a clinical setting.[14] The study of knowledge utilization and implementation is a direct outgrowth of the movement toward evidence-based or evidence-informed healthcare. Research to demonstrate efficacy of a new treatment is often completed in idealized patients, and this research needs to be repeated with usual patients to confirm that the same treatment will make a difference in everyday practice settings on usual patients.

Informal Communities of Practice

The concept of a community of practice (CoP) refers to the process of social learning that occurs when people who have a common interest in some subject or problem collaborate over an extended period to share ideas, find solutions, and build innovations. Do you have a wound care CoP?

A previous version of Wikipedia noted, *"The term [community of practice] was first used in 1991 by Jean Lave and Etienne Wenger [to describe] situated learning as part of an attempt to 'rethink learning' at the Institute for Research on Learning. In 1998, the theorist Etienne Wenger extended the concept and applied it to other contexts, including organizational settings...Some of the aims and goals of a community of practice include: the design of more effective knowledge-oriented organizations, creating learning systems across organizations, improving education and lifelong learning, rethinking the role of professional associations and a design of a world in which people can reach their full potential...[a community of practice is] a group of individuals participating in a communal activity, and experiencing/continuously creating their shared identity through engaging in and contributing to the practices of their communities."*

Following are questions to ponder:
• Do you participate in one or more CoP?
• Can you describe their membership and essential components?
• How could you optimize your participation to maximize your social learning and improve your wound care knowledge?
• Could and should you foster a CoP?

Local to Global, Micro to Macro

Persons with chronic wounds do not always receive the expert professional healthcare that they require. There is a social responsibility to increase collaboration within interprofessional teams on

Concept	Strength	Weakness	Threats	Opportunities	Next Steps: Personal Portfolio
Wound care knowledge					
Patient and circle of care					
Interprofessional team relations and new partnerships					
Caring clinician and personal growth					
Continuous professional development/ lifelong learning					
Knowledge transfer projects					
Community of practice					

Figure 3. Personal scorecard.

community, national, and international levels. The World Health Organization (WHO) document, "Transformative Scale Up of Health Professional Education,"[15] highlights the active strategies of healthcare personnel, especially in developing countries, including Sub-Saharan Africa where millions of people are without health services. More providers are needed, and these providers require training that is more relevant to the population's health needs. Education of individual professions needs to include a greater emphasis on interprofessional communication and collaboration. There is also a gap between the needs of private and public healthcare systems and the social responsibility to these countries that must be balanced with improved personal finances that accompany immigration to a developed country. Policies from the WHO will be welcomed to assist developing countries (national authorities) in working with local communities, development partners, and educational institutions.

Conclusion

This chapter can be a starting point for your personal journey to improve outcomes for people with chronic wounds. Figure 3 presents a personal scorecard for you to copy and update on a regular basis for your personal self-assessment and evaluation of the journey. This is also a way to identify personal needs and plan your future educational portfolio. We challenge you to be:

- More effective communicators and collaborators with your patients and their circle of care
- Patient-centered (Do you practice the 4-E model?)
- Better distillers of *wound care knowledge* through:
    - Examining the evidence base presented in this book
    - Reviewing guidelines with good methodological quality
    - Seeking the opinions of others in your own personal network in order to develop your *wound care expertise*
    - Building your own wound care network or *community of practice* within or outside your organization or workplace.

Have you also personally:
- Become a more dedicated *interprofessional*

team member by listening, sharing, and collaborating with passion and commitment
- Developed a *knowledge translation* strategy for your workplace to improve the efficacy, efficiency, and effectiveness of your care
- Improved your *personal caring?*

Regarding your current physical, psychological, spiritual, and mental scorecard:
- Where are your strengths and weaknesses, and can you improve?
- Do you have an action plan?

Can you be more effective in your commitment to *continuous professional development and lifelong learning*? Do you learn personally from a situational *continuous professional development* model, or do you still rely on conferences and formal educational opportunities to obtain continuing education credits as your major method of learning?

In closing, we challenge you to complete your own personal scorecard and to construct your personal learning portfolio. We urge you to reach out to patients, families, and caregivers in order to build the trust and the confidence that heal wounds, patients, and lives.

We wish you every success in *International Interprofessional Wound Caring!*

Diane L. Krasner
George T. Rodeheaver
R. Gary Sibbald
Kevin Y. Woo

References

1. World Union of Wound Healing Societies. *Principles of Best Practice: Minimising Pain at Wound Dressing-related Procedures.* A Consensus Document. London, UK: MEP Ltd; 2004.
2. Osterberg L, Blaschke T. Adherence to medication. *N Engl J Med.* 2005;353(5):487–497.
3. Snyder RJ. Venous leg ulcers in the elderly patient: associated stress, social support, and coping. *Ostomy Wound Manage.* 2006;52(9):58–68.
4. Benner P. *From Novice to Expert: Excellence and Power in Clinical Nursing Practice.* Menlo Park, CA: Addison-Wesley Publishing Co; 1984.
5. Winter GD. Formation of the scab and the rate of epithelization of superficial wounds in the skin of the young domestic pig. *Nature.* 1962;193:293–294.
6. Sibbald RG, Williamson D, Orsted HL, et al. Preparing the wound bed—debridement, bacterial balance, and moisture balance. *Ostomy Wound Manage.* 2000;46(11):14–37.
7. Sibbald RG, Orsted H, Schultz GS, Coutts P, Keast D; International Wound Bed Preparation Advisory Board;

Canadian Chronic Wound Advisory Board. Preparing the wound bed 2003: focus on infection and inflammation. *Ostomy Wound Manage.* 2003;49(11):23–51.

8. Sibbald RG, Goodman L, Woo KY, et al. Special considerations in wound bed preparation 2011: an update©. *Adv Skin Wound Care.* 2011;24(9):415–436.

9. Woo K, Ayello EA, Sibbald RG. The edge effect: current therapeutic options to advance the wound edge. *Adv Skin Wound Care.* 2007;20(2):99–117.

10. Price P. The challenge of outcome measure in chronic wounds. *J Wound Care.* 1999;8(6):306–308.

11. Sackett DL, Straus SE, Richardson WS, Rosenberg W, Haynes RB. *Evidence-based Medicine: How to Practice and Teach EBM.* 2nd ed. Edinburgh, Scotland: Churchill Livingstone; 2000.

12. Tuckman BW. Developmental sequence in small groups. *Psychol Bull.* 1965;63:384–399.

13. Keller VK, Carroll JG. A new model for physician-patient communication. *Patient Educ Couns.* 1994;23(2):131–140.

14. Greenhalgh T, Robert G, Macfarlane F, Bate P, Kyriakidou O. Diffusion of innovations in service organizations: systematic review and recommendations. *Milbank Q.* 2004;82(4):581–629.

15. World Health Organization. Transformative Scale Up of Health Professional Education. Available at: http://www.who.int/hrh/resources/transformative_education/en/index.html. Accessed January 8, 2011.

CHAPTER 3

Science of Wound Healing: Translation of Bench Science into Advances for Chronic Wound Care

Linda Cowan, PhD, ARNP, FNP-BC, CWS;
Joyce Stechmiller, PhD, ACNP-BC, FAAN;
Priscilla Phillips, PhD;
Gregory Schultz, PhD

Objectives

The reader will be challenged to:

- Assess the basic concepts of molecular regulation in normal wound healing and identify common alterations that may lead to chronic wounds
- Analyze evidence for state-of-the-art approaches to correct molecular imbalances in chronic wounds
- Formulate basic concepts regarding the implication of biofilms in contributing to chronic inflammatory states of nonhealing wounds
- Identify potential diagnostic tools that may assist the clinician in rapid detection of important biomarkers indicating impaired wound healing.

Introduction

Traditionally, most acute skin wounds heal without clinically significant complications, and the resulting scar tissue functions similarly enough to unwounded skin that the repaired wound does not cause substantial problems. However, some acute skin wounds fail to heal in an expected or predicted manner and become chronic, which invariably leads to a wide range of complications, including infection, poor quality of life, increased risk of lower limb amputation, and, ultimately, death from systemic sepsis. Although much is understood about the basic science of normal skin wound healing, only recently has research begun to unravel the molecular and cellular reasons why some wounds fail to heal. Fortunately, these discoveries are constantly being translated into new therapies that selectively target the bacterial, molecular, and cellular abnormalities that impair healing, correct imbalances, and convert the chronic wound into a healing wound.

Overview of Normal Skin Wound Healing

The process of normal healing within acute skin wounds involves a distinct 4-phase sequence that results in the creation of a scar: hemostasis, inflammation, repair, and remodeling (Plate 8, page 344).[1-3] During the initial hemostasis phase, fibrinogen is proteolytically converted to fibrin by thrombin, leading to formation of the fibrin clot, which stimulates platelets to degranulate, releasing numerous growth factors and proinflammatory cytokines

Cowan L, Stechmiller J, Phillips P, Schultz G. Science of wound healing: translation of bench science into advances for chronic wound care. In: Krasner DL, ed. *Chronic Wound Care: The Essentials*. Malvern, PA: HMP Communications; 2014:17–28.

in the wound. These important regulatory molecules chemotactically draw in neutrophils and macrophages, initiating the inflammatory phase. As shown in Plate 9 (page 344), a key function of the inflammatory cells is to engulf invading bacteria and fungi and kill them by generating reactive oxygen species (ROS) inside the endosomes. A second key function of inflammatory cells is to secrete proteases, including the matrix metalloproteinases (MMPs) and elastase, which remove (debride) extracellular matrix (ECM) molecules like collagen that were damaged during the injury.[4] Inflammation continues to increase, reaches a maximum by about 5 to 7 days after injury, and, in the absence of continued inflammatory stimulation, decreases to low levels by about 14 days after injury. Acute inflammation stimulates the wound to enter into the repair phase, which is characterized by proliferation and migration of fibroblasts from the adjacent uninjured dermis into the provisional fibrin wound matrix, where the fibroblasts synthesize large amounts of new collagen and other ECM proteins that replace the fibrin matrix.[5] Vascular endothelial cells in the surrounding vasculature also proliferate and migrate into the fibrin matrix to form new capillaries (neovascularization) that provide essential nutritional support for the rapidly metabolizing fibroblasts. Epithelial cells from the edge of the injury and especially from the stem cell niches in the hair follicles and sweat glands proliferate and migrate across the new scar matrix that is being generated by the fibroblasts. Some fibroblasts in the wound matrix differentiate into myofibroblasts and contract the newly forming scar matrix, reducing the wound area by ~20% in human skin wounds. When the epithelial cells have resurfaced the wound, the first 3 phases of wound healing are completed, but the initial scar matrix is not static. Over the next 6 to 12 months, the initial scar matrix is slowly remodeled by proteases that remove the highly irregular scar tissue, which is replaced by new collagen that is organized into a much more normal, basket-weave structure found in uninjured dermis.[4]

Normal skin wound healing is a highly integrated process that involves platelets, inflammatory cells, fibroblasts, epithelial cells, and vascular endothelial cells. The actions of these wound cells are closely regulated by key proteins including pro- and anti-inflammatory cytokines, growth factors, receptors, proteases, inhibitors, and ECM proteins that dictate the activities of these cells. As normal wound healing proceeds, the regulatory proteins and the responses of the individual cells interact ultimately to result in repair of the injury.

Overview of Molecular and Cellular Abnormalities in Chronic Wounds

All chronic wounds begin as acute wounds, but acute wounds become chronic wounds when they fail to progress through the sequential phases of healing as expected.[4,6] A key question to ask is, are there common molecular and cellular patterns in chronic wounds that indicate the stage of the wound healing sequence where most chronic wounds stall? The simple answer is yes. Cellular and molecular data from numerous clinical studies suggest that most chronic wounds get "stuck" in a prolonged inflammatory phase that is due to the presence of both planktonic (free flowing) and biofilm bacteria in the wound (Figure 1).[7,8] The bacteria stimulate production of proinflammatory cytokines like tumor necrosis factor-alpha (TNF-α) and interleukin 1 (IL-1), which act as chemotactic factors (chemical messengers) to recruit neutrophils, macrophages, and mast cells into the wound. The inflammatory cells that are drawn into the wound secrete proteases (MMPs, neutrophil elastase, and plasmin) and ROS in an attempt to kill bacteria and detach biofilm colonies that are tightly attached to the wound bed. However, because bacterial biofilms are tolerant to ROS as well as antibodies and even antiseptics, the biofilms persist and continue to stimulate inflammation. This results in chronically elevated levels of proteases and ROS that eventually begin to destroy essential proteins that are necessary for healing, including growth factors, their receptors, and ECM proteins. These "off-target" effects of proteases and ROS combine to reduce cell proliferation, migration, and generation of functional scar matrix.[1,9-11] The "biological sum" of this prolonged inflammatory state is a distorted molecular and cellular wound environment that prevents wound healing. In the simplest terms, the molecular and cellular environment between acute

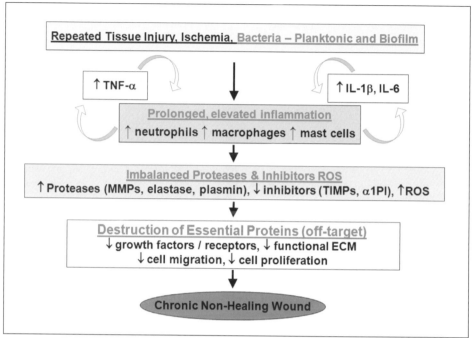

Figure 1. Molecular and cellular pathology of chronic wounds. Acute wounds that become critically colonized by planktonic and biofilm bacteria develop chronic inflammation that is characterized by high levels of proteases and ROS that destroy "off-target" proteins that are essential for healing, resulting in a chronic wound.

healing wounds and chronic wounds is totally different. As shown in Figure 2, these "imbalances" must be corrected by clinical therapies or the wound will not progress to healing. Strategies designed to reverse these imbalances would be expected to promote healing, and indeed, innovative new treatments are being developed and tested, and some have already been shown to clinically improve healing of chronic wounds. Of utmost importance is attention to evidence-based wound care, adequate wound bed preparation, appropriate management of underlying disease, and correction of other contributing factors (such as too much or too little moisture, excessive friction and shear, and inadequate nutrition) that may impair wound healing.[4]

Repeated Tissue Injury

Clinical observations indicate that acute wounds that develop into chronic wounds are frequently subjected to repeated episodes of tissue injury leading to ischemia, such as prolonged

pressure in spinal cord-injury patients (pressure ulcers), vasculopathies (venous leg ulcers), or blunt trauma that occurs on plantar foot surfaces of people with diabetic neuropathy.[4,6] This causes the epidermis to break down, generating an open wound that quickly becomes colonized with planktonic bacteria.

Bacterial Bioburden and Biofilms

Decades of clinical and laboratory research have conclusively shown that high concentrations of planktonic bacteria found in clinically infected wounds can impair wound healing, primarily by stimulating inflammation and by secreting exotoxins, proteases, and virulence factors that impair inflammatory cell functions and break down host tissue to promote dissemination of the bacteria and to provide nutrients for the rapidly proliferating bacteria. Historically, many nonhealing wounds were not reported to have high levels of planktonic bacteria when assessed by standard clinical microbiology as-

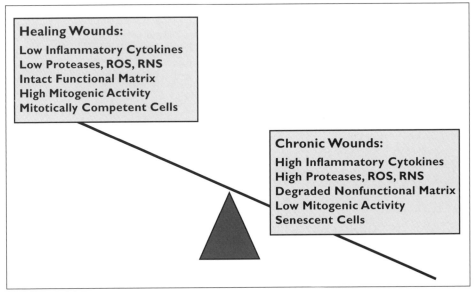

Figure 2. Imbalanced molecular and cellular environments of healing and chronic wounds. The molecular and cellular environment of acute healing wounds is dramatically different than that of chronic wounds and must be "rebalanced" to approximate the environment of healing wounds before healing can progress. Adapted with permission from Mast BA, Schultz GS. Interactions of cytokines, growth factors, and proteases in acute and chronic wounds. *Wound Repair Regen*. 1996;4(4):411.

says. However, serial aggressive debridement and systemic and topical treatments designed to reduce bacterial bioburden were frequently found to improve healing. This led to the concept of *critical colonization*, which was an attempt to recognize that something about the bioburden was impairing healing (Plate 10, page 345). New data suggest that the critical factor determining wound bioburden is usually the presence of bacteria in polymicrobial biofilm communities.[5]

A *biofilm* is a community of microorganisms surrounded by an extracellular polymeric matrix (EPM), which attaches to a surface.[12] Recent studies demonstrate that biofilms are becoming a significant component of infections in humans.[12-14] The Centers for Disease Control and Prevention and the National Institutes of Health project that biofilms are associated with 65% of nosocomial (hospital-acquired) infections and up to 80% of all human infections in the United States. In addition, treatment of biofilm-associated infections costs billions of dollars and results in hundreds of thousands of

deaths annually in the United States.[12] Both acute and chronic wounds are susceptible to the development of biofilms within the wound bed.

Open wounds provide a perfect environment for opportunistic organisms, such as bacteria, to reside and reproduce. Analyses of the microflora of chronic wounds (such as pressure and diabetic foot ulcers) demonstrate a phenomenon known as *chronic wound pathogenic biofilms*.[12-14] Typical mechanisms by which biofilms impede wound healing progress involve heightening the level of inflammation; increasing the amount of ROS and proteases in the wound bed; stimulating overly aggressive immune responses; producing detrimental exogenous toxins within the wound environment; and impairing normal chemokine signalling pathways.[15] Aerobic organisms within biofilms use oxygen and help to create anaerobic niches within the biofilm matrix that support the development of anaerobes within the biofilm.[12] Importantly, the presence of biofilms in a wound may affect the wound healing process without visible clinical signs of infection. However, there may be indications of bacterial imbalance (eg, change in wound color or odor together with the presence of devitalized tissue and ischemia).[15]

Studies suggest that certain bacterial groups, which by themselves are considered essentially harmless (such as *Corynebacterium spp*), tend to form symbiotic communities with other bacteria and fungi in chronic wounds. These polymicrobial groups in biofilms are termed **functional equivalent pathogroups** because they have been shown to have functionally detrimental effects on wound healing similar to other well known pathogens, such as *Staphylococcus aureus*.[12] In addition, biofilm colonies may extend 2 mm beneath the wound bed and into surrounding healthy tissue, making them difficult to eradicate by many traditional bedside debridement methods. Treatment options to consider include debridement and the use of a broad-spectrum topical antimicrobial agent directly after debridement to control the planktonic bacterial load and to reduce the progression into biofilms. Importantly, recent data indicate that mature biofilm communities can re-establish in wounds within 3 days following debridement.[5] If control of microbial progression from planktonic to mature biofilms is not achieved, a change from an early stage biofilm to a polymicrobial "complex" mature wound biofilm may develop and ultimately lead to a compromised state.[15]

Biofilm experts suggest that traditional culturing methods, which involve inoculating a culture medium with a cotton swab sample obtained from the patient, are insufficient to identify true components of the polymicrobial mature biofilm colonies.[12,15] The exact microbial composition of biofilms is largely undetectable by traditional cotton swab culture techniques due to the protective polymeric coating that biofilms produce. This self-protective coating encapsulates the colony and is also impervious to most systemic and topical antimicrobials/antibiotics. Other limitations of the traditional clinical swab sampling approach include the following:
- Cotton swab cultures typically query only the most common aerobic organisms
- Culture results are often unavailable for 2 to 3 days
- The culture is naturally biased toward identifying only those cultivable bacterial species

that are easily cultured under standard laboratory conditions on standard growth media.[12]

Recent literature suggests that the polymerase chain reaction (PCR) assay is a cost-effective, rapid, and more sensitive method to detect microbial pathogens (particularly biofilm microbes) in clinical specimens. The diagnostic value of PCR may be clinically superior to traditional swab cultures as well as other modern options, such as pyrosequencing techniques. Pyrosequencing essentially generates millions of short ~100 nucleotide sequences, and software scans the entire bacterial and fungal DNA databases for matches of DNA sequences. Thus, pyrosequencing can identify all bacterial and fungal species present in a biopsy, but it is more expensive and requires about a week to generate the data. The PCR identification of bacteria and fungi in wound biopsies is a more focused and limited approach that uses primer sequences that "probe" for unique DNA sequences of ribosomal RNAs. This real-time PCR testing specifically probes for ~30 bacteria and fungi species in a wound sample. However, it is less expensive and rapid (costs ~$100 and is completed in less than 24 hours).[15]

Elevated Proinflammatory Cytokines

Closely linked to the bacterial bioburden in a wound is the proinflammatory cytokine profile. In general, fluids from acute healing wounds tend to have an early peak of major proinflammatory cytokines, TNF-α and IL-1β, and their natural inhibitors, P55 and IL-1 receptor antagonist, within the first few days after injury, which corresponds to the rapid increase in inflammatory cells in the acute wound.[16] The levels of proinflammatory cytokines begin to decrease after 6 to 7 days as the inflammatory stimuli in acute wounds decrease. However, in a study of chronic leg ulcers, the levels of inflammatory cytokines, IL-1β, IL-6, and TNF-α were significantly higher than in acute healing wounds, and as the chronic ulcers began to heal, the levels decreased.[8] These findings indicate that chronic wounds have persistently elevated levels of proinflammatory cytokines, but as chronic wounds heal, the molecular environment changes to a less proinflammatory wound environment.

Elevated Proteases

Another major concept to emerge from wound fluid analyses is that levels of proteases, especially MMPs and neutrophil elastase, are much higher in chronic wounds than in acute wound fluids.[6,16,17] During the early phase of acute wound healing, the average level of protease activity in mastectomy fluids was found to be low, suggesting that protease activity is tightly controlled during the early phase of wound healing.[9] However, in chronic wounds, the average level of protease activity was found to be approximately 116-fold higher than in acute mastectomy wound fluids. Furthermore, as chronic venous ulcers began to heal, the levels of protease activity decreased.[9] Similar results were reported for fluids or biopsies of chronic pressure ulcers, where levels of MMP-2, MMP-9, and MMP-1 were 10 to 25 times higher than levels in acute surgical wound fluids.[18,19] Levels of the tissue inhibitors of metalloproteinases (TIMPs), which are the natural inhibitors of MMPs, were found to be decreased in wound fluids from chronic venous ulcers compared to acute mastectomy wound fluids.[20]

In nonhealing chronic pressure ulcers, MMP-8, the neutrophil-derived collagenase, was elevated, indicating that there may be a persistent influx of neutrophils releasing MMP-8 and elastase, which could contribute to the destruction of ECM proteins and growth factors that are essential for healing.[21] Chronic venous ulcers were found to have 10-fold to 40-fold higher levels of neutrophil elastase activity and to have degraded α1-antitrypsin. Elevated MMP-2 and MMP-9 levels in chronic venous ulcers also were observed to coincide with degradation of fibronectin in the wound bed.[22,23] Fibronectin is an important multidomain adhesion protein that is present in the ECM and granulation tissue and is important in promoting epithelial cell migration. Proteases in chronic wound fluids were shown to rapidly degrade exogenously added growth factors, such as transforming growth factor-alpha (TGF-α), epidermal growth factor (EGF), or platelet-derived growth factor (PDGF), using *in-vitro* laboratory tests. In contrast, exogenously added growth factors were stable when added to acute surgical wound fluids.[1,9–11]

Reduced Mitogenic Activity of Chronic Wound Fluids

Another key concept that emerged from laboratory analysis demonstrates that the mitogenic activity of chronic wound fluids is dramatically less than levels in acute wound fluids. For example, fluids from chronic leg ulcers did not stimulate DNA synthesis of cells in culture, while acute wound fluids strongly stimulate proliferation of cells in culture. Furthermore, when acute and chronic wound fluids were combined, the mitotic activity of acute wound fluids was inhibited.[7,24,25] These results show that the proteases in chronic wound fluid degrade growth factors that are normally present in acute wound fluids, and without the essential actions of these growth factors, wound healing will not progress.

Factors Affecting Cell Senescence

In chronic wounds, the capacity of the wound cells to respond to cytokines and growth factors is altered. Research suggests that fibroblasts (cells that manufacture collagen and perform other essential functions in wound healing) have a diminished response to growth factors in chronic wounds. For example, fibroblast cultures established from chronic venous leg ulcers proliferated slowly and formed less dense confluent cultures when compared to normal fibroblast cultures established from uninjured dermis.[26] In another study of chronic venous leg ulcers that were present for more than 3 years, fibroblasts proliferated poorly in response to PDGF added to the culture medium and rapidly approached senescence compared to fibroblasts cultured from venous ulcers that had been present for less than 3 years.[27]

The molecular environments of acute and chronic wounds are dramatically different (Figure 2). Healing wounds have low bacterial bioburden and no biofilms, low levels of inflammatory cytokines, low levels of proteases, high levels of growth factors, and cells that divide rapidly in response to growth factors. The molecular and cellular environment of chronic wounds is exactly the opposite. Chronic wounds have high levels of bacterial biofilms, elevated levels of inflammatory cytokines, high levels of proteases, low levels of growth factors, and cells that are approaching senescence.[27–29] With this in mind, new treatment strategies should be designed to re-establish in

Table I. TIME and wound bed preparation assessment tool.	
TISSUE	Debridement assessment: • Color assessment • Tissue perfusion • TCP02 (color Doppler angiography)
INFECTION	Wound bed and surrounding skin: • Temperature • Odor • Color • pH
MOISTURE	Assess maceration or desiccation, leg volume transepidermal water loss (TEWL)
EDGE	2D evaluation • Acetate tracing • Digital photography • Digital tools and PC software • 3D evaluation • Probes, molds • Scanning systems

Adapted with permission from Dowsett C, Ayello E. TIME principles of chronic wound bed preparation and treatment. *Br J Nurs.* 2004;13(15):S16–S23.

chronic wounds the balance of bacterial bioburden, cytokines, growth factors, proteases, their natural inhibitors, and competent cells found in healing wounds. Chronic wounds fail to heal because of molecular and cellular abnormalities in the wound environment. For example, studies have shown altered signaling pathways and levels of gene expression (eg, elevated c-myc and beta-catenin, altered intracellular localization of EGF receptor) that reflect the stalled migration of keratinocytes at the edge of chronic wounds.[30] Several innovative approaches to identifying and managing chronic wounds are being developed and are based on identifying and correcting these types of molecular and cellular abnormalities.

Innovative Approaches for Correcting Molecular Abnormalities of Chronic Wounds

Debridement. Clearly, proper wound debridement is a key element of wound bed preparation. This was demonstrated by Steed et al[29] who performed a clinical study that showed that healing of chronic diabetic foot ulcers (treated at 10 different centers) was closely correlated with the frequency of debridement. The benefit of wound debridement was seen in both patients who received standard care and patients who were treated with topical PDGF. It is possible that frequent sharp debridement of diabetic ulcers may reduce the level of inflammation in the wound by mechanically removing biofilms as well as by converting the chronic wound into a pseudo-acute wound molecular environment. Therefore, appropriate wound debridement should be considered a vital component in the care of patients with chronic diabetic foot ulcers.

TIME to heal wounds. A second category of approaches to correcting the molecular imbalance in chronic wounds is targeted at the elevated levels of inflammatory cytokines. The simplest approach to correcting this condition is to prepare the wound bed using debridement and moisture control. This concept has been more thoroughly described in an article that unites wound bed preparation under a *TIME* acronym that stands for **T**issue debridement, **I**nfection/inflammation, **M**oisture balance, and **E**dge effect (Plate 11, page 345). Correctly applying the concepts of wound bed preparation to the care of a patient's wound requires a tool that helps assess when each of the 4 components has been optimized. As shown in Table 1, assessment of the TIME components involves good clinical judgment and objective measurements of wound parameters, as described by Dowsett and Ayello.[31]

Proteases. Another important clinical approach to correcting molecular imbalances in chronic wounds is to lower the levels of MMPs and other proteases. Several therapeutic approaches are currently used. Innovative wound dressings that contain denatured collagen (gelatin) and oxidized regenerated cellulose (Promogran, Systagenix Wound Management, Quincy, Massachusetts) are available. The gelatin in the dressing acts as a substrate sink for proteases, especially MMPs, and has been shown to reduce levels of protease activities in fluids from chronic human wounds measured *in vitro*.[32] One study of chronic diabetic plantar surface ulcers found that 31% of 51 patients treated with Promogran added to conventional dressings had complete wound closure compared with 28% of 39 patients treated with conventional dressings (*P* = .12).[33] Analysis of healing rates in subcategories of patients suggested that the effect of Promogran was more dramatic in healing in ulcers of less than 6 months' duration.

Another clinical approach that has been used to correct elevated levels of proteases, especially MMPs, is applying topical protease inhibitors. One study investigated topical treatment of diabetic foot ulcers with doxycycline.[34] Doxycycline is a member of the tetracycline family of antibiotics and is an effective inhibitor of metalloproteinases, including MMPs and the TNF-α converting enzyme (TACE).[35] A randomized controlled trial of 1% topical doxycycline treatment of patients with chronic diabetic foot ulcers found that all 4 ulcers treated daily with doxycycline in a carboxymethyl cellulose vehicle healed in less than the 20-week treatment period, while only 1 of 3 ulcers treated with vehicle healed in 20 weeks. Importantly, no adverse events attributable to the doxycycline treatment occurred.[34]

Other methods of wound care can be used to lower levels of proteases in wound beds. For example, negative pressure wound therapy (NPWT) removes wound fluid containing high levels of proteases from the wound bed while drawing fresh plasma that contains protease inhibitors (α2 macroglobulin, α1-antitrypsin) into the wound bed.[36] In addition, dressings that absorb large amounts of wound exudate, especially dressings that contain highly charged polymers (eg, negatively charged polyacrylic acid or carboxymethylated cellulose or positively charged polyquats), can ionically bind the charged protease proteins and sequester the proteases in the matrix of the dressing, thus sparing the proteins in the wound bed that are essential for healing.[37]

Optimal use of advanced therapies to reduce the elevated levels of proteases would ideally depend on actually measuring the levels of proteases in a patient's wound. Thus, clinicians may find a rapid, point-of-care (POC) detector that measures levels of MMP activities in a wound fluid sample useful. Two prototype MMP detectors are currently under final development. Both MMP detectors would enable clinicians to assess the level of MMP protease activity in wound fluid samples collected at the bedside in approximately 10 minutes. One device utilizes lateral flow strip (LFS) technology like that used in early pregnancy test kits that are performed at home on urine samples. This LFS detector for MMPs produces a line on the test strip when MMP activities in a wound fluid sample are low and no line on the test strip when the MMP activities are high, which is opposite from how LFS detectors typically indicate if a biomarker is present in a sample. A second prototype MMP detector generates a fluorescent signal that is proportional to the level of MMP activities in wound fluid that is collected on a swab and added to the MMP substrate solution. Gibson et al[38] used the fluorescence POC detector prototype to measure MMP levels in samples of acute and chronic wound fluids collected by swabs at the bedside. After 10 minutes of reaction, MMP levels were almost 6 times higher in chronic wounds (n = 6) than the average level measured in acute wounds (n = 3). Assessing the level of MMPs in wounds should help clinicians determine if the level of proteases is so high that healing would not likely occur and could help clinicians determine if the wound should be debrided and treated with dressings that reduce protease activities and/or reduce bacterial bioburden.

Growth factors. The application of recombinant growth factors to the wound is another approach to correcting the abnormal molecular environment of chronic wounds. Several clinical studies have reported improved healing of various types of chronic wounds with recombinant human growth factors and cytokines, including PDGF,[39,40] keratinocyte growth factor-2 (KGF-2),[41] transforming growth factor beta (TGF-β),[42] basic fibroblast growth factor (bFGF),[43,44] and granulocyte-macrophage colony-stimulating factor (GM-CSF).[43] It is important to recognize that growth factors can only function well in chronic wounds when the environment is similar to that found in acute wounds. In other words, growth factors cannot convert a chronic wound to an acute wound and do not function in a necrotic, inflamed, protease-laden wound. Thus, the principles of wound bed preparation must be used in conjunction with topical growth factor treatments.

A logical extension of the principles of wound bed preparation is to combine therapies that address more than one aspect of TIME. Indeed, combining topical growth factor treatment (Regranex®, Healthpoint, Ltd., Fort Worth, Texas) with protease inhibiting dressings (Fibracol Plus® collagen-alginate, Systagenix Wound Management, Quincy, Massachusetts, or Oasis® small intestinal submucosa, Healthpoint, Ltd.) rapidly healed 34 of 36 chronic wounds that had failed to heal by other wound care techniques, including when these therapies were used alone.[45] However, combining therapies should be used with caution because some combinations of topical treatments can inactivate or impair active components of one or more of the treatments.[46] For example, combining microbicidal dressings that contain PHMB, ionic silver, or iodine with Santyl® debriding ointment reduces the enzymatic activity of the collagenase enzyme in the Santyl.[47]

Conclusion

Wound healing occurs through 4 phases. These phases are sequentially regulated by the actions of cytokines, growth factors, ECM proteins, and proteases. If an acute wound fails to move through a phase of healing, molecular imbalances will occur, leading to a chronic wound. Chronic wounds

---

Take Home Messages for Practice

- Moist wound healing is evidence-based. Avoid using products or therapies in chronic full-thickness wounds that dry out the wound bed at any time. Remember, balance is important. Keeping the wound bed moist but not too moist (as evidenced by periwound maceration or dressings that need to be changed more than 2 or 3 times per day) is sometimes a challenge.

- Always attempt to include the patient's preferences, values, and any unique patient limitations (cognitive, physical, and psychosocial/emotional) in your treatment plan. For example, a patient or his or her caregiver is not likely to be compliant with a daily treatment plan that requires him or her to manually "milk" and discard bloody drainage from tubing left in a surgical wound if he or she faints at the sight of blood.

- Start with the simple and most cost-effective products and therapies for chronic wound care that address TIME principles. Always recheck wound progress within 2 weeks of starting or changing wound treatments. If wound healing is the goal (not palliative wounds) and no improvement is seen within 2 to 4 weeks of initiating a wound treatment, 1) verify that all TIME principles are being addressed, 2) verify patient/caregiver understanding/compliance with treatment orders, 3) assess and address comorbid conditions that may impair wound healing (unrelieved friction/shear/pressure; inadequate nutrition), and 4) consider tissue biopsy to rule out other pathology (eg, malignancy, pyoderma gangrenosum). If all of these factors have been satisfactorily addressed, consider changing wound treatment modalities, possibly including the initiation of advanced therapies.

---

are characterized by bacterial biofilms, elevated inflammatory cytokines and proteases, low levels of mitogenic activity, and senescent cells that are unable to respond to growth factors. Healing of chronic wounds occurs as the molecular environment of the wound shifts to the environment of an acute wound. New therapies are designed to correct the molecular abnormalities of chronic wounds and correspond to the principles of wound bed preparation.

Self-Assessment Questions

1. Which of the following is NOT a reason why PCR as a diagnostic tool may be more desirable than standard swab cultures for measuring bacterial strains present in a biofilm?
   A. Results are obtained quicker than standard culture techniques
   B. It identifies more strains with greater accuracy
   C. The test can be done at the bedside like a rapid strep test
   D. It may be more cost effective

2. What does the M stand for in the TIME acronym approach to wound management?
   A. Manage nutrition
   B. Manage moisture
   C. Manage edema
   D. Manage infection

Answers: 1-C, 2-B

References

1. Bennett NT, Schultz GS. Growth factors and wound healing: Part II. Role in normal and chronic wound healing. *Am J Surg.* 1993;166(1):74–81.
2. Bennett NT, Schultz GS. Growth factors and wound healing: biochemical properties of growth factors and their receptors. *Am J Surg.* 1993;165(6):728–737.
3. Lawrence WT. Physiology of the acute wound. *Clin Plast Surg.* 1998;25(3):321–340.
4. Doughty DB, Sparks-DeFriese B. Wound-healing physiology. In: Bryant RA, Nix DP, eds. *Acute and Chronic Wounds.* 4th ed. St. Louis, MO: Elsevier Mosby; 2010:63–82.
5. Wolcott RD, Rumbaugh KP, James G, et al. Biofilm maturity studies indicate sharp debridement opens a time-dependent therapeutic window. *J Wound Care.* 2010;19(8):320–328.
6. Mast BA, Schultz GS. Interactions of cytokines, growth factors, and proteases in acute and chronic wounds. *Wound Repair Regen.* 1996;4(4):411–420.
7. Harris IR, Yee KC, Walters CE, et al. Cytokine and protease levels in healing and non-healing chronic venous leg ulcers. *Exp Dermatol.* 1995;4(6):342–349.
8. Trengove NJ, Bielefeldt-Ohmann H, Stacey MC. Mitogenic activity and cytokine levels in non-healing and healing chronic leg ulcers. *Wound Repair Regen.* 2000;8(1):13–25.
9. Trengove NJ, Stacey MC, MacAuley S, et al. Analysis of the acute and chronic wound environments: the role of proteases and their inhibitors. *Wound Repair Regen.* 1999;7(6):442–452.
10. Tarnuzzer RW, Schultz GS. Biochemical analysis of acute and chronic wound environments. *Wound Repair Regen.* 1996;4(3):321–325.
11. Yager DR, Chen SM, Ward SI, Olutoye OO, Diegelmann RF, Cohen IK. Ability of chronic wound fluids to degrade peptide growth factors is associated with increased levels of elastase activity and diminished levels of proteinase inhibitors. *Wound Repair Regen.* 1997;5(1):23–32.
12. Dowd SE, Wolcott RD, Sun Y, McKeehan T, Smith E, Rhoads D. Polymicrobial nature of chronic diabetic foot ulcer biofilm infections determined using bacterial tag encoded FLX amplicon pyrosequencing (bTEFAP). *PLoS One.* 2008;3(10):e3326.
13. James GA, Swogger E, Wolcott R, et al. Biofilms in chronic wounds. *Wound Repair Regen.* 2008;16(1):37–44.
14. Smith DM, Snow DE, Rees E, et al. Evaluation of the bacterial diversity of pressure ulcers using bTEFAP pyrosequencing. *BMC Med Genomics.* 2010;3:41.
15. Cowan T. Biofilms and their management: from concept to clinical reality. Presented at the Second Annual Journal of Wound Care Lecture in Manchester Town Hall in Manchester, England, March 10, 2011.
16. Schreml S, Szeimies R, Prantl L, Landthaler M, Babilas P. Wound healing in the 21st century. *J Am Acad Dermatol.* 2010;63(5):866–881.
17. Yager DR, Nwomeh BC. The proteolytic environment of chronic wounds. *Wound Repair Regen.* 1999;7(6):433–441.
18. Yager DR, Zhang LY, Liang HX, Diegelmann RF, Cohen IK. Wound fluids from human pressure ulcers contain elevated matrix metalloproteinase levels and activity compared to surgical wound fluids. *J Invest Dermatol.* 1996;107(5):743–748.
19. Rogers AA, Burnett S, Moore JC, Shakespeare PG, Chen WY. Involvement of proteolytic enzymes—plasminogen activators and matrix metalloproteinases—in the pathophysiology of pressure ulcers. *Wound Repair Regen.* 1995;3(3):273–283.
20. Bullen EC, Longaker MT, Updike DL, et al. Tissue inhibitor of metalloproteinases-1 is decreased and activated gelatinases are increased in chronic wounds. *J Invest Dermatol.* 1995;104(2):236–240.
21. Ladwig GP, Robson MC, Liu R, Kuhn MA, Muir DF, Schultz GS. Ratios of activated matrix metalloproteinase-9 to tissue inhibitor of matrix metalloproteinase-1 in wound fluids are inversely correlated with healing of pressure ulcers. *Wound Repair Regen.* 2002;10(1):26–37.
22. Wysocki AB, Staiano-Coico L, Grinnell F. Wound fluid from chronic leg ulcers contains elevated levels of me-

talloproteinases MMP-2 and MMP-9. *J Invest Dermatol.* 1993;101(1):64–68.

23. Grinnell F, Zhu M. Fibronectin degradation in chronic wounds depends on the relative levels of elastase, alpha1-proteinase inhibitor, and alpha2-macroglobulin. *J Invest Dermatol.* 1996;106(2):335–341.

24. Bucalo B, Eaglstein WH, Falanga V. Inhibition of cell proliferation by chronic wound fluid. *Wound Repair Regen.* 1993;1(3):181–186.

25. Katz MH, Alvarez AF, Kirsner RS, Eaglstein WH, Falanga V. Human wound fluid from acute wounds stimulates fibroblast and endothelial cell growth. *J Am Acad Dermatol.* 1991;25(6 Pt 1):1054–1058.

26. Agren MS, Eaglstein WH, Ferguson MW, et al. Causes and effects of the chronic inflammation in venous leg ulcers. *Acta Derm Venereol Suppl (Stockh).* 2000;210:3–17.

27. Trengove NJ, Langton SR, Stacey MC. Biochemical analysis of wound fluid from nonhealing and healing chronic leg ulcers. *Wound Repair Regen.* 1996;4(2):234–239.

28. Schultz GS, Sibbald RG, Falanga V, et al. Wound bed preparation: a systematic approach to wound management. *Wound Repair Regen.* 2003;11 Suppl 1:S1–S28.

29. Steed DL, Donohoe D, Webster MW, Lindsley L. Effect of extensive debridement and treatment on the healing of diabetic foot ulcers. Diabetic Ulcer Study Group. *J Am Coll Surg.* 1996;183(1):61–64.

30. Stojadinovic O, Brem H, Vouthounis C, et al. Molecular pathogenesis of chronic wounds: the role of beta-catenin and c-myc in the inhibition of epithelialization and wound healing. *Am J Pathol.* 2005;167(1):59–69.

31. Dowsett C, Ayello E. TIME principles of chronic wound bed preparation and treatment. *Br J Nurs.* 2004;13(15):S16–S23.

32. Cullen B, Smith R, McCulloch E, Silcock D, Morrison L. Mechanism of action of PROMOGRAN, a protease modulating matrix, for the treatment of diabetic foot ulcers. *Wound Repair Regen.* 2002;10(1):16–25.

33. Veves A, Sheehan P, Pham HT. A randomized, controlled trial of Promogran (a collagen/oxidized regenerated cellulose dressing) vs. standard treatment in the management of diabetic foot ulcers. *Arch Surg.* 2002;137(7):822–827.

34. Chin GA, Thigpin TG, Perrin KJ, Moldawer LL, Schultz GS. Treatment of chronic ulcers in diabetic patients with a topical metalloproteinase inhibitor, doxycycline. *WOUNDS.* 2003;15(10):315–323.

35. Stechmiller J, Cowan L, Schultz G. The role of doxycycline as a matrix metalloproteinase inhibitor for the treatment of chronic wounds. *Biol Res Nurs.* 2010;11(4):336–344.

36. Stechmiller JK, Kilpadi DV, Childress B, Schultz GS. Effect of Vacuum-Assisted Closure Therapy on the expression of cytokines and proteases in wound fluid of adults with pressure ulcers. *Wound Repair Regen.* 2006;14(3):371–374.

37. Edwards JV, Yager DR, Cohen IK, et al. Modified cotton gauze dressings that selectively absorb neutrophil elastase activity in solution. *Wound Repair Regen.* 2001;9(1):50–58.

38. Gibson D, Cowan LJ, Stechmiller JK, Schultz GS. Initial clinical assessment of a point of care device to rapidly measure MMP activities in wound fluid swab samples. Presented at the 25th Annual Conference of the Southern Nursing Research Society in Jacksonville, FL, February 16–19, 2011.

39. Steed DL. Clinical evaluation of recombinant human platelet-derived growth factor for the treatment of lower extremity diabetic ulcers. Diabetic Ulcer Study Group. *J Vasc Surg.* 1995;21(1):71–81.

40. Smiell JM, Wieman TJ, Steed DL, Perry BH, Sampson AR, Schwab BH. Efficacy and safety of becaplermin (recombinant human platelet-derived growth factor-BB) in patients with nonhealing, lower extremity diabetic ulcers: a combined analysis of four randomized studies. *Wound Repair Regen.* 1999;7(5):335–346.

41. Robson MC, Phillips TJ, Falanga V, et al. Randomized trial of topically applied repifermin (recombinant human keratinocyte growth factor-2) to accelerate wound healing in venous ulcers. *Wound Repair Regen.* 2001;9(5):347–352.

42. Robson MC, Phillip LG, Cooper DM, et al. Safety and effect of transforming growth factor-beta(2) for treatment of venous stasis ulcers. *Wound Repair Regen.* 1995;3(2):157–167.

43. Robson MC, Hill DP, Smith PD, et al. Sequential cytokine therapy for pressure ulcers: clinical and mechanistic response. *Ann Surg.* 2000;231(4):600–611.

44. Robson MC, Phillips LG, Lawrence WT, et al. The safety and effect of topically applied recombinant basic fibroblast growth factor on the healing of chronic pressure sores. *Ann Surg.* 1992;216(4):401–408.

45. Carson SN, Travis E, Overall K, Lee-Jahshan S. Using Becaplermin Gel with collagen products to potentiate healing in chronic leg wounds. *WOUNDS.* 2008.

46. Cowan L, Phillips P, Liesenfeld B, et al. Caution: when combining topical wound treatments, more is not always better. *Wound Practice & Research.* 2011;19(2):60–64.

47. Shi L, Ermis R, Kiedaisch B, Carson D. The effect of various wound dressings on the activity of debriding enzymes. *Adv Skin Wound Care.* 2010;23(10):456–462.

CHAPTER 4

Wound Assessment and Documentation

Lia van Rijswijk, MSN, RN, CWCN; Morty Eisenberg, MD, MScCH, CCFP, FCFP

Objectives

The reader will be challenged to:

- Evaluate commonly assessed wound characteristics
- Explain the rationale for assessing different wound characteristics
- Analyze the purpose of wound assessment in clinical practice.

Introduction

Appreciation of the wound healing process, factors that may affect it, and the number of products available to manage wounds has increased dramatically during recent years. However, a significant portion of wound healing knowledge is based on the results of laboratory studies, while knowledge about the efficacy and clinical effectiveness of many wound care interventions remains limited or even nonexistent. As a result, clinicians not only must remain up-to-date about newly available evidence-based guidelines of care, they also must carefully monitor the outcome of all interventions.[1] Optimal patient and wound assessment practices not only guide all decisions of care, they also are crucial to assessing clinical outcomes.[2-4] At the same time, general education on the topic remains limited; many commonly used wound assessment terms remain poorly defined; and confusion about assessment and staging is common. This may explain why many clinicians continue to feel insecure about the process itself.[5]

Fortunately, we know which indices of wound healing are most appropriate to monitor outcomes in clinical practice. Generally, it is better to regularly assess using the same possibly less-than-perfect tool than not to assess at all. Every plan of care and intervention, as well as the clinician's ability to determine the effectiveness of care, is based on a complete patient history, assessment, and regular follow-up assessments.[6]

This chapter will focus on the practical application of available research as it pertains to the clinical assessment and documentation of nonsutured, mostly chronic wounds. The assessment of wound pain is reviewed in Chapter 9.

van Rijswijk L, Eisenberg M. Wound assessment and documentation. In: Krasner DL, ed. *Chronic Wound Care: The Essentials*. Malvern, PA: HMP Communications; 2014:29–46.

Assessment:
What it is and What it is Not

Verbs commonly used to describe the process of follow-up care include *assess, evaluate, monitor*, or *inspect*. It is important not to use them interchangeably, because their use affects the level of knowledge required to implement the process. To monitor or inspect means to watch, keep track of, or check, usually for a special purpose.[7] To evaluate — to determine the significance of an observation through appraisal and study — requires specific skills and knowledge. Similarly, to collect, verify, organize, and determine the importance of data (eg, to assess) is impossible without specific skills and an understanding of the condition involved.[6,7] For example, the plan of care for a home-bound patient may include 2 visits per week; once a week, the home health aide will change the dressing and monitor the patient and wound for signs of improvement, infection, or deterioration, and once a week, the registered nurse will change the dressing and complete a wound assessment to quantify progress. In the United States, for nurses, the type of assessment a nurse can perform is determined by statutory law (State Nurse Practice Acts): in most cases, registered nurses assess and evaluate; licensed practical nurses or licensed vocational nurses monitor and inspect.

Clinical Wound Assessment Rationale

Goals of care and wound care plans of care. The *patient history* and *wound assessment findings* are the foundation for developing the individual's goals of care and wound care plan of care, which will guide treatment. For example, a patient history will help determine if healing or palliation should be the goal of care, and a wound history can provide important insights about the need for further diagnostic testing. If pressure redistribution is needed, a patient history and assessment will determine if frequent turning is appropriate and feasible. Subsequent follow-up assessments designed to monitor and evaluate outcome(s) will determine whether the wound is moving in the direction of the ultimate outcome, the *goal of care*.[2–4]

Developing a realistic and clearly defined goal of care is particularly important when managing patients with chronic wounds because these patients often have a number of concomitant conditions that may affect the healing process or the wound care plan. A chronic wound presents a considerable burden to patients, caregivers, and, frequently, healthcare professionals.[8] If the goals of care are not realistic or not clearly defined, patients and caregivers may become discouraged. Research suggests that it is important for clinicians to communicate and provide information about wound healing expectations with patients.[9] Defining short-term as well as long-term goals of care may help. For example, the overall goal of care for a full-thickness wound with necrotic tissue may be complete healing, but the short-term goal of care could be to reduce pain and obtain a healthy granulating wound bed. In addition to developing realistic long-term and short-term goals of care, it helps to remember that even seemingly unstable patterns may result in a desired outcome, providing one does not lose sight of it.

Outcome and treatment effectiveness. In recent years, considerable efforts have been made to discover and test *physical, chemical, and biological markers of normal or abnormal healing*. Many studies have shown a correlation between molecular and cellular abnormalities in wound fluid and nonhealing.[10,11] If future research shows that these chemical abnormalities are the cause, not the effect, of nonhealing, tests may be developed to help clinicians diagnose chronic wounds and offer alternative approaches to treatment. No cause-and-effect relationship has been established thus far, and laboratory tests that yield valid, reliable, and clinically useful information to assess healing are not available. Decades of research have shown that regular clinical assessments can help clinicians determine whether the wound is moving in the direction of the goal of care or desired outcome. The effectiveness of interventions — that is, their ability to produce the decided, decisive, or desired effect — cannot be ascertained unless baseline assessment data are compared to follow-up data. By extension, the cost to obtain the desired effect — the cost-effectiveness of care — also cannot be calculated without comparing standardized assessment data. In addition to monitoring the effectiveness of the plan of care, regular reassessments may help motivate patients and caregivers. Systematically gathered assessment and reassessment data will also help clinicians devel-

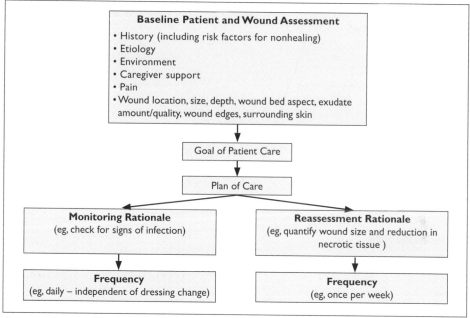

Baseline Patient and Wound Assessment
- History (including risk factors for nonhealing)
- Etiology
- Environment
- Caregiver support
- Pain
- Wound location, size, depth, wound bed aspect, exudate amount/quality, wound edges, surrounding skin

Goal of Patient Care

Plan of Care

Monitoring Rationale
(eg, check for signs of infection)

Reassessment Rationale
(eg, quantify wound size and reduction in necrotic tissue)

Frequency
(eg, daily – independent of dressing change)

Frequency
(eg, once per week)

Figure 1. Reassessment and monitoring frequency and rationale.

op a treatment outcome database. The gathered data can be reviewed, analyzed, and compared to outcomes reported in the literature to develop or modify wound care guidelines and individual wound care plans of care. Because experiential outcome data is limited, this type of information is crucial when trying to develop care plans and pathways.[12,13] In summary, wound assessment and reassessment guidelines are a necessary and integral part of the individual patient's wound care plan of care as well as a tool to accumulate much needed outcome data on chronic wound care.[13,14]

Clinical Wound Assessment Frequency

After gathering baseline or admission assessment data, clinicians have to decide *how often and why the wound should be reassessed*. The latter seems obvious, but in some patient care settings, it is not unusual to encounter orders for twice daily wound assessments without any rationale for doing so. *Overall patient condition, wound severity, patient care environment, goal,* and *overall plan of care* affect the reassessment and monitoring frequency and rationale (Figure 1). For example, when a patient has a systemic condition that may increase the risk of infection,

the wound may require more frequent monitoring and assessments. Dressing/treatment selection also may be affected by reassessment frequency. For example, if a wound must be reassessed daily, it should not be covered with a dressing that is designed to remain in place for a number of days. However, with the possible exception of mechanical debridement using wet-to-dry gauze, there is no evidence to support using products that require daily (or more frequent) removal, and moisture-retentive dressings are recommended for all healable wounds.[2-4,15-18] Therefore, daily wound assessments should be the exception, not the rule. Since the goals of wound care and dressing choices are based on wound characteristics, such as amount of wound exudate, wound depth, and amount of necrotic tissue, these variables should be monitored or formally assessed each time a moisture-retentive dressing is changed.[16,19] Wound monitoring should occur based on patient and wound factors, independent of dressing change needs. Depending on the patient care setting and risk factors for complications, the *condition of the dressing, wound pain,* and *temperature and condition of the surrounding skin* can be monitored as frequently as needed without re-

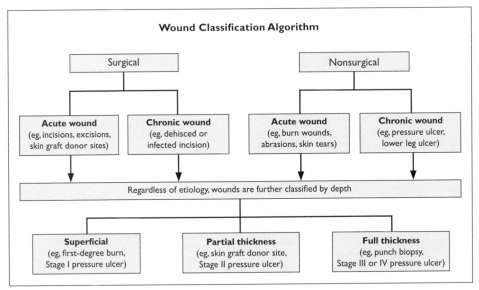

Figure 2. Wound classification algorithm.

moving the dressing.[6,20] When a chronic wound is progressing well, in most patient care settings, daily monitoring (without changing the dressing) and regular assessment (at least weekly) are generally recommended.[11–13,20]

Assessing the Wound

General wound classification. The first step in the patient and wound assessment process is to *diagnose and classify the wound*. For this purpose, most wounds can be classified as belonging in one of two general categories. The first category is related to the *cause* (surgical or nonsurgical) and whether the wound is chronic or acute (Figure 2). Despite evolving definitions of the term *chronic wound*, the following continues to be widely used: *a wound that has failed to proceed through an orderly and timely process to produce anatomic and functional integrity or a wound that has proceeded through the repair process without establishing a sustained anatomic and functional result.*[21] Other definitions include a 3-month timeframe for restoration of anatomic and functional integrity.[22] Clinicians should always consider the possibility that a nonsurgical wound is not caused by pressure or by venous or arterial insufficiency. These so-called *atypical ulcers*, for example, wounds caused by inflammatory or

metabolic disease, vasculopathy, malignancy, deep infections, or drug reactions, do not meet the general definition of chronic wounds. Similarly, the etiology of some wounds cannot be determined until further testing is done. Regardless, *acute wounds* generally heal more expediently than chronic — or atypical — wounds. Hence, the goals of care are different. Similarly, because superficial and partial-thickness wounds can be expected to take less time to heal and are less likely to develop complications than full-thickness wounds, the second general category is based on *initial wound depth.*[23]

With the exception of the *Clinical, Etiology, Anatomy, Pathophysiology (CEAP) classification system for venous disease*, where all open wounds are classified as class 6 active ulcers,[24,25] most wound classification/staging systems are based on wound depth.[4,26,27] Information about the validity and reliability of these systems is limited. However, their use (eg, pressure ulcer staging) is standard practice in many patient care settings, and the presence of a deeper (more severe) wound is usually associated with worse outcomes and longer healing times than less severe wounds.[13,28] In addition, *diabetic foot ulcer classification systems*, such as the *Wagner Classification* or *University of Texas Wound Classification System*, include other wound-associated variables, such as *the presence of infection, ischemia, and a combination of infection and ischemia*. Therefore, use of these systems may help clinicians perform a more complete wound assessment, particularly at baseline.[25,29]

Choosing a wound assessment method. Clinical wound assessment is not an exact science. It is primarily rooted in clinical observation and hampered by ongoing confusion about commonly used wound-related terms and definitions.[5,19,30] Regardless of the method chosen, the *assessment process*, defined as *collecting, verifying, and organizing data*, will always require the talents of a skilled professional. Since communication, including communicating wound assessment data, is such an integral part of being able to track progress toward achieving the goal of care, standardization of the terminology and techniques used is crucial.

Reliability and validity. Reliability and validity are important clinical concerns. When 2 or more people make the same assessment (*reliability*), it is important that the assessments are similar. For example, with respect to wound measurements, specifying which position the patient should be in when the wound is measured and which type of tape measure or tracing device should be used will greatly increase reliability. The *validity* of an assessment, its ability to assess what it is supposed to, can be increased by choosing the appropriate method. For example, assessing wound depth by looking at a photograph is not as valid as measuring actual depth.

Qualitative, descriptive, and quantitative methods. A wound assessment method can be descriptive, qualitative, or quantitative. The use of descriptive and qualitative methods alone (eg, the wound has improved and is smaller than last week) is not acceptable for determining a plan of care or evaluating outcomes. For some wound variables, clinicians have no choice but to describe the observation (eg, wound odor), but if a valid and reliable quantitative method exists, it should be used in order to facilitate communication and continuity of care.

Prepare to assess. A wound assessment cannot be performed if loose debris, particulate matter, or dressing residue is present. Therefore, *wound cleansing* is an important early step in the wound assessment process. For assessment pur-

poses, rinsing the wound with saline will usually suffice. However, when particulate matter is adherent to the wound bed, other forms of debridement may be necessary, including irrigation at safe pressures (between 4 and 15 pounds per square inch).[2-4]

Assessing and measuring wound depth. Wound depth assessment and measurement are important because they affect the goal and wound care plan of care (treatment modality) and help monitor treatment effectiveness. Deep wounds take longer to heal than partial-thickness wounds.[13] It is important to differentiate *staging* (which is a description of depth) from *measuring* the actual depth of the wound. When a wound has sufficient depth (eg, a stage III pressure ulcer), recording ulcer stage during the first assessment does not replace the need for measuring actual depth. If a wound is covered with eschar, wound depth cannot be assessed. In these instances, document "unable to stage" or "unable to assess wound depth" and explain why.[4] Also, the exact depth of wounds with sinus tracts or tunnels may be difficult to assess because the bottom of the tunnel cannot be seen. These wounds can be classified as full-thickness (Table 1), and the amount of wound care product needed to fill the tract or tunnel can be used as a gauge for determining the extent of tissues involved.

Many wounds do not fit into simple depth categories and contain areas of partial-thickness and full-thickness dermal involvement. When using a pressure ulcer or foot ulcer staging system, the stage corresponding with the deepest area of the wound should be documented. Similarly, a wound containing areas of partial- and full-thickness dermal involvement is classified as a full-thickness wound.

Burn wounds are classified based on *depth* and *area*. For example, partial-thickness wounds are classified as superficial or deep second-degree burns, and wound area is defined as total body surface area involved. As mentioned, classification systems for diabetic foot ulcers also include a description of wound depth. Pressure ulcer staging systems, on the other hand, are solely based on the depth of tissue injury. Assessing the extent of dermal involvement can be particularly difficult because dermal thickness varies with age (thin at birth and after the

Table 1. Staging and describing the extent of tissue damage

Structures Involved	Examples of Wounds, Commonly Used Wound Descriptions, Classification, or Staging Systems
• Epidermis (stratum corneum, granulosum, spinosum, and germinativum)	Superficial wound Category/stage I pressure ulcer* Grade 0 (or 0) diabetic foot ulcer** First-degree burn
• Epidermis • Dermis (hair follicles, apocrine and sebaceous glands, blood and lymph vessels, nerve endings)	Partial-thickness wound Shave biopsy abrasion Skin graft donor site Category/stage II pressure ulcer* Grade 1 (or I) diabetic foot ulcer** Category Ib, IIa, IIb, and III skin tear*** Second-degree burn
• Epidermis • Dermis • Subcutaneous tissue/superficial fascia (fat, fibrous and elastic tissue, deeper blood vessels)	Full-thickness wound Punch biopsy Penetrating wound Category/stage III pressure ulcer* Grade 2 (or I) diabetic foot ulcer** Category Ia skin tear*** Third-degree burn
• Epidermis • Dermis • Subcutaneous tissue • Deep fascia/underlying structures (muscle, tendon, bone)	Full-thickness wound Dehisced surgical wound Category/stage IV pressure ulcer* Grade 3 (or II/III) diabetic foot ulcer** Third-degree (sometimes called fourth-degree) burn

*European Pressure Ulcer Advisory Panel and National Pressure Ulcer Advisory Panel. Prevention and treatment of pressure ulcers: quick reference guide. Washington, DC: National Pressure Ulcer Advisory Panel; 2009. **Wagner FW Jr. The dysvascular foot: a system for diagnosis and treatment. *Foot Ankle.* 1981;2(2):64–122 or (text in parentheses) Lavery LA, Armstrong DG, Harkless LB. Classification of diabetic foot wounds. *Ostomy Wound Manage.* 1997;43(2):44–53. ***Payne RL, Martin ML. Defining and classifying skin tears: need for a common language. *Ostomy Wound Manage.* 1993;39(5):16–20.

fifth decade of life), sex (thicker in men than in women), and anatomical location (ranging from less than 1 mm on the eyelids to greater than 4 mm on the back).[31]

Another limitation is that few wound classification systems have been tested for validity and reliability, which causes problems with accuracy when used in clinical practice.[32,33] Finally, staging systems were not designed to capture changes that occur during the healing process, and they should be used to facilitate admission diagnostic procedures only. Just as we do not change the admission assessment of a deep second-degree burn to a superficial second-degree burn when it is healing, pressure ulcers should not be downstaged or backstaged as they heal.

If there is sufficient depth, all wounds, including pressure ulcers, should be measured at the initial and follow-up assessments.

How To

Assessing and measuring wound depth,

undermining, and tunneling. When trying to assess and describe the extent of tissue damage, it may be helpful to find *markers of wound depth*. For example, islands of epithelium in the wound bed may be indicative of a superficial or partial-thickness wound (Table 1). When underlying structures, such as fascia or tendon, are visible, the wound extends down through the dermis and can be classified as full-thickness. The presence of fibrin slough on the wound bed is usually indicative of a full-thickness injury. It helps to remember that dermal thickness ranges from approximately 1 mm to 4 mm; thus, most wounds that are deeper than 4 mm involve subcutaneous tissue and can be classified as full-thickness wounds.[31] Finally, document if the wound bed is irregular, for example: "Lateral aspect of wound extends through subcutaneous tissue. Proximal aspect of the wound contains dermis." The depth of full-thickness wounds is most commonly measured and quantified by gently inserting a sterile swab into the wound at a 90° angle or perpendicular to the surrounding skin. Find the deepest point and put a gloved forefinger on the swab at skin level. Remove the swab and place it next to a measuring guide, calibrated in centimeters.[34] The presence or absence of *undermining*, a space between the surrounding skin and wound bed, and tunneling also can be determined in this manner. The depth of a *tunnel* or *pocket* of undermining can be measured using the same technique as described for wound depth. The validity and reliability of this method depends on clinician skills and documentation.

First, determine if you need assistance to help the patient remain in the position required to perform the assessment and make sure that you have all the equipment (eg, ruler, pen, paper) at hand. Second, the value of the measurement for evaluating change (reliability) also depends on documenting how (patient position) and where (eg, most lateral area) in the wound it was obtained. If tunneling or undermining is present, estimate and record the percentage of the wound margin involved and the location. If it is difficult to describe where the measurement was obtained, draw a picture of the wound and mark the area or use a "clock" system. For example, for all assessment findings, the area of the wound closest to the patient's head is 12 o'clock. There are no limi-

tations on how many depth measurements can be made, and it may be helpful to take 2 or 3 measurements in different areas to get a clear picture of the wound dimensions. Taking multiple measurements close together and recording the average may improve accuracy. Insertion of any object into the wound may cause trauma, and if cotton swabs are used, particles can remain in the wound bed. A variety of disposable wound probes with or without attached foam tips and ruled measurement sticks are commercially available and, unlike cotton swabs, will not deposit particulates in the wound bed. Technological advances also have led to the development and increased availability of handheld devices designed to scan and measure wound size and depth and to calculate volume.[35-37] If valid and reliable, these devices may help standardize assessment and documentation practices. In clinical practice, at this time, wound volume is rarely included as an important wound assessment variable. Measuring wound volume is complicated, and calculating it based on area and depth is generally unreliable.[37] Most importantly, it does not help clinicians decide which treatment to use and it has not been shown to predict treatment outcome.

Regardless of how depth is measured, once a method has been chosen for a particular wound, *standardizing the procedure is crucial to evaluate whether the wound is moving in the direction of the goal of care.*

Assessing wound area/size. Measuring and recording wound size upon admission are crucial to helping clinicians develop the goal of care and patient care plan. First, initial wound size affects healing time. Large wounds take more time to heal than small wounds.[14,38] Second, ongoing wound measurements quantify change in wound area/size to help answer the question, "Is the wound healing?" In fact, percentage reduction in wound size during the first 2 to 4 weeks of care has consistently been found to be an independent predictor of whether a chronic wound is going to heal. These observations have been made for diabetic foot ulcers,[39] venous leg ulcers,[40,41] and full-thickness pressure ulcers.[14,38] Given the consistency and strength of this evidence, it is recommended that clinicians reevaluate the plan of care if a chronic wound does not exhibit a size reduction of 20% to 50% after 2 to 4 weeks of care.[2-4,16,17]

Table 2. Commonly used methods to measure wounds in the clinic

Method	Description	Advantages	Disadvantages	Comments
Tape measure or ruler	• Length (longest area of tissue breakdown) and width (longest measurement perpendicular to the length) are measured using a disposable measuring guide/ruler calibrated in centimeters • Record length, width, method of measurement, patient position at time of assessment	• Easy • Inexpensive • Fast • Good inter-rater and intra-rater reliability • Provides a clinically reliable record of changes in wound size over time	• May be difficult to determine wound edge • Length x width usually does not provide actual wound size • Reliability decreases with increasing wound size • Method may not be suitable for research purposes	• Good correlation between ruler measurements, tracings, and perimeter measurements has been found
Tracing	• Disposable acetate sheet, measuring guide, or plastic bag is held over the wound while tracing the edges with a permanent, fine-tip marker; add location markers (eg, head, toes), date, patient number • Clean the sheet or remove contaminated side of plastic bag/measuring guide • Attach tracing to chart and/or calculate area using 1.0-cm or 0.5-cm grid paper* • Record area, method of obtaining and calculating measurement, patient position at time of measurement	• Easy • Expense is determined by materials used • Fast • Excellent interrater and intrarater reliability	• May be difficult to see wound margins • If transparency does not contain grid, tracing has to be copied to grid paper to calculate area • Manual counting of squares on grid paper may cause over- or underestimation of actual area	• Tracings can be a valuable part of patient records and changes in wound area can easily be compared

* Some measuring guides incorporate a 1.0-cm or 0.5-cm grid. See Figure 3.

How To

The most commonly used techniques for measuring wound area/size in the clinical setting include **tape measurements** and **tracings** (Table 2, Figure 3). Both measurement methods have advantages and disadvantages (Table 2), and their accuracy depends to a large extent on defining and recognizing the wound edge — a well documented challenge.[30] Before developing and implementing a wound measurement protocol, the following limitations should be considered. *All 2-dimensional measurement techniques only provide an index of wound area.* Even though length x width calculations provide valuable information about the progress of a wound, the ac-

tual number obtained when multiplying length and width measurements is accurate only if the wound has a regular geometric shape. Ruler-based measurements are less accurate for irregular or large wounds.[42] In addition, research shows that measuring the longest measurement of the wound (length) followed by the longest measurement perpendicular to the length (width) yields more reliable results than using the "clock" method (head-to-toe = length and side-to-side = width).[43] As with other assessments, *patient position at the time of measurement*, *recording how the measurements were obtained* (see measuring wound depth), and *method consistency* are important. For example, if patient positioning limita-

CHRONIC WOUND CARE: The Essentials

tions necessitate moving the surrounding skin in order to visualize and measure the wound (as may be the case with wounds in the gluteal cleft area), this should be documented. In these instances, wound measurements can vary considerably and short-term (eg, weekly) comparisons are unlikely to be valid. Fortunately, research also has shown that when using paper tape or a grid transparency, wound measurements take approximately 1 minute to complete.[44]

Some devices that measure wound depth also measure wound area,[35–37] and in addition to tape measures and acetate tracings (Figure 3), devices that use electronic or computerized planimetry and digital photography using computerized planimetry are also available. These methods of measurement show improved accuracy and high interrater and intrarater reliability,[45,46] although measurements are more accurate for large than for small wounds.[47]

Color photographs, most commonly used for documentation, also can be used to measure wound area/size, as long as the wound is not on a curved surface.[48] Photographs can be taken using a regular 35-mm or digital camera with a linear measurement scale next to the wound and/or at a standard distance. Similar to regular wound

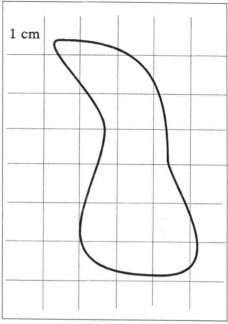

Figure 3. Using a 1.0-cm grid to determine wound size, count the crosspoints that fall completely within the ulcer. This ulcer measures 13 cm². When using a 0.5-cm grid, count the crosspoints and divide the number by 4.

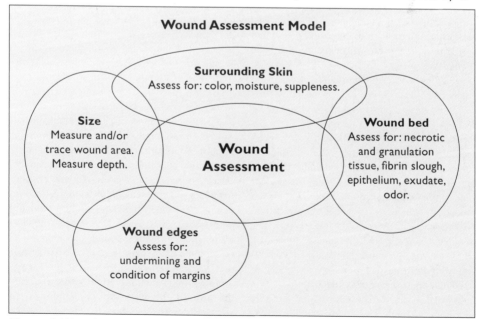

Figure 4. Wound assessment model. ©1994 Krasner and van Rijswijk.

measurement methods, the accuracy of the measurement depends to a large extent on the definition and identification of the wound edge.[49] In addition, **standard photographs** or **digital images** can be a useful addition to the patient chart (see documentation) and digital images can be used for telemedicine. Although specialty cameras with grid film or photography using ruler measurement have reasonable degrees of accuracy, **stereophotogrammetry**, using a video camera and special computer software, has been found to be precise.[50] Despite limitations, photographs may help wound care experts assess wounds, including estimating wound size, when a bedside assessment cannot be performed.[45] The equipment needed to utilize these measuring techniques may not be readily available or prove too costly in the clinical setting. For the most part, manual measurements are most practical and economical. Better still, after measuring the wound, a simple calculation ([(baseline area − current area) / baseline area] x 100%) will provide the clinician with an estimate of percent reduction in wound area since the start of treatment, which will help answer the question, "Is the wound healing?"[2,4,14,38–41]

Assessing the wound bed. After cleansing and measuring the dimensions of the wound, the appearance of the wound bed needs to be assessed and documented (Figure 4) because wound bed appearance affects both the goal and the wound care plan of care (treatment modality) and helps monitor treatment effectiveness.[2–5,16–18] Research using a tool that includes rating the predominant tissue type in a wound (eg, granulation tissue, slough, necrotic tissue) has shown this tool to be sensitive to change in tissue type and correlates well with overall improvement.[51] In another pressure ulcer healing instrument study, change in tissue type was predictive of outcome (healing) but not as important as the presence of pockets (undermining) or change in wound area.[52] At this time, many wound assessment recommendations are based on limited levels of evidence. However, more evidence is likely to become available with increasing research of wound healing instruments and wound care algorithms that typically include several wound assessment variables.

In order to develop a wound care plan of care and monitor its effect in clinical practice, simply noting the presence or absence of granulation tissue, necrotic tissue, and fibrin slough is insufficient because this method will not capture changes in the wound bed until the process is complete (eg, completely free of necrotic tissue). Also, as previously mentioned, confusion about wound terminology and qualitative descriptors remains an important concern and potential impediment to optimal wound assessment.[5,19,30,49] Hence, clear descriptions and, if possible, quantification are important because many wounds contain a combination of granulation and necrotic tissue or fibrin slough (Figure 5).

Estimating tissue percentage range (eg, less than 25% necrotic tissue or 25%–50% necrotic tissue) was first studied as part of the **Pressure Sore Status Tool**, later revised as the **Bates-Jensen Wound Assessment Tool (BWAT)**.[53] Subsequent research has shown that, in clinical practice, percentage description of necrotic tissue/fibrin slough is a valid concept for determining which type of dressing to use and whether debridement is needed and has prospective validity when used in wound assessment tools.[5,13,15]

How To

After cleansing the wound, carefully inspect all aspects of the wound bed and estimate what percentage of the wound bed is covered with necrotic tissue, granulation tissue, and newly formed epithelium. The latter can be visible on the wound edges and in the wound bed of partial-thickness or superficial wounds. Necrotic tissue can be described as dry or moist and may vary in color from black to yellow, gray, tan, or brown. Soft, yellow necrotic tissue is often described as fibrin slough. The amount and aspect of granulation tissue should be estimated and described (Figure 5). Healthy granulation tissue has a pebbled texture and is shiny red or pink. Depending on anatomical location, it is not uncommon for muscle tissue, tendon, ligaments, or bone to be visible in deep wounds. This, too, should be noted. In persons with diabetic foot ulcers, for example, the ability to probe to bone is considered predictive of osteomyelitis and, although not very specific, further diagnostic tests should be considered.[54]

Assessing the wound edges and surrounding skin. In addition to assessing the extent and depth of undermining, the condition of the **wound edges** should be noted. Both assessments

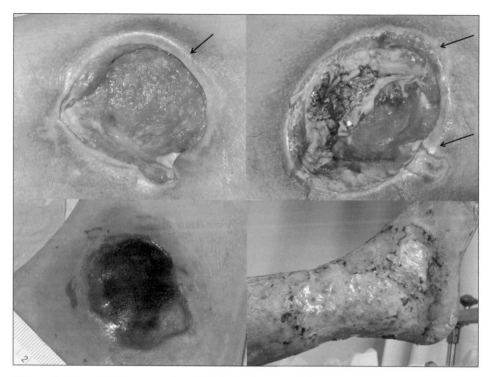

Figure 5. Wound bed presentations. Clockwise from top left:
a) Full-thickness wound contains 95% healthy granulation tissue. Note rolled wound edge and area of undermining (arrow).
b) Full-thickness wound containing 50% necrotic tissue (including slough). Note rolled wound edges and areas of breakdown suggesting undermining.
c) Wound depth cannot be assessed; > 80% of wound bed covered with dry necrotic tissue. Note erythema of surrounding skin and evidence of recent bleeding suggesting trauma/inflammation.
d) Wounds containing 100% necrotic tissue (fibrin slough). Unable to assess depth.

influence the patient course and wound care plan of care. For example, when wound edges are undermined, the application of a primary wound filler dressing to reduce wound dead space is usually required,[2,15] and pressure ulcers with undermining and pockets may take longer to heal than ulcers without undermining.[52] Similarly, in one venous ulcer study, the absence of a healing wound edge with evidence of re-epithelization was a predictor of increased time to healing.[55]

The condition of the *surrounding skin* also may provide important information about the status of the wound and the effects of treatment. Surrounding skin assessment includes evaluating *color*, *induration*, *edema*, and *suppleness* (Figure 4). If the surrounding skin is white/pale, it may be macerated, suggesting that wound exudate has overwhelmed the dressing or that moisture from the outside (eg, urine) was able to penetrate the dressing. Redness of the surrounding skin may be suggestive of unrelieved pressure or prolonged inflammation.[2] Inflammation/vasodilation will cause an increase in skin temperature. A temperature difference between the skin immediately surrounding and a short distance from the wound can be assessed using the back of the hand or finger. Also, *redness, tenderness, warmth, and swelling of the surrounding skin are the classic clinical signs of infection.*[56] Results of one study in patients with venous ulcers showed a significant correlation between a 2°F increase in surrounding skin temperature and clinical signs of wound infection.[57] Digital infrared thermometers, such as the one used in this study, could help provide early warning signs of wound infection. However, clinicians should be aware of the many environmental and patient-related factors that can influence the accuracy of these thermometers.[57] As with wound bed assessments, it is important to remember that most wound edge and surrounding skin assessment information is based on expert opinion and consensus.

How To

After cleansing the wound, examine the *distinctness, degree of attachment to the wound base, color, and thickness of the wound edge*. If it is difficult to see where the wound ends and the surrounding skin starts, re-epithelization may be taking place, and this observation should be charted. Thick ("rolled") and unattached wound margins, commonly described as *epibole* or "*closed wound edges*," are believed to hinder the normal migration of epithelial cells across the wound bed. When observed, this is usually an indication that the wound has been present for some time and that the newly formed epithelial cells have migrated down and around the wound edge because they did not find moist, healthy, granulation tissue to resurface in the wound bed. Callus formation around the wound in a person with a diabetic foot ulcer may be an important indicator of unrelieved pressure.

Irritation of the surrounding skin, which also may impair wound healing, can result from contact with feces or urine, from a reaction to the dressing or tape used, or from a reaction to frequent or inappropriate dressing/tape removal. In patients with darkly pigmented skin, skin color changes (eg, a difference between the patient's usual skin color and the color of the skin surrounding the wound) should be noted.[4] *Signs of maceration include pale, white, or grey periwound skin*, and in patients with leg ulcers, the surrounding skin may exhibit signs of *capillary leakage* (hemosiderin pigmentation, lipodermatosclerosis) or *ischemia* (absence of hair growth; cool, clammy skin).[3,25] Assessing and documenting *suppleness* of the surrounding skin is important because overly moist as well as overly dry skin (commonly seen in pa-

tients with impaired peripheral perfusion) is more prone to injury. *Induration* (an abnormal firmness of the tissues) and *edema* are assessed by gently pressing the skin within approximately 4 cm of the wound edge. Document the location and the extent (in centimeters) of induration and edema as well as pitting or nonpitting characteristics. In one study that evaluated a pressure ulcer assessment instrument, the presence of induration was associated with delayed healing.[58]

Assessing exudate and odor. The type and amount of wound exudate should be assessed because these characteristics provide important information about wound status and the most appropriate treatment.[59] Change in the amount of exudate also may be a sign of healing.[58] However, at this time, no reliable and valid wound exudate assessment tool exists. Some suggestions include rating/describing the amount of moisture in the wound bed and the condition of the surrounding skin.[16,53] Other suggestions include using the type of dressing needed to control exudate as a "yardstick," eg, wounds with scant exudate are those that can be covered with a nonabsorptive dressing for up to 7 days.[55] Clinically, rating the amount of wound exudate will be useful only if a description of each rating is provided. The content and construct validity of the following descriptors, but not their prospective validity or reliability, has been established.[5,15,53] When the wound is dry, there is no exudate. A moist wound contains scant or small amounts of exudate — enough to keep the wound moist but not wet. A moderately exuding wound is wet/saturated and a highly exuding wound is bathing in fluid. In addition to amount, the type of exudate should be described. Most commonly, exudate type is recorded as *serous* (clear fluid without blood, pus, or debris); *serosanguineous* (thin, watery, pale red to pink fluid); *sanguineous or bloody* (bloody, bright red); and *seropurulent or purulent* (thick, cloudy, yellow, or tan).[53] Regardless of which assessment is chosen, consistent and clear descriptions will help achieve the goal of wound assessment to monitor progress.

Traditionally, the presence of *wound odor* (and pus) was used to diagnose infection. Hence, when moisture-retentive dressings were first used, the odor that inevitably accompanied their removal was sometimes mistaken for infection. All wounds, particularly after they have been occluded, will emit an odor, and as with all wound assessment variables, cleansing is important prior to assessing odor. Necrotic wounds tend to have an offensive odor, and wounds infected with anaerobic bacteria tend to produce a distinct acrid or putrid smell.[60] *Pseudomonas* infection often produces a characteristic fruity or sweet odor. Odor is a subjective assessment and cannot be quantified. However, a descriptive odor assessment can provide important information, because a change in the type or amount of odor may be indicative of a change in wound status. As with all assessment parameters, standardizing what to assess, how to assess, and how to document it will increase their usefulness. Odor assessments can include a ***description of the odor*** (eg, sweet, like fresh blood, putrid) as well as a ***description of the amount of odor*** (eg, filled the room, could only smell it immediately following dressing removal, disappeared when dressing was discarded).

How To

Using the information provided, adopt an existing or develop a ***wound exudate and odor assessment instrument*** that meets the requirements of the clinical practice site. Combined with other wound assessments, consistent use will help guide topical wound care decisions and monitor outcomes.

Clinical wound assessment for signs of infection. All wounds are contaminated with a variety of organisms. Determining when these organisms have invaded the tissues and multiplied to cause cellular injury (infection) can be very challenging in patients with chronic wounds. The classic clinical signs of infection — redness, tenderness, warmth, swelling of the surrounding skin, the presence of pus, and skin anesthesia or sloughing[56] — are usually easy to identify in acute wounds. In chronic wounds, however, unrelieved pressure, chronic inflammation, and allergic reactions to dressings also can cause redness, tenderness, warmth, and swelling of the surrounding skin. At the same time, signs of infection in chronic wounds are often blunted. In one study, 7 of 20 persons with diabetic foot ulcers and no clinical symptoms of infection had biopsy-confirmed osteomyelitis.[54] Thus, infections in chronic wounds can easily be overdiagnosed or underdiagnosed. For example, when wound care

specialists were asked to diagnose infection by looking at the photographs of 120 nonhealing wounds, the percentage of correctly diagnosed infections ranged from 37% to 90%, indicating great variability and low reliability.[61]

For chronic wounds, the following variables for assessing wound infection have been proposed: ***increasing pain; the presence of erythema, edema, warmth, purulent exudate, sanguinous exudate, serous exudate, and delayed healing; discoloration of granulation tissue; friable granulation tissue; pocketing at the base of the wound; foul odor; and wound breakdown***.[60,62] Not surprisingly, given the complexity of chronic wound healing, in a study of persons with diabetic foot ulcers, none of these individual wound variables predicted actual microbial load, but a composite of these variables did have some diagnostic validity.[62] In another study, an examination of basically the same wound variables in patients with leg or foot ulcers showed that wounds with debris, increased exudate, and friable tissue were 5 times more likely to have scant or light bacterial growth, whereas wounds with elevated temperature were 8 times more likely to have moderate or heavy bacterial growth.[63] While direct evidence remains sparse, the literature is consistent in that a combination of the aforementioned wound observations should raise concerns about the possibility that a chronic wound is infected. Specifically, most evidence-based guidelines of care include recommendations to assess the patient and review the patient's history for risk of infection and at least 4 signs of clinical infection, for example:

- Inflammation, increased pain, increased exudate, or pyrexia[64]
- Increase in amount or change in characteristics of exudate, decolorization and friability of granulation tissue, undermining, abnormal odor, epithelial bridging (a bridge of epithelial tissue across a wound bed) at the base of the wound, or sudden pain[65]
- Elevated temperature, purulent exudate, foul purulent wound exudate, increasing wound pain, cellulitis, increasing wound size, undermining of the wound, or peripheral wound induration[15,16]
- Erythema, edema, odor, purulent or foul-smelling exudate, increase in ulcer pain and exudate, fever, or friable or irregular granulation tissue.[2]

In addition to some of these variables, the EPUAP/NPUAP guideline includes an increase in the amount of necrotic tissue as a possible sign of infection.[4] If the wound is not healing and the aforementioned wound changes are observed, most guidelines recommend a *quantitative tissue, swab, or bone culture* be obtained, providing this approach is consistent with the patient goal of care.[2,4] At all times, it is crucial to remember that a patient's overall health condition affects his or her risk of infection, confirming the observation of Louis Pasteur (1822–1895) that "the germ is nothing — the milieu [the environment within] is everything."

How To

Following the patient and wound assessment, recommendations described together with careful documentation and evaluation of findings will result in prompt recognition of wound changes or a lack of progress that could signal the presence of infection. If baseline patient and wound assessment findings or a change in the patient's overall health condition suggests an increased risk of infection, consider increasing the frequency with which the wound is assessed. If an infection is suspected, additional diagnostic tests — including quantitative tissue, swab, or bone biopsy for culture — should be ordered.

Documentation evaluation and wound healing instruments. All wound and patient assessment variables must be carefully documented and evaluated. The assessments provide the (documented) foundation for the plan of care (treatment modality), but in order to evaluate the effectiveness of the wound care plan of care, assessments must be reviewed over time. For example, measuring the wound on a regular basis is useless unless wound area and percent change are calculated weekly or once every 2 weeks. Many facilities utilize separate wound assessment forms that facilitate evaluation of the observations. As long as wound assessment protocols are clearly defined and changes in all observations are consistently reviewed, the overall goal of clinical wound assessments can be met.

For documentation purposes, regular or digital wound photographs can be taken to serve as a permanent record. Prior to developing a wound photograph guideline, it is important to carefully review the guideline rationale and all procedures. Compliance with the Health Insurance Portability and Accountability Act in the United States and other regulatory and legal standards is essential. Healthcare institutions and systems often have photography guidelines that must be followed by individual practitioners. A wound photograph guideline should include descriptions on what to include in the photograph (labels), how to maximize clinical information in the photograph itself, and whether or not the photograph should be accompanied by a written report.[66,67]

Meeting the second objective of wound assessment — to monitor treatment effectiveness — may be facilitated by using a wound healing instrument. Most are not designed to guide care and cannot replace the need to assess the wound variables discussed. However, their use will not involve additional patient care procedures as long as the wound assessment definitions used in the setting's wound care protocol are similar to those used in the wound assessment instrument. For example, almost all instruments used to measure healing contain wound size, wound bed aspects, and exudate as variables for assessment. Hence, these observations can all be simply transferred to a wound healing instrument. A careful review of 10 different wound healing instruments concluded that the use of wound healing instruments cannot be generally endorsed but that the *BWAT (previously Pressure Sore Status Tool)* and *PUSH (Pressure Ulcer Scale for Healing)* have been validated to the greatest extent for use with different types of chronic wounds.[68] In addition, content and prospective validity of BWAT variables also has been established,[5,13,15] and additional research using the PUSH tool for use in a variety of chronic wounds[51] and the *DESIGN-R instrument* for pressure ulcer monitoring has been conducted.[52] In light of increased emphasis on standardized documentation and outcomes evaluations, it can be anticipated that research using these instruments will continue providing clinicians with the data they need to develop and implement evidence-based guidelines for wound assessment and documentation.

Conclusion

Wound assessments are the foundation for establishing patient goals and wound care plans of care and are the only means of determining the effectiveness of interventions. Regular reassessments also may motivate patients and caregivers and will help clinicians develop their own treatment outcome database. Knowledge about the appropriateness, validity, and reliability of commonly used assessment terms and methods to describe wounds, develop wound care plans of care, and ascertain outcomes has increased substantially in recent years. While much remains unknown, application of existing knowledge will help clinicians provide evidence-based care and optimize outcomes in all patient care settings.

Take Home Messages for Practice

- A thorough wound assessment includes a complete patient evaluation.
- Treatment is predicated on the results of the wound assessment.
- In clinical practice, consistency of assessment methods used is key.

Self-Assessment Questions

1. Commonly assessed wound characteristics include:
   A. Wound depth, wound size, tissue type, etiology, and tissue perfusion
   B. Wound depth, tissue perfusion, surrounding skin condition, and wound odor
   C. Tissue type, amount of exudate, wound depth, surrounding skin condition, wound etiology, and contamination
   D. Tissue type, amount of exudate, wound depth and size, odor, surrounding skin condition, and wound edges

2. Wound size is an important characteristic to assess on a regular basis because:
   A. It helps clinicians select the right dressing
   B. Documentation of wound size affects reimbursement rates
   C. Change in wound size is a predictor of healing
   D. A change in wound size correlates with a change in patient status

3. The process of wound assessment can best be defined as:
   A. Collecting, verifying, and organizing information about the wound for the purpose of evaluating the effectiveness of the plan of care
   B. Watching and tracking changes in the wound for the purpose of documenting its status
   C. Keeping track of information about the wound so as to facilitate communication
   D. Collecting wound status information for the purpose of selecting the most appropriate treatment modalities

Answers: 1–D, 2–C, 3–A

References

1. van Rijswijk L, Gray M. Evidence, research, and clinical practice: a patient-centered framework for progress in wound care. *Ostomy Wound Manage.* 2011;57(9):26–38.
2. Association for the Advancement of Wound Care (AAWC). Association for the Advancement of Wound Care guideline of pressure ulcer guidelines. Malvern, PA: Association for the Advancement of Wound Care (AAWC); 2010.
3. Registered Nurses Association of Ontario (RNAO). Assessment and management of venous leg ulcers: guideline supplement. Toronto, ON: Registered Nurses Association of Ontario (RNAO); 2007.
4. National Pressure Ulcer Advisory Panel, European Pressure Ulcer Advisory Panel. Pressure ulcer treatment recommendations. In: Prevention and treatment of pressure ulcers: clinical practice guideline. Washington, DC: National Pressure Ulcer Advisory Panel; 2009:51–120.
5. Beitz JM, van Rijswijk L. A cross-sectional study to validate wound care algorithms for use by registered nurses. *Ostomy Wound Manage.* 2010;56(4):46–59.
6. van Rijswijk L. Frequency of reassessment of pressure ulcers. *Adv Wound Care.* 1995;8(4):suppl 19–24.
7. *Merriam-Webster's Collegiate Dictionary.* 11th ed. Springfield, MA: Merriam-Webster, Inc; 2010.
8. van Rijswijk L. The language of wounds. In: Krasner DL, Rodeheaver GT, Sibbald RG, eds. *Chronic Wound Care: A Clinical Source Book for Healthcare Professionals.* 4th ed. Malvern, PA: HMP Communications; 2007:25–28.
9. Spilsbury K, Nelson A, Cullum N, Iglesias C, Nixon J, Mason S. Pressure ulcers and their treatment and effects on quality of life: hospital inpatient perspectives. *J Adv Nurs.* 2007;57(5):494–504.
10. Schultz GS, Wysocki A. Interactions between extracellular matrix and growth factors in wound healing. *Wound Repair Regen.* 2009;17(2):153–162.
11. Karim RB, Brito BL, Dutrieux RP, Lassance FP, Hage JJ. MMP-2 assessment as an indicator of wound healing: a feasibility study. *Adv Skin Wound Care.* 2006;19(6):324–327.

12. Ennis WJ, Meneses P. Wound healing at the local level: the stunned wound. *Ostomy Wound Manage.* 2000;46(1A Suppl):39S–48S.

13. Bolton L, McNees P, van Rijswijk L, et al; Wound Outcomes Study Group. Wound-healing outcomes using standardized assessment and care in clinical practice. *J Wound Ostomy Continence Nurs.* 2004;31(2):65–71.

14. Polansky M, van Rijswijk L. Utilizing survival analysis techniques in chronic wound healing studies. *WOUNDS.* 1994;6(5):150–158.

15. Beitz JM, van Rijswijk L. Using wound care algorithms: a content validation study. *J Wound Ostomy Continence Nurs.* 1999;26(5):238–249.

16. ConvaTec. SOLUTIONS wound care algorithm. Princeton, NJ: ConvaTec; 2008. Available at: www.guideline.gov.

17. Steed DL, Attinger C, Colaizzi T, et al. Guidelines for the treatment of diabetic ulcers. *Wound Repair Regen.* 2006;14(6):680–692.

18. Centers for Medicare & Medicaid Services. OASIS-C Process-Based Quality Improvement Manual. Baltimore, MD: Centers for Medicare & Medicaid Services; 2010.

19. Beitz JM, van Rijswijk L. Developing evidence-based algorithms for negative pressure wound therapy in adults with acute and chronic wounds: literature and expert-based face validation results. *Ostomy Wound Manage.* 2012;58(4):50–69.

20. van Rijswijk L, Lyder CH. Pressure ulcer prevention and care: implementing the revised guidance to surveyors for long-term care facilities. *Ostomy Wound Manage.* 2005 Apr;Suppl:7–19.

21. Lazarus GS, Cooper DM, Knighton DR, et al. Definitions and guidelines for assessment of wounds and evaluation of healing. *Arch Dermatol.* 1994;130(4):489–493.

22. Mustoe TA, O'Shaughnessy K, Kloeters O. Chronic wound pathogenesis and current treatment strategies: a unifying hypothesis. *Plast Reconstr Surg.* 2006;117(7 Suppl):35S–41S.

23. Clark RA. Cutaneous tissue repair: basic biological considerations. I. *J Am Acad Dermatol.* 1985;13(5 Pt 1):705–725.

24. Eklöf B, Rutherford RB, Bergan JJ, et al; American Venous Forum International Ad Hoc Committee for Revision of the CEAP Classification. Revision of the CEAP classification for chronic venous disorders: consensus statement. *J Vasc Surg.* 2004;40(6):1248–1252.

25. Bolton L, Corbett L, Bernato L, et al; Government and Regulatory Task Force, Association for the Advancement of Wound Care. Development of a content-validated venous ulcer algorithm. *Ostomy Wound Manage.* 2006;52(11):32–48.

26. Doupis J, Veves A. Classification, diagnosis, and treatment of diabetic foot ulcers. *WOUNDS.* 2008;20(5):117–126.

27. Lavery LA, Armstrong DG, Harkless LB. Classification of diabetic foot wounds. *Ostomy Wound Manage.* 1997;43(2):44–53.

28. Oyibo SO, Jude EB, Tarawneh I, Nguyen HC, Harkless LB, Boulton AJ. A comparison of two diabetic foot ulcer classification systems: the Wagner and the University of Texas wound classification systems. *Diabetes Care.* 2001;24(1):84–88.

29. Frykberg RG, Zgonis T, Armstrong DG, et al; American College of Foot and Ankle Surgeons. Diabetic foot disorders. A clinical practice guideline (2006 revision). *J Foot Ankle Surg.* 2006;45(5 Suppl):S2–S66.

30. Van Poucke S, Nelissen R, Jorens P, Vander Haeghen Y. Comparative analysis of two methods for wound bed area measurement. *Int Wound J.* 2010;7(5):366–377.

31. Odland GF, Short JM. Structure of the skin. In: Thomas B, Arndt KA, Fitzpatrick WH, eds. *Dermatology in General Medicine.* New York, NY: McGraw-Hill Book Co; 1971.

32. Defloor T, Schoonhoven L, Katrien V, Weststrate J, Myny D. Reliability of the European Pressure Ulcer Advisory Panel classification system. *J Adv Nurs.* 2006;54(2):189–198.

33. Buntinx F, Beckers H, De Keyser G, et al. Inter-observer variation in the assessment of skin ulceration. *J Wound Care.* 1996;5(4):166–170.

34. Krasner D. Wound measurements: some tools of the trade. *Am J Nurs.* 1992;92(5):89–90.

35. Hammond CE, Nixon MA. The reliability of a hand-held wound measurement and documentation device in clinical practice. *J Wound Ostomy Continence Nurs.* 2011;38(3):260–264.

36. Romanelli M, Magliaro A. Objective assessment in wound healing. In: Kirsner RS, Falabella AF, eds. *Wound Healing.* Boca Raton, FL: Taylor & Francis Group; 2005:671–679.

37. Little C, McDonald J, Jenkins MG, McCarron P. An overview of techniques used to measure wound area and volume. *J Wound Care.* 2009;18(6):250–253.

38. Edsberg LE, Wyffels JT, Ha DS. Longitudinal study of Stage III and Stage IV pressure ulcer area and perimeter as healing parameters to predict wound closure. *Ostomy Wound Manage.* 2011;57(10):50–62.

39. Sheehan P, Jones P, Caselli A, Giurini JM, Veves A. Percent change in wound area of diabetic foot ulcers over a 4-week period is a robust predictor of complete healing in a 12-week prospective trial. *Diabetes Care.* 2003;26(6):1879–1882.

40. Kantor J, Margolis DJ. A multicentre study of percentage change in venous leg ulcer area as a prognostic index of healing at 24 weeks. *Br J Dermatol.* 2000;142(5):960–964.

41. van Rijswijk L. Full-thickness leg ulcers: patient demographics and predictors of healing. Multi-Center Leg Ulcer Study Group. *J Fam Pract.* 1993;36(6):625–632.

42. Keast DH, Bowering CK, Evans AW, Mackean GL, Burrows C, D'Souza L. MEASURE: a proposed assessment framework for developing best practice recommendations for wound assessment. *Wound Repair Regen.* 2004;12(3 Suppl):S1–S17.

43. Bryant JL, Brooks TL, Schmidt B, Mostow EN. Reliability of wound measuring techniques in an outpatient wound center. *Ostomy Wound Manage.* 2001;47(4):44–51.

44. Liskay AM, Mion LC, Davis BR. Comparison of two devices for wound measurement. *Dermatol Nurs.* 1993;5(6):437–441,434.

45. Houghton PE, Kincaid CB, Campbell KE, Woodbury MG, Keast DH. Photographic assessment of the appearance of chronic pressure and leg ulcers. *Ostomy Wound Manage.* 2000;46(4):20–30.

46. Sugama J, Matsui Y, Sanada H, Konya C, Okuwa M,

Kitagawa A. A study of the efficiency and convenience of an advanced portable Wound Measurement System (VISITRAK). *J Clin Nurs*. 2007;16(7):1265–1269.

47. Shaw J, Hughes CM, Lagan KM, Bell PM, Stevenson MR. An evaluation of three wound measurement techniques in diabetic foot wounds. *Diabetes Care*. 2007;30(10):2641–2642.

48. Plassman P, Melhuish JM, Harding KG. Methods of measuring wound size: a comparative study. *WOUNDS*. 1994;6(2):54–61.

49. Terris DD, Woo C, Jarczok MN, Ho CH. Comparison of in-person and digital photograph assessment of stage III and IV pressure ulcers among veterans with spinal cord injuries. *J Rehabil Res Dev*. 2011;48(3):215–224.

50. Langemo DK, Melland H, Hanson D, Olson B, Hunter S, Henly SJ. Two-dimensional wound measurement: comparison of 4 techniques. *Adv Wound Care*. 1998;11(7):337–343.

51. Hon J, Lagden K, McLaren AM, O'Sullivan D, Orr L, Houghton PE, Woodbury MG. A prospective, multicenter study to validate use of the PUSH in patients with diabetic, venous, and pressure ulcers. *Ostomy Wound Manage*. 2010;56(2):26–36.

52. Matsui Y, Furue M, Sanada H, et al. Development of the DESIGN-R with an observational study: an absolute evaluation tool for monitoring pressure ulcer wound healing. *Wound Repair Regen*. 2011;19(3):309–315.

53. Bates-Jensen BM, Vredevoe DL, Brecht ML. Validity and reliability of the Pressure Sore Status Tool. *Decubitus*. 1992;5(6):20–28.

54. Schwegler B, Stumpe KD, Weishaupt D, et al. Unsuspected osteomyelitis is frequent in persistent diabetic foot ulcer and better diagnosed by MRI than by 18F-FDG PET or 99mTc-MOAB. *J Intern Med*. 2008;263(1):99–106.

55. Falanga V, Saap LJ, Ozonoff A. Wound bed score and its correlation with healing of chronic wounds. *Dermatol Ther*. 2006;19(6):383–390.

56. Stevens DL, Bisno AL, Chambers HF, et al; Infectious Diseases Society of America. Practice guidelines for the diagnosis and management of skin and soft-tissue infections. *Clin Infect Dis*. 2005;41(10):1373–1406.

57. Fierheller M, Sibbald RG. A clinical investigation into the relationship between increased periwound skin temperature and local wound infection in patients with chronic leg ulcers. *Adv Skin Wound Care*. 2010;23(8):369–379.

58. Bates-Jensen BM. The Pressure Sore Status Tool a few thousand assessments later. *Adv Wound Care*. 1997;10(5):65–73.

59. Baranoski S. Wound assessment and dressing selection. *Ostomy Wound Manage*. 1995;41(7A Suppl):7S–12S.

60. Cutting KF, Harding KG. Criteria for identifying wound infection. *J Wound Care*. 1994;3(4):198–201.

61. Lorentzen HF, Gottrup F. Clinical assessment of infection in nonhealing ulcers analyzed by latent class analysis. *Wound Repair Regen*. 2006;14(3):350–353.

62. Gardner SE, Hillis SL, Frantz RA. Clinical signs of infection in diabetic foot ulcers with high microbial load. *Biol Res Nurs*. 2009;11(2):119–128.

63. Woo KY, Sibbald RG. A cross-sectional validation study of using NERDS and STONEES to assess bacterial burden. *Ostomy Wound Manage*. 2009;55(8):40–48.

64. Australian Wound Management Association Inc., New Zealand Wound Care Society Inc. Australian and New Zealand Clinical Practice Guideline for Prevention and Management of Venous Leg Ulcers. Port Melbourne, VIC, Australia: Cambridge Publishing; 2011.

65. Institute for Clinical Systems Improvement (ICSI). Pressure ulcer prevention and treatment. Health care protocol. Bloomington, MN: Institute for Clinical Systems Improvement (ICSI); 2010.

66. Phillips K. Incorporating digital photography into your wound care practice. *Wound Care Canada*. 2006;4(2):16–18.

67. Knowlton SP, Brown G. Legal aspects of wound care. In: Baranoski S, Ayello EA, eds. *Wound Care Essentials: Practice Principles*. 3rd ed. Ambler, PA: Lippincott Williams & Wilkins; 2012.

68. Pillen H, Miller M, Thomas J, Puckridge P, Sandison S, Spark JI. Assessment of wound healing: validity, reliability and sensitivity of available instruments. *Wound Practice and Research*. 2009;17(4):208–217.

Wound Cleansing, Wound Irrigation, Wound Disinfection

George T. Rodeheaver, PhD;
Catherine R. Ratliff, PhD, APRN-BC, CWOCN, CFCN

Objectives

The reader will be challenged to:

- Differentiate between wound cleansing, wound irrigation, and wound debridement
- Identify nontoxic wound cleansing solutions
- Select the appropriate devices for irrigating wounds
- Analyze which antimicrobials are toxic to wounds (antiseptics) and which are safe for wounds (antibiotics).

Introduction

Wound cleansing is one of the most important components of an effective wound management protocol. Optimal wound healing cannot occur until all pro-inflammatory material and foreign bodies have been removed from the wound. In its broadest sense, wound cleansing can encompass aggressive debridement of all devitalized tissue, extensive use of fluids for cleansing, and selective use of topical antimicrobial agents to control bacterial contamination and colonization. Each of these steps is essential for obtaining a clean, vital wound that has the greatest potential for healing at an optimal rate. However, in its strictest meaning, wound cleansing is the use of fluids to gently remove loosely adherent contaminants and devitalized material from the wound surface. If the materials cannot be removed gently with fluids, more specific mechanical techniques are required. These mechanical techniques are termed debridement. For further information on debridement, refer to Chapter 6.

The benefits of obtaining a clean wound must be weighed against the trauma to the wound that results from the cleansing. Wound cleansing is a mechanical process that traumatizes the wound. The practitioner must always attempt to minimize wound trauma during wound cleansing. By definition, the wound is already a traumatic insult to the body's integrity, and any additional trauma inflicted in attempts to manage the wound will only delay the reparative process. If contaminants cannot be removed with gentle wound cleans-

Rodeheaver GT, Ratliff CR. Wound cleansing, wound irrigation, wound disinfection. In: Krasner DL, ed. *Chronic Wound Care: The Essentials.* Malvern, Pa: HMP Communications, 2014:47–62.

ing, more specific debridement technique should be employed.

Wound trauma incurred during wound cleansing can be chemical, mechanical, or both. Mechanical trauma occurs when the mechanical forces of scrubbing and high-pressure irrigation must be absorbed by the delicate wound tissue. Chemical trauma occurs when the fluids used to cleanse wounds contain chemicals that are toxic to the wound tissue. A philosophy to consider is: "Don't do to a wound what you wouldn't do to your own eye." Few caregivers treat someone else's wound as sensitively as they would treat their own eyes. Yet the sensitive care required for your eye is exactly the quality of care required for wounds to optimize their potential for rapid resolution.

Wound Cleansing

Cleansing solutions. Wound cleansing is the process of using fluids to gently remove inflammatory contaminants from the wound surface. In the majority of cases, water or saline is sufficient for cleansing the wound surface. Because of the limited contact time between the wound and the cleansing solution, it is not essential that the solution be isotonic (0.9% sodium chloride). No differences have been noted in the rates of infection and healing between the use of tap water and sterile normal saline in the cleansing of acute and chronic wounds.[1,2] Tap water can be used for cleansing if it comes from a properly treated drinking supply. An acceptable saline solution can be made by adding 1 teaspoon of salt to 1 quart of boiling water (8 teaspoons per gallon). Any water with known or suspected contaminants should not be used for this purpose.

When enhanced cleansing efficacy is needed, a commercial wound cleanser can be used. Commercial wound cleansers contain surface-active agents to improve removal of wound contaminants. Surface-active agents (surfactants) by the nature of their chemical structure and chemical charge help break the bonds of the foreign bodies to the wound surface. The strength of their chemical reactivity is directly proportional to their cleansing capacity and toxicity to cells. Therefore, cleansing capacity needs to be balanced against toxicity to wound healing cells.

Surfactants can be categorized according to

their chemical charge in solution (cationic, anionic, or nonionic). Most surfactants with charges and many nonionic surfactants have been shown to be toxic to cells, delay wound healing, and inhibit the wound's defenses against infection.[3-7] *Since the US Food and Drug Administration (FDA) does not critically scrutinize the safety and efficacy of wound cleansers, it is the responsibility of the practitioner to select a wound cleansing solution that has been documented by independent testing to be safe for use in open wounds.*

Documentation of safety is difficult, since standardized tests for wound cleansers have not been established. However, tests that directly compare wound cleansers under controlled conditions can provide useful information on relative safety. A study has ranked the relative toxicity of several commercial wound cleansers based on their relative toxicity to white blood cells.[8] Polymorphonuclear leukocytes (PMNs) were isolated from rabbit blood, exposed for 30 minutes to increasing 1:10 dilutions of the test solutions, then assayed for viability (Trypan blue dye exclusion) and functionality (phagocytic efficiency). The extent of dilution required to provide viability and functionality similar to PMNs exposed to Hanks' Balanced Salt Solution alone was used as the basis of an index of toxicity. If a wound cleansing solution required a 1:1,000 dilution to eliminate its toxicity, then its toxicity index was 1,000. The results showed that there was a wide range in the relative toxicity indices (10 to 10,000) for the cleansers tested. In general, the relative toxicity indices for wound cleansers were 10 to 1,000, while those for skin cleansers were 10,000. Cleansers that are formulated to remove fecal contamination from intact skin (skin cleansers) are stronger and thus more toxic than cleansers that are meant to be used in wounds. Skin cleansers should never be used in wounds.

In a subsequent study, additional wound cleansers with and without the presence of an antiseptic were tested.[9] The toxicity indices for the wound cleansers ranged from 10 to 1,000 without the presence of an antiseptic (Table 1). However, when an antiseptic was added to the wound cleanser, the toxicity index, in general, increased to 10,000. The benefit of adding the antiseptic to the wound cleanser has not been documented.

The relative toxicity values listed in Table 1 are

Table 1. Relative toxicity indices of nonantimicrobial and antimicrobial wound cleansers

Product (nonantimicrobial)	Manufacturer	Toxicity Index
Dermagran®	Derma Sciences, Inc	10
Shur-Clens®	Conva Tec®	10
Biolex™	Bard Medical Division, CR Bard Inc	100
Cara-Klenz™ Wound & Skin Cleanser	Carrington Laboratories Inc	100
Saf-Clens® Chronic Wound Cleanser	ConvaTec®	100
Clinswound™	Sage Laboratories, Inc	1,000
Constant-Clens™ Dermal Wound Cleanser	Sherwood Medical-Davis & Geck	1,000
Curaklense™ Wound Cleanser	Kendall Healthcare Products Co	1,000
Curasol™	Healthpoint Medical	1,000
Gentell Wound Cleanser™	Gentell	1,000
Sea-Clens® Wound Cleanser	Coloplast Sween Corp	1,000
Ultra-Klenz™ Wound Cleanser	Carrington Laboratories, Inc	1,000
Product (antimicrobial)	**Manufacturer**	**Toxicity Index**
Clinical Care® Dermal Wound Cleanser	Care-Tech® Laboratories, Inc	1,000
Dermal Wound Cleanser	Smith & Nephew United, Inc	10,000
MicroKlenz™ Antimicrobial Wound Cleanser	Carrington Laboratories, Inc	10,000
Puri-Clens™ Wound Deodorizer & Cleanser	Coloplast Sween Corp	10,000
Restore™	Hollister Inc	10,000
Royl-Derm™	Acme United Corp	10,000
SeptiCare™ Antimicrobial Wound Cleanser	Sage Laboratories, Inc	10,000

Reprinted with permission from WOUNDS 1997;9(1):15–20. Copyright ©1997, HMP Communications.

based on the results of in-vitro testing, and their clinical relevance has not been determined. In addition, the values of relative toxicity should not be used as a guide for diluting the commercial wound cleanser. The commercial wound cleanser should be used at its recommended strength. The toxicity index is only a guide to help in the selection of a commercial wound-cleansing agent. A similar in-vitro test of cleanser toxicity was conducted using fibroblasts.[10] Monolayers of cultured fibroblasts were exposed to dilutions of the various cleansers for 15 minutes, and cell viability was determined by cell uptake of fluorescein diacetate. The results were similar to those reported in Table 1.

A third study utilized human fibroblasts, red blood cells, and white blood cells as test cells for several wound cleansers.[11] This study involved Constant-Clens™ (Kendall Healthcare, Mansfield, Mass), Shur-Clens®, Saf-Clens™ (ConvaTec, Princeton, NJ), Cara-Klenz™, and Ultra-Klenz™ (Carrington Laboratories, Irving, Tex). The relative results were somewhat differ-

ent than those shown in Table 1. Constant-Clens was found to be the most biocompatible cleanser tested, and Shur-Clens was found to be the least biocompatible. Analysis of the Shur-Clens tested indicated that it did not meet the manufacturer's specification on pH, which accounted for its unexpected toxicity. The relative results for the other cleansers were similar to those reported in Table 1.

In a more recent study, the toxicity index of several skin and wound cleansers was evaluated using both fibroblasts and keratinocytes.[12] In this study, the cell monolayers were exposed to the test solutions for 30 minutes and their viability determined by an MTS assay. The definition of toxicity index was identical to that of previous reports. Their results in general agreed with those in Table 1 but contained the results for several agents not included in Table 1. The reader is encouraged to review the article.

Scrubbing devices. Use of a scrubbing device, such as a cloth, sponge, or brush, can enhance the efficacy of wound cleansing solutions.

Whenever these devices are used, the user must realize that mechanical trauma is being imparted to the wound. It is essential to minimize this trauma by using nonabrasive devices and as little force as necessary to achieve appropriate cleansing. If the desired cleansing is not achieved with moderate force, other means of wound cleansing should be considered. One should not try to cleanse the wound by increasing the force applied to the scrubbing device.

Saline has minimal ability to reduce the frictional forces encountered by the wound tissue from a scrubbing device. The surfactant properties of commercial wound cleansers significantly reduce the coefficient of friction between a scrubbing device and the wound tissue.[13]

The coarseness of the scrubbing device should be as low as possible while still providing cleansing action. Wounds scrubbed with coarse sponges were shown to be significantly more susceptible to infection than less traumatized wounds scrubbed with a smoother sponge.[13]

Wound Irrigation

Wound cleansing can also be accomplished by irrigating the wound with fluid. The hydraulic forces generated by the stream of fluid act on the debris on the wound surface and flush it from the wound. In order to remove the wound debris, the force of the irrigation stream has to be greater than the adhesion forces holding the debris to the wound surface. Therefore, it would be logical to assume that increasing the pressure of the irrigation stream would increase the cleansing efficiency of the irrigation process.

Several studies have documented that increasing the pressure of the irrigating stream enhances removal of bacteria and soil from wounds.[14-16] Pressures up to 25 pounds per square inch (psi) were more effective than lower pressures, especially the low pressure produced by a bulb syringe. The efficacy of bacterial removal at 15 psi was significantly greater than that achieved at 10 psi. However, increasing the irrigation pressure to 20 psi or 25 psi did not significantly improve upon the result obtained with 15 psi.

Irrigation devices that delivered fluid streams at pressures of 70 psi were developed for dental hygiene in the early 1960s. It was not long before surgeons suspected that these devices might provide benefit in cleansing contaminated orificial wounds[17] and traumatic wounds in general.[18-20] The use of the mechanical irrigation device at various pressures from 10 psi to 70 psi was shown to be significantly more effective in removing bacteria and debris from wounds when compared to irrigation with a bulb syringe.[20-22] The use of 70 psi was also found to be more effective in removing wound debris than 25 psi or 50 psi.[20] Using quantitative tissue biopsies, irrigation at 50 psi was shown to more effectively remove bacterial contamination than gravity irrigation from a height of 60 cm to 65 cm or irrigation by bulb syringe.[23,24]

Some results suggest that the pressure of the irrigating stream is the important component, not whether it is pulsatile or continuous. Experimental studies comparing pulsatile or continuous stream irrigation have not documented the superiority of the pulsatile stream.[14,21,22] In addition, these high-pressure, pulsatile, irrigation devices are expensive, cumbersome, and difficult to keep sterile. A more practical and convenient way to produce pressurized irrigation is to deliver the irrigant from a syringe through a needle or catheter. It has been shown that delivery of saline from a 35-mL syringe through a 19-gauge needle delivers a stream of irrigant to the wound surface at 8 psi.[25] Plastic tubing or angiocatheters that do not have a point but have the same bore size as a 19-gauge needle would deliver the same pressure of irrigation fluid but would be safer than the needle due to the potential hazard of accidental needle sticks. When compared to irrigation with a bulb syringe, irrigation with a 35-mL syringe and 19-gauge needle resulted in significantly enhanced removal of bacteria and a significantly reduced incidence of wound infection. This experimental benefit has been confirmed in a human study.[26] Three hundred and thirty-five patients who presented to the emergency department with traumatic wounds of less than 24 hours duration were randomly assigned to wound cleansing by standard bulb syringe (controls, low pressure) or a 12-cc syringe and 22-gauge needle (experimental, 13 psi). Two hundred and seventy-seven patients (83%) returned for wound evaluation; of these, 117 were in the control group and 151 were in the experimental group. In the control group, 27.8% of the wounds were inflamed and 6.9% were infected. In the experimental group, 16.8% of the wounds were inflamed and 1.3% were infected. *There was a statistically significant decrease in both wound inflammation and wound infection for wounds cleansed with syringe and needle irrigation (13 psi) compared to wounds cleansed with bulb syringe (0.05 psi).*

Other combinations of syringes and catheter sizes can also be utilized. In general, as the size of the syringe increases, the pressure decreases, because the force applied to the plunger is distributed over a larger cross-sectional area. For example, with a 19-gauge needle, the pressures generated by 6-, 12-, and 35-mL syringes are 30 psi, 20 psi, and 8 psi, respectively. In contrast, increasing the size of the needle increases the pressure because there is greater flow. For example, with a 35-mL syringe, the pressures generated with a 25-, 21-, and 19-gauge needle are 4 psi, 6 psi, and 8 psi, respectively.

Delivery of saline at increased pressure has been made more convenient with the availability of devices that insert directly into an IV bag. These systems usually involve a syringe and tubing with a valve that allows for ejection of the fluid under pressure and then the refilling of the syringe by pulling back the plunger. This is a quick and easy way to achieve bedside wound irrigation.

Other convenient devices are tapered tips on squeezable bottles that when squeezed yield pressurized irrigation. The tips can be purchased separately and placed on the bottles of sterile saline. Some products are sold with the irrigation tips already in place. The user controls the exact pressure generated by these devices, and therefore, the pressures have not been reported.

Recently, irrigation of wounds has been made more convenient by the introduction of battery-powered, disposable, pulsatile, irrigation systems (Stryker® Instruments, Kalamazoo, Mich; Davol Inc, Cranston, RI; Zimmer, Inc, Dover, Ohio) to remove larger amounts of wound debris. These self-contained, sterile systems insert into an IV bag and pump the sterile saline through a choice of tips at elevated irrigation pressures. The fluid is delivered in a pulsatile stream through the tips. The tips are single orifice or multiple orifices and deliver different spray patterns from streams to showers. The spray tips also contain a suction cone and a vacuum line so that the irrigation

fluid can be contained and aspirated into a vacuum canister. The impact pressure generated by these new devices is currently being determined. Preliminary results indicate that the manufacturers are aware of the concern about exceeding 15 psi and have engineered their devices to deliver irrigation fluid below this level. Since these devices are relatively new, clinical reports of their performance are limited.[27–30] However, in a recent in-vivo animal study, the benefits of pulsed lavage irrigation compared to bulb syringe in reducing wound bacterial levels were quantitated.[31]

These devices may be considered as an alternative to whirlpool therapy because they provide suction to remove the irrigation fluid and all of the loosened wound debris. For the patient with a chronic wound who is unresponsive, has cardiopulmonary compromise, or has venous insufficiency and is not a candidate for whirlpool therapy, pulsatile lavage with suction may be an effective alternative. In a comparison of pulsatile irrigation and whirlpool therapy, Haynes et al[32] found pulsatile irrigation to be more effective. Wounds treated with pulsatile irrigation developed new healthy granulation tissue at a rate of 12.2% per week compared to 4.8% per week for similar wounds treated with whirlpool. In addition to being an alternative to whirlpool therapy, these pulsatile irrigation systems also minimize cross contamination because they are disposable, decrease treatment time because of their ease and convenience, and increase wound healing and decrease hospital stays because of efficacy of cleansing. These benefits suggest that disposable pulsatile irrigation systems may be cost effective. Additionally, these devices are versatile, since the pressure, tip configuration, and frequency of irrigation can be personalized to provide the best outcome for each patient and wound. Environmental contamination is possible with these devices, and infection control precautions should be used routinely.[33]

Pressurized irrigation can also be accomplished by applying pressure to the IV bag of a standard irrigation set up.[34–36] In this situation, a standard blood pressure cuff is wrapped around the IV bag and inflated to the desired pressure. Increasing or decreasing the pressure on the cuff will adjust the pressure of the exiting irrigation stream. However, applying 15 mmHg pressure to the blood pressure cuff does not mean that the fluid exiting the tip is at 15 psi. Quantitative testing with standardized equipment (type of cuff, size of IV bag, design of irrigation tip, etc) would be required to establish the direct correlation between cuff pressure and irrigation pressure.

A pressurized canister is another concept for conveniently delivering pressurized saline to the wound. It is claimed that the saline is delivered in a 19-gauge stream at 8 psi. Data to support this claim are not available. A clinical study comparing this product to the bulb syringe procedure suggested that the pressurized canister was effective in cleansing debris and bacteria from the wound in less time and with less expense than the bulb syringe procedure.[37] The study demonstrated that the pressurized canister needed to be 6 inches from the wound, and the stream must contact the wound at a 45-degree angle to minimize splashing. Similar results were reported in another study comparing the pressurized canister to a 30-mL syringe with a 20-gauge IV catheter.[38]

A common problem with all of these innovative techniques for delivering pressurized irrigation fluid is that the manufacturers do not know what impact pressure their system delivers to the wound surface. In the report by Singer et al,[34] the pressure the authors measured was within the system, not the exiting fluid impact pressure. The studies by Weller[37] and Chisholm et al[38] claim to deliver a pressure of 8 psi, but this value is unsubstantiated.

When using pressurized irrigation, the practitioner should always be concerned about splashing the irrigation fluid out of the wound. It is essential to wear protective clothing, gloves, and eyewear during the irrigation procedure because of the significant risk of viral contamination from contact with such fluid. In addition, the use of splash shields on the irrigation device or over the wound is also recommended. These splash shields have been shown to significantly reduce environmental splatter.[39] For large cavity wounds, it may be practical to seal the wound with a transparent film dressing and irrigate through the film to prevent splashing.[40]

Another complication of high-pressure irrigation is dispersion of fluid into the adjacent tissue or along tissue planes.[17,41,42] The extent of this dispersion is related to the magnitude of the pressure. Fluid dispersion into wound tissue was significantly greater for a 70-psi irrigation stream than for an 8-psi irrigation stream.[41] When a single orifice tip was used to irrigate wounds in dogs, the irrigation fluid extensively penetrated the tissue, especially when the pressure was increased above 30 psi.[42] When a multijet tip (shower head) was utilized, irrigating fluid was not forced into the surrounding tissue. The influence of pressure on tissue penetration was further clarified by a study that compared irrigation at 15 psi to irrigation at 20 psi.[16] Following irrigation of partial-thickness wounds on the backs of rats with saline containing 1% aniline blue dye, full-thickness wound biopsies were excised, and the depth of penetration into the skin was quantitated. When the wound was exposed to 20 psi, the irrigation stream penetrated the entire thickness (100%) of skin. In contrast, irrigation with saline at 15 psi only resulted in superficial (10%–15%) penetration of the wound tissue. These results strongly suggest that soft tissue wounds should not be irrigated with fluids delivered at greater than 15 psi.

The efficacy of high-pressure irrigation in removing bacteria decreases with the age of the wound. For acute wounds treated in the emergency room, most bacteria are surface contaminants and are more easily removed than bacteria within the tissue. As the wound ages without appropriate control of wound bacteria, the bacteria invade the tissue and cannot be removed without antibiotics or surgical debridement. Daily irrigation of infected experimental wounds with high-pressure irrigation was ineffective in significantly reducing the mean level of bacteria within the wound tissue.[43] These results would suggest that irrigation alone will not reduce the level of bacteria within the tissue of chronic wounds. In this situation, surgical debridement or, alternately, topical antibiotics should be considered.

Despite the ability of Saxe et al[43] to obtain significant reduction in bacterial levels in their animal experiment, the benefit of irrigation has been reported in 1 study involving chronic wounds. Diekmann[44] used a dental irrigating device on its lowest setting (6 psi) to irrigate pressure ulcers on 8 patients twice a day for 2 weeks. Eight other patients with similar type pressure ulcers received standard care. Wounds treated with pressurized irrigation had a mean decrease in wound area of

51%, while the mean decrease in wound area of the control wounds was only 13%. The large standard deviation and small number of wounds in each sample made the difference not statistically significant. These results are encouraging and support the contention that clean wounds heal faster than unclean wounds.

Another form of wound irrigation is the whirlpool bath that contains a pump that generates pressurized streams of water in the bath through jets. The use of whirlpool is recommended for chronic wounds that contain thick exudate, slough, or necrotic tissue. Wound cleansing is enhanced in the whirlpool because of the extended time of contact between the wound and the fluid. This extended soaking time saturates and softens the wound debris and facilitates its removal. The aggressiveness of the irrigation process can be controlled by how close the wound is placed to a jet. The impact pressure generated by the jets has not been determined. The practitioner and the patient should know when maximal acceptable pressure has been achieved.

Using bacteria as a marker for cleansing action, 2 studies have demonstrated that whirlpool is an effective cleansing technique.[45,46] These studies indicated that a 20- to 30-minute immersion with agitation followed by 30 seconds of rinsing at maximum force tolerated was the most effective cleansing technique. Feedar and Kloth[47] recommend whirlpool twice daily in conjunction with interim wound dressings to facilitate debridement of necrotic tissue. However, once the wound has been cleansed of foreign debris, the trauma to the newly exposed healing tissue outweighs the benefits of the whirlpool. Therefore, clean, granulating wounds should not be exposed to whirlpool therapy.

The Cochrane collaboration conducted a review of wound cleansing studies on wound cleansing for pressure ulcers and found no large scale randomized, controlled trial.[48] Only 1 study demonstrated a statistically significant difference in outcomes for wounds cleansed with saline spray containing aloe vera, silver chloride, and decyl glucoside (Vulnopur) compared to isotonic saline. No statistically significant improved healing rate was seen when water was compared to saline. One study compared different cleansing techniques, but no statistically significant change

in healing was seen with or without whirlpool.

Wound Disinfection

All chronic wounds are colonized with bacteria. Unless the patient is severely immunocompromised, these bacteria can be controlled with the host's resistance and best clinical practice based on standard, physiologically sound management procedures. The single most important parameter in reducing the level of bacterial colonization in the chronic wound is removal of all devitalized material. Bacteria thrive in devitalized tissue and exudate. Aggressive debridement and thorough cleansing are the physiologically sound procedures for disinfecting wounds. Bacteria do not normally survive in clean, healthy tissue.

A chronic wound that has been converted to a clean wound by physiologically sound procedures should show signs of healing within 2–4 weeks.[49-51] If healing is not apparent, the treatment plan needs to be critically reviewed to ensure that pressure relief, adequate nutrition, acceptable blood supply, and proper wound dressings are being provided. If all of these factors have been evaluated and the wound is not healing, high levels of bacterial colonization or organisms could be establishing critical colonization in the wound tissue, and this bacterial damage may be inhibiting the healing process.

Although the influence of bacteria on healing is controversial, it seems obvious that viable bacteria in a wound would be competing with the wound healing cells for nutrients and oxygen. Bacteria would also be elaborating metabolic wastes, reactive enzymes, and toxins. All of these agents would be inflammatory, and prolonged inflammation retards wound healing.

Several well controlled clinical studies have documented that patients with pressure ulcers and venous ulcers with high bacterial levels (> 1.0×10^5) do not heal.[52-57] Other studies involving leg ulcers have reported that healing occurred despite high levels of bacteria.[58-61] However, these studies did not report the rate of wound healing. Wound healing can occur in the presence of high levels of bacteria, but it is probable that healing would have occurred much faster if the level of bacterial critical contamination had been reduced.

In addition to the level of bacteria involved in

Table 2. Partial list of antiseptic agents that have been used in the false hope of killing bacteria without killing wound cells

Acetic acid
Alcohols
Aluminum salts
Boric acid
Chlorhexidine
Formaldehyde
Gentian violet
Hexachlorophene
Hydrogen peroxide
Hypochlorite
Iodine, povidone-iodine
Merthiolate
Permanganate
Silver nitrate

Reprinted with permission from *WOUNDS* 1997;9(1):15–20. Copyright ©1997, HMP Communications.

critical colonization and contamination, the species of bacteria present may also be important. Several of the bacterial studies identified specific species of organisms present in the nonhealing wounds and found a strong correlation with the gram-negative organisms, such as Proteus mirabilis, Pseudomonas aeruginosa, Escherichia coli, and Bacteroides species.[52–54] These studies indicated that Proteus species may be more deleterious to wound healing than the other gram-negative organisms. Clinical experience has documented that beta-hemolytic streptococci are always a significant concern in the wound regardless of their number. In addition, anaerobic organisms become an important part of the microbial population as the wound deteriorates. Synergy is known to occur between aerobic and anaerobic bacteria in chronic wounds, which increases their pathological effect.[62]

When high levels of bacteria in the wound are suspected as the cause of nonhealing, a quantitative culture needs to be obtained. Quantitative cultures are different than standard swab cultures, since extreme effort is made to thoroughly cleanse the wound surface of contaminants and then obtain a specified volume, weight, or surface area of wound material for analysis. Quantitative cultures can be tissue biopsies, needle aspirates, or standardized quantitative swabs.[63] Tissue bi-

opsy—removal of a piece of tissue with a scalpel or punch biopsy and quantification of the number of organisms per gram of tissue—has been the gold standard with which other methods of monitoring tissue bacteria have been compared.[64] Needle aspiration utilizes a 22-gauge needle and 10-cc syringe inserted into the tissue to aspirate fluid that subsequently can be quantified in colony forming units per volume of fluid.[65] Quantitative swab culture was first described by Levine et al[66] and consists of cleansing the wound with saline followed by rotating the end of a cotton tip applicator over a 1 cm^2 surface area of the wound with sufficient pressure to express fluid from underlying tissue. Serial dilutions are made and spread on agar plates, and results are expressed as organisms per swab or by categorizing from scant to heavy bacterial growth.

Although tissue biopsy is the gold standard, there is excellent correlation between the results of tissue biopsies and quantitative swabs, even when semiquantitative results have been utilized.[66,67] Any microbiology laboratory can perform a semiquantitative analysis of a swab obtained under controlled conditions. The important component is obtaining the sample according to a specified protocol.[68] It is important to remember that rather than trying to determine the exact number of organisms, you are determining if there is a high level ($> 1.0 \times 10^5$) of bacteria in the wound that may be responsible for impaired healing. In chronic wound specimens, Bill et al[69] have demonstrated a 79% correlation between quantitative swabs and tissue biopsies in identifying the wounds with greater than 10^5 organisms. In a subsequent study, the same group showed a 79% correlation between quantitative and semiquantitative swabs of chronic wounds.[70]

To reduce a harmful level of increased bacterial burden, a short course of a topical antimicrobial agent should be considered if the wound is clean, further debridement and cleansing are not required, and nutritional status is adequate to support healing. The agents of choice are topical antiseptics or topical antibiotics. Do not use antiseptics in wounds to reduce bacteria in clean wound tissue. Unlike antibiotics that can selectively kill bacteria without harming tissue, antiseptics do not have a selective antibacterial mechanism and thus damage all cells upon contact. ***Therefore, the*** *repeated use of uncontrolled antiseptics in chronic wounds may cause such damage to the cells essential for wound repair that optimal wound healing is delayed.*

The scientific literature is replete with documentation of the ability of antiseptics to rapidly kill high levels of bacteria. These favorable results are obtained by exposing bacteria suspended in fluid directly to the antiseptic solution. Thus, there is direct contact between the bacteria and the antiseptic, and the results are optimized. However, a test tube of fluid does not represent a chronic wound. When wound exudate, necrotic tissue, or blood is added to the test tube, the effectiveness of the antiseptics is significantly reduced, if not completely eliminated.

Antiseptics are used primarily as prophylactic agents for killing bacteria on the surface of tissue because of their inability to effectively penetrate tissue. In order to be effective as a therapeutic agent, an antiseptic has to penetrate into critically colonized tissue in an active form with sufficient concentration to provide antimicrobial activity. Antiseptics actively bind to many organic substrates present in the wound because of their chemical reactivity.[71-73] Thus, antiseptics, when used at clinically appropriate concentrations, might never reach the bacteria in the wound tissue with effective antimicrobial activity. In 1919, after extensive experimentation, Fleming[72] summarized his results as follows: "This would seem to indicate clearly that it is impossible to sterilize a wound with an antiseptic, even if it were possible to keep the antiseptic solution in the wound for a long time without dilution..."

No controlled clinical study has been able to refute Fleming's conclusion that topical antiseptics offer little benefit in reducing the number of bacteria that reside within wound tissue. The benefit that most authors report when evaluating antiseptics as part of a wound management study is most likely due to another aspect of the wound management protocol, such as debridement. Most wound bacteria reside in necrotic tissue. When more aggressive debridement is instituted as part of a clinical study, the bacterial burden in the wound is reduced, and the wound improves. In uncontrolled studies, the improvement in the wound has been inappropriately ascribed to the utilization of antiseptics.

Numerous reports in the literature describe the benefits of different antiseptics (Table 2). However, when all of these reports were reviewed for scientific validity, none of them truly validated the ability of an antiseptic agent alone to decontaminate a pressure ulcer.[74]

A more recent literature review from 2004 confirms that clinical results involving antiseptics are confusing.[75] Some recent reviews suggest that the history associated with uncontrolled antiseptic solutions should not prevent clinicians from considering antiseptics that have been reformulated in more effective and safer delivery systems.[76,77] By controlling the release of the antiseptic, they may reduce toxicity but they also may reduce killing capacity. This is a complex issue, and each report should be read critically to determine safety versus efficacy.

Even the clinical standard, povidone-iodine, does not have well controlled studies to validate its efficacy. Several published studies indicate that the use of povidone-iodine decreases bacterial levels and promotes healing.[78-82] None of these studies were controlled by treating a similar group of patients the same way but with saline rather than povidone-iodine. When such a study was conducted, povidone-iodine was shown to be ineffective.[83] The use of povidone-iodine continues to be controversial. A recent analysis of the literature concluded that the "outcome supports the continued use of PVP-I with caution."[84]

Another formulation of bound iodine is cadexomer iodine.[85] In this situation, the iodine is trapped in a 3-dimensional spherical microbead starch lattice. The iodine is at a concentration of 0.9% (w/w). Cadexomer iodine (CI) is available as a powder, ointment, gel, or paste. One key property of CI is its high absorption capacity: 1 g CI can absorb up to 7 mL of water or body fluid. As CI absorbs fluid, it slowly releases iodine. It would be difficult to differentiate the clinical benefits of absorption versus the benefits of iodine because of CI's ability to absorb wound exudate, bacteria, toxins, etc.

Most of the clinical efficacy studies involving CI have compared the product to standard care.[85] In most of those studies, CI was shown to be beneficial in controlling exudate, cleansing the wound, reducing bacterial levels, and improving healing. The benefits of CI's absorption properties versus the presence of iodine were not differentiated. When a clinical study was conducted comparing CI directly to another absorbing bead product without iodine, there was no significant difference in healing or control of bacteria.[86]

Dakin's solution (0.5% sodium hypochlorite) is another antiseptic solution that is commonly used to treat chronic wounds. Alexis Carrel established the popularity of Dakin's solution in his miraculous treatment of open war wounds in World War I.[87] However, under those conditions, any agent would have proven beneficial. Despite its long history of clinical use, no controlled studies have documented its antimicrobial efficacy compared to standard practice. The clinical benefit of Dakin's solution is probably due to its ability to dissolve necrotic tissue.[88] Removal of necrotic tissue would be correlated with a reduction in the level of bacteria in the wound and an improvement in healing. In this situation, Dakin's solution is acting as a chemical debriding agent and as such should be discontinued when the necrotic tissue has been removed. Dakin's solution should never be used to pack a clean wound.

Acetic acid is another agent that has a long history of clinical use. The activity of acetic acid is probably due only to its physiologically unacceptable low pH.89 Because *Pseudomonas* species are extremely sensitive to acidic environments, topical acetic acid (5%) has been shown to be of benefit in 2 uncontrolled trials where Pseudomonas infections were present.[90,91]

Hydrogen peroxide is another agent that has an undocumented reputation as an effective antiseptic agent. Hydrogen peroxide has little antimicrobial activity, but it is very effective in dissolving blood clots. Therefore, under the right condition where blood clots or hematomas are present, hydrogen peroxide acts as an effective chemical debriding agent, not as an antiseptic. The American Medical Association reviewed the literature on hydrogen peroxide and concluded that it had little bactericidal effect in tissue but that its effervescence might provide some mechanical benefit in loosening debris and necrotic tissue in the wound.[92]

Silver in the form of 0.5% silver nitrate solution was used extensively in the care of burn wounds[93] in the late 1960s and early 1970s. For maximum effectiveness, the dressings had to be saturated ev-

ery 2 hours, a process that is time consuming, and silver stained everything black. These issues were resolved with the introduction of silver sulfadiazine cream.[94] This cream still needs to be manually removed and reapplied twice daily.

Adding silver to dressings has revolutionized the wound care market. Regardless of how the silver is added, by nanocrystalline silver metal or complexes of silver salts, the active agent is the silver cation. Almost every type of dressing previously available is now available with silver. The challenge to the clinician is to determine if all of the *in vitro* results characterizing the various dressings have any relevance to clinical benefit. After evaluating numerous parameters of dressing performance including silver content, rate of silver release, and antibacterial activity, Parsons et al[95] concluded that the dressing should be selected on standard clinical parameters rather than on a dressing's silver content or release kinetics. However, in order to obtain effective antimicrobial kill, Warriner and Burrell[96] reported that a minimum concentration of 30–40 mg/L of Ag+ had to be generated in the local wound fluid.

As with other antiseptics delivered by controlled-release vehicles, the true benefit of the presence of silver has to be evaluated in human wounds. Recent reviews have indicated that clinical evidence of benefit for silver-containing dressings is lacking.[97–99] (See Chapter 8) Even when benefit is claimed, the clinician has to read the report carefully to document that the claimed benefit did not actually come from the dressing itself. ***Do not forget that these new dressings with silver were FDA approved as devices not drugs. As devices, dressings cannot make a therapeutic claim for a released active ingredient; otherwise, they would be drug-delivery vehicles.***

Conclusion

Although no scientifically valid documentation exists, practitioners continue to use antiseptics in wounds because of tradition. This tradition must stop. Antiseptics are toxic chemicals that, when used in clean wounds, do more harm than good. The volume of literature that documents the extreme toxicity of these agents is overwhelming. It includes *in-vitro* tests[100–102] as well as *in vivo* tests in animals[100,103–106] and humans.[107,108]

Accepting the fact that traditional concentrations of antiseptic solutions are too toxic for wound care, some practitioners have assumed that diluting the antiseptic will dilute its toxicity to wound healing cells while maintaining its toxicity to bacteria. Certain reports in the literature support this contention by finding a "magic" dilution of antiseptic that kills bacteria but not wound healing cells.[100,109] These reports are misleading, because the antiseptic agents were tested in test tubes with saline that contained no wound materials, such as exudate or tissue.[110] Although the basis for diluting antiseptics appears dubious, the process is fully encouraged. If everyone that continues to use antiseptics would dilute them 1:1,000 or 1:10,000, they would see a significant improvement in wound healing because they significantly reduced the toxicity of the topical antiseptic agent they were using.

Another way of controlling the toxicity of antiseptic solutions is to control the dose of antiseptic exposed to the wound by using controlled delivery vehicles or dressings instead of solutions.[77] The clinician has to be aware that by reducing the level of antiseptic present in the wound, the antiseptic will be less effective in killing the bacteria. Because antiseptics do not have a specific mechanism for killing bacteria, it stands to reason that an antiseptic level sufficient to kill bacteria should also kill important wound healing cells.

When an antimicrobial agent is deemed necessary to reduce bacterial levels within the wound, a topical antibiotic should be utilized. The use of topical antibiotic therapy has been the mainstay of burn care for the past 2 decades. Some topical antibiotics that have been used for chronic wounds are listed in Table 3. None of these agents are commonly used systemically in clinical practice. Clinically utilized systemic antibiotics should not be used topically on chronic wounds because of the risk for selecting out resistant strains of bacteria. Although Bendy et al[52] documented the success of topical gentamicin in reducing bacterial levels and promoting healing in pressure ulcers, there are other topical antibiotics that will do a similar job without developing strains of bacteria that are resistant to clinically essential systemic antibiotics.

The use of topical antibiotics in chronic wounds has not been reported often in the literature. Despite the limited number of studies

Table 3. Topical antibiotics that have been utilized to control bacteria in chronic wounds

Mafenide acetate
Metronidazole
Mupirocin
Nitrofurazone
Polysporin
Silver sulfadiazine

that have been reported, the results have been impressive. The use of silver sulfadiazine cream in heavily contaminated pressure ulcers resulted in reduction of bacterial levels to less than 10^5 organisms per gram of tissue in all treated ulcers within 3 weeks.[83] In another study, 10 patients with putrid-smelling ulcers and positive cultures for anaerobic organisms were treated twice daily with metronidazole gel.[111] After 5 days of treatment, all odor was eliminated, and repeat cultures were negative for anaerobic organisms. A review of antimicrobial treatments for diabetic foot ulcers concluded that the "evidence is too weak to recommend any particular antimicrobial agent."[112]

Topical antibiotics can be effective when used against sensitive organisms. When in doubt about the sensitivity of the organisms in the wound to the antibiotic being used, consult your micro-

Take-Home Messages for Practice
- Effective wound cleansing is essential for effective wound healing.
- The benefits of wound cleansing must always be balanced against the harm inflicted upon the wound.
- Select biocompatible wound cleansers and utilize them in a nontraumatic manner.
- When irrigating wounds, keep the irrigation pressure below 15 psi.
- Do not use antiseptic agents in clean wounds.
- For nonhealing, clean wounds that contain high levels of bacteria, consider a 2-week trial of topical antibiotic.
- Newer delivery systems that provide controlled release of antiseptics may provide benefit in wounds, but this has to be proven in well controlled trials.

biologist. Well defined tests for determining the sensitivity of wound organisms to topical antibiotic preparations exist.[113,114] In general, topical antibiotics should not be used for more than 2 weeks, and patients must be monitored for any signs of reaction to the antibiotic.

Controlling wound colonization or critical colonization with topical antimicrobials is a complex issue.[62] The primary concern with the use of topical antibiotics is the selection or development of more resistant bacteria. This concern is so predominant that the authors of the European Wound Management Association (EWMA) Position Document on Management of Wound Infection chose not to discuss the use of topical antibiotics.[115] This concern can be minimized with short exposure to high doses of effective antibiotics approved for topical use. Even the use of antiseptics is not devoid of resistance selection or development.[116] This is especially concerning now that controlled-release dressings are reducing the dose of antiseptic present in the wound. Low levels of antimicrobial agents are the primary causation of selection or development of bacterial resistance.

Self-Assessment Questions

1. For a pressure ulcer containing adherent necrotic tissue, slough, and viscous exudate, what is the best wound care protocol?
   A. Scrub wound vigorously to remove debris
   B. Pack with gauze soaked in Dakin's solution and change every 8 hours
   C. Debridement in conjunction with frequent wound irrigation
   D. Cover with occlusive dressing for several days

2. For a clean pressure ulcer containing moderate exudate, which is the least desirable treatment?
   A. Irrigation with isotonic saline
   B. Irrigation with a skin cleanser
   C. Irrigation with a nontoxic wound cleanser
   D. Irrigation with a wound cleanser containing an antiseptic

3. Which of the following devices is the most appropriate for irrigating a wound with viscous exudate?
   A. Saline from the bottle (0 psi)

B. Bulb syringe (2 psi)
C. 30-cc syringe with a 19-gauge catheter (8 psi)
D. Water Pik at high setting (> 15 psi)

4. For a clean pressure ulcer with high bacterial levels, which is the best topical agent to use for a short time?
   A. Iodophor solution
   B. Dakin's solution
   C. Hydrogen peroxide solution
   D. Silver sulfadiazine cream

Answers: 1-C, 2-B, 3-C, 4-D

References
1. Beam JW. Wound cleansing: water or saline? *J Athl Train.* 2006;41(2):196–197.
2. Valente JH, Forti RJ, Freundlich LF, Zandieh SO, Crain EF. Wound irrigation in children: saline solution or tap water? *Ann Emerg Med.* 2003;41(5):609–616.
3. Rydberg B, Zederfeldt B. Influence of cationic detergents on tensile strength of healing skin wounds in the rat. *Acta Chir Scand.* 1968;134(5):317–320.
4. Bettley FR. The toxicity of soaps and detergents. *Br J Dermatol.* 1968;80(10):635–642.
5. Custer J, Edlich RF, Prusak M, Madden J, Panek P, Wangensteen OH. Studies in the management of the contaminated wound. V. An assessment of the effectiveness of pHisoHex and Betadine surgical scrub solutions. *Am J Surg.* 1971;121(5):572–575.
6. Edlich RF, Schmolka IR, Prusak MS, Edgerton MT. The molecular basis for toxicity of surfactants in surgical wounds. 1. EO:PO block polymers. *J Surg Res.* 1973;14(4):277–284.
7. Bryant CA, Rodeheaver GT, Reem EM, Nichter LS, Kenney JG, Edlich RF. Search for a nontoxic surgical scrub solution for periorbital lacerations. *Ann Emerg Med.* 1984;13(5):317–321.
8. Foresman PA, Payne DS, Becker D, Lewis D, Rodeheaver GT. A relative toxicity index for wound cleansers. *WOUNDS.* 1993;5(5):226–231.
9. Hellewell TB, Major DA, Foresman PA, Rodeheaver GT. A cytotoxicity evaluation of antimicrobial and non-antimicrobial wound cleansers. *WOUNDS.* 1997;9(1):15–20.
10. Burkey JL, Weinberg C, Brenden RA. Differential methodologies for the evaluation of skin and wound cleansers. *WOUNDS.* 1993;5(6):284–291.
11. Wright RW Jr, Orr R. Fibroblast cytotoxicity and blood cell integrity following exposure to dermal wound cleansers. *Ostomy Wound Manage.* 1993;39(7):33–40.
12. Wilson JR, Mills JG, Prather ID, Dimitrijevich SD. A toxicity index of skin and wound cleansers used on in vitro fibroblasts and keratinocytes. *Adv Skin Wound Care.* 2005;18(7):373–378.
13. Rodeheaver GT, Smith SL, Thacker JG, Edgerton MT, Edlich RF. Mechanical cleansing of contaminated

245.

14. Madden J, Edlich RF, Schauerhamer R, Prusak M, Borner J, Wangensteen OH. Application of principles of fluid dynamics to surgical wound irrigation. *Curr Topics Surg Res.* 1971;3:85–93.

15. Rodeheaver GT, Pettry D, Thacker JG, Edgerton MT, Edlich RF. Wound cleansing by high pressure irrigation. *Surg Gynecol Obstet.* 1975;141(3):357–362.

16. Foresman PA, Etheridge CA, Thacker JG, Rodeheaver GT. Influence of a Pulsatile Irrigation System on Bacterial Removal from and Tissue Injury to Contaminated Wounds (unpublished research report). Charlottesville, Va: University of Virginia Health Sciences Center; 1989.

17. Bhaskar SN, Cutright DE, Gross A. Effect of water lavage on infected wounds in the rat. *J Periodontal.* 1969;40(11):671–672.

18. Gross A, Bhaskar SN, Cutright DE, Beasley JD 3rd, Perez B. The effect of pulsating water jet lavage on experimental contaminated wounds. *J Oral Surg.* 1971;29(3):187–190.

19. Gross A, Cutright DE, Bhaskar SN. Effectiveness of pulsating water jet lavage in treatment of contaminated crushed wounds. *Am J Surg.* 1972;124(3):373–377.

20. Grower MF, Bhaskar SN, Horan MJ, Cutright DE. Effect of water lavage on removal of tissue fragments from crush wounds. *Oral Surg Oral Med Oral Pathol.* 1972;33(6):1031–1036.

21. Green VA, Carlson HC, Briggs RL, Stewart JL. A comparison of the efficacy of pulsed mechanical lavage with that of rubber-bulb syringe irrigation in removal of debris from avulsive wounds. *Oral Surg Oral Med Oral Pathol.* 1971;32(1):158–164.

22. Stewart JL, Carlson HC, Briggs RL, Green VA. The bacteria-removal efficiency of mechanical lavage and rubber-bulb syringe irrigation in contaminated avulsive wounds. Oral Surg Oral Med Oral Pathol. 1971;31(6):842–848.

23. Hamer ML, Robson MD, Krizek TJ, Southwick WO. Quantitative bacterial analysis of comparative wound irrigations. Ann Surg. 1975;181(6):819–822.

24. Brown LL, Shelton HT, Bornside GH, Cohn I Jr. Evaluation of wound irrigation by pulsatile jet and conventional methods. *Ann Surg.* 1978;187(2):170–173.

25. Stevenson TR, Thacker JG, Rodeheaver GT, Bacchetta C, Edgerton MT, Edlich RF. Cleansing the traumatic wound by high pressure syringe irrigation. *JACEP.* 1976;5(1):17–21.

26. Longmire AW, Broom LA, Burch J. Wound infection following high-pressure syringe and needle irrigation. *Am J Emerg Med.* 1987;5(2):179–181.

27. Loehne H. Pulsatile lavage with concurrent suction. In: Sussman C, Bates-Jensen BM, eds. Wound Care: A Collaborative Practice Manual for Physical Therapists and Nurses. Gaithersburg, Md: Aspen Publishers; 1998:389–403.

28. Cicione M. Making waves. Case Review. 1998;July/August:26–29.

29. Ho C, Burke DT, Kim HJ. Healing with hydrotherapy. Adv Directors Rehabil. 1998;7(5):45–49.

30. Morgan D, Hoelscher J. Pulsed lavage: promoting comfort and healing in home care. *Ostomy Wound Manage.*

2000;46(4):44–49.

31. Svoboda SJ, Bice TG, Gooden HA, Brooks DE, Thomas DB, Wenke JC. Comparison of bulb syringe and pulsed lavage irrigation with use of a bioluminescent musculoskeletal wound model. *J Bone Joint Surg Am.* 2006;88(10):2167–2174.

32. Haynes LJ, Brown MH, Handley BC, et al. Comparison of Pulsavac and sterile whirlpool regarding the promotion of tissue granulation. *Phys Ther.* 1994;74(5 Suppl):S4.

33. Maragakis LL, Cosgrove SE, Song X, et al. An outbreak of multidrug-resistant Acinetobacter baumannii associated with pulsatile lavage wound treatment. *JAMA.* 2004;292(24):3006–3011.

34. Singer AJ, Hollander JE, Subramanian S, Malhotra AK, Villez PA. Pressure dynamics of various irrigation techniques commonly used in the emergency department. *Ann Emerg Med.* 1994;24(1):36–40.

35. Vadodaria SJ, Parekh DB. An irrigation system for large-wound toileting. *Ann Plast Surg.* 1990;25(2):152–153.

36. Leslie LF, Faulkner BC, Woods JA, et al. Wound cleansing by irrigation for implant surgery. *J Long Term Eff Med Implants.* 1995;5(2):111–128.

37. Weller K. In search of efficacy and efficiency. An alternative to conventional wound cleansing modalities. *Ostomy Wound Manage.* 1991;37:23–28.

38. Chisholm CD, Cordell WH, Rogers K, Woods JR. Comparison of a new pressurized saline canister versus syringe irrigation for laceration cleansing in the emergency department. *Ann Emerg Med.* 1992;2(11):1364–1367.

39. Pigman EC, Karch DB, Scott JL. Splatter during jet irrigation cleansing of a wound model: a comparison of three inexpensive devices. *Ann Emerg Med.* 1993;22(10):1563–1567.

40. Chernofsky MA, Murphy RX Jr, Jennings JF. A barrier technique for pulsed irrigation of cavitary wounds. *Plast Reconstr Surg.* 1993;91(2):365–366.

41. Wheeler CB, Rodeheaver GT, Thacker JG, Edgerton MT, Edlich RF. Side-effects of high pressure irrigation. *Surg Gynecol Obstet.* 1976;143(5):775–778.

42. Carlson HC, Briggs RL, Green VA, Stewart JL. Effect of pressure and tip modification on the dispersion of fluid throughout cells and tissues during the irrigation of experimental wounds. *Oral Surg Oral Med Oral Pathol.* 1971;32(2):347–355.

43. Saxe A, Goldstein E, Dixon S, Ostrup R. Pulsatile lavage in the management of postoperative wound infections. Am Surg. 1980;46(7):391–397.

44. Diekmann JM. Use of a dental irrigating device in the treatment of decubitus ulcers. Nurs Res. 1984;33(5):303–305.

45. Niederhuber SS, Stribley RF, Koepke GH. Reduction of skin bacterial load with use of the therapeutic whirlpool. Phys Ther. 1975;55(5):482–486.

46. Bohannon RW. Whirlpool versus whirlpool rinse for removal of bacteria from a venous stasis ulcer. *Phys Ther.* 1982;62(3):304–308.

47. Feedar JA, Kloth LC. Conservative management of chronic wounds. In: Kloth LC, McCulloch JM, Feddar JA, eds. Wound Healing: Alternatives in Management. Philadelphia, Pa: FA Davis; 1990.

48. Moore ZE, Cowman S. Wound cleansing for pressure ul-

cers. *Cochrane Database Syst Rev*. 2005;(4):CD004983.

49. Robson MC, Phillips LG, Thomason A, et al. Recombinant human platelet-derived growth factor-BB for the treatment of chronic pressure ulcers. *Ann Plast Surg*. 1992;29(3):193–201.

50. Robson MC, Phillips LG, Thomason A, Robson LE, Pierce GF. Platelet-derived growth factor BB for the treatment of chronic pressure ulcers. *Lancet*. 1992;339(8784):23–25.

51. van Rijswijk L. Full-thickness pressure ulcers: patient and wound healing characteristics. *Decubitus*. 1993;6(1):16–21.

52. Bendy RH Jr, Nuccio PA, Wolfe E, et al. Relationship of quantitative wound bacterial counts to healing of decubiti: effect of topical gentamicin. *Antimicrobial Agents Chemother (Bethesda)*. 1964;10:147–155.

53. Lookingbill DP, Miller SH, Knowles RC. Bacteriology of chronic leg ulcers. *Arch Dermatol*. 1978;114(12):1765–1768.

54. Daltrey DC, Rhodes B, Chattwood JG. Investigation into the microbial flora of healing and non-healing decubitus ulcers. *J Clin Pathol*. 1981;34(7):701–705.

55. Sapico FL, Ginunas VJ, Thornhill-Joynes M, et al. Quantitative microbiology of pressure sores in different stages of healing. *Diagn Microbiol Infect Dis*. 1986;5(1):31–38.

56. Lyman IR, Tenery JH, Basson RP. Correlation between decrease in bacterial load and rate of wound healing. *Surg Gynecol Obstet*. 1970;130(4):616–621.

57. Margraf HW, Covey TH Jr. A trial of silver-zinc-allantoinate in the treatment of leg ulcers. *Arch Surg*. 1977;112(6):699–704.

58. Gilchrist B, Reed C. The bacteriology of chronic venous ulcers treated with occlusive hydrocolloid dressings. *Br J Dermatol*. 1989;121(3):337–344.

59. Alper JC, Welch EA, Ginsberg M, Bogaars H, Maguire P. Moist wound healing with a vapor permeable membrane. *J Am Acad Dermatol*. 1983;8(3):347–353.

60. van Rijswijk L, Brown D, Friedman S, et al. Multicenter clinical evaluation of a hydrocolloid dressing for leg ulcers. *Cutis*. 1985;35(2):173–176.

61. Eriksson G, Eklund AE, Kallings LO. The clinical significance of bacterial growth in venous leg ulcers. *Scand J Infect Dis*. 1984;16(2):175–180.

62. Bowler PG, Duerden BI, Armstrong DG. Wound microbiology and associated approaches to wound management. *Clin Microbiol Rev*. 2001;14(2):244–269.

63. Stotts NA. Determination of bacterial burden in wounds. *Adv Wound Care*. 1995;8(4 Suppl):46–52.

64. Robson MC, Heggers JP. Bacterial quantification of open wounds. *Mil Med*. 1969;134(1):19–24.

65. Lee PC, Turnidge J, McDonald PJ. Fine-needle aspiration biopsy in diagnosis of soft tissue infections. *J Clin Microbiol*. 1985;22(1):80–83.

66. Levine NS, Lindberg RB, Mason AD Jr, Pruitt BA Jr. The quantitative swab culture and smear: a quick, simple method for determining the number of viable aerobic bacteria on open wounds. *J Trauma*. 1976;16(2):89–94.

67. Thomson P, Taddonio T, Tait M, et al. Correlation between swab and biopsy for the quantification of burn wound microflora. International Congress on Burn Injuries Program and Abstract Book. 1990;8:381.

68. Cuzzell JZ. The right way to culture a wound. *Am J Nurs*. 1993;93(1):48–50.

69. Bill TJ, Ratliff CR, Donovan AM, Knox LK, Morgan RF, Rodeheaver GT. Quantitative swab culture versus tissue biopsy: a comparison in chronic wounds. *Ostomy Wound Manage*. 2001;47(1):34–37.

70. Ratliff CR, Rodeheaver GT. Correlation of semi-quantitative swab cultures to quantitative swab cultures from chronic wounds. *WOUNDS*. 2002;14(9):329–333.

71. Zamora JL, Price MF, Chuang P, Gentry LO. Inhibition of povidone-iodine's bactericidal activity by common organic substances: an experimental study. *Surgery*. 1985;98(1):25–29.

72. Fleming A. The action of chemical and physiological antiseptics in a septic wound. *Br J Surg*. 1919;7:99–129.

73. Lacey RW. Antibacterial activity of povidone towards nonsporing bacteria. *J Appl Bacteriol*. 1979;46(3):443–449.

74. Morgan JE. Topical therapy of pressure ulcers. *Surg Gynecol Obstet*. 1975;141(6):945–947.

75. Cooper R. A review of the evidence for the use of topical antimicrobial agents in wound care. Available at: http://www.worldwidewounds.com/2004/february/Cooper/Topical-Antimicrobial-Agents.html. Accessed February 13, 2007.

76. Drosou A, Falabella A, Kirsner R. Antiseptics on wounds: an area of controversy. *WOUNDS*. 2003;15(5):149–166.

77. White RJ, Cutting K, Kingsley A. Topical antimicrobials in the control of wound bioburden. *Ostomy Wound Manage*. 2006;52(8):26–58.

78. Connell JF Jr, Rousselot LM. Povidone-iodine. Extensive surgical evaluation of a new antiseptic agent. *Am J Surg*. 1964;108:849–855.

79. Gilgore A. The use of povidone-iodine in the treatment of infected cutaneous ulcers. *Curr Ther Res*. 1978;24(7):843–848.

80. Lee BY, Trainor FS, Thoden WR. Topical application of povidone-iodine in the management of decubitus and stasis ulcers. *J Am Geriatr Soc*. 1979;27(7):302–306.

81. Sugarman B. Infection and pressure sores. *Arch Phys Med Rehabil*. 1985;66(3):177–179.

82. Michael J. Topical use of PVP-I (Betadine) preparations in patients with spinal cord injury. *Drugs Exp Clin Res*. 1985;11(2):107–109.

83. Kucan JO, Robson MC, Heggers JP, Ko F. Comparison of silver sulfadiazine, povidone-iodine and physiologic saline in the treatment of chronic pressure ulcers. J Am Geriatr Soc. 1981;29(5):232–235.

84. Banwell H. What is the evidence for tissue regeneration impairment when using a formulation of PVP-I antiseptic on open wounds? *Dermatology*. 2006;212(Suppl 1):66–76.

85. Sundberg J, Meller R. A retrospective review of the use of cadexomer iodine in the treatment of chronic wounds. *WOUNDS*. 1997;9(3):68–86.

86. Moss C, Taylor AEM, Shuster S. Comparison of cadexomer iodine and dextranomer for chronic venous ulcers. *Clin Exp Dermatol*. 1987;12(6):413–418.

87. Carrel A, Dehelly G. The Treatment of Infected Wounds. New York, NY: Hoeber; 1917.

88. Taylor HD, Austin JH. The solvent action of antiseptics on necrotic tissue. *J Exp Med*. 1918;27(1):155–164.

89. Leveen HH, Falk G, Borek B, et al. Chemical acidification of wounds. An adjuvant to healing and the unfavorable action of alkalinity and ammonia. *Ann Surg.* 1973;178(6):745–753.

90. Phillips I, Lobo AZ, Fernandes R, Gundara NS. Acetic acid in the treatment of superficial wounds infected by Pseudomonas aeruginosa. *Lancet.* 1968;1(7532):11–13.

91. Milner SM. Acetic acid to treat Pseudomonas aeruginosa in superficial wounds and burns. *Lancet.* 1992;340(8810):61.

92. AMA Drug Evaluation. 10th ed. Chicago, Ill: American Medical Association; 1994:620–621.

93. Moyer CA, Brentano L, Gravens DL, Margraf HW, Monafo WW Jr. Treatment of large human burns with 0.5 per cent silver nitrate solution. *Arch Surg.* 1965;90(6):812–867.

94. Fox CL Jr. Silver sulfadiazine—a new topical therapy for Pseudomonas in burns. Therapy of Pseudomonas infection in burns. *Arch Surg.* 1968;96(2):184–188.

95. Parsons D, Bowler PG, Myles V, Jones S. Silver antimicrobial dressings in wound management: a comparison of antibacterial, physical, and chemical characteristics. *WOUNDS.* 2005;17(8):222–232.

96. Warriner R, Burrell R. Infection and the chronic wound: a focus on silver. *Adv Skin Wound Care.* 2005;18(Suppl 1):2–12.

97. Bolton L. Are silver products safe and effective for chronic wound management? *J Wound Ostomy Continence Nurs.* 2006;33(5):469–477.

98. Tomaselli N. The role of topical silver preparations in wound healing. *J Wound Ostomy Continence Nurs.* 2006;33(4):367–380.

99. Bergin SM, Wraight P. Silver based wound dressings and topical agents for treating diabetic foot ulcers. *Cochrane Database Syst Rev.* 2006;(1):CD005082.

100. Lineaweaver W, Howard R, Soucy D, et al. Topical antimicrobial toxicity. *Arch Surg.* 1985;120(3):267–270.

101. Cooper ML, Laxer JA, Hansbrough JF. The cytotoxic effects of commonly used topical antimicrobial agents on human fibroblasts and keratinocytes. *J Trauma.* 1991;31(6):775–784.

102. Teepe RG, Koebrugge EJ, Lowik CW, et al. Cytotoxic effects of topical antimicrobial and antiseptic agents on human keratinocytes in vitro. *J Trauma.* 1993;35(1):8–19.

103. Branemark PI, Ekholm R. Tissue injury caused by wound disinfectants. *J Bone Joint Surg Am.* 1967;49(1):48–62.

104. Brennan SS, Leaper DJ. The effect of antiseptics on the healing wound: a study using the ear chamber. *Br J Surg.* 1985;72(10):780–782.

105. Cotter JL, Fader RC, Lilley C, Herndon DN. Chemical parameters, antimicrobial activities, and tissue toxicity of 0.1 and 0.5% sodium hypochlorite solutions. *Antimicrob Agents Chemother.* 1985;28(1):118–122.

106. Brennan SS, Foster ME, Leaper DJ. Antiseptic toxicity in wounds healing by secondary intention. *J Hosp Infect.* 1986;8(3):263–267.

107. Becker GD. Identification and management of the patient at high risk for wound infection. *Head Neck Surg.* 1986;8(3):205–210.

108. Viljanto J. Disinfection of surgical wounds without inhibition of normal wound healing. *Arch Surg.* 1980;115(3):253–256.

109. Heggers JP, Sazy JA, Stenberg BD, et al. Bactericidal and wound-healing properties of sodium hypochlorite solutions: the 1991 Lindberg Award. *J Burn Care Rehab.* 1991;12(5):420–424.

110. Rodeheaver G. Commentary. *Diabetes Spectrum.* 1992;5(6):349–350.

111. Witkowski JA, Parish LC. Topical metronidazole gel. The bacteriology of decubitus ulcers. *Int J Dermatol.* 1991;30(9):660–661.

112. Nelson EA, O'Meara S, Golder S, Dalton J, Craig D, Iglesias C; DASIDU Steering Group. Systematic review of antimicrobial treatments for diabetic foot ulcers. *Diabet Med.* 2006;23(4):348–359.

113. Rodeheaver GT, Gentry S, Saffer L, Edlich RF. Topical antimicrobial cream sensitivity testing. *Surg Gynecol Obstet.* 1980;151(6):747–752.

114. Nathan P, Law EJ, Murphy DF, MacMillan BG. A laboratory method for selection of topical antimicrobial agents to treat infected burn wounds. *Burns.* 1978;4:177–187.

115. European Wound Management Association (EWMA). Position Document: Management of Wound Infection. London, UK: MEP Ltd; 2006.

116. Gilbert P. Avoiding the resistance pitfall in infection control: does the use of antiseptic products contribute to the spread of antibiotic resistance? *Ostomy Wound Manage.* 2006;52(10A Suppl):1S–7S.

CHAPTER 6

Wound Debridement

Dot Weir, RN, CWON, CWS;
Pamela Scarborough, PT, DPT, MS, CDE, CWS, CEEAA;
Jeffrey A. Niezgoda, MD, FACHM, MAPWCA, CHWS

Objectives
The reader will be challenged to:
- Discuss the contribution that debridement makes to wound-bed preparation
- Distinguish the types of debridement used in wound-care practices today
- Differentiate selective from nonselective debridement
- Analyze who would and would not be candidates for debridement in your clinical practice.

Introduction

The word debridement first came from the French *desbrider*, meaning, "to unbridle." It was probably first used as a medical term by surgeons working several hundred years ago in war zones, who recognized that grossly contaminated soft-tissue wounds had a better chance of healing if the affected tissue was surgically removed.[1]

Wound debridement has evolved and is now recognized as a key component of preparing a wound bed for healing.[2-7] The presence of necrotic or devitalized tissue on the surface of a wound prevents accurate assessment of the extent of tissue destruction, inhibiting clinicians' abilities to correctly stage or classify wounds using standard assessment tools.

During the normal cascade of events leading to wound repair, inflammatory cells, such as neutrophils and macrophages, are activated to remove devitalized tissue, participate in antimicrobial defense, and facilitate the beginning of the repair process. The alteration in this and subsequent cellular activities creates an environment leading to wound chronicity and, ultimately, a milieu of increasing necrotic burden.

The term necrotic burden has been frequently used to describe dead or devitalized tissue, excess exudate, and high levels of bacteria found on the surface of many chronic, non-healing wounds. In addition to the evident nonviable tissue, resident cells, such as fibroblasts and keratinocytes, may be phenotypically altered and no longer responsive to certain signals, including growth factors. This state is described by the term cellular senescence.[7,8]

Weir D, Scarborough P, Niezgoda JA. Wound debridement. In: Krasner DL, ed. Chronic Wound Care: The Essentials. Malvern, Pa: HMP Communications, 2014:63–78.

Necrotic or devitalized tissue impedes wound management and healing in several ways:

- Devitalized tissue may mask or mimic signs of infection
- Necrotic tissue serves as a source of nutrients for bacterial cells, thus contributing to the risk of critical colonization or infection
- Devitalized tissue acts as a physical barrier to healing and may impede normal matrix formation, angiogenesis, or granulation tissue development and epidermal resurfacing
- The presence of necrotic or devitalized tissue contributes to the stimulus to produce inflammatory cytokines leading to the overproduction of matrix metalloproteases (MMPs).[7–9]

The Decision to Debride

The overall condition of the patient and individual goals of care must be considered in the decision to debride. In most cases, a terminally ill patient with an intact eschar would not be a candidate for debridement. The result of such an action may be a larger, potentially more painful wound requiring more extensive topical care with little-to-no opportunity for healing due to the patient's severely compromised condition. The patient's general state of health, nutritional status, and medications must also be considered. The patient on anticoagulants, for example, may need to be debrided with a less invasive technique than sharp or surgical debridement or would be more safely debrided in a controlled setting, such as the operating room or hospital clinic, than at the bedside, in the home, or in the long-term care setting. Furthermore, access to adequate anesthesia, whether topical, regional, or general, must be considered for all patients with wounds in sensate areas.

Most chronic wounds require some type of debridement. Debridement is not just a singular event; rather, it is a combination of modalities to achieve a clean, healthier wound bed, as well as a repeated intervention to continuously stimulate and revive the surface cells, keeping the wound in a state of "readiness to heal."[8] Chronic wounds have underlying pathogenic abnormalities that cause necrotic tissue to form and the necrotic/cellular burden to accumulate. To manage this recognized impediment to wound healing, *the practice standard of "maintenance" debridement is recognized and accepted. This includes repeated debridement sessions that continue until the wound can sustain a healthy functional wound bed.*[2] Steed et al[9] found that diabetic foot ulcers that were debrided sharply on a routine basis healed more consistently than ulcers that were not well debrided and maintained.

The decision to debride should be carefully considered in certain wound etiologies. Prior to performing debridement of any type in the lower extremity, vascularity must be assessed. Stable, noninfected heel or lower-extremity ulcers in the presence of impaired circulation[10] usually should not be debrided unless they show signs of infection (erythema, fluctuance, separation from the edge with drainage, purulence)[11] (Plates 12–14, Page 346). Palpating the pedal pulse of patients with lower-extremity wounds is inadequate to assess blood flow. Patients with diabetes who have lower-extremity wounds may need formal noninvasive assessment (digital toe pressures and wave forms, transcutaneous oxygen studies, or ultrasound arterial evaluations) to determine blood flow due to the propensity of the more proximal vessels to calcify. Maintaining a dry, stable eschar often leads to the eschar demarcating and separating slowly as epithelial migration occurs from the edge. With certain etiologies, such as pyoderma gangrenosum, it is well known that debridement may actually result in a worsening of the wound or pathergy.

Types of Debridement

Globally, debridement falls into 2 categories, selective and nonselective.[12] With selective debridement, only nonviable tissue is removed, while with nonselective techniques, both viable and nonviable tissue may be targeted. Debridement is also commonly classified or categorized by the method or the mechanism of action of the various techniques utilized to eliminate abnormal tissue from the wound bed.

The types of debridement currently used in clinical practice include sharp (instrument/surgical, laser, and hydrosurgical), mechanical (whirlpool, pulsed lavage, and low-frequency ultrasound), enzymatic, autolytic, and biotherapy or maggot debridement therapy (MDT). Clinicians may choose 1 or a combination of 2 or more methods over the course of the management of a wound to achieve and maintain a clean wound bed.

Sharp

Sharp debridement refers to the use of instruments or devices capable of excising or cutting away necrotic tissue and surface debris (Plate 15, Page 346). The instruments include, but are not limited to, forceps or pickups, scalpels, curettes, scissors, and rongeurs. While the instruments may be disposable or reusable, those found in the average suture-removal kit are generally not strong or sharp enough to adequately accomplish wound debridement. Further, sharp debridement may be accomplished using devices, such as the laser or high-powered parallel waterjet (Versajet®, Smith & Nephew, Largo, Fla).

Instrument Debridement

Sharp instrument debridement is a fast method of removing the necrotic burden. This intervention can often achieve a clean wound base in one treatment, particularly if the procedure is performed in the operating room. Conservative sharp debridement may also be performed in serial sessions, potentially combined with another form of debridement ultimately resulting in a clean wound.

The clinician performing instrument debridement should have adequate training and skill competencies. The practitioner's basic healthcare training does not necessarily indicate adequate competency to perform instrument debridement. Certain physicians, such as surgeons and podiatrists, are the best prepared. Others, particularly nurses, physical therapists, and physician extenders, such as nurse practitioners and physician assistants, should undergo additional didactic and skills lab training, plus a further hands-on preceptorship, before performing routine sharp debridement. Evidence of completion of such training should be maintained in the clinician's employee file. Knowledge of one's particular licensure practice act is paramount before performing this procedure.[3] Some states prohibit certain levels of healthcare practitioners from performing debridement of living tissue and restrict their practice to the debridement of devitalized tissue. Clarification of the limitations on your professional practice by your state-specific practice board is reasonably prudent practice.

As previously mentioned, many chronic wounds require maintenance debridement, even if the wound has been surgically prepared previously. This is typically accomplished with sharp instruments, such as a curette, and is minimally excisional by removing the immediate wound surface. The goal is always to enhance wound healing by reducing or eliminating bacteria and biofilms, as well as senescent cells. Additionally, maintenance debridement enables the clinician to assess and address the wound edges. Epiboly, or the growth of keratinocytes down the edge of a wound, results in a closed wound edge with cells less likely or unable to migrate out and resurface the wound.

The patient must be adequately prepared for sharp debridement. Informed consent should be obtained, particularly if operative debridement will be performed. The facility or agency protocol will dictate consent policies that should be followed. Prior to sharp/surgical debridement, the wound site should be prepared by adequate cleansing to remove exudate, residue, and any loose debris, which may have accumulated since the previous dressing change. The choice to use an antimicrobial cleanser or solution depends on the presence or absence of infection, the appearance of surface contamination or presumed colonization, and the patient's own host defenses. Because transient local bacteremia may occur with sharp/surgical debridement, the immunocompromised patient may be best managed with prophylactic systemic antibiotics in preparation for the procedure.

Adequate pain management before, during, and after the procedure is imperative. Premedication can help to reduce anxiety and discomfort related to cleansing and preparing the wound for debridement. Topical or local anesthetics should be employed after adequate cleansing to reduce or eliminate procedural pain. Lastly, the practitioner needs to plan for post-procedural pain with adequate orders for pain control after the procedure is completed. For further information, see Chapter 9.

Patients must understand the reason for the sharp/surgical debridement. The clinician should keep in mind that, to the average person, scabs are good and are to be left alone. To enhance patient cooperation and decrease anxiety during procedures, a non-rushed explanation of basic wound-bed preparation at the patient's level of comprehension should be undertaken. Describing the difference between a scab and necrotic tissue and the detrimental effects of the necrotic tissue to overall wound healing will assist patients in understanding why they will benefit from debridement. Lastly, patients must feel that they are in control. Assure them that if the procedure is too painful and they are unable to tolerate the discomfort, the procedure will be stopped. This will go a long way toward establishing patient trust and willingness to consent to future procedures.

The decision to perform sharp surgical debridement in the operating room is largely based on the extent and depth of the anticipated debridement and the need to accomplish the procedure under controlled conditions (pain, bleeding, asepsis). Other factors may include:

- Emergent procedures, such as in the case of infected wounds or patient sepsis
- The need for a higher degree of asepsis, such as with the presence or potential presence of tendon, bone, or joints
- The need for extensive bone debridement
- The need for adequate anesthesia
- Wounds involving extensive undermining, sinus tracts, or tunneling
- The potential for excessive bleeding
- The patient's anxiety or stress related to the procedure.

In addition to the use of instruments, the operating room provides an environment for the use of devices that accomplish debridement into deeper tissues more rapidly than with instruments. These include the use of laser and the high-powered waterjet.

Laser Debridement

The term laser is an acronym for light amplification by the stimulated emission of radiation.[13] Laser debridement, a form of surgical sharp debridement, uses focused beams of light to cauterize, vaporize, or slice through tissue. It is an operative procedure that likely is used less frequently than other forms of debridement.

There are several light sources available for lasers: argon, CO_2, neodymium yttrium aluminum garnet (Nd:YAG), and tunable. The emission of light at different wavelengths enables the laser to target different types of body tissues, depending on the part of the tissue that absorbs the light. When laser energy hits tissue, ablation occurs. The intense heat of laser light causes water within a cell to boil. After the water boils, it expands and ruptures the cell wall, vaporizing the cell contents and creating a small amount of steam as a by-product.[13]

Water readily absorbs CO_2 laser energy, which makes this kind of laser energy inefficient in fluid-filled cavities. CO_2 energy, however, is considered one of the most efficient and precise cutting lasers on the market. The argon laser works best on pigmented tissue and is absorbed easily within the hemoglobin-rich retinal surface. The contact YAG lasers are better at coagulation than other lasers, such as the CO_2 laser, which only works on smaller vessels and, therefore, would be ineffective in controlling significant bleeding. Different laser sources are used in different situations depending on the type of tissue involved, extent of the necrosis, location of the wound, and the goal of the procedure. Due to the potential risk of injury to adjacent tissue, the use of laser energy for debridement is a highly skilled procedure not available in all settings. Newer work with pulsed versus continuous laser beams has reduced the risk of negative effects.[13]

Hydrosurgical Debridement

The high-powered parallel waterjet (Versajet®) is a newer surgical debridement tool that precisely removes tissue using a high-energy water beam. This US Food and Drug Administration (FDA)-approved medical device has the ability to focus a high-powered stream of water into a high-energy cutting implement. The saline used in the waterjet is enclosed in a sterile circuit that passes through a small but highly powerful pump. The saline is directed through high-pressure tubing into a hand piece where it is directed into a 180-degree turn and forced through a nozzle 0.005" in diameter. The energized saline emerges in a focused beam of up to 15,000 psi. The saline beam is directed parallel to the wound so that the cutting mechanism is a highly controlled form of tangential excision. If the handset is positioned in an oblique position, irrigation and tissue removal are accomplished. The surgeon can further regulate the excising effect of the waterjet by adjusting its pressure and velocity via 10 power settings. As the water speed increases, the excising effect on the unwanted tissue increases. This cutting action provides the surgeon control over the wound surface.[14,15]

This form of surgical debridement is reported to be less effective in pressure ulcers covered with dry eschar. The preferred approach is to sharply remove the eschar and then use the waterjet to debride the underlying necrotic tissue. Consequently, all of the necrotic tissue, fibrinous debris, and granulation tissue can be removed with no injury to the healthy underlying collateral tissue. Surgeons can perform more aggressive wound debridement while simultaneously removing less surrounding tissue.[14,15] Granick et al[14] reported improved patient outcomes, fewer required surgeries, and lower costs related to achieving a well-prepared wound bed for more rapid time to surgical closure or application of effective topical therapies (Plate 16, Page 346).

Mechanical Debridement

The term mechanical debridement refers to the use of some external force to dislodge and remove debris and necrotic burden from the wound surface. Because of the nature of the mechanical force, this method is considered to be primarily nonselective. Mechanical methods include various forms of hydrotherapy, wet-to-dry or wet-to-moist dressings, and low-frequency ultrasound.

Hydrotherapy

Hydrotherapy, the use of fluids for cleansing and debridement, includes whirlpool, pulsatile lavage with suction, irrigation, and jet lavage.

Whirlpool

Whirlpool is considered a nonspecific form of mechanical debridement that facilitates cleansing by immersing the patient's body part in a tub or tank while a turbine agitates the water. Whirlpool treatment is no longer a highly favored mechanical debridement treatment modality for a variety of reasons. The risk of infection from cross-contamination and aerosolization are dangers that must be considered.[5]

In most instances, whirlpool is an inappropriate modality for chronic venous insufficiency leg ulcers and diabetic foot ulcers. Chronic venous leg ulcers are already "wet" due to their highly exudative nature. Whirlpool creates the potential to exacerbate the often macerated condition of the tissue surrounding the wound. In addition, McCulloch and Boyd[16] demonstrated that the legs of patients with chronic, venous-insufficiency ulcers immersed in the whirlpool longer than 5 minutes with the leg in the customary dependent position resulted in increased venous hypertension and vascular congestion leading to limb edema.

In the case of the neuropathic foot with or without an ulcer in patients with diabetes, the prolonged exposure to water during whirlpool macerates the skin, leaving the foot more susceptible to injury. Additionally, the warm water contributes to the anhydrotic condition frequently existing with this patient population by washing away the already diminished body oils that assist in protecting the skin.[17]

Whirlpool therapy may not be available or practical in all healthcare settings because of the equipment required and the need to transport the patient to the area of the facility where the tanks are located.[18] Because of infection control issues related to aerosolization, portable tanks taken to patient rooms is a practice that has been eliminated in many settings. Finally, the cost effectiveness of whirlpool is questionable due to its labor intensive nature.

Pulsatile Lavage with Suction

Pulsatile lavage with suction (PLWS) has reduced or eliminated the use of whirlpool in many practices. This modality is highly effective in dislodging necrotic tissue and, although technically nonselective, can be of great benefit with judicious placement of the tips dispersing the pulsating irrigant. In addition, this modality has simultaneous suction, which removes the irrigant, exudate, and debris from the wound bed (Plate 17, Page 346).[19] This method of debridement is one of the few that can function in tracts, tunnels, and extensive undermining. Pressure settings should be below 15 psi to prevent driving bacteria into underlying soft tissue and to prevent damage to granulation tissue if present in the wound bed.[10] Personal protective equipment (PPE) is necessary for the provider. In addition, treatment should be delivered in an enclosed private treatment area to avoid contamination by aerosolization.[20] Recently, a flexible polyurethane protective shield to cover the wound area and instrumentation has been developed to assist in preventing or minimizing the aerosolization associated with PLWS. Research has not been done on this protective shield to demonstrate if aerosolization is completely contained when using PLWS. It is essential that the clinician be experienced when treating complex wounds, such as those with fistulas, exposed cavity linings, and ones with long tunnels in body cavities.[19,21]

Jet Lavage

Jet Lavage (Jetox™, DeRoyal Industries, Powell, Tenn) is a wound-cleansing and debridement modality combining compressed oxygen with a small amount of saline, which delivers a constant stream to the surface of the wound. This modality converts the saline and oxygen into microdroplets, which are then accelerated to supersonic speeds and sprayed on the treatment area gently removing only the necrotic tissue layer, without damaging the viable layer underneath. It has been reported to have a beneficial effect for patients with painful wounds because of a desensitizing effect created by the combination of the spray with air or oxygen.[22]

The force delivered to the wound surface is dependent upon the rate of the flow of the oxygen. The recommended ranges are from 9 L/min–15 L/min, which delivers the saline at 4 psi–12 psi, respectively.[22] This is certainly adequate for effective wound cleansing as well as dislodgement and removal of loose surface debris. The latex-free disposable units make this modality useful in all practice settings including home care.

Wound Irrigation

Wound irrigation may be used to clean wounds and perform minimal debridement of loose tissue. It is recommended that a 35-mL syringe with a 19-gauge needle or angiocatheter or available prepackaged systems be used to deliver the optimal pressure to adequately cleanse the wound without harming healthy tissue.[10] This form of hydrotherapy is ineffective on firmly attached fibrin or slough and eschar due to lack of enough force to dislodge the necrotic tissue from the wound bed.

It is worth mentioning again that due to the aerosolization effects of hydrotherapy modalities, particularly pulsed lavage, jet lavage, and forceful irrigation, the clinician should wear PPE including gloves, fluid proof aprons or gowns, hair covers, masks, and face/eye shields. Upon completion of the procedure, flat surfaces in the room should be wiped down according to the infection-control standards of the facility or agency.

Wet-to-Dry Dressings

The dressing technique commonly referred to as either wet-to-dry or wet-to-moist has been documented and most likely remains the most common form of not only debridement but also dressing used in the United States today.[23] The name carries a bit of irony in that rarely is the gauze dressing placed into the wound bed in a "wet" level of hydration. Rather, the most commonly discussed procedure is to wet open-weave gauze, squeeze or wring it out until it is just moist, and open and place it into the wound bed so that a layer of the gauze is in intimate contact with the wound surface. The proposed mechanism of action is that as the gauze dries and is subsequently removed from the wound bed, it will be adherent to the wound surface and the necrotic tissue will be torn from the wound as the dressing is removed.

This nonselective form of debridement is unquestionably one of the more controversial issues in wound management. The technique carries many disadvantages that overshadow most potential benefits. For example:

1. The procedure is nonselective as a form of debridement and will indiscriminately remove any tissue with which it is in contact
2. Gauze does not have to completely dry to cause trauma to the wound surface—the very absorption of exudate off of the wound surface will cause fibers to become imbedded into the wound tissue and, consequently, adhere on removal[24]
3. Wet-to-dry dressings often cause pain when removed
4. The gauze is often over packed, causing increased detrimental pressure to the wound, increasing the likelihood of further tissue necrosis
5. Exposed structures, such as bone or tendon,

will likely dry out using this procedure.

Additionally, wet-to-dry dressings may impede wound healing due to local tissue cooling, disruption of angiogenesis by dressing removal, and increased infection risk from frequent dressing changes, strike through, and prolonged inflammation.[25] Wet-to-dry dressings are also labor intensive and costly.

With all of the negatives aside, when performed properly, debridement using this technique can be a relatively quick and often effective method of removing devitalized tissue in a wound bed that is completely covered with necrotic tissue. It is important that adequate, ambient, wound fluid is present to prevent surface desiccation. Additionally, in the presence of massively large wounds, moistened gauze is often the only packing material choice to reasonably, cost-effectively pack into a large defect of space. However, once granulation tissue begins to form in the wound bed, it is imperative that the clinician shift from the wet-to-dry technique to one that will not damage the new, fragile tissue in the wound bed.

Ultrasound

The medical use of ultrasound is not a new concept in medicine. The use of ultrasound to treat many disorders began to appear in the literature[26] as early as 1949. Therapeutic ultrasound delivers energy through mechanical vibrations in the form of sound waves at frequencies above detection by the human ear (> 20 kHz). Historically, ultrasound is commonly associated with diagnostic imaging in which high-frequency ultrasound waves with minimal physiological effects are utilized. In addition, high-frequency therapeutic ultrasound (in the 1 MHz–3 MHz range) has been used in physical therapy, physical medicine, and rehabilitation and sports medicine for many years for treatment of soft-tissue injuries and wounds.[27] Recently, low-frequency ultrasound has been added as an energy to impact tissues in the wound bed.

Ultrasound therapy in general provides therapeutic effects related to the energy created by the sound wave on the tissues at which the energy is directed. The effects are labeled thermal and nonthermal. Thermal effects occur as ultrasound travels through body tissue with a certain percentage being absorbed, resulting in the generation of heat and thermal energy. The degree of absorption depends on the nature of the tissue, the extent of blood flow, and the frequency of the sound wave used.[29] Thermal effects are generally created by high-frequency ultrasound using the 1 MHz–3 MHz range of sound waves creating increased blood flow, reduction in muscle spasm, increased extensibility of collagen fibrils, and a pro-inflammatory response.[27]

Nonthermal effects include cavitation and acoustic streaming and are the primary effects created by low-frequency ultrasound.[28-40] Cavitation is described as the formation of miniscule gas bubbles in tissue fluids. The expansion and contraction in size of these bubbles occur in tandem with the variations in the ultrasound field-pressure levels. At certain amplitudes of the sound waves, the bubbles implode; this implosion results in the formation of tiny shock waves, the vibration of which causes changes in the permeability of cell membranes. These locally generated shock waves in turn liquefy necrotic tissue, other wound debris, and associated biofilm. Research has shown that such implosion-related shock waves destroy the bacterial cell walls.[29-31] It has been demonstrated that this process interrupts the metabolism of the bacteria and essentially kills them without damaging host cells.

The second effect of low-frequency ultrasound is acoustic streaming, which initiates a unidirectional movement in fluid in an ultrasound field, causing a temporary disturbance in the cell membrane. This activity causes biochemical effects including an increase in cell-membrane permeability,[34,35] increased protein synthesis,[36,37] mast cell degranulation,[38] increased growth-factor production,[39] and enhanced nitric-oxide synthetase-mediated cellular mechanisms.[28,40] All of the aforementioned effects of low-frequency ultrasound ultimately stimulate cell activity and thereby enhance clinical outcomes.[41,42]

There are 2 different types of systems for low-frequency ultrasound: contact and non-contact. Refer to Table 1 for a comparison of these technologies.

Ultrasound-assisted wound therapy (UAW), contact low-frequency ultrasound, has been utilized as a wound debridement and cleansing technique for years in the United Kingdom, Russia, and Germany. This technique of wound debridement has many advantages: the results can be as immediate as sharp or surgical debridement; it generally requires only topical anesthesia, is selective for nonviable or necrotic tissue, and can be effectively used for excisional debridement. Ultrasound-assisted wound therapy is bactericidal at the surface, penetrates into surrounding tissues, and can be performed in a variety of settings by trained personnel. Ultrasound-assisted wound therapy procedures allow therapy at the bedside and can be utilized at the time of surgery to provide adjunctive therapy during incision and drainage procedures.

When using contact low-frequency ultrasound-assisted wound treatment devices, the probe is in intimate contact with the wound bed tissues. These devices currently include Misonix SonicOne™ (Medline Industries, Mundelein, Ill) and Sonoca 180 (Söring Inc, Fort Worth, Tex). The built-in lavage system may provide further reduction of cell debris and bacteria to more effectively cleanse the wound site.

Ultrasound-assisted wound treatment has been proven to eradicate surface and adjacent tissue colonization of bacteria; therefore, individuals with a history of frequent cellulitis caused by multiple resistant bacteria may benefit from the reduced need for systemic antibiotics. Collaborative work done by Pierson and Niezgoda[33] emphasizes the benefits of UAW treatment. Brooke Army Medical Center isolated 25 highly antibiotic-resistant *Acinetobacter ssp* (primarily *A baumannii*) from wounded soldiers returning from Iraq. Using a previously described protocol for an *in-vitro* model, the bacterial suspension was set to a 0.5 McFarland standard and then serially diluted to approximately 100,000 CFU/mL. Initial colony counts were taken prior to sonocation. Test solutions were treated with sonocation at 60% output in 10-second bursts, followed by 50-second cool-down periods, until a total of 120 seconds of sonication was achieved. Aliquots were taken and plated after each 20 seconds of sonocation. Bacterial death was measured by both colony counts after 24 hours of growth and acridine orange staining using a standard protocol. After UAW treatment, a significant log decrease in bacterial load was noted with less than 5% viable bacteria identified after a 120-second treatment.

Contact ultrasonic-assisted wound therapy utilizes low-frequency pulsed ultrasound directed to the wound surface and surrounding tissues via an ultrasound probe. Wound-irrigation fluid is directed through an opening in the probe's tip to administer the fluid directly to the wound surface to serve as a coupling medium, coolant, wound lavage, or flush and topically treat the wound base (Plate 18, Page 346).

Indications for the use of UAW include but are not limited to:
- Locally infected wounds
- Wounds with impaired circulation
- Wounds with the need for debridement, irrigation, and topical treatment
- Pressure ulcers, diabetic foot ulcers, lower-extremity diabetic ulcers, and venous ulcers

Contraindications for the use of UAW include:
- Untreated advancing cellulitis with signs of systemic response
- Wounds with metal components, such as joint replacements, plates, and screws, or implanted electronic devices within the treatment field
- Uncontrolled pain.

The treatment setting for use of UAW therapy is dependent upon availability of the equipment and trained personnel and potentially includes 3 areas. The hospital outpatient clinic is the primary treatment location. With the portability of the equipment, the treatment could also be utilized at the bedside in the acute care and intermediate care setting and in the operating room at the time of surgical incision and drainage, dressing changes, or debridement. The high cost of individual ultrasound units and attachments prohibits providing multiple departments with the equipment.

Noncontact, nonthermal therapeutic ultrasound (MIST Therapy™ System, Celleration®, Eden Prairie, Minn) produces low-intensity (0.1 W/cm^2–0.5 W/cm^2), low-frequency (40 kHz) ultrasound to promote wound healing through cleansing and maintenance debridement that gradually removes yellow slough, fibrin, tissue exudate, and bacteria. Noncontact, nonthermal therapeutic ultrasound achieves debridement through multiple sessions over an extended period of time. It can be used on a variety of wounds including, but not limited to, acute, traumatic, chronic, and dehisced wounds. Noncontact, nonthermal therapeutic ultrasound delivers

Table 1. Summary of low-frequency ultrasound technologies

Features	Misonix SonicOne™	Sonoca 180™	MIST Therapy™
Frequency	22.5 kHz	20–80 kHz	40 kHz
Intensity	Variable (auto gain control)	Variable 40%–100%	Preset (based on wound size)
Mode	Continuous or pulsed	Continuous	Continuous
Fluid delivery	Sterile-saline vapor	Sterile-saline vapor	Sterile-saline mist
Controls	Foot pedal	Foot pedal	Button on hand piece
Treatment time	Usually 2–5 min	Usually 2–5 min	Wound size dependent 3–20 min
Wound-bed contact	Yes (autoclavable metal probes)	Yes (autoclavable metal probes)	No (disposable applicator)
Aerosolization	Yes	Yes	No
Debridement capability	Immediate	Immediate	Maintenance
Selective	Yes	Yes	Yes

Table information adapted. Courtesy of Luther Kloth, PT, MS, FAPTA, CWS, FACCWS.

continuous ultrasonic energy via an atomized saline solution to the wound bed without direct contact of the device to the body or the wound. The mist acts as a conduit for transmitting ultrasonic energy to the treatment site. This therapy is also believed to promote wound healing through the processes of cavitation and micro streaming, the effects of which were described earlier in this section. Four clinical studies have evaluated the safety and efficacy of noncontact, low-frequency therapeutic ultrasound in patients with a variety of wounds, including recalcitrant pressure ulcers, chronic lower-extremity leg and foot ulcers, and diabetic foot ulcers. Among these, a randomized, controlled, double-blind trial demonstrated improved healing of recalcitrant diabetic foot ulcers compared with a sham procedure in patients receiving standard wound-care therapy.[43] Treatments are typically administered 3 times per week for 3 to 20 minutes (average 5 minutes) each depending on wound size. The compact, portable treatment device consists of a generator, transducer, and single-use disposable applicator that utilize prepackaged sterile-saline bottles. A new single-use disposable applicator is used for each treatment session to ensure generation of a sterile mist.

To use the low-frequency therapeutic ultrasound system, practitioners must remove dressings, discard contaminated materials, and clean the device with the germicidal wipe provided. The applicator is held perpendicular to the wound and moved in slow even strokes vertically across the wound in multiple passes, then repeated in horizontal passes. The recommended distance between the leading edge of the applicator and the wound is approximately 0.5 cm–1.5 cm (0.2 in–0.6 in). Placing an absorbent pad beneath the area of the patient being treated will absorb any saline run-off.

The outcomes of the use of low-frequency ultrasound in wound care may include:
• Wound debridement producing a wound bed with reduced adherent nonviable tissue
• Decreased pain related to the process of decreased bacterial colonization and reversal of the inflammatory state with reduced pH
• Stimulation of granulation tissue formation
• Reduced infection rate
• Reduction of systemic antibiotic use
• Decreased time to closure.

Autolytic Debridement

Autolytic debridement is the use of the body's

own available wound fluid to loosen and liquefy necrotic tissue. This fluid contains endogenous proteolytic enzymes, such as collagenase, and inflammatory cells, such as macrophages and neutrophils, which enter the wound site during the normal inflammatory process. In the presence of adequate vascular supply, leukocyte function, and level of neutrophils, the use of moisture-retentive dressings creates an environment providing prolonged contact of this wound fluid with necrotic tissue. This contact softens and ultimately liquefies the devitalized tissue leaving the healthy tissue not only unharmed but also sequestered in an environment conducive to wound healing.

The process of autolytic debridement is slower than other methods, requiring multiple dressing applications, and can often take weeks to accomplish. It is frequently used in combination with other types of debridement, such as pulsatile lavage with suction or instrument debridement. While slower, it is usually a pain-free type of debridement as long as the patient can tolerate the dressings changes. The absence of pain can reduce the stress and anxiety caused by other faster forms of debridement. It also can be accomplished with basic technical skills.

It is important that all members of the healthcare team, the patient, and family members are aware of how the autolytic debridement process is accomplished. Monitoring the fluid collection beneath the selected dressing is essential to prevent prolonged exposure of intact skin, which could lead to moisture-associated skin damage, such as maceration or denudation. Additionally, the collection of fluid containing dead cells, cellular debris, and bacteria, as well as the odor that frequently accompanies this fluid, may lead to the fear that the wound is infected, despite the absence of other clinical indicators. Culture of this material would likely reveal bacteria that are present in the fluid but not pathogenic to the wound, possibly leading to treatment with antibiotics that are not warranted or needed. The wound surface should be thoroughly and safely irrigated or cleansed before an assessment for clinical signs of infection is carried out.

Autolytic debridement can be utilized to debride wounds of all types regardless of etiology. It is frequently the method of choice in the home or long-term care setting where access to other

more aggressive forms of debridement may not be feasible or available. The only real contraindication is the infected wound in which faster removal of the devitalized tissue and aggressive drainage and cleansing of the wound surface are critical. See Chapter 5 for further information.

Enzymatic Debridement

As described previously, autolytic debridement is a form of enzymatic or chemical debridement, using the body's naturally occurring enzymes to degrade devitalized tissue. The addition of a topical preparation to specifically target necrotic tissue therapeutically "ramps-up" this process and is generally referred to as chemical or enzymatic debridement. Like autolysis, enzymatic debridement is also an effective alternative to the more expensive and aggressive methods of debridement in settings, such as home or long-term care.

The concept of using proteolytic enzymes to digest necrotic tissue as an adjunct in the treatment of complex wounds is rather old and probably stems from observing the ageless healing techniques of natives in tropical countries. As an example, for wounds, eczema, warts, and ulcers, these natives seem to have utilized the papain-rich material obtained by scratching the skin of the green fruit of the papaw tree *(Carica papaya).*[8] Further, the natives would occasionally expose the wounds to urine and wrap them in green leaves from the same plant. These 3 naturally occurring materials contain the chemical compounds papain, urea, and chlorophyll, which are components of commercial preparations available in certain countries today, papain-urea and papain-urea-chlorophyllin copper.[44]

Papain-Urea Combinations

While no longer available in the U.S., papain is used to attack and break down any protein containing cysteine residues, making it rather nonselective because most proteins contain cysteine residues. Collagen contains no cysteine residues and, therefore, is unaffected by papain. The addition of urea facilitates the proteolytic action of papain. Urea alters the 3-dimensional structure of proteins, disrupts their hydrogen bonds, and exposes the activators of papain by solvent action. Urea also contributes to the reduction of disulfide bridges. As the disulfide bridges are reduced, cysteine residues become exposed, making them more susceptible to the action of papain. Papain and urea combined are probably twice as effective as papain alone.[8] Papain-urea is also active within a broad pH range (3.0–12.0), making it effective for nonspecific bulk debridement. It is also more rapidly effective in breaking down dense necrotic tissue, such as eschar, and devitalized deeper wounds, such as pressure ulcers.

The nonselective nature of this enzymatic preparation is thought to stimulate a prominent inflammatory response, and as a result, there is often pain ranging from mild and transitory to considerable associated with its use. However, in early studies conducted in the 1950s, when chlorophyllin was added to the papain/urea combination, the inflammatory response was reduced considerably. Chlorophyllin derivatives appear to neutralize the breakdown products of the papain/urea combination in addition to reducing malodors. Chlorophyllin-copper complex inhibits the hemagglutinating and inflammatory properties of protein degradation products in the wound, including the products of enzymatic digestion. Its mechanism of action is postulated to be prevention of agglutinated erythrocytes, thus, decreasing thrombus formation, fibrin deposition, and plugging of capillaries and lymphatic vessels.[8,45–47]

The effects of chlorophyllin on viable tissue are not clearly understood; however, it is thought that adding this ingredient to the papain/urea combination has no detrimental effect. Published studies and abstracts on the use of papain-urea-chlorophyllin-copper complex have shown that chlorophyllin, in combination with papain/urea, neutralizes inflammatory products of the enzymatic process.[45–47] Data suggest that papain-urea-chlorophyllin-copper complex may have a stimulatory effect on granulation tissue and possibly angiogenesis.[8]

An advantage to using the combination of papain/urea may be when the patient requires fast bulk debridement, is not a candidate for surgical/sharp debridement, and/or has deep pressure ulcers with loss of sensation.[8] Disadvantages are the nonselective nature of this debridement process, which may harm healthy tissue and cause inflammation and discomfort to the patient in the absence of chlorophyllin-copper complex.

The recommended use of a papain-urea preparation is a daily or twice daily application depending upon the amount and nature of the necrotic tissue as well as the amount of exudate produced. The ointment is applied directly to the tissue and covered with an appropriate dressing. Cross-hatching of dry or dense eschar or tissue is recommended to facilitate contact and penetration of the ointment and to hasten the debridement process (Plate 19, Page 346). Protection of the surrounding skin with a moisture barrier product can prevent discomfort or denudation of the intact skin from the exudate resulting from the debridement process.

Papain-urea with chlorophyllin copper is generally recommended for use in wounds exhibiting a combination of necrotic and viable tissues to continue the debridement process while protecting and promoting the growth of the healthier viable tissues.

The use of hydrogen peroxide or preparations containing the salts of heavy metals, such as silver, is discouraged with the papain-urea combinations, as these agents may inactivate the activity of the papain.

Collagenase

The only enzymatic debriding agent available in the U.S. at this time is collagenase. Collagenases belong to a family of extracellular MMPs that occur naturally in many tissues and cells in the body.[12,48,49] Considering that 70%–80% of the skin consists of collagen, the action of collagenases is important in the cleaning and remodeling of wounds. Collagenases are the only enzymes that can *specifically* cleave native collagen.[8,46,48]

Topical collagenase is a bacterial collagenase derived from *Clostridium histolyticum*. Reported to be most active in a pH range of 6–8, topical collagenase is specific to native and denatured collagen and is resistant to breakdown by other proteases.[8,48,49] This enzyme cleaves collagen (specifically type I and type III) into small peptides, converting it to gelatin, upon which less specific enzymes can then act.[8,48,50,51] Collagenase is thought to promote debridement by digesting collagen bundles that anchor nonviable collagen strands to the wound bed.[8,48,49] Until these fibers are severed, debridement cannot take place and granulation tissue formation is slowed, preventing the wound from re-epithelizing. Collagenase does not break down viable collagen. There are several theories as to why, such as, mucopolysaccharide sheaths, pH gradients within the wound bed, and absence of water. Collagenase has no known effect on viable tissue and is not associated with increased patient discomfort.[8]

The recommended use of collagenase is daily within the area of the wound and more often if the dressing becomes soiled. The ointment is applied directly to the tissue and covered with an appropriate dressing. Cross-hatching of dry or dense eschar or tissue is recommended to facilitate contact and penetration of the ointment and to hasten the debridement process. Protection of the surrounding skin with a moisture-barrier product can prevent discomfort or denudation of the intact skin from the exudate resulting from the debridement process. If a wound infection is suspected, use of Polysporin® Powder (bacitracin/polymyxin B sulfate, Pfizer, New York, NY) on the wound surface prior to application of the collagenase ointment has been studied and found to be effective in reducing bacterial burden.[52]

The use of enzymatic agents for the debridement of necrotic tissue is not new. Pharmaceutical agents for this use[53] have been available since the 1950s. As with autolytic debridement, the only real contraindication is the infected wound in which faster removal of the devitalized tissue and aggressive draining and cleansing of the wound surface are critical (see Chapter 5 for further information). Ongoing use in the healing chronic wound has and is being studied, and the use for maintenance debridement and continued use for prolonged periods of time may be warranted.[8] Necrotic tissue as a clinically visible component of the wound leads clinicians to think of debridement as a single event or single phase in the healing process. While initial debridement is important to remove that particular barrier to healing, maintenance debridement is necessary to keep the ongoing necrotic tissue from accumulating. Apoptosis, or programmed cell death, is a reoccurring process in wounds, resulting in a cycle of adequate blood flow or decreased edema with periods of borderline ischemia and increasing edema.[8] As a result, maintenance debridement becomes necessary, and continued use of less aggressive enzymatic agents, such as collagenase or papain-urea with

chlorophyllin copper, may accomplish this and, as a result, promote the proliferation of healthier granulation tissue.

Biotherapy

Biotherapy, also referred to as biosurgery or MDT, is the purposeful use of maggots in wound care.

Historically, maggots have been known for centuries to help heal wounds. Many military surgeons noted that soldiers whose wounds became infested with maggots had a much lower mortality rate and cleaner, faster healing wounds than did soldiers with similar wounds that were not infested. During the late 1920s, William Baer, an orthopedic surgeon at Johns Hopkins University, began to systematically treat, study, and publish case studies of patients with applications of maggots to their wounds.[54] Larval therapy was successfully and routinely performed by thousands of physicians until mid-1940, when its use was supplanted by the new antibiotics and surgical techniques that were developing in World War II. Maggot therapy was occasionally used during the 1970s and 1980s, but only when antibiotics, surgery, and modern wound care failed to control the deteriorating wound. Resurgence in the use of maggots has occurred in the past 10 years, as more widespread acceptance among the medical community as well as patients has occurred.

Maggots have 3 proposed actions: debridement, antimicrobial, and facilitation of wound healing. They are indicated for debriding non-healing necrotic skin and soft-tissue wounds, including pressure ulcers, venous ulcers, neuropathic foot ulcers, and nonhealing traumatic or post-surgical wounds.[54]

Maggots selectively debride by feeding on the necrotic tissue, cellular debris, and exudate in wounds. The maggot secretes collagenases, trypsin-like, and chymotrypsin-like enzymes, which breakdown the necrotic tissue into a semi-liquid form that the creatures can ingest.[55]

To attach to tissue and provide locomotion, maggots use a pair of mandibles or hooks (Plate 20, Page 347). The maggot also uses these hooks during feeding to disrupt membranes and thus facilitate the penetration of their proteolytic enzymes.[56] Additional debridement may be facilitated by the maggots crawling about within the wound, dislodging small amounts of necrotic material.

Studies have shown biosurgery using maggots to be an effective and rapid treatment for the debridement of chronic wounds.[57] A Cochrane review of randomized, controlled trials (RCTs) comparing larval therapy to conventional debridement concluded that while "the evidence is insufficient to support a firm conclusion of efficacy of larval therapy in any chronic or acute wound, appropriately powered, prospective RCTs are warranted."When these RCTs are conducted, it is hoped that maggot therapy will be compared to a hydrogel under a moisture-retentive dressing, a modality with significant evidence of debriding efficacy during 14 days of use.[58]

The ability of maggots to kill or prevent the growth of a range of potentially pathogenic bacteria has been the subject of a number of studies. Marked antimicrobial activity has been detected against *Streptococcus* A and B and *Staphylococcus aureus* with some activity detected against *Pseudomonas* sp and a clinical isolate of a resistant strain of S aureus (MRSA).[59,60]

Growth of granulation tissue has been reported to be faster with better wound-healing rates using maggot therapy. One study suggests a possible mode of action for facilitating wound healing is the increase in tissue oxygenation that takes place when using maggot therapy.[61] Sherman et al[62] demonstrated that maggot therapy enhanced the closure rate of pressure ulcers in spinal cord injury patients.

In 2004, the FDA approved the production and marketing of Medical Maggots (Monarch Labs, Irvine, Calif) as a medical device for the following indications: debriding nonhealing necrotic skin and soft-tissue wounds, including pressure ulcers, venous stasis ulcers, neuropathic foot ulcers, and nonhealing traumatic or post-surgical wounds.

The technique for application and use of MDT is not difficult but is specific. Maggots themselves cannot be disinfected. The eggs are chemically disinfected with Lysol, sodium hypochlorite, or another agent, and then placed in sterile containers so that the newly hatched maggots remain disinfected. The wound bed is cleansed and prepared, and the surrounding skin should be dried thoroughly and protected with a skin-barrier wipe. The wound is "picture-framed" by build-

ing 1 or 2 layers of hydrocolloid or pectin skin barrier strips. Commonly, practitioners will apply a skin contact cement (ie, Skin Bond Cement®, Smith & Nephew, Largo, Fla). The maggots are applied to the wound with 5 to 8 maggots per cm² of wound surface area,[54] and a closed mesh or veil dressing is applied, adhered to the cemented edged barrier. This prevents "migration" of the maggots outside of the wound area. The wound should be further dressed with gauze or other absorbent materials due to the increased exudate that generally results. The dressing is left in place for 48 to 72 hours, removing the maggots as they become satiated and move to the surface of the dressing. One or 2 cycles are applied each week. The total duration of treatment will depend on the size and character of the wound, the clinical response, and the overall goals of therapy.[54] Instrument debridement of thick, dry eschar or tough fibrous tissue prior to initiation of MDT will hasten the effect and shorten the treatment time (Plates 21–24, Page 347).

Conclusion

Regardless of the type or technique used, effective wound debridement is paramount to achieving adequate wound-bed preparation and ultimately wound healing and has become a standard of care among wound care providers. Once the decision to debride is made, the methodology used is dependent upon the patient's plan of care, the overall goals of therapy, the urgency of the need, the setting in which the care is being provided, the skill level of the care providers, and access to the modalities. Adequate wound debridement is essential for successful outcomes in the management of chronic wounds and is critically important to create a wound environment in

Take-Home Messages for Practice
- Debridement is an essential component of preparing a wound for healing. Each patient's individual plan of care must be evaluated and debridement selected within the context of the overall goals of care.
- The choice of debridement method is dependent upon the urgency of the need, the patient condition, and available resources.

which to achieve the desired benefits of modern advanced wound therapies, such as growth factors and bioengineered tissues.

Self-Assessment Questions

1. The presence of necrotic tissue in a wound can inhibit healing in the following ways EXCEPT:
   A. Necrosis can mimic or be a source of infection
   B. Necrotic tissue contributes to a prolonged inflammatory response
   C. Necrotic tissue may reduce protein stores
   D. Necrotic tissue can impede migration of healthy cells

2. The most appropriate method of debridement for a patient who is septic or with an infected wound is:
   A. Wet-to-dry dressings
   B. Surgical
   C. Pulsed lavage with suction
   D. Enzymatic

3. Personal protective equipment is required with the following debridement procedure
   A. Wet-to-dry dressings
   B. Pulsed lavage with suction
   C. Autolytic
   D. Maggot debridement

4. Autolytic debridement liquefies necrotic tissue utilizing naturally occurring:
   A. Red blood cells
   B. Hormones
   C. Leukocytes and enzymes
   D. Growth factors

Answers: 1-C, 2-B, 3-B, 4-D

References

1. Debridement. Available at: http://www.answers.com/topic/debridement. Accessed March 18, 2007.
2. Enoch S, Harding K. Wound bed preparation: the science behind the removal of barriers to healing. *WOUNDS*. 2003;15(7):213–229.
3. Myers B. Debridement. In: Myers B, ed. Wound Management: Principles and Practice. Upper Saddle River, NJ: Prentice Hall; 2004:65–87.
4. Zacur H, Kirsner RS. Debridement: rationale and therapeutic options. *WOUNDS*. 2002;14(7 Suppl E):2E–7E.
5. Ramundo JM. Wound debridement. In: Bryant RA, Nix DP, eds. Acute and Chronic Wounds: Current Management Concepts. 3rd ed. Saint Louis, Mo: Mosby Elsevier; 2007:176–192.
6. Calianno C, Jakubek P. Wound bed preparation: laying the foundation for treating chronic wounds, part 1. *Nursing*. 2006;36(2):70–71.
7. Ayello EA, Dowsett C, Schultz GS, et al. TIME heals all wounds. Nursing. 2006;34(4):36–42.
8. Falanga V. Wound bed preparation and the role of enzymes: a case for multiple actions of therapeutic agents. *WOUNDS*. 2002;14(2):47–57.
9. Steed DL, Donohoe D, Webster MW, Lindsley L. Effect of extensive debridement and treatment on the healing of diabetic foot ulcers. Diabetic Ulcer Study Group. *J Am Coll Surg*. 1996;183(1):61–64.
10. Bergstrom N, Bennett MA, Carlson CE, et al. Clinical Practice Guuidelines Number 15: Treatment of Pressure Ulcers. Rockville, Md: US Department of Health Care Policy and Research. Agency for Health Care Policy and Research; 1994. AHCPR Publication 95-0653.
11. Wahl LM, Wahl SM. Inflammation. In: Cohen IK, Diegelmann RF, Lindblad WJ, eds. Wound Healing: Biochemical & Clinical Aspects. Philadelphia, Pa: WB Saunders Co; 1992:77–95.
12. Falanga V. Classifications for wound bed preparation and stimulation of chronic wounds. *Wound Repair Regen*. 2000;8(5):347–352.
13. Andersen K. Laser technology: a surgical tool of the past, present and future. *AORN J*. 2003;78(5):794–807.
14. Granick MS, Jacoby M, Noruthrun S, Datiashvili RO, Ganchi PA. Clinical and economic impact of hydrosurgical debridement on chronic wounds. *WOUNDS*. 2006;18(2):35–39.
15. Mosti G, Mattaliano V. The debridement of chronic leg ulcers by means of a new, fluidjet-based device. *WOUNDS*. 2006;18(8):227–237.
16. McCulloch JM, Boyd VB. The effects of whirlpool and the dependent position on lower extremity volume. *J Orthop Sports Phys Ther*. 1992;16(4):169–173.
17. American Diabetes Association. Consensus Development Conference on Diabetic Foot Wound Care in Boston, Mass, April 7–8, 1999.
18. Ayello EA, Cuddigan JE. Debridement: controlling the necrotic/cellular burden. *Adv Skin Wound Care*. 2004;17(2):66–78.
19. Loehne HB. Wound debridement and irrigation. In: Kloth LC, McCulloch JM, eds. Wound Healing: Alternatives in Management. 3rd ed. Philadelphia, Pa: FA Davis Co; 2002:203–231.
20. Loehne HB, Street SA, Gaither B, Sherertz RJ. Aerosolization of microorganisms during pulsatile lavage with suction. Presented at the 15th Annual Symposium on Advanced Wound Care & 12th Annual Medical Research Forum on Wound Repair in Baltimore, Md, April 27–30, 2002.
21. Ayello EA, Cuddigan JE. Jump-start the healing process. Nursing Made Incredibly Easy! 2003;1(2):18–27.
22. Jetox™-HDC. Available at: http://www.deroyal.com/divisions/Featured%20Products/jetoxhdc/. Accessed March 28, 2007.
23. Armstrong MH, Price P. Wet-to-dry gauze dressings: fact and fiction. *WOUNDS*. 2004;16(2):56–62.

24. Weir D, Bohanan BG, Hockenbrocht GP, Moulavi DL. Improved wound packing and debridement: evaluation of a new fabric sponge. *WOUNDS*. 1992;4(6):216–226.

25. Ovington LG. Hanging wet-to-dry dressings out to dry. *Home Health Nurs*. 2001;19(8):28–34.

26. Nyborg WL. Biological effects of ultrasound: development of safety guidelines. Part I: personal histories. *Ultrasound Med Biol*. 2000;26(6):911–964.

27. Speed CA. Therapeutic ultrasound in soft tissue lesions. *Rheumatology*. 2001;40(12):1331–1336.

28. Suchkova VN, Baggs RB, Sahni SK, Francis CW. Ultrasound improves tissue perfusion in ischemic tissue through a nitric oxide dependent mechanism. *Thromb Haemost*. 2002;88(5):865–870.

29. Young S. Ultrasound therapy. In: Kitchen S, ed. Electrotherapy: Evidence-Based Practice. 11th ed. New York, NY: Churchill Livingstone; 2002:211–230.

30. Ballard K, Charles H. Ultrasound therapy. *Nurs Times*. 2001;97(24):58–59.

31. Schoenbach SF, Song IC. Ultrasonic debridement: a new approach in the treatment of burn wounds. Plast Reconstr Surg. 1980;66(1):34–37.

32. Scherba G, Weigel RM, O'Brien WD Jr. Quantitative assessment of the germicidal efficacy of ultrasonic energy. Appl Environ Microbiol. 1991;57(7):2079–2084.

33. Pierson T, Niezgoda JA, Learmonth S, Blunt D, McNabb K. Effects of low frequency ultrasound applied in vitro to highly antibiotic resistant acinetobacter isolates recovered from soldiers returning from Iraq. Presented at the 18th Annual Symposium on Advanced Wound Care in San Diego, Calif, April 21–24, 2005.

34. Dyson M. Non-thermal cellular effects of ultrasound. Br J Cancer. 1982;45(Suppl V):165–171.

35. Dyson M. Therapeutic applications of ultrasound. In: Nyborg WL, Ziskin MC, eds. Biological Effects of Ultrasound. Clinics in Diagnostic Ultrasound. New York, NY: Churchill Livingstone; 1985:121–133.

36. Harvey W, Dyson M, Pond JB, Grahame R. The stimulation of protein synthesis in human fibroblasts by therapeutic ultrasound. *Rheumatol Rehabil*. 1975;14(4):237–241.

37. Webster DF, Pond JB, Dyson M, Harvey W. The role of cavitation in the in vitro stimulation of protein synthesis in human fibroblasts by ultrasound. *Ultrasound Med Biol*. 1978;4(4):343–351.

38. Fyfe MC, Chahl LA. Mast cell degranulation: a possible mechanism of action of therapeutic ultrasound. Ultrasound Med Biol. 1982;8(Suppl 1):62–65.

39. Young SR, Dyson M. Macrophage responsiveness to therapeutic ultrasound. *Ultrasound Med Biol*. 1990;16(8):809–816.

40. Altland OD, Dalecki D, Suchkova VN, Francis CW. Low-intensity ultrasound increases endothelial cell nitric oxide synthase activity and nitric oxide synthesis. *J Thromb Haemost*. 2004;2(4):637–643.

41. Stanisic M, Provo B, Larson D, Kloth L. Wound debridement with 25 kHz ultrasound. *Adv Skin Wound Care*. 2005;18(9):484–490.

42. Breuing KH, Bayer L, Neuwalder J, Orgill DP. Early experience using low frequency ultrasound in chronic wounds. *Ann Plast Surg*. 2005;55(2):183–187.

43. Ennis WJ, Foremann P, Mozen N, Massey J, Conner-Kerr T, Meneses P. Ultrasound therapy for recalcitrant diabetic foot ulcers: results of a randomized, double-blind, controlled, multi-center study. MIST Ultrasound Diabetic Study Group. *Ostomy Wound Manage*. 2005;51(8):24–39.

44. Brett DW. Chlorophyllin—a healer? A hypothesis for its activity. *WOUNDS*. 2005;17(7):190–195.

45. Miller EW. Decubitus ulcers treated with papain-urea-chlorophyllin ointment. *NY State J Med*. 1956;56(6)1446–1448.

46. Miller JM, Howard F. The interaction of papain, urea and water-soluble chlorophyllin in a proteolytic ointment for infected wounds. *Surgery*. 1957;43(6):939–948.

47. Morrison JE, Casali JL. Continuous proteolytic therapy for decubitis ulcers. *Am J Surg*. 1957;93(3):444–448.

48. Jung W, Winter H, Knowl AG. Considerations for the use of clostridial collagenase in clinical practice. *Clin Drug Invest*. 1998;15(3):245–252.

49. Sibbald GR, Williamson D, Orsted HL, et al. Preparing the wound bed—debridement, bacterial balance and moisture balance. *Ostomy Wound Manage*. 2000;46(11):14–35.

50. Staiano-Coico L, Higgins PJ, Schwartz SB, et al. Wound fluids: a reflection of the state of healing. *Ostomy Wound Manage*. 2000;46(Suppl 1A):85S–93S.

51. Pilcher BK, Dumin JA, Sudbeck BD, et al. The activity of collagenase-1 is required for keratinocyte migration on a type 1 collagen matrix. *J Cell Biol*. 1997;137(6):1445–1457.

52. Boxer AM, Gottesman N, Bernstein H, Mandl I. Debridement of dermal ulcers and decubiti with collagenase. *Geriatrics*. 1969;24(7):75–86.

53. Burke JF, Golden T. A clinical evaluation of enzymatic debridement with papain-urea-chlorophyllin ointment. *Am J Surg*. 1958;95(5):828–842.

54. Sherman RA. Maggot debridement in modern medicine. *Infect Med*. 1998;15(9):651–656.

55. Ziffren SE, Heist HE, May SC, Womack NA. The secretion of collagenase by maggots and its implication. *Ann Surg*. 1953;138(6):932–934.

56. Thomas S, Jones M, Shutler S, Andrews A. Wound care. All you need to know about maggots. *Nurs Times*. 1996;92(46):63–70.

57. Sherman RA. Maggot therapy for treating diabetic foot ulcers unresponsive to conventional therapy. *Diabetes Care*. 2003;26(2):446–451.

58. Bolton L. Maggot therapy [evidence corner]. *WOUNDS*. 2006;18(9):A19–A22.

59. Thomas S, Andrews AM, Hay NP, Bourgoise S. The antimicrobial activity of maggot secretions: results of a preliminary study. *J Tissue Viability*. 1999;9(4):127–132.

60. Freidman E, Shaharabany M, Ravin S, et al. Partially purified antibacterial agent from maggots displays a wide range of antibacterial activity. Presented at the 3rd International Conference on Biotherapy in Jerusalem, Israel, May 24–27, 1998.

61. Wollina U, Liebold K, Schmidt WD, Hartmann M, Fassler D. Biosurgery supports granulation and debridement in chronic wounds—clinical data and remittance spectroscopy measurement *Int J Dermatol*. 2002;41(10):635–639.

62. Sherman RA, Wyle FA, Vulpe M. Maggot debridement therapy for treating pressure ulcers in spinal cord injury patients. *J Spinal Cord Med*. 1995;18(2):71–74.

CHAPTER 7

Cofactors in Impaired Wound Healing

Nancy A. Stotts, RN, EdD, FAAN;
Deidre D. Wipke-Tevis, RN, PhD;
Harriet W. Hopf, MD

Objectives

The reader will be challenged to:

- Examine the major cofactors associated with impaired healing in chronic wounds
- Analyze the wound healing impairment caused by various cofactors
- Assess the mechanisms by which the major factors impair healing.

Introduction

Healing of chronic wounds is a complex process that requires the interaction of many factors for normal repair. Healing is the restoration of structure and function after tissue injury. In acute wounds, healing progresses in an established sequence and in a broad but accepted timeframe.[1] When this sequence or timeframe is interrupted or altered for any reason, the result is a chronic wound. The rate of healing in such wounds is slower and not as predictable. Impairment in healing is manifest as a delay in the rate of healing and/or the development of wound-related complications.

Many factors are associated with impaired healing of chronic wounds. These factors vary to some extent by the nature of the wound. A complete list of the factors related to impaired healing across all populations would be long and not very meaningful. There are, however, factors related to healing that cross the various wound populations. Assessing these factors will allow the practitioner to screen patients and address the major and most common factors known to impair healing in chronic wounds. Thus, this chapter describes the major factors in impaired healing of chronic wounds, the effect of each factor on wound healing, and the mechanism by which each is thought to lead to impairment. Common factors that impair wound healing include *old age, insufficient oxygenation/perfusion, malnutrition, increased bioburden, old wound tissue, excess pressure, psychophysiological stress, concomitant conditions*, and *adverse effects of therapy* (Table 1). Identification of these factors is critical

Stotts NA, Wipke-Tevis DD, Hopf HW. Cofactors in impaired wound healing. In: Krasner DL, ed. *Chronic Wound Care: The Essentials.* Malvern, PA: HMP Communications, 2014:79–86.

Table I. Cofactors in impaired healing

Old age

Insufficient oxygenation/perfusion

Malnutrition

Increased bioburden

Old wound tissue

Excess pressure

Psychophysiological stress

Concomitant conditions

Adverse effects of therapy

to healing of chronic wounds, as correction of impediments to healing generally leads to healing. Conversely, if an impediment is not recognized and corrected, the wound is unlikely to heal.

Age

Age has been associated with impaired healing, as there are differences in healing in the fetus, child, adult, and the elderly. Fetal wound healing occurs without an inflammatory response.[2] Wound healing and contraction occur more rapidly in childhood than in adulthood. As adulthood progresses, dermal vascularity decreases, collagen density decreases, the basement membrane flattens, fragmentation of elastin occurs, and the number of mast cells decreases. As people age, the entire healing process occurs more slowly, including the inflammatory response.[3]

Although the elderly experience these physiological changes, their rate of healing remains within a normal range or only slightly delayed in the absence of chronic disease.[4] Yet the elderly are more likely to have chronic illnesses, such as cardiovascular disease, pulmonary disease, and diabetes, and because of this association, age is often noted as a cofactor in impaired healing. Differentiating which dimensions of impaired healing in the elderly are due to concomitant disease and which are due to aging is the subject of ongoing research.

Low Oxygen and Perfusion

Low oxygen levels and *decreased perfusion* are often related to impaired healing, as well as increased risk of infection. Oxygen is needed for

collagen formation; the rate and quality of collagen are decreased when sufficient oxygen is not present. Angiogenesis (replacement of injured blood vessels) and epithelization are similarly impaired in hypoxic wounds. In addition, hypoxia inhibits resistance to infection. When neutrophils and macrophages ingest foreign material and microorganisms, more oxygen is consumed than during their resting state. Lack of sufficient oxygen slows leukocyte activity, decreases superoxide release and, therefore, bacterial killing, and often is associated with wound infection.[5,6]

Although *hemoglobin* carries much of the oxygen content in the blood, dissolved oxygen is most important for wound healing, because wounds depend on diffusion from relatively scarce capillaries for oxygenation. Thus, anemia does not result in impaired healing unless the anemia is severe (hematocrit < 18%). Wound oxygen tension is not decreased when subjects are anemic as long as the subjects have adequate circulating intravascular volume.[7] Cardiac output increases to compensate for the decreased oxygen content, and that, combined with decreased viscosity, increases wound blood flow sufficiently to increase wound temperature by 1.5°C to 2°C and to maintain normal wound oxygen. Clinical studies have confirmed and extended these early findings: levels of hydroxyproline, a major component of collagen, are not decreased in subjects with anemia.[8,9] Data indicate that anemia is not a cofactor in impaired healing unless the anemia is sufficient to impair cardiac output or the patient does not have sufficient circulating volume.

Smoking tobacco clearly impairs wound healing via several mechanisms. The triad of nicotine, carbon monoxide, and hydrogen cyanide from smoking are thought to interact to produce deleterious effects.[10] Nicotine acts as a potent vasoconstrictor, increases platelet adhesiveness, and enhances the risk of microvascular thrombosis and ischemia. Carbon monoxide binds with hemoglobin and aggravates the situation, reduces available sites for oxygen carrying, and lowers oxygen saturation. Hydrogen cyanide inhibits the enzyme systems necessary for oxidative metabolism and the cellular transport of oxygen. Thus, a major adverse effect of smoking is the creation or worsening of wound hypoxia.[11]

Hypovolemia (ie, the lack of adequate intravascular volume) has also been associated with impaired healing.[12,13] With hypovolemia, circulating volume is insufficient to transport oxygen and nutrients to the tissues; if the state is prolonged, cellular activities needed for healing are diminished. Unfortunately, even supplemental oxygen does not increase tissue oxygen levels when tissues are hypoperfused.[12] Hypovolemia that is clinically obvious (eg, hypoxemia, thirst, decreased urine output, or hypotension) is treated with supplemental fluid. A more difficult situation occurs when subclinical hypovolemia or underhydration is present. Subclinical hypovolemia is defined as the presence of decreased intravascular volume with no overt clinical signs and symptoms. Subclinical hypovolemia can be detected by measuring capillary refill time at the forehead (< 3 sec) or prepatellar knee (< 5 sec) or by measuring cutaneous (skin) oxygen levels, a more precise, though more complex and expensive, method.

Subclinical hypovolemia has been well documented in the surgical population. In examining the effects of various levels of inspired oxygen on tissue and wound oxygenation, researchers found tissue hypoxia in a subset of the study sample.[12] Treatment with a bolus of fluid resolved the hypoxia, and the authors concluded that subclinical hypovolemia had been present. It is important to note that no signs or symptoms were present that would have allowed the clinician to diagnose the hypovolemia. Follow-up studies showed that fluid titration based on subcutaneous oxygen levels led to higher tissue oxygen levels and greater quantities of hydroxyproline being synthesized in surgical patients in the early postoperative period than when fluid was administered based on a traditional fluid formula.[13] In the chronic wound population, subclinical hypovolemia has been identified in pilot work with elderly nursing home residents with pressure ulcers.[14] Fluid administration for subclinical hypovolemia, however, has potential deleterious effects. Although inadequate hydration is much more common than fluid overload, care must be taken to maximize intravascular volume without causing fluid overload. Vasoconstriction caused by pain, psychophysiologic stress, or cold cannot be overcome by fluid administration. Thus, cold and vasoconstricted patients are at higher risk of fluid overload. Conversely, patients who are warm and well perfused will tolerate high volumes of fluid

infusion, resulting in higher tissue oxygen levels and lower infection rates.[5]

Malnutrition

Either *inadequate intake of nutrients* or *preexisting malnutrition* has the potential to delay healing or result in infection. While most wounds heal regardless of nutritional status, severe protein-calorie malnutrition or specific nutritional deficits that are symptomatic can impair healing.[15] Providing adequate nutrition to all persons with injuries should be a therapeutic goal so that wound healing can occur within an optimal environment.[5]

Most wound healing abnormalities are associated with protein-calorie malnutrition rather than depletion of a single nutrient.[16] Nonetheless, *inadequate quantities of specific nutrients* can impact healing. Deficiencies of protein result in decreased fibroblast proliferation, reduced proteoglycan and collagen synthesis, decreased angiogenesis, and disrupted collagen remodeling. Protein requirements increase with healing. Provision of arginine and glutamine supplements (nonessential amino acids) has produced mixed results. Of these, arginine has shown the most significant wound healing effects, specifically increasing the inflammatory response in patients with diabetes.[16] Recent intake rather than remote intake of nutrients is more important in supporting collagen deposition and healing.

With *insufficient carbohydrate intake*, body protein is catabolized for energy. Protein, thus, is diverted from repair to provide the glucose needed for cellular maintenance. This adaptation process is especially important in fighting infection, as leukocytes require glucose for phagocytosis. *Fat inadequacy* is seen only in prolonged starvation or severe hypermetabolic states, and deficiencies of the fat-soluble vitamins (A, D, E, and K) may develop in these situations. Lack of vitamin A can result in an inadequate inflammatory response, while an excess of it may cause an excess inflammatory response; both impair healing.[16] *Thiamine (B1) deficiency* results in decreased collagen formation, while pantothenic acid (B5) deficiency results in decreased tensile strength and fewer fibroblasts. Inadequate vitamin C may result in lysis of collagen exceeding synthesis, meaning new wounds may have delayed collagen formation, and old wounds may break-down. Levels of vitamin E in excess of the recom-mended 100 IU daily may result in retardation of healing and fibrosis.

Zinc, *iron*, *copper*, and **manganese** are needed in small quantities for normal collagen formation. Data strongly suggest that zinc deficiencies im-pair healing, and repletion in states of deficiency returns healing to its normal rate. Supplementing those with normal zinc levels has not been shown to augment healing. Zinc deficiencies are seen in the elderly as well as those with chronic metabol-ic stress, excessive wound drainage, and persistent diarrhea. Regarding copper, impaired healing has been seen with decreased copper stores, although somewhat more rarely. Iron deficiency is primar-ily a problem in infants and may impair collagen formation. Severe iron deficiency also results in impaired healing because of its role in hydroxyl-ation of proline and lysine to make collagen. Of these mineral deficiencies, iron deficiency is most often detected and treated.[16]

Most studies that examine nutrition and chronic wounds address the pressure ulcer pop-ulation.[17] Review articles indicate that research has not demonstrated a cause-and-effect rela-tionship between nutritional status or intake and the development or healing of pressure ulcers. Nonetheless, provision of adequate nutrition, es-pecially protein, is important in optimizing host status to tissue tolerance and healing of existing ulcers. Additionally, data indicate that nutritional deficiencies are present in a portion of venous ulcer patients.[18] Further work is needed to con-firm these findings.

Bioburden

Bioburden, the metabolic load imposed by bacteria on tissue, is often a cofactor in impaired healing.[19,20] Wounds that have impaired healing are more susceptible to infection, and infected or heavily contaminated wounds demonstrate im-paired healing. *All wound surfaces are contami-nated* with bacteria, yet it is rare that the organ-isms on the wound surface cause the infection. Nonetheless, contamination is important, because the organisms compete with new tissue for nu-trients and oxygen, and their byproducts are del-eterious to the normal physiological balance of the healing wound. Overall, contamination pre-disposes the patient to delayed healing and sets up an environment for infection to develop.

Wound infection is present when microorgan-isms invade tissue. Diagnosis usually is based on clinical signs, ie, the presence of pus, warmth, pain, erythema, and induration. In immunocompro-mised persons and those with neuropathy, often the only sign of infection is a change in sensation around the wound. Also, in some chronic wounds, poorly granulating tissue may be a sign of infec-tion.[20] Wound infection in the elderly presents as decreased cognitive function or functional status, requiring the provider to investigate to find the source of the problem.[14]

Wound culture is performed to identify the specific organism(s) and identify an antibiotic to which the organism(s) is(are) sensitive. **Qualita-tive** wound cultures are not useful in diagnosing wound infection, because all wounds are con-taminated to some degree. **Quantitative** culture (either of a tissue biopsy or a carefully obtained swab) may be more reliable but is not available at most hospitals. A wound that contains $\geq 10^5$ organisms per gram of tissue is unlikely to heal without treatment because of excessive bacterial burden. The exception to this criterion is with beta hemolytic streptococcus where fewer organ-isms (10^3 organisms per gram of tissue) are re-quired to produce infection.[19,20]

Host resistance and the local environment are important in determining whether a contami-nated wound becomes infected. Normal, healthy tissue is resistant to microorganisms. In fact, con-tamination by a small number ($\leq 10^2$) of organ-isms per gram of tissue will activate leukocytes and has been seen as a factor that supports rather than impairs healing.[14]

Local environmental factors that contribute to bacterial proliferation and the development of impaired healing include the presence of devital-ized tissue, dirt in the wound, an abscess distant from the site of the injury, and a hematoma or large wound space.[20] Super-infection from con-tamination, regardless of whether from stool, urine, or another wound site, is also associated with infection in pressure ulcers.[17]

Old Tissue

Old tissue is a factor recently recognized as an impediment to healing. In studies of recombinant growth factors, debridement of old tissue from chronic wounds was shown to enhance healing.[21] This supports clinical experience that radical debridement of tissue is essential to effective treatment of chronic wounds. While the exact mechanism by which old tissue impairs healing is not entirely understood, debridement involves removal of senescent fibroblasts, inflammatory cells, and old scar tissue, implicating these factors in the impairment. It is not clear, however, exactly when tissue converts to "old" tissue; further research should clarify this issue.

Excess Pressure

Pressure, *shear*, and *friction* are cofactors in all types of chronic wounds. They are most often associated with *pressure ulcers*[17] but also are significant factors in the majority of chronic wounds. Little documentation exists to support this triad as contributing to chronic wounds, but clinical experience supports these as important factors in impaired healing. In the *venous ulcer population*, this problem is seen in the shear and friction that occur when compression stockings or bandages are utilized. Friable epithelial tissue may be disrupted under the stocking or bandage, especially along the previously intact skin of the shin, over the bony prominences of the ankle, and around the edge of the ulcer. Shear and friction occur most often during stocking application or removal and with ambulation. Clinically, this problem is most often seen in the elderly who have limited strength and manual dexterity. Often, coexisting arterial disease is present in the patient with venous ulcers. Inappropriate application of compression stockings and/or bandages may result in additional damage due to ischemia.

In persons with *neuropathic ulcers*, it is well accepted that excess pressure that is not perceived and that continues beyond tissue tolerance causes damage and prevents repair.[5] In the pressure ulcer population, data show that low pressures for long periods of time or high pressures for short periods produce pressure ulcers.[17] Controversy exists over what level of pressure causes vessel occlusion that leads to ischemia and necrosis.

Psychophysiological Stress

Stress has been identified as a potential cofactor in impaired healing. The proposed mechanism is through stimulation of the sympathetic nervous system, with the outflow of vasoactive substances and subsequent vasoconstriction. Increased cortisol levels also have been implicated, as steroids are known to impair wound healing. The major stressors that have been investigated in this category are *psychological stress*, *pain*, and *noise*. Stress has been linked with pressure ulcer development in patients transferred from acute care to long-term care, using cortisol as an objective measure of stress. Although the numbers are small, and the ulcers are not severe, data show that subjects with higher cortisol levels developed ulcers, while subjects with lower cortisol levels did not develop ulcers. Relaxation and guided imagery also are related to healing in persons with wounds. Stress, measured with cortisol levels, and inflammation were reduced with relaxation and imagery. These data suggest that available therapies might be used to decrease the sympathetic nervous system response to stress and thus support healing in persons with wounds.[22] Further research is needed to establish the direct effect on healing.

Intuitively, *pain* is thought to be an important issue in the development and healing of chronic wounds. For example, a recent large database study found that the presence of pain upon admission to a nursing home was associated with pressure ulcer development within the first 6 months after admission. Data do not indicate, however, if pain is a cofactor in healing impairment.[23] Pain reduction using transcutaneous electrical nerve stimulation (TENS) and music has been shown to be effective in reducing pain in persons with open wounds.[22] Unfortunately, healing was not an outcome measure when evaluating these treatments. It would seem logical that a reduction in pain would mitigate vasoconstriction thus increasing wound perfusion and supporting wound healing. Whether this is true remains to be established.

Noise is another stressor that results in a systemic cardiovascular response that may affect repair. Noise has been shown to increase epinephrine levels and later *in-vitro* leukocyte function. In addition, intermittent noise has been shown to decrease healing in an animal model.[22] However, studies have not specifically addressed this issue in the chronic wound patient population.

Concomitant Conditions

A myriad of concomitant conditions is associated with impaired healing. Major conditions include **peripheral vascular disease, diabetes mellitus, pulmonary disease, cardiac disease, conditions that result in immunocompromise,**[4,5] and **specific treatments,** including **surgery.**[24]

Persons with **vascular disease** are at risk for impaired healing. In arterial disease, the cause is accepted as tissue hypoxia due to arteriosclerotic disease. In venous disease, back pressure from venous hypertension and edema is thought to contribute to impaired healing. **Persons with diabetes** mellitus are at risk for impaired healing. Glucose control is essential for normal healing, and high glucose levels are often seen in diabetes, especially during periods of physiological stress and repair. High glucose levels result in impaired leukocyte function and increased risk of infection. Diabetes also appears to reduce growth factors and growth factor receptors in wounds. Lack of sensation is a serious problem in the more advanced states of diabetes where Charcot foot and neuropathy occur. When persons lack normal protective sensation, initial damage may occur without the person being aware of it. In addition, an existing wound may be exacerbated by excess pressure and mechanical or thermal damage in persons who lack sensation.[4] Unfortunately, it is common to see persons with multiple concomitant conditions, such as a person with a venous leg ulcer and coexistent arterial disease and diabetes.

Immunocompromised patients include persons who are HIV-positive, those with cancer, the malnourished, those receiving immunosuppressive agents, and the aged. Persons who are immunocompromised are unable to mount an adequate inflammatory response or the response is delayed. With immunocompromise, all phases of healing are delayed, and patients may be at risk for infection or wound disruption.[22]

Adverse Effects of Treatment

Iatrogenic effects of therapy also may result in impaired healing. Thus, treatment for pathologies may be a cofactor in healing impairment. Examples of such treatments are **radiation therapy, chemotherapy, steroid therapy,** and **anti-inflammatory drugs.**[22]

Radiation disrupts cell mitosis at the time of the treatment and has ongoing effects for the individual's life. These include obliterative arteritis and fibrosis that result in woody, hypoxic skin that does not heal well after injury. The dose and dose rate, along with the patient's genetics, determine the extent of damage and the speed at which it occurs. Bone marrow is the organ most sensitive to radiation exposure. The effects of radiation are seen immediately in terms of the number and various circulating cell types. Recovery depends on the dose of radiation and the half-life of the various cells.

Chemotherapy is designed to interrupt the cell cycle. It affects cells while they are dividing. This is accomplished in most anticancer drugs by damaging DNA or preventing DNA repair. Hormonal anticancer agents prevent binding of hormones, while others antagonize receptors to inhibit tumor growth. The primary effects of chemotherapy on healing are experienced during the treatment period and immediately after treatment.

A newly introduced form of cancer treatment is the use of **antiangiogenic agents (eg, bevacizumab),** which block new blood vessel formation around the tumor by binding to a particular growth factor. Although these agents have the potential to impair wound healing, the pathway for wound angiogenesis and tumor angiogenesis appears to be somewhat different, and these agents have not caused the wound healing problems many anticipated.[25]

Steroids impair all phases of healing by suppressing the inflammatory response, reducing immunocompetent lymphocytes, decreasing antibody production, and diminishing antigen processing. Clinical signs of inflammation are suppressed. If steroids are administered at the time of injury, their impact is greater than if they are administered several days after injury because of their effect on the inflammatory response that accompanies the initial injury. When the initial inflammatory response is decreased, all subsequent phases of healing are delayed, and the risk of infection is increased. Other medications, such as nonsteroidal anti-inflammatory agents, phenylbutazone, and vitamin E, disrupt the normal healing process. Their effects are primarily anti-inflammatory and, thus, are seen early after injury.[5]

Conclusion

Healing in individuals with chronic wounds is a complex process. One cannot simply dress the wound and expect healing to occur. It is important to assess the individual for the presence of each of the potential cofactors described in this chapter. Typically, evaluation of cofactors for impairment is integrated into the initial history and physical and should be an integral part of the ongoing holistic patient assessment. Early identification of the cofactors for impaired healing allows the practitioner to make a differential diagnosis, initiate appropriate referrals, and develop a comprehensive plan of care. Management of local and systemic cofactors that impact repair will mitigate their adverse effects and facilitate healing of chronic wounds.

Take-Home Messages for Practice

- A thorough history is the basis for determining factors present that may impair healing.
- It is important to assess the scientific evidence for the manifestation of specific factors on healing for patients with wounds.
- Current scientific knowledge about the mechanisms by which specific cofactors impair healing should be utilized when evaluating patients with wounds.

Self-Assessment Questions

1. Factors associated with impaired healing are:
   A. Warm temperature and low perfusion
   B. Warm temperature and high perfusion
   C. Cold temperature and high perfusion
   D. Cold temperature and low perfusion

2. Factors that contribute to impairment in healing due to infection are:
   A. Albumin of 4.5 g/dL
   B. Abscess distant from the wound
   C. 10^3 organisms per gram of tissue
   D. Healthy tissue

3. Anemia is a risk factor for impaired healing when:
   A. People are smokers
   B. Diabetes mellitus is present

C. Intravascular volume is low
D. Chemotherapy is utilized

Answers: 1-D, 2-B, 3-C

References

1. Lazarus GS, Cooper DM, Knighton DR, et al. Definitions and guidelines for assessment of wounds and evaluation of healing. *Arch Dermatol.* 1994;130(4):489–493.
2. Yang GP, Lim IJ, Phan TT, Lorenz HP, Longaker MT. From scarless fetal wounds to keloids: molecular studies in wound healing. *Wound Repair Regen.* 2003;11(6):411–418.
3. Gosain A, DiPietro LA. Aging and wound healing. *World J Surg.* 2004;28(3):321–326.
4. Enoch S, Price P. Cellular, molecular and biochemical differences in the pathophysiology of healing between acute wounds, chronic wounds and wounds in the aged. Available at: http://www.Worldwidewounds.com/2004/august/Enoch/pathophysiology-Of-Healing.html. Accessed April 23, 2006.
5. Ueno C, Hunt TK, Hopf HW. Using physiology to improve surgical wound outcomes. *Plast Reconstr Surg.* 2006;117(7 Suppl):59S–71S.
6. Hunt TK, Hopf H, Hussain Z. Physiology of wound healing. *Adv Skin Wound Care.* 2000;13(2 Suppl):6–11.
7. Hopf HW, Viele M, Watson JJ, et al. Subcutaneous perfusion and oxygen during acute severe isovolemic hemodilution in healthy volunteers. *Arch Surg.* 2000;135(12):1443–1449.
8. Jonsson K, Jensen JA, Goodson WH 3rd, et al. Tissue oxygenation, anemia, and perfusion in relation to wound healing in surgical patients. *Ann Surg.* 1991;214(5):605–613.
9. Hopf HW, Hunt TK. Does — and if so, to what extent — normovolemic dilutional anemia influence postoperative wound healing? *Chirurgische Gastroenterologie.* 1992;8:148–150.
10. Sorensen LT, Hemmingsen U, Kallehave F, et al. Risk factors for tissue and wound complications in gastrointestinal surgery. *Ann Surg.* 2005;241(4):654–658.
11. Jensen JA, Goodson WH, Hopf HW, Hunt TK. Cigarette smoking decreases tissue oxygen. *Arch Surg.* 1991;126(9):1131–1134.
12. Chang N, Goodson WH 3rd, Gottrup F, Hunt TK. Direct measurement of wound and tissue oxygen tension in postoperative patients. *Ann Surg.* 1983;197(4):470–478.
13. Hartmann M, Jonsson K, Zederfeldt B. Effect of tissue perfusion and oxygenation on accumulation of collagen in healing wounds. Randomized study in patients after major abdominal operations. *Eur J Surg.* 1992;158(10):521–526.
14. Stotts NA, Hopf HW. Facilitating positive outcomes in older adults with wounds. *Nurs Clin North Am.* 2005;40(2):267–279.
15. Albina JE. Nutrition in wound healing. *JPEN J Parenter Enteral Nutr.* 1994;18(4):367–376.
16. Arnold M, Barbul A. Nutrition and wound healing. *Plast Reconstr Surg.* 2006;117(7 Suppl):42S–58S.
17. Thomas DR. Prevention and treatment of pressure ul-

cers. *J Am Med Dir Assoc.* 2006;7(1):46–59.

18. Wipke-Tevis DD, Stotts NA. Nutritional risk, status, and intake of individuals with venous ulcers: a pilot study. *J Vasc Nurs.* 1996;14(2):27–33.

19. Healy B, Freedman A. Infections. *BMJ.* 2006;332(7545):838–841.

20. Frantz RA. Identifying infection in chronic wounds. *Nursing.* 2005;35(7):73.

21. Attinger CE, Janis JE, Steinberg J, et al. Clinical approach to wounds: debridement and wound bed preparation including the use of dressings and wound-healing adjuvants. *Plast Reconstr Surg.* 2006;117(7 Suppl):72S–109S.

22. Stotts NA. Impaired wound healing. In: Carrieri-Kohlman VK, Lindsey AM, West CM, eds. *Pathophysiological*

Phenomena in Nursing: Human Responses to Illness. 3rd ed. Philadelphia, PA: WB Saunders; 2003:331–347.

23. Newland PK, Wipke-Tevis DD, Williams DA, Rantz MJ, Petroski GF. Impact of pain on outcomes in long-term care residents with and without multiple sclerosis. *J Am Geriatr Soc.* 2005;53(9):1490–1496.

24. Khuri SF, Henderson WG, DePalma RG, et al; for the Participants in the VA National Surgical Quality Improvement Program. Determinants of long-term survival after major surgery and the adverse effect of postoperative complications. *Ann Surg.* 2005;242(3):326–343.

25. Zondor SD, Medina PJ. Bevacizumab: an angiogenesis inhibitor with efficacy in colorectal and other malignancies. *Ann Pharmacother.* 2004;38(7-8):1258–1264.

CHAPTER 8

Infections in Chronic Wounds

Stephan Landis, MD, FRCPC; **Siobhan Ryan**, MD, FRCPC;
Kevin Y. Woo, PhD, RN, FAPWCA;
R. Gary Sibbald, BSc, MD, MEd, FRCPC (Med, Derm), MACP, FAAD, MAPWCA

Objectives

The reader will be challenged to:

- Differentiate the concepts of wound contamination, colonization, critical colonization, and infection
- Distinguish infection in a chronic wound based upon bedside clinical assessment
- Analyze microbial culture results to identify specific multiresistant organisms
- Select appropriate empiric antimicrobial therapy for increased superficial bacterial burden and deep infection in chronic wounds
- Manage the presence of MRSA in a chronic wound.

Introduction

Early recognition and management of increased bacterial burden and infection is vital during the ongoing care of a chronic wound. Bacterial damage will cause wound deterioration, delaying wound healing and increasing the risks of further morbidity and mortality. The appropriate use of antimicrobial agents is an ongoing challenge in this field. Interestingly, 1 in 4 persons with chronic wounds are receiving antibiotics at any one time, and 60% have received systemic antibiotics within the previous 6 months.[1] This increased use of antibiotics is related to the clinical uncertainty associated with diagnosing and managing infection in chronic wounds.

The basic principles of wound management have evolved from the use of lint, animal grease and honey in Ancient Egyptian times (1600 BCE) to moist wound healing techniques that were first described in the 1960s. Unfortunately, some of the basic principles surrounding diagnosis and management of infection have been forgotten resulting in the indiscriminate use of antibiotics. This has promoted the development of antimicrobial resistance, particularly with methicillin-resistant *Staphylococcus aureus* (MRSA).

Definitions and Concepts

All chronic wounds contain microorganisms acquired either from the host or from the external environment. *Microorganisms interact with chronic ulcers at 4 levels: wound contamination, colonization, critical colonization, and infection.*[2]

Landis S, Ryan S, Woo KY, Sibbald RG. Infections in chronic wounds. In: Krasner DL, ed. *Chronic Wound Care: The Essentials.* Malvern, Pa: HMP Communications, 2014;87–110.

1. *Contamination* refers to the presence of non-replicating microorganisms on the wound surface but the bacteria do not evoke any clinical host response.
2. *Colonization* refers to the presence of replicating microorganisms attached superficially to the surface wound tissue without any detectable host injury. Some common colonizing flora are: *Corynebacteria* sp, coagulase negative *staphylococci*, and *viridans streptococci*. However, wound colonizers are not necessarily harmful and have been shown to accelerate wound healing. Wound healing occurs predictably beneath a moist occlusive dressing in the presence of a moderate nonpathogenic bacterial burden of normal skin flora.
3. *Critical colonization* involves a replicating microbial burden in the wound surface compartment. Wound healing is delayed or arrested[3] in additional to other subtle clinical signs of host injury.
4. *Wound infection* refers to the presence of multiplying microorganisms within the deep compartment of a wound. Explicit clinical signs are usually detectable to indicate host injury. Although various factors can influence the development of a wound infection, the common factors are described in the following relationship:

$$\text{Probability of infection} = \frac{(\text{micro burden}) \times (\text{virulence})}{(\text{host resistance})}$$

Microorganisms invade host tissues when the level of microbial burden or virulence has reached a level where host responses are overwhelmed. Of these 3 factors contributing to the probability of infection, reduced host resistance is frequently overlooked while much attention has been placed on microbial burden and virulence.

Determinants of Chronic Wound Infection

The ability of the host to resist microbial interference is the most important determinant of chronic wound infection and involves many different local and systemic components. These components include:

Size and location of the wound. Larger wounds are at greater risk of infection than smaller wounds and are associated with heavy microbial burdens. The location of a wound may determine the risk of wound infection. For example, a diabetic neurotrophic or neuroischemic ulcer over a bony deformity on a plantar surface or a pressure ulcer over a chronically soiled sacrum or perineal site are both more susceptible to infection than a localized pressure ulcer over the scapula.

Age of the wound. Chronic wounds of long duration (more than 6 weeks) are more likely to become infected involving deep tissue structures and bone. It is important to recognize that chronic wounds often have a polymicrobial flora (eg, gram-positive and gram-negative aerobes and anaerobes).[4]

Vascular perfusion. Inadequate local vascular supply leading to poor tissue oxygenation will favor microbial proliferation, increase the risks of infection and reduce the likelihood of healing. In fact, wounds are generally deemed healable if tissue oxygen partial pressures are > 40 mmHg, and difficult to heal if below 20 mmHg.[5] Up to 30% of diabetic neuroischemic foot ulcers will not heal in patients with an ankle-systolic pressure of < 50 mmHg or an ankle-brachial index < 0.3.[6] Clinicians should maintain a high index of suspicion because infection is more likely to be covert when tissue perfusion is poor.

Presence of devitalized tissue or foreign bodies. Devitalized tissues including eschar and slough are food source for bacteria. The presence of devitalized tissues thus increases the risk for the development of infection. The presence of foreign bodies, such as orthopedic prostheses, surgical mesh, sutures, or dressing materials can harbor microorganisms and thus predispose an individual to infection.

Systemic and Personal Factors

Behavioral determinants. Some individuals may have difficulty adhering to the treatment plan due to a lack of understanding, poor motivation, and depression. Poor personal hygiene, alcohol abuse, and smoking may also interfere with wound healing. Wound infection rates are 6 times higher in smokers than in nonsmokers.[7]

Among individuals who are having difficulty maintaining adequate nutritional intake, wound healing falters and the risk of infection increases when serum albumin levels are consistently below 2.5–3.0 g/dL.

Social determinants. Education and socioeconomic background must be taken into account to determine the healability of wounds. For example, individuals may not have the resources to purchase appropriate offloading devices that are essential for healing diabetic neurotrophic or neuroischemic foot ulcers.

Associated co-morbidities. Underlying conditions, such as poorly controlled diabetes mellitus (HgbA1c > 0.84), increase the risk of infection through hyperglycemia and inadequate neutrophil function especially with HgbA1c levels above 0.12 or 12%.[8] Chronic renal and liver impairment, as well as immune suppressing therapies, (eg, corticosteroid therapy, cytotoxic chemotherapies), and chronic viral infections (eg, human immunodeficiency virus infection, hepatitis B and C) increase the risk of wound infection. Conditions, including venous insufficiency, congestive heart failure, hepatic insufficiency and cor pulmonale, are associated with peripheral edema states that will reduce local host defense and increase the risk of infection.

Pathogenesis of Infection in Chronic Wounds

Microorganisms. Intact skin is the best defense mechanism for preventing microbial invasion. It not only serves as a barrier but also inhibits pathogen colonization through normal surface host flora, and promotes the antimicrobial effects of epidermal lipids. Few pathogens can breach this first line of defense. Once the skin barrier is compromised, microbial contamination and colonization occurs. The ecology of wounds is complex and most chronic wounds host polymicrobial flora, containing a range of 1.6 to 4.4 bacterial species per ulcer.[9] Whether or not infection ensues depends upon which microorganisms are involved, how likely they are to produce disease, and how effectively the host can resist invasion. Interestingly, almost 90% of ulcers without clinical signs of infection still contain more than 1 species of bacteria.[10] Bacteria possess numerous virulence strategies to help tip the balance in favor of host infection. These include:

1. The presence of *adhesins* that allow bacteria

to attach themselves to the host
2. The presence of *cell capsules* that protect the bacteria from phagocytosis
3. The production of *bacterial biofilm structures* that provide a shield over the expanding bacterial colonies.[11]

Microorganisms need not invade host tissue directly to impair wound healing. They produce a wide array of enzymes and toxins at the wound surface that can affect host immunity. The concept of bacterial synergy recognizes the importance of interspecies interactions.[12] The growth of gram-negative organisms and anaerobes may be enhanced by the presence of facultative bacteria providing exchangeable microbial growth factors.[13] Although, the concept of synergy has not been conclusively proven in chronic wounds, there are good examples of microbial cooperation in other conditions, including necrotizing soft tissue infections.

Staphylococcus aureus is a common pathogen found in chronic wounds. It has the ability to produce many enzymes that have been associated with disease production. These bacterial associated enzymes include: *catalase* that blocks phagocyte-mediated killing; *hyaluronidase* that breaks down connective tissue matrix; *beta-lactamase* that imparts penicillin resistance; and *nucleases or lipases* that disrupt cells leading to abscess formation. A variety of extracellular toxins are also produced and include: *alpha toxin*, that lyses the host cells (eukaryotic) but not bacterial cytoplasmic membranes; *beta toxin*, that degrades sphingomyelin, and breaks down cells (erythrocytes, leukocytes, and fibroblasts); *gamma toxin*, that breaks down erythrocytes; sigma toxin that has a surfactant effect; and *leukocidin*, that may induce granulocytopenia. In the extreme situation, the production of *toxic shock syndrome toxin* (TSST) induces a catastrophic multisystem disorder leading to the rapid development of shock and death through its activity as a super antigen.

Other microorganisms, such as *streptococci*, have active cell surface virulence factors, such as *capsular polysaccharide, peptidoglycan, lipoteichoic acid*, and *M-protein*, that promote bacterial resistance and avert phagocytosis.

Anaerobes favor the relatively hypoxic environment of the chronic ulcer[14] and are frequently overlooked as major microbial players in wound infection. Frequent anaerobic wound colonizers include: *Bacteroides, Peptostreptococcus,* and *Prevotella* species. They may not be identified on routine wound swab sampling because anaerobic culture and isolation techniques are more complex, labor-intensive and costly. In 9 wound surveys (1976–1999) involving wounds of diverse etiologies, a total of 3,116 microbial isolates were described using sensitive isolation techniques; 1,399 of the 3,116 organisms or 45% of the bacterial isolates involved the presence of anaerobes.[15]

Host Defense Factors

Acute wounds follow a predictable cascade that can be described by the following acronym: **V-I-P-E-R**. This cascade induces a vascular phase (**V**) with initial vasoconstriction, platelet activation, and rapid fibrin plugging. The inflammatory phase (**I**) that follows, typically a pronounced increase in blood flow to the site of injury, as well as increased vascular permeability, with a rapid mobilization of phagocytic cells, complement and antibody. Cytokine and growth factor release act in unison to sequester and remove microorganisms, foreign debris, bacterial toxins, and enzymes. The proliferative phase (**P**) overlaps with the inflammatory phase to produce new tissue substrate and granulation. This occurs through neovascularization, angiogenesis, matrix material deposition, and subsequent epithelial migration (**E**) to establish a new skin barrier. The final remodeling phase (**R**) of new skin tissue then occurs over several months.

While this host cascade progresses in a predictable manner in acute wounds, the healing sequence is stalled or arrested in the inflammatory (**I**) or proliferative (**P**) phases, with the development of infection. Thus an acute wound becomes chronic. Host injury occurs in a wound infected with a virulent population of microorganisms. Under most circumstances, the host will try to maintain a balance of colonizing flora and keep pathogenic flora in check through a wide array of defense mechanisms. However, this balance is upset within the chronic wound. Infection stimulates an inflammatory response leading to a persistent influx of neutrophils. Neutrophils release damaging substances such as cytolytic enzymes, free oxygen radicals, and inflammatory mediators. Eventually, localized thrombosis and vasocon-

stricting metabolites lead to tissue hypoxia. These tissue-damaging events can promote ongoing bacterial proliferation, ie, anaerobes, and further tissue destruction. As the immune response becomes increasingly self destructive in chronic infection, an adaptive down regulation of the immune response develops, particularly in overwhelming infection. The wound-bacterial relationship requires a very fine balance where the host tries to fend off pathogenic microorganisms while attempting to limit immunological injury and foster healing.

Numerous studies have indicated that the presence of chronic infection delays wound healing and reduces tissue tensile strength, particularly in the proliferative phase (**P**). This occurs because of over-exuberant small vessel angiogenesis with ongoing thrombosis of larger vessels leading to localized tissue hypoxia. Fibroblasts in chronically-infected wounds are reduced in number, have reduced metabolic activity, and form weak collagen in disorganized patterns. There is also increased collagenolytic activity in these wounds. Thus the patterns of development of granulation tissue are markedly influenced by infection in the proliferative phase (**P**). Granulation tissue within an infected wound tends to be pale or gray, and is sometimes described as looking more like "cooked meat" rather than the healthy firm pink "raw hamburger" granulation base required for healing. This tissue is often edematous with marked friability and increased tendency to bleed easily. The epithelization phase (**E**) has also been shown to be impaired where granulation tissue displays the features of bacterial damage.

Diagnosis: Bedside Assessments

The assessment of infection in a chronic wound is a bedside skill. There is no gold standard for the diagnosis of this condition. What does bedside clinical assessment tell us about the recognition of infection in chronic wounds?

Over the ages, acute wound infection has been described by *the 4 classic signs of inflammation: rubor (vasodilatation), calor (increased temperature), dolor (painful cytokine-mediated stimulation of nociceptive nerve fibers and nerve damage), and tumor (increased vessel permeability leading to edema). Sometimes the presence of purulent exudate is added to support the diagnosis of infection.*

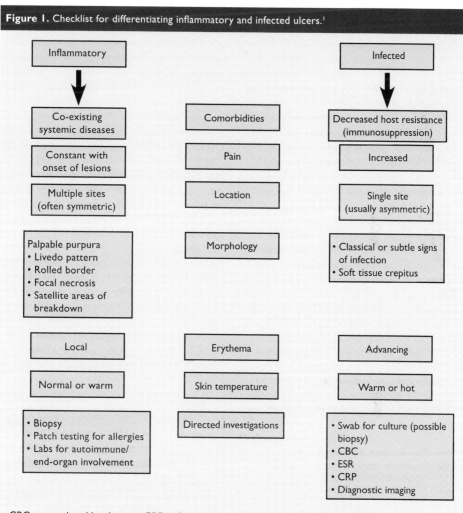

Figure 1. Checklist for differentiating inflammatory and infected ulcers.[1]

Inflammatory		Infected
Co-existing systemic diseases	Comorbidities	Decreased host resistance (immunosuppression)
Constant with onset of lesions	Pain	Increased
Multiple sites (often symmetric)	Location	Single site (usually asymmetric)
Palpable purpura • Livedo pattern • Rolled border • Focal necrosis • Satellite areas of breakdown	Morphology	• Classical or subtle signs of infection • Soft tissue crepitus
Local	Erythema	Advancing
Normal or warm	Skin temperature	Warm or hot
• Biopsy • Patch testing for allergies • Labs for autoimmune/ end-organ involvement	Directed investigations	• Swab for culture (possible biopsy) • CBC • ESR • CRP • Diagnostic imaging

CBC = complete blood count; CRP = C-reactive protein; ESR = erythrocyte sedimentation rate

The mean sensitivity of these signs in the diagnosis of chronic wound infection is low at 0.38.[16]

On the other hand, signs associated with chronic wounds also include: *delayed healing, increased serous drainage/inflammation, increased tenderness, friable/bleeding granulation tissue, foul odor, and increased wound breakdown with increased size and satellite areas of new ulceration.* Using these criteria, we note that the corresponding sensitivity rises to 0.62, an increase of more than 60%.[16] Microbiological data is used to supplement and support the clinical diagnosis rather than make the diagnosis.

Severe infection in a chronic wound is seldom subtle, particularly when local microbial invasion leads to a systemic inflammatory response with a "sepsis syndrome." This is characterized by fever, chills, rigors, hypotension, and in the extreme, multiorgan dysfunction. Infection of moderate severity often may lack systemic features, but most chronic wounds in this situation will show a rim of periwound cellulitis with increased erythema, swelling, and an increase in local temperature at the wound edges. Infections consisting primarily of gram-positive organisms typically have purulent exudate. The exudate in mixed infections, particularly where gram negatives are present, is often less purulent. Bacterial leukocidins, phospholipases, and toxins rapidly destroy neutrophils, producing watery exudates, sometimes referred to as "dishwater pus." The presence of a noxious odor is associated with the presence of anaerobic bacteria, but it is an insensitive sign, and noted in only about half of chronic wounds infected with anaerobes. Some chronic wound infections are of mild severity. These represent so-called "covert" infections, where the host is being sufficiently harmed to the point that healing does not take place. In these cases, the pathogen is sufficiently contained so that typical inflammatory changes are absent, and may represent "critical colonization."

Infection must be considered in any chronic wound that fails to show signs of progressive healing despite favorable conditions. We need only to recall the clinical signs associated with chronic wound infection, described above. However, most clinical signs have pitfalls. When cellulitis is localized solely to subdermal lymphatics, there may be few superficial findings, except increased pain.

Alternatively, noninfectious processes can produce an inflammatory response that can mimic infection including a condition called pyoderma gangrenosum. Tissue destruction with "sterile" pus composed of a massive neutrophil infiltrate in the skin may be evident. An acute Charcot foot can also be confused with cellulitis, when there is erythema, swelling, and warmth over recent small bony fractures. Inexperienced clinicians may over-diagnose infection in ischemic limbs displaying characteristic dependent rubor. The key clinical difference is that this ischemic rubor will blanche within 1 minute of elevating the limb above the level of the heart, while inflammatory rubor will only partially diminish if there is true tissue infection. Chronic venous insufficiency, venous thrombosis, and lipodermatosclerosis have all been confused with cellulitis in an edematous leg. Infection and inflammation[1] are compared and contrasted in Figure 1.[1]

Increased Bacterial Burden and Infection

Bacteria can delay healing in a chronic wound through damage in a superficial or deep compartment. Topical treatment is usually adequate if bacterial damage is superficial, systemic therapy is often indicated if deep bacterial damage is suspected. In this section we will take the signs and symptoms listed above and assign them to the superficial or the deep dermal compartment. Some signs may be present with infection at both levels. Superficial damage can be documented through the mnemonic NERDS:[17] **N**onhealing, **E**xudate that has increased, **R**ed friable granulation, **D**ebris on the surface, and **S**mell (Figure 2).

Deep infection often requires systemic treatment. Clinicians need to triangulate looking for 2 or 3 signs. Odor and increased exudate are in both the superficial and deep clusters of the characteristic signs and additional criteria are needed to determine if bacterial damage is superficial, deep or both. The term STONES[17] refers to the increased wound **S**ize, increased surrounding skin **T**emperature, the probing or exposed **O**s, **N**ew or satellite areas of breakdown, the 3 "**E**"s (**E**rythema, **E**xudate, and **E**dema) along with **S**mell. These 2 paradigms represent a theoretical framework to study the effects of various antimicrobial agents, but require further validation and modification.

Bacterial Loads, Types, and How To Collect Them

Quantitative bacteriology (bacterial burden). As bedside wound evaluation of infection may lack adequate clinical diagnostic sensitivity, the assessment of bacterial burden has become an important adjunctive procedure.

Skin and subcutaneous tissue are remarkably impervious to bacterial challenges. In 1956, Elek[18] showed that the subcutaneous injection of S aureus in young, healthy volunteers produced no signs of infection until the inoculum was $>10^5$ (1.0×10^6 or higher) colony forming units (CFUs) per mL. Since then a large number of studies have tried to determine the specific bacterial quantitative threshold that best predicts the probable occurrence of soft tissue infection. Bendy et al[19] demonstrated that pressure ulcers were more likely to heal if bacterial burdens fell to $< 1.0 \times 10^6$ CFUs per mL. Krizek et al[20] demonstrated that skin grafting would often fail if there were $> 1.0 \times 10^6$ CFUs per gram of tissue in the wound bed. Wound closures tended to fail if wound beds contained $> 1.0 \times 10^6$ CFUs per gram of tissue. Noyes et al[21] confirmed that wound exudate must carry bacterial burdens of

Figure 2. The mnemonic "NERDS" for the diagnosis of superficial, increased bacterial burden.

Letter		KEY INFORMATION	Comments
N	Nonhealing wound 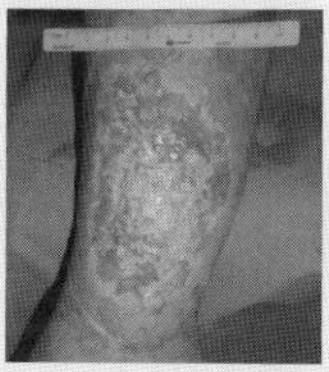	• The wound is nonhealing despite appropriate interventions (healable wound with the cause treated and patient centered concerns addressed) • Bacterial damage has caused an increased metabolic load in the chronic wound creating a pro-inflammatory wound environment that delays healing	• To determine a healing trajectory the wound size should decrease 30% after 4 weeks of appropriate treatment to heal by week 12. • If the wound does not respond to topical antimicrobial therapy consider systemic antimicrobial and biopsy after 4–12 weeks to rule out an unsuspected diagnosis such as vasculitis, Pyoderma gangrenosum, or malignancy
E	Exudative wound 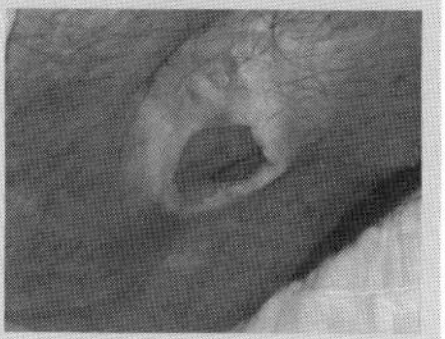	• An increase in wound exudate can be indicative of bacterial imbalance and leads to periwound maceration • Exudate is often clear before it becomes purulent or sanguineous Increased exudate needs to trigger the clinician to assess for subtle signs of infection	• Increased exudate needs to trigger the clinician to assess for subtle signs of infection • Protect periwound area using the LOWE© memory jogger (Liquid film forming acrylate; Ointments; Windowed dressings; External collection devices) for skin barrier for wound margins
R	Red and bleeding wound 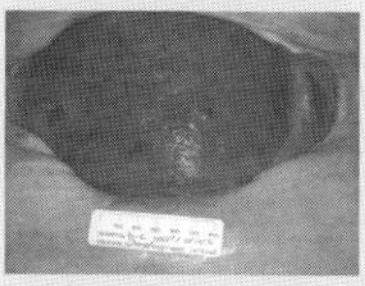	• When the wound bed tissue is bright red with exuberant granulation tissues and bleeds easily, bacterial imbalance can be suspected.	• Granulation tissue should be pink and firm. The exuberant granulation tissue that is loose and bleeds easily reflects bacterial damage to the forming collagen matrix and an increased vasculature of the tissue.
D	Debris in the wound 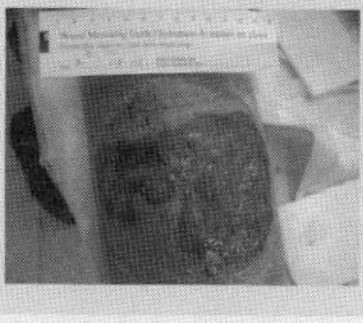	• Necrotic tissue and debris in the wound is a food source for bacterial and can encourage a bacterial imbalance. New debris indicates the wound surface is hostile to cells.	• Necrotic tissue in the wound bed will require debridement in the presence of adequate circulation • Debridement choice needs to be determined based on wound type, clinician skill, and resources
S	Smell from the wound 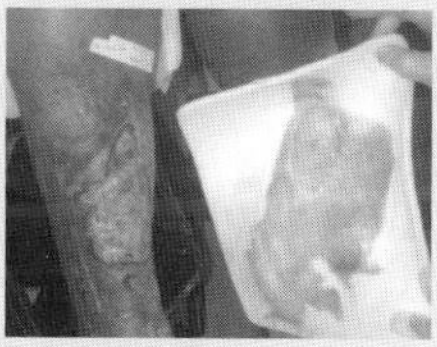	• Smell from bacterial byproducts caused by tissue necrosis associated with the inflammatory response is indicative of wound related bacterial damage. Pseudomonas has a sweet characteristic smell /green color and anaerobes have a putrid odor due to the breakdown of tissue.	• Clinicians need to differentiate the smell of bacterial damage from the odor associated with the interaction of exudate with different dressing materials particularly some hydrocolloids. Odor may come from superficial or deep tissue damage and this should not be relied on along with exudate alone as the only signs of increased superficial bacterial burden.

© Sibbald and Ayello 2006.
Used with permission

Table 1. Practical techniques for assessing infection in chronic wounds

Technique	Description	Laboratory processing	Strength	Limitations	Indications
Qualitative swab	Irrigate the wound, then rotate the tip of a swab over a defined area	Inoculated into media for identification of organisms	Identify organisms without relative quantitative counts	No quantitative data Prone to contamination with surface colonizers	Common practice for initial/routine bacteriological assessment
Semiquantitative swab	Rotate the tip of swab over a defined area on the wound bed	Inoculated and streaked into 4 quadrants on standard media	Quick Cheap Reproducible Correlates with quantitative biopsy	Reduced specificity Prone to contamination with surface colonizers	Should become standard of practice if further data confirm its applicability
Wound fluid aspiration	Irrigate wound with up to 10 cc of saline or water, then aspirate fluid with needle and syringe	Inoculated and streaked into 4 quadrants on standard media	Cheap Reproducible May correlate with quantitative biopsy	Sampling error Invasive	Deep abscess without surface connection
Quantitative biopsy	Wound is cleaned and biopsy taken from granulation tissue without debris	Weighed, serial dilutions, plating and incubation then permit enumeration and identification of colonies. Colony counts are calculated.	Determines quantitatively the concentration of microorganisms within the tissue	Invasive procedure Biopsy sites maybe slow to heal or bleed Costly Time consuming	Application usually reserved for research settings

> 1.0 x 10^6 CFUs per mL in order to produce invasive infection. These studies have generally agreed with Elek's findings. Large populations of bacteria are required to produce sufficient toxin and proteolytic enzymes in order to overcome host resistance and damage living tissue. In the presence of a foreign body, infection was established with a lower infective dose. In fact, infection associated with a foreign body, took place with a bacterial dose reduction of 4-logs.

There are several methods to quantify bacteria in a chronic wound and each method has its advantages and pitfalls as outlined below (Table 1).

1. *Quantitative biopsy.* Quantitative biopsy has been considered the gold standard for measuring bacterial burden in a wound (Table 1). Comparing paired burn wound biopsies, results from quantitative biopsies that contained >10^5 CFUs per gram of tissue were correlated to histological evaluation of bacterial invasion into soft tissue.[22] However, the study has been criticized for using only a small part of the wound. Overall, while quantitative biopsy may be valid in the diagnosis of infection in burn wounds, little is known about its utility in chronic wounds. The utility of quantitative techniques are limited by observations that many chronic wounds, colonized with normal skin flora, will heal even in the

presence of > 10^6 CFUs per gram of tissue if host resistance is dominant over bacterial damage. Other chronic wounds may not heal if virulent pathogens, such as beta hemolytic streptococci, are present even at much lower concentrations. In addition, this technique has limited clinical application because of increased costs, labor and time requirements, need for expert technical processing, risks of bacteremia from an invasive biopsy, and potentially unnecessary local tissue trauma.

2. *Quantitative swab technique.* The quantitative swab technique (exact quantity of dilutant, serial dilutions) is a research tool for assessing both the quality and quantity of microbial flora in soft tissue. It closely approximates findings obtained from quantitative biopsy, but like biopsy technique, it is time consuming and expensive. Also, it has not been extensively studied in chronic wounds.[23]

3. *Semiquantitative swab technique.* Although semiquantitative techniques of bacterial assessment have been described in chronic wounds, these require further validation. The semiquantitative swab has been developed to obtain an extra degree of quantification from the routine culture swab. To ensure that the pathogen causing the infection is cultured, it is recommended that the wound be irrigated with normal saline until all visible debris has been washed away. Healthy granulation tissue is selected for the swab site. The Levine technique (see below) has been validated in burn patients with paired quantitative biopsies. Plate counts > 30 CFUs identified all patients with > 10^5 CFUs per gram of tissue on quantitative biopsy. Most laboratories do not report wound swabs in semiquantitative fashion, as the technique has not been extensively described in the literature and has been validated only in burn patients. Also, results are dependent upon the means by which the culture is obtained. Inadequate wound bed preparation may invalidate results. The area where the swab comes into contact with the wound surface is of critical importance: the greater the area swabbed, the greater the number of organisms obtained. It is not clearly established how much wound surface area should be sampled for a semiquantitative swab to most closely reflect the quantitative wound biopsy. Gardner et al[24] have recommended the Levine method for ob-

taining a bacterial swab as being most closely associated with results of quantitative biopsies. This method selects a central area of wound with a granulation base and recommends pressing the swab over 1 cm^2 of the wound surface just enough to produce exudate on the surface. The swab is then rotated 360 degrees and placed in the transport media. The swab needs to be processed in the laboratory in a timely fashion where the contents are plated on the Petri dish in 4 serial dilutions representing the 4 quadrants. The quadrant growth responds to a 1+ to 4+ scale or may be reported as scant, light, moderate or heavy growth. Swabs should not contain debris or dried exudate from the wound surface. In this example, 4+ or heavy growth was equated to 10^5 growth. Although this semiquantitative approach is a promising and more practical alternative to quantitative wound biopsy, it requires further study in chronic wounds.

Qualitative Bacteriology (Bacterial Species)

Microorganisms isolated from chronic wounds have varying degrees of pathogenicity, depending upon whether they represent normal or acquired flora. Highly virulent microorganisms rarely exist as "benign colonizers" and should be treated regardless of numbers. These may include: *Mycobacteriaceae, B anthracis* (anthrax bacillus), toxin-producing *Corynebacterium diphtheriae, Erysipelothrix* spp, *Treponema* spp, *Brucella* spp, chronic *herpes simplex* infection (immunocompromised hosts), invasive dimorphic fungi (*Coccidioides* spp, *Blastomyces* spp, *Histoplasma* spp), and some parasitic organisms (eg, *leishmaniasis*).

The flora of a chronic wound generally evolves in a predictable fashion, according to the duration of the wound. In principle, during the first 4 weeks, wounds are colonized by gram-positive organisms, initially with normal skin flora, followed by *enterococci*, beta hemolytic *streptococci*, and *S aureus*. Group B beta hemolytic *streptococci* are the most common *streptococci* in diabetic foot infections and are commonly associated with *S aureus* as co-pathogens. ***The pathogenicity of many microorganisms is enhanced in the setting of polymicrobial infection through the concept of bacterial synergism.*** When present together in a wound, group B beta hemolytic *streptococci* and *S aureus* possess an enhanced ability to lyse cell membranes.

After the first 4 weeks, facultative anaerobic gram-negative rods, such as enteric lactose-fermenting bacilli, colonize chronic wounds. The most common examples include: *Proteus* spp, *Escherichia coli*, and *Klebsiella* spp.

As time progresses, common obligate anaerobic flora, such as *Bacteroides* and *peptostreptococcus* spp, join the polymicrobial environment of the chronic wound. They may often outgrow other flora by at least 1-log in numbers. Some anaerobes can be virulent, and may reflect the causes of microbial infection, where routine cultures are reported as "negative" or "no growth." It is important to recall that partial oxygen tissue pressures in the middle of chronic, nonhealing ulcers may be ischemic with levels as low as 5 to 20 mmHg, creating the ideal growth environment for fastidious anaerobic bacteria.[25] The synergistic relationships and interactions between anaerobes and aerobic flora in a chronic ulcer infection may be more important than the individual microorganisms themselves.

Finally, the wound becomes colonized with nonlactose fermenting gram-negative aerobic rods, such as *Pseudomonas* spp, *Stenotrophomonas* spp, and *Acinetobacter* spp. These microorganisms are typically waterborne, and can contaminate the wound from regular footwear or during bathing.

Thus, a chronic wound develops an increasingly complex microflora. Older wounds tend to have larger surface areas and deeper tissue layer involvement. For this reason, osteomyelitis, or bony infection within a chronic wound has a statistically greater chance of anaerobic polymicrobial participation than chronic wounds without osteomyelitis.

The role of common skin colonizers with low virulence is often unclear. Pathogens, such as *Enterococcus* spp or fungal *Candida* spp, usually do not require treatment when cultured as part of a polymicrobial infection. However, if the microorganisms are isolated in sufficient numbers in the absence of other pathogens, and in a wound with signs of clinical infection, then they should be treated with antimicrobial agents.

The long-term persistence of a chronic wound tends to occur in sicker patients and is associated with frequent and prolonged hospitalization. These patients are exposed to multiple antibiotics, and are at risk for the development of antimicrobial-resistant pathogens, such as MRSA.

The diagnosis of osteomyelitis is an important aspect of chronic wound management, since chronic wounds currently account for the largest proportion of chronic osteomyelitis in medical practice. The development of osteomyelitis in a chronic wound occurs because of contiguous spread of infection from overlying soft tissues to deeper regions of underlying bone and joints as part of ongoing ulcer enlargement. Diabetic foot ulcers are the most likely to develop underlying osteomyelitis. The longer an ulcer has been present and the larger its size, then the more likely it is to be complicated by osteomyelitis.

The most practical test for chronic osteomyelitis is to have exposed bone, or alternatively palpate or probe the wound with a sterile gloved finger and/or a blunt instrument.

In the context of a diabetic neuropathic foot ulcer, Grayson et al[26] calculated an 89% positive predictive value of underlying osteomyelitis if bone is directly encountered. Where osteomyelitis is suspected but bone cannot be probed, a plain x-ray may show the typical changes of osteomyelitis such as osteolysis, bony sclerosis, periosteal elevation, and bone fragmentation.[27] If such changes are not seen, the x-ray should be repeated in 2 to 3 weeks when radiographic abnormalities are likely to become evident. The use of magnetic resonance imaging (MRI) and radionuclide scanning is less clear, particularly as these tests have less specificity and are of greater expense when compared to high level of clinical suspicion, bedside assessment and plain radiography. To document and follow the progress of osteomyelitis, the use of a laboratory determination of the Erythrocyte Sedimentation Rate (ESR) or C Reactive Protein (CRP) level can be useful. An ESR level above 40 without another cause or an elevated CRP protein may be useful clinically. The CRP may normalize at a faster rate than the ESR with the resolution of osteomyelitis.

Specimen Collection, Transport, and Culture (Table 1)

The simplest and most commonly used method for assessing the presence of infection in a chronic wound is the nonquantitative swab. If properly performed, the swab should provide an accurate qualitative assessment of microbial wound flora.

Before obtaining a bacterial swab culture, the wound bed should be adequately prepared to remove nonrepresentative surface colonizing microorganisms. This is accomplished by applying saline compresses or irrigating the wound, and then performing superficial debridement if necrotic eschar or slough is present on the wound surface.

Qualitative results are better if actual tissue curettings are sent for culture. If isolated collections of abscess fluid are available, then these should be aspirated in a capped syringe and sent for microbial culture. The results of the semiqualitative swab will adequately guide antimicrobial therapeutic choices in the majority (93%) of diabetic foot infections.[28]

The irrigation-aspiration technique[29] has been described for use in infected pressure ulcers. After irrigating the ulcer bed twice with saline, at least 2.5 mL of residual fluid is aspirated and sent for aerobic and anaerobic cultures. This technique has a high correlation with paired skin punch biopsy results. The main limitation however remains that the swab technique does not provide quantitative measures.

The rapid slide technique described by Heggers et al[30] assesses bacterial burden prior to carrying out primary or delayed secondary closure. It may be useful in determining if there is significant microbial load in a chronic wound. However, it is rarely performed on a routine basis, since it does not permit a qualitative assessment and needs to be paired with qualitative swab data. The reproducibility of this technique has not been extensively published.

Other techniques, such as the agar contact plate, the contact sponge technique, and the capillary gauze technique, have been devised to quantify microbial load in chronic wounds. These techniques are all limited by the fact that they primarily evaluate wound surface flora, and can be nonspecific with a discrepancy compared with the organisms isolated from tissue samples.

Expeditious transport of specimens to the microbiology laboratory is critical for all of the techniques described above. Given that a significant practice of wound care occurs in the community, it is necessary that effective and practical means

of transport of diagnostic specimens is available to community practitioners. Currently aerobic transport media will support the survival of typical aerobes that are found in chronic wounds, while preventing excessive microbial overgrowth. On the other hand, anaerobic flora will not tolerate a prolonged transport time in most routine aerobic media. Ideally, swabs obtained for anaerobic culture should be inoculated onto pre-reduced, anaerobically-sterilized transport media.

Treatment of Chronic Wound Infection

Treating a chronic wound infection involves systematically identifying and correcting the underlying cause of the wound and addressing aberrant host factors that lead to the development of infection in the first place. This might include:
1. Relieving local pressure
2. Managing stress factors
3. Controlling edema
4. Stopping smoking
5. Improving glycemic control
6. Revascularizing ischemic tissues
7. Improving nutrition
8. Lowering immunosuppressive therapy where feasible
9. Discontinuing potentially offending drugs.

Wound bed preparation (sharp wound debridement and wound bed cleansing) can produce a rapid reduction in bacterial burden because the majority of organisms on the wound surface are removed.

Approach to Antimicrobial Use

It is important to differentiate antiseptics, disinfectants and antibiotics. *Antiseptics* refer to topical agents that are applied to skin, mucous membranes, or inanimate objects to prevent the growth and reproduction of microorganisms, but do not usually kill the organisms. *Disinfectants* are chemical substances that kill microorganisms on organic or inanimate surfaces and are generally harmful to humans. *Antibiotics* are drugs that slow the growth or kill microorganisms, but are generally harmless to the host when used topically or systemically.

There is little, if any, role for disinfectant use in the treatment of wounds. For further information, see Chapter 5.

Antiseptics. Antiseptic use must be selective and applications should be based on reasonable evidence or expert opinion. Historically, common agents such as hydrogen peroxide and aniline dyes (gentian violet, mercurochrome) have been used, although there is no evidence they are efficacious. *Hydrogen peroxide* de-sloughs only during its short effervescent phase, and may harm healthy granulation tissue. *Gentian (crystal) violet* is a topical antifungal with an additional narrow gram-positive but poor gram-negative antiseptic action. It is a potential carcinogen and may produce irritation locally including chemical burns and even ulceration particularly on mucous membranes. This substance can induce tattoo type staining of healing skin.

Mercurochrome's antiseptic effect was discovered in 1919, and used primarily for minor injuries. Its antimicrobial efficacy for chronic wounds has not been established. This agent was removed from the "generally recognized as safe" list by the FDA in 1998, because of theoretical concerns over mercury poisoning especially if used in large quantities.

Diluted acetic acid or vinegar (standard vinegar at 5% is usually diluted to 0.5% to avoid excessive burning and stinging) is a popular adjunctive short-term topical treatment in superficial wound infections with *Pseudomonas* spp, as well as other aerobic gram-negative bacilli. *Pseudomonas aeruginosa*, in particular, is prone to develop quick antimicrobial resistance to most topical and systemic agents. A simple treatment like acetic acid for local superficial infections is preferable. The low pH and particular sensitivity of *Pseudomonas* spp to vinegar means that infections may be effectively treated, even if used with a topical compress for 10 to 15 minutes per day. Dilute vinegar soaks are also effective in odor control[31] (anti-anaerobic activity) and have been used in the palliation of distal gangrene in patients with vascular insufficiency, who either refuse surgery or where surgery is contraindicated. Topical acetic acid may be effective for superficial compartment *Pseudomonas* related bacterial damage but systemic agents are often required if deep infection develops. Two systemic agents or a topical and systemic agent should be used in combination due to a trend of developing frequent antimicrobial resistance. Acetic acid, even in usual concentrations, is cy-

totoxic and its use should be limited to patients where the reduction of bacterial burden is more important than its tissue toxicity. For further information, see Chapter 5.

Iodine preparations are potent broad-spectrum antiseptics. Expert opinion favors less toxic iodine dressings for short-term use in healable wounds where microbial burden is high in the superficial wound compartment (eg, cadexomer iodine). In chronic, nonhealable wounds with or without infection, an iodine solution can be ordered combining moisture and bacterial reduction (topical povidone iodine). In a nonhealable wound, debridement should be conservative, removing only loose slough and emphasizing bacterial reduction as more important than tissue toxicity.

Chlorhexidine and its derivative polyhexamethylene biguanide (PHMB) also have a broad spectrum of action along with relatively low tissue toxicity and a good tissue residual effect. Over the next few years, safer iodine and chlorhexidine products will be combined with moist interactive dressings to treat an increased bacterial burden in the superficial wound compartment and serve as an alternative to silver.

For millennia, silver has been recognized for its antimicrobial properties, where it is effective against a broad range of aerobic, anaerobic, gram-negative, gram-positive bacteria, yeast, viruses, as well as methicillin-resistant *Staphylococcus aureus* (MRSA) and vancomycin-resistant *Enterococcus* (VRE).[32] Silver may also have specific pro-healing and anti-inflammatory properties.[33] Silver has an advantage over many of the other traditional wound antimicrobials because it works on at least 3 different bacterial related metabolic processes:

1. Blocks transport of nutrients into bacterial cell walls by binding to peptidoglycans that are absent in mammalian cells
2. Denatures microbial proteins especially those involved in respiration in the bacterial mitochondria
3. Binds to microbial DNA inactivating translation of proteins and replication of DNA.

Silver requires ionization in an aqueous media to exert its antimicrobial effect. For this reason, ointments and creams should not be used under silver dressings or on the immediate wound margin where the material can leak into the aqueous

Table 2. Empiric antibiotic therapy for chronic wound infection.

	Complex	Simple
Ulcer type	Diabetic, Sacral/trochanteric (deep), malignant	Venous leg, Other
Common microflorae	*S aureus*, streptococci, skin flora, anaerobes, aerobic gram-negatives bacilli, *Pseudomonas* spp	*S aureus*, streptococci, skin flora
↓ Clinical presentation	↓ Empiric antibiotic options: dose, route, and duration	
Mild: Superficial No systemic response No osteomyelitis Ambulatory management	• Amoxicillin/clavulanate 500/125 mg PO TID x 14 days • Clindamycin 300-450 mg QID + Ciprofloxacin 500 mg PO BID (or moxifloxacin 400 mg OD) x 14 days • Linezolid (MRSA) 600 mg PO BID x 14 days	• Cephalexin 500 mg PO QID x 14 days • Clindamycin 300 mg PO TID x 14 days
Moderate: Superficial to deep +/- systemic response No osteomyelitis Ambulatory or in-patient management	• Clindamycin 600 mg PO TID + Ciprofloxacin 500 mg PO BID x 14days • Clindamycin 600 mg PO TID + Ceftriaxone 1g/IV Q24H x 2–12 wks • Vancomycin (MRSA) 1g/IV Q12H x 14 days • Linezolid (MRSA) 600 mg IV BID x 14 days	• Clindamycin 600 mg PO TID + Ciprofloxacin 500 mg PO BID x 14 days • Clindamycin 600 mg PO TID + Ceftriaxone 1g/IV Q24H x 2–12 wks
Severe: Deep Systemic response **+/- Osteomyelitis** Limb/life threatening In-patient management **Prolonged oral therapy (2–12 weeks) is required if bone or joints are involved**	• Clindamycin 600 mg PO TID + Ceftriaxone 1g/IV Q24H x 14 days • Piperacillin/tazobactam 4.5g/IV Q8H x 14 days • Clindamycin 600 mg PO TID + Gentamicin 5 mg/kg/IV Q24H x 14 days • Imipenem 500 mg/IV Q6H x 14 days • Meropenem 1g/IV Q8H x 14 days • Vancomycin (MRSA) 1g/IV Q12H x 14 days • Linezolid (MRSA) 600 mg/IV BID x 14 days	• Clindamycin 600 mg PO TID + Ceftriaxone 1g/IV Q24H x 14 days • Piperacillin/tazobactam 4.5 g/IV Q8H x 14 days

wound environment and interfere with the silver ionization process.

There are several advantages to the new modern silver dressings over silver sulfadiazine cream. Silver sulfadiazine cream became available in the late 1960s but it does not provide autolytic debridement or moisture balance. There is a relatively small amount of the silver in the ionized form and much larger amounts of the silver metal are absorbed systemically than with the new silver dressings. Silver sulfadiazine cream can cause local argyria or dermal deposition leading to a slate blue grey discoloration but silver dressings have only been associated with periwound keratin staining that can be easily removed or dissipates with shedding of the scale. The new silver dressings also combine sustained release with moisture balance. In some dressings with calcium alginate components silver dressings provide autolytic debridement. Silver dressings should be judged by their moisture balance properties and the level of silver released. Table 3 presents silver products commonly used in wound management. The dressings are divided into low, medium and high release products. If a low release product is not clinically effective after a 2- to 4-week trial then a medium or high release product should be substituted or the increased bacterial burden needs to be treated systemically.

Sibbald et al[34] investigated the original Acticoat burn dressing in 29 stalled chronic wounds. Quantitative biopsies were performed for bacterial culture at the beginning and end of the 4-week study with a number of patients converting to a healing trajectory. This study did not demonstrate a change in the deep tissue quantitative bacterial biopsies and the improvements in these patients are most likely due to improved surface compartment critical colonization. A number of patients had a dramatic reduction in local wound pain. A minority of patients experienced local burning and stinging immediately after application due to a probable rapid diffusion of the silver ions. If the dressing is soaked in water for a longer period of time, subjects are less likely to experience the burning with dressing application.

The same researcher[35] investigated stalled venous ulcers and the use of Acticoat 7™ (Smith & Nephew, Largo, Fla) dressing applied at weekly intervals. This 15-patient case series was a pilot study of 4-layer elastic bandage application with each patient acting as their own control. The subjects were biopsied at baseline and an average of 6 weeks later for quantitative bacterial burden and histology. There was a dramatic healing response with 4 of the 12 patients that completed the study; healing in an average of 9 weeks. There was a decrease in *Staphylococcus aureus* counts in the second paired quantitative bacterial biopsies and this was associated with healing. Histology demonstrated an anti-inflammatory action with a decrease in neutrophil infiltrates associated with healing. This same anti-inflammatory action has not been documented to date with the lower release silver products.

The only randomized controlled trials (RCT) with silver dressings in chronic wounds have been performed with a medium release silver foam dressing[36] (Contreet®, Coloplast, Humlebaek, Denmark). In an efficacy study, patients with venous disease and mixed arterial and venous disease were randomized to receive either compression with the moderate silver releasing foam compared to a foam dressing alone (Allevyn™, Smith & Nephew, Largo, Fla). The patient's stalled wounds also had an increased exudate, increased pain, odor or abnormal granulation tissue in the superficial wound compartment. At the 4 week mark, there was a 45% reduction in wound size in the silver foam group compared to a 25% reduction in the ulcer size for the foam comparator ($P = 0.05$). In addition there were fewer patients with odor and there was better exudate management with less leakage. A similar RCT[37] compared the same silver foam dressing, enrolling 619 patients from 80 wound clinics around the world. In this study the silver foam was compared to the best clinical practice in the wound care center enrolling the patients with venous, mixed venous and arterial ulcers, with a small number of patients enrolled with foot and pressure ulcers. The relative reduction in ulcer size was 50% for the silver foam dressing compared to 34% for the local best practices ($P < 0.01$) and there was a significant and accelerated decrease in odor and a decrease in ulcer leakage.

Antibiotics (Table 2)

Antibiotics may be delivered topically or systemically (oral or parenteral). In a systematic re-

Table 3. Silver preparations used in wound management.

Preparation	Delivery Mechanism	Product Name	Benefits	Disadvantages
Silver salts				
Silver nitrate	0.5% solutions in burn wounds	Silver nitrate solution	• Easy to use • High cytotoxicity	• Staining • May lead to electrolyte imbalance • Short half-life
Silver sulfadiazine	1% in carrier cream-chronic wounds and burns	Flamazine, Silvadene, SSD cream (+) Contradictory values on silver release rate in literature	• Easily available • Wide clinical acceptance though controlled studies using Silvadene are rare	• Cytotoxic (in vitro) • Tends to leave heavy deposits of foreign matter (termed a pseudoeschar) in the wound bed • Pain associated with removal of pseudoeschar. • Neutropenia possible. • Staining of tissue known to occur • Short half-life • High incidence of sulpha allergy • May need a secondary dressing especially as product tends to "melt" being petrolatum- based
Silver amorphous hydrogel	Silver chloride	SilvaSorb Gel (+)	Low cytotoxicity, broad spectrum antimicrobial that delivers time-released silver for 3 days	May need secondary dressing
Silver sodium chloride polyacrylate sheets	Silver chloride	• SilvaSorb Sheet • SilvaSorb Perforated • SilvaSorb Cavity (+)	Low cytotoxicity, broad spectrum antimicrobial that delivers time-released silver for 7 days. Donates moisture or absorbs up to 5 times their weight in exudate	Absorbs well, but slowly
Silver-calcium-sodium phosphates	Co-extruded in polymer matrix (film) for superficial wounds with limited exudate	• Arglaes Film • Arglaes Island (+)	Residual antimicrobial activity lasts up to 7 days	Limited absorption of fluid for film version. Good absorption from island version with calcium alginate pad

Table 3. Silver preparations used in wound management. *(Continued)*

Preparation	Delivery Mechanism	Product Name	Benefits	Disadvantages
Silver salts				
Silver chloride site disc	Polyacrylate silver chloride	SilvaSorb Site (+)	Protection for vascular and nonvascular percutaneous tubes. Delivers silver for 7 days. Translucent, flexible, low profile	Not self adhesive, and similar to other site dressings, needs a secondary adhesive product for securement
Silver salt/calcium alginate powder	Polymer silver chloride in alginate powder	Arglaes powder (+)	• Low cytotoxicity silver • Antimicrobial activity up to 5 days with fluid management • Virtually any size, shape, or depth of wound managed easily with this product	Needs a secondary dressing for coverage
Silver calcium alginate/carboxymethylcellulose dressing		Maxorb Extra Ag (sheet or rope) (+) Silvercel (sheet or rope) (+)	Low cytotoxicity delivers silver for 4 days for superior absorption and fluid handling, vertical wicking and 1-piece removal	Product not differentiated by color from nonsilver alginate, may cause stocking and tracking problems
Silver salt/ collagen		Covalon ColActiveAg (+)	Added benefit of collagen in dressing	Secondary dressing is required
Silver-sodium carboxy-methylcellulose dressing	Dressing containing 1.2% ionic silver released via ion exchange	Aquacel Ag (+)	Provides fluid lock to prevent excess wound fluid from macerating surrounding skin, good vertical wicking	May need to be rehydrated if sticks to wound.
Silver salt containing foam	Highly exudating chronic wounds	Contreet Foam (++) Optifoam Ag Mepilex Ag (++)	Provides bacterial balance in a foam dressing 2nd generation foam that allows partial fluid lock high absorption	Similar to all foams may give back moisture leading to irritation and potential maceration of the surrounding skin
Silver salt combined with hydrocolloid	Chronic wounds with increased bacterial burden	Contreet HC (+)	Provides odor control under hydrocolloid dressing	Limited fluid absorption
Metallic silver				
Silver charcoal	Silver incorporated into charcoal for odor control	Actisorb (0)	Silver kills organisms which are trapped onto the charcoal. Deodorizing properties as odor molecules bind to charcoal. Product also traps endotoxins	Poor absorption properties. Product cannot be cut as charcoal particles will leak out

Table 3. Silver preparations used in wound management. *(Continued)*

Preparation	Delivery Mechanism	Product Name	Benefits	Disadvantages
Nanocrystalline sliver				
Silver coated fabric	Burns Chronic wounds	Acticoat burn (+++)	Equivalent to silver nitrate in burns with less frequent dressing changes, anti-inflammatory	• May need to add moisture or pre-soak dressing • Staining of the wound • May cause burning and stinging on application
Silver coating - 3 layers	Leg ulcers and other chronic wounds for up to 7 days wear time	Acticoat 7 (+++)	Sustained release of bactericidal concentrations of silver over 7 days Useful for weekly compression therapy in venous ulcers	May provide higher initial release of silver compared to other dressings in this class
Silver coated fabric with calcium alginate core	Moderately exudating chronic wounds	Acticoat Absorbent (+++)	Provides rapid and high absorption and haemostasis	Potential of staining of wound

© Sibbald 2006 (adapted from Sibbald, 2004; Orsted & Sibbald, 2005)
Ionized silver levels: 0 none; + low; ++ moderate; +++ high
Used with permission.

view, O'Meara et al[38] examined the clinical improvement and cost-effectiveness of topical and systemic antimicrobial agents in the prevention and healing of chronic wounds. They concluded that there was insufficient evidence to support the therapeutic role of these agents in wound healing in the absence of increased bacterial burden or infection.[37] The use of topical antibiotics has been long debated, as they are often used too liberally, for too long a period of time, raising concerns about the development of antimicrobial resistance, contact dermatitis, and host sensitization. Clear guidelines for the use of topical agents do not exist, although expert opinion offers some direction. Studies assessing the efficacy and cost-effectiveness of antimicrobial agents in the treatment of chronic wounds are fraught with inconsistencies, so results are difficult to compare. Controlled trials support the use of topical mupirocin for the treatment of impetigo, caused by Group A beta hemolytic *Streptococcus* or *S aureus*. There is extensive burn experience describing

the efficacy of topical silver sulfadiazine. This formulation reduces bacterial numbers to < 10^5 CFUs per gram of tissue in pressure ulcers and is associated with enhanced wound healing.

However, topical antibiotics may be redundant if used in combination with systemic antibiotic therapy. On the other hand, topical agents may be inadequate for soft tissue infection with significant microbial invasion. The main indications for topical antibiotic use would be for superficial wound infection, or critical colonization, where there is impaired wound healing, pale friable granulation tissue, or suspected or proven high microbial burden, without periwound cellulitis (NERDS and not STONES as described above and in Figures 2 and 3).

There is a much lower tolerance for suspected infections of neurotrophic or neuroischemic foot ulcers in persons with diabetes because of the attendant risks of limb- and life-threatening sepsis. Hence, the clinical threshold to initiate early use of antibiotics is accepted in diabetic ulcers,

Figure 3. The mnemonic "STONES" for the diagnosis of deep compartment infection.[16]

Letter		KEY INFORMATION	Comments
S	Size is bigger 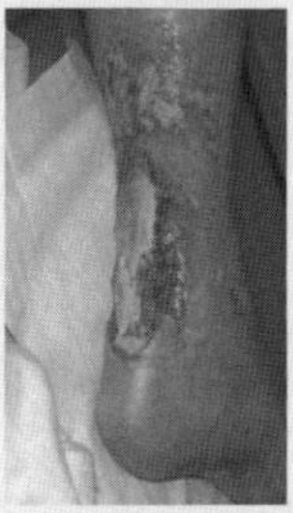	• Size as measured by the longest length and widest width at right angles to the longest length. Only very deep wounds need to have depth measured with a probe	• Clinicians need to have a consistent approach to measurement • An increased size from bacterial damage is due to the bacteria spreading from the surface to the surrounding skin and the deeper compartment. This indicates that a combination of bacterial number and virulence has overwhelmed the host resistance
T	Temperature increased 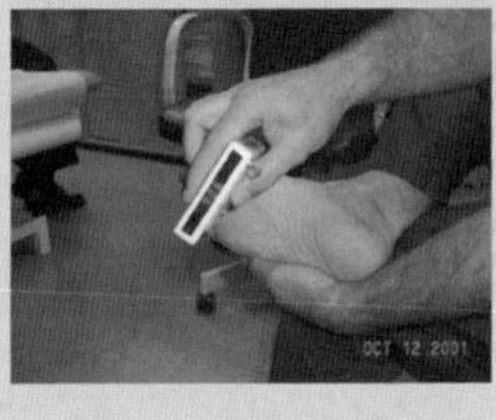	• With surrounding tissue infection there is an increased temperature. This may be performed crudely by touch with a gloved hand or by using an infrared thermometer or scanning device, there is > 3°F difference in temperature between 2 mirror image sites.	It is important to distinguish between infection and the other 2 potential causes of temperature change: • A difference in vascular supply (decreased circulation is colder) • Inflammatory conditions are not usually as warm but they can demonstrate a marked increase temperature with extensive deep tissue destruction (Acute Charcot joint)
O	Os (probes to or exposed bone) 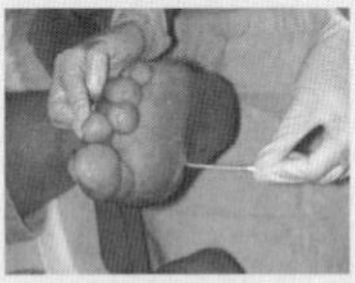	• There is a high incidence of osteomyelitis if there is exposed bone or you can probe to the bone in a person with a neurotrophic foot ulcer	• x-rays and bone scans are less reliable for diagnosis of osteomyelitis with loss of bone mass that occurs with neuropathy (pelvis x-rays may be more reliable)
N	New areas of breakdown 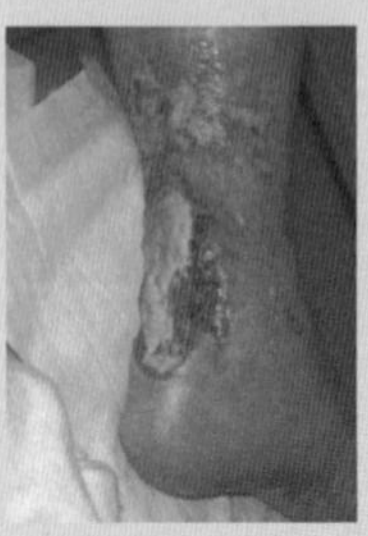	• Note the satellite areas of skin breakdown that are separated from the main ulcer. • It is important to remember this may be due to not correcting the cause of the wound, infection, or local damage	• Search for the cause of the satellite areas of breakdown and the need to correct the cause • Check for local damage and consider infection, increased exudate, or other sources of trauma

Figure 3. The mnemonic "STONES" for the diagnosis of deep compartment infection.[16]

Letter		KEY INFORMATION	Comments
E	Exudate, Erythema, Edema 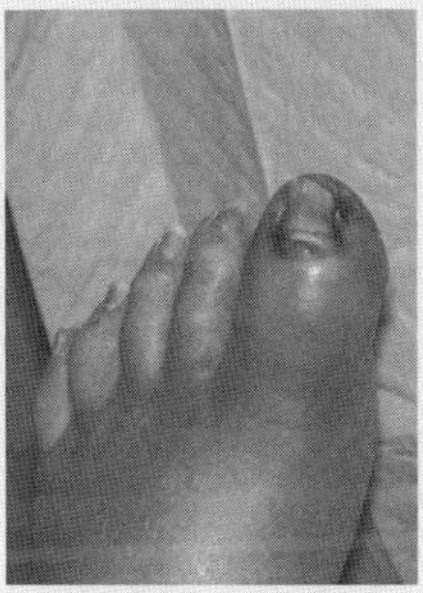	• All of the features here are due to the inflammatory response. With increased bacterial burden, exudate often increases in quantity and transforms from a clear or serous texture to frank purulence and may have a hemorrhagic component. The inflammation leads to vasodilatation (erythema) and the leakage of fluid into the tissue will result in edema.	• For exudate control we need to determine the cause and then match the absorbency of the dressing (none, low, moderate, heavy) to amount of exudate from the wound • Assess surrounding skin to evaluate for maceration. Refer to the enabler LOWE© (Liquid film forming acrylate, Ointments; Windowed dressings; External collection devices) • For erythema and edema control, the cause or the tissue infection needs to be treated
S	Smell 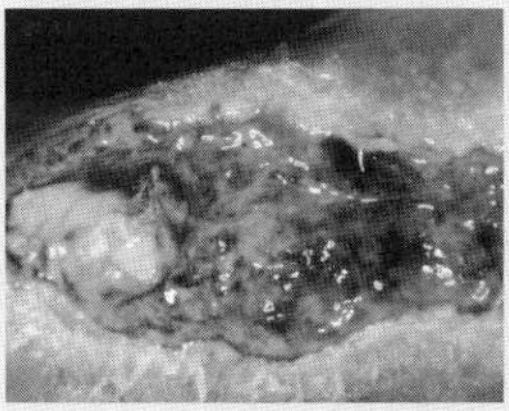	• Bacteria that invade tissue have a "foul" odor. There is an unpleasant sweet odor from *Pseudomonas*. Gram-negative organisms and anaerobe organisms can cause a putrid smell from the associated tissue damage	• Make sure the smell is from organisms and not the normal distinct odor from the interaction of exudate with some of the dressing material • Systemic antimicrobial agents are indicated that will treat the causative organisms and devitalized tissue should be aggressively debrided in wounds with the ability to heal

© Sibbald and Ayello 2006.
Used with permission

as compared to suspected infections in chronic venous or pressure ulcers. Broad-spectrum agents are advocated as treatment because of the polymicrobial nature of diabetic foot infections, but there is insufficient evidence to recommend 1 specific regimen over any other. Clinicians should remember that diabetes can be classified as a relative immunodeficiency state and that host resistance is lower with advantage to the bacteria. The inflammatory response may be muted especially in patients with high blood sugars and an Hgb A1c above 0.12.

For other chronic wounds with infection of the deeper compartments, using systemic oral or parenteral antibiotic therapy would be more appropriate. Antimicrobial therapy should be individualized as described in Table 2. Once microbial culture data are available, antimicrobial therapy can be modified with a step down approach to

oral treatment, usually once the patient has been afebrile for 48 hours and sufficient improvement in clinical signs have occurred.

Most studies of limb- or life-threatening infection arising from infection in a chronic wound have used a 2-week treatment course of parenteral antibiotics, followed by a variable course of oral therapy, depending upon the extent of infection.[39] When associated osteomyelitis is present, oral antimicrobial therapy should be continued for 3 to 4 months, in addition to any appropriate surgical intervention.[40]

For further information on the use of antimicrobials, see Chapter 5.

Approach to Multiresistant Microorganisms

With increasing frequency, chronic wounds are becoming colonized and infected with micro-

Figure 4. Flow chart for the management of wound positive for MRSA.

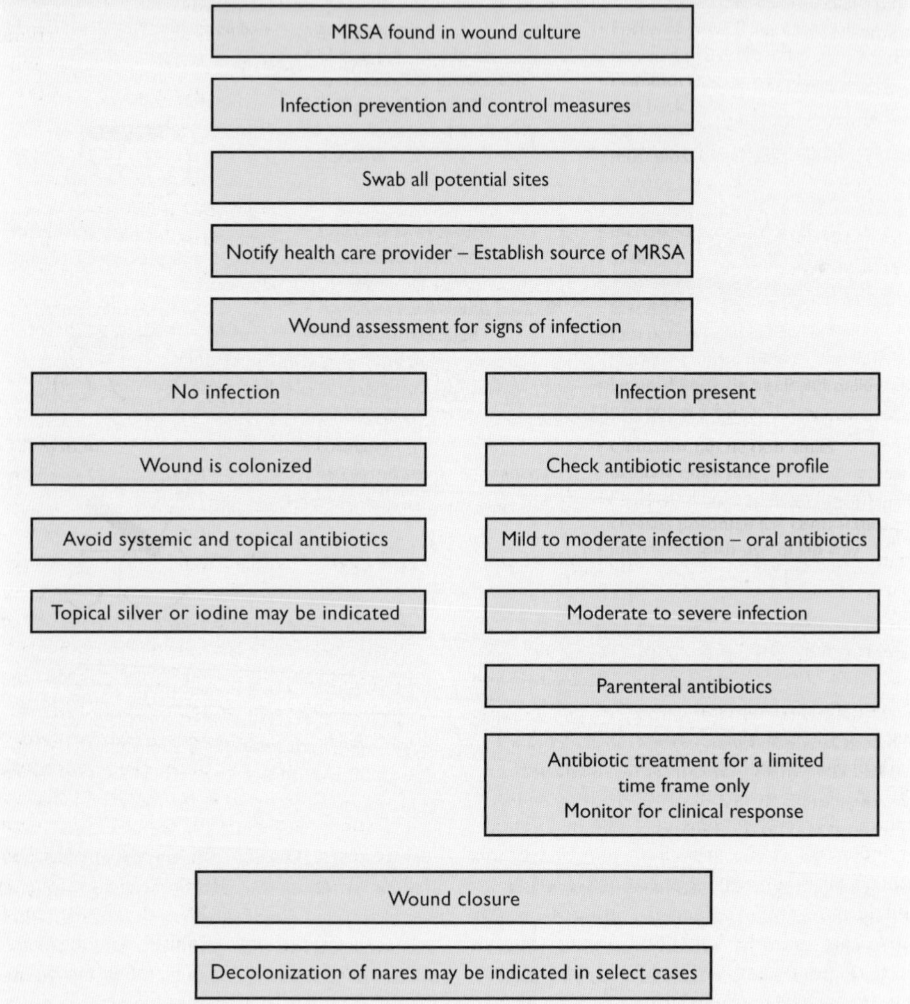

```
          ┌──────────────────────────────────────┐
          │      MRSA found in wound culture       │
          └──────────────────────────────────────┘

          ┌──────────────────────────────────────┐
          │ Infection prevention and control measures │
          └──────────────────────────────────────┘

          ┌──────────────────────────────────────┐
          │         Swab all potential sites        │
          └──────────────────────────────────────┘

          ┌──────────────────────────────────────┐
          │ Notify health care provider – Establish source of MRSA │
          └──────────────────────────────────────┘

          ┌──────────────────────────────────────┐
          │   Wound assessment for signs of infection   │
          └──────────────────────────────────────┘
```

No infection	Infection present
Wound is colonized	Check antibiotic resistance profile
Avoid systemic and topical antibiotics	Mild to moderate infection – oral antibiotics
Topical silver or iodine may be indicated	Moderate to severe infection
	Parenteral antibiotics
	Antibiotic treatment for a limited time frame only Monitor for clinical response

```
          ┌──────────────────────────────────────┐
          │             Wound closure              │
          └──────────────────────────────────────┘

          ┌──────────────────────────────────────┐
          │ Decolonization of nares may be indicated in select cases │
          └──────────────────────────────────────┘
```

CBC = complete blood count; CRP = C-reactive protein; ESR = erythrocyte sedimentation rate

organisms that are resistant to the more standard choices of antibiotics. Wounds should always be assessed for clinical signs of infection, as indicated above, and where necessary appropriate antibiotic therapy should be initiated. However, when an infected wound is unresponsive to treatment, then the possibility of infection with a resistant or unusual microorganism should be considered. Wound swabs or biopsy will help to identify the causative agent. As well, a high index of suspicion

should be maintained, if the patient presents with 1 or more factors that may predispose them to colonization or infection with a resistant microorganism.

Common risk factors for the presence of methicillin-resistant *Staphylococcus aureus* (MRSA) in a chronic wound include:

1. Recent hospitalization
2. Transfer from a chronic care facility
3. Recent incarceration

4. Long-term antibiotic therapy

5. Crowded social conditions.

However, in cases of skin and soft tissue infections with community-acquired MRSA (CA-MRSA), easily identifiable risk factors may not be present.[41] The approach to management of the patient with a chronic wound who is positive for MRSA involves the same basic steps as the approach to a wound that is positive for a microorganism that is sensitive to treatment with beta-lactam agents or similar agents. A flow chart outlining the approach to the patient with a chronic wound who is positive for MRSA is found in Table 4.

Once a wound is noted to be positive for MRSA, infection prevention and control measures should be rigorously observed to prevent the spread of the microorganism to other wound care patients and providers (see Table 4). Hospitals, long-term care facilities, ambulatory care centers, and home care programs all have specific protocols for infection prevention and control that may vary, but nevertheless usually involve universal and/or contact precautions. Consistent hand hygiene and hand-washing by health care professionals is the single most important factor in reducing the spread of MRSA,[42] and in general, other nosocomial infections.

Patients with a chronic wound positive for MRSA may well carry the microorganism in multiple body sites including the nose, rectum, perineum or axillae, as well as, at the insertion sites of percutaneous lines, indwelling catheters and feeding tubes. If possible, percutaneous or indwelling catheters, and other unnecessary indwelling devices should be removed. It is helpful if the patient's direct health care providers are notified of the patient's wound status, so that appropriate long term management can be arranged. As well, this sentinel source may help to determine the origin of the MRSA, which might potentially reduce further spread to other patients.

Wounds positive for MRSA should be examined for signs of infection. If there is no indication of infection, then systemic and topical antibiotics should be avoided. Systemic antibiotics are required only if clinical features of infection are present. They have no role in infection prophylaxis.

Topical antibiotics to be specifically avoided include mupirocin, fusidic acid, clindamycin, eryth-

romycin, and gentamicin. These agents will induce microbial resistance if used long term in a chronic wound. In a Canadian study, more than 50% of the isolates from skin and soft tissue infections were shown to have high level resistance to mupirocin. MRSA resistance to mupirocin has been described and is believed to have developed during long term treatment of chronic ulcers.[43] Since topical mupirocin may be of benefit in some patients for decolonization of MRSA from the nares, further microbial resistance to this antibiotic would be detrimental to long term patient care.

Topical antimicrobials that contain either silver[44] or iodine in a less toxic form, such as cadexomer,[45] are useful in the management of wounds that are colonized with MRSA, and may reduce the potential evolution to wound infection.

If a wound is positive for MRSA and clinical signs of infection are present, then these signs should be identified and documented. In the case of mild to moderate infection, then oral antibiotics should be used. The health care practitioner should familiarize him/herself with local patterns of antibiotic resistance of MRSA strains, so that the appropriate antibiotic choices can be made.

Where MRSA is susceptible, using 2 of the following 3 antibiotics for a limited period is indicated: *doxycycline, trimethoprim-sulfamethoxazole* or *rifampin*, or using a single antibiotic (*linezolid*), may also be used. In a recent study of community-acquired MRSA, 100% of the isolates from skin and soft tissue infections were susceptible to trimethoprim-sulfamethoxazole and this agent may be used alone.[46] Although an expensive agent, linezolid, an oxazolidinone, is an appropriate alternative to vancomycin in patients with impaired renal function, poor venous access, or inability to tolerate glycopeptides. Linezolid is also limited by its association with anemia and myelodepression, and its use should be reserved for severe refractory MRSA infections. Although many MRSA stains remain sensitive to fluoroquinolones, resistance is merging due to overuse of fluoroquinolones. A mild to moderate wound infection with MRSA should be treated for 2 to 3 weeks with the indicated antibiotics, following which the patient's wound should be assessed to determine if the infection has resolved. If signs of infection have improved but not cleared, then a repeat 2- to 3-week course of antibiotics is probably indicated. Long-term use of antibiotics in patients with wounds containing multiresistant microorganisms is felt to contribute to further antimicrobial resistance.

If the wound shows signs of moderate to severe infection, then parenteral therapy with either *vancomycin* or *linezolid* is indicated, provided that the microorganism is sensitive to these agents. A pre-determined period of treatment with antibiotics should be outlined first, and then the patient must be re-assessed to determine if the infection has resolved. Repeating the bacterial culture with a swab may show continued presence of MRSA in the wound. Hence, the goal of treatment is to resolve the clinical infection, but not necessarily the full eradication of the microorganism from the wound. So, as soon as infection in a chronic wound has resolved, then the antibiotic should be stopped.

Once the wound has closed, then decolonization of the nares may be attempted, if warranted. This should be done, if there are no other sites of carriage of MRSA. Current approaches to decolonization are controversial.[47] Generally, this is achieved through topical *mupirocin* applied to the nasal vestibule twice daily for 5 days, as well as daily body bathing with *chlorhexidine*. Repeated use of mupirocin may be needed, but a risk of *mupirocin resistant* MRSA (MR-MRSA) exists. Nasal decolonization may be more successful in those patients with limited risk factors for recurrence of the carrier state, and for otherwise healthy wound care providers. There is no clear evidence to show that it will be successful. For further information, the reader is referred to the Centers for Disease Control and Prevention ([CDC]: http://www.cdc.gov) and the Association for Professionals in Infection Control (http://www.apic.org).

Conclusion

Infection is a frequent problem in chronic wounds, delaying healing and contributing to adverse outcomes. A diagnosis of chronic wound infection must be made with a holistic review of the patient, and it is important to understand the relationships between microbial burden, virulence and host resistance. A systematic evaluation of the wound should be supported by microbial cultures where indicated. There is no gold standard test for the identification of infection.

The semiqualitative swab taken from an appropriately prepared wound surface still remains the current standard of practice for microbial assessment although the diagnosis of surface increased bacterial burden or deep infection should be made on clinical criteria. Wound debridement and cleansing are probably as important as topical antibiotic use in the treatment of wound infection and reducing microbial burden. Topical agents may be considered in wounds with covert or mild infection without significant tissue invasion, but this is based at best upon expert opinion. Evidence of tissue invasion requires the empiric use of systemic oral or parenteral antibiotics, that are chosen based upon the severity of infection and the duration of the chronic wound with bacterial swab results used to identify multiresistant

---

Take-Home Messages for Practice

• The likelihood of developing infection in a chronic wound is directly proportional to the presence of a critical number of disease-producing microorganisms, and inversely related to the host's ability to resist microbial invasion

• The assessment of infection in a chronic wound remains a bedside skill, where a high index of suspicion, clinical acumen and supportive microbiological information offer the best tools for successful management

• Antimicrobial agents are initially begun on an empiric basis, until more definitive microbiological data are available. Wounds present for less than 1 month should be covered for gram-positive organisms. Wounds present for greater than 1 month duration or in persons with immunosuppression require broad coverage with gram-positive, gram-negative, and anaerobic organisms. Generally, the more extensive the infection and the longer the duration then specific treatment based on bacteriological data is required

• Multiresistant microorganisms, such as MRSA, can complicate current chronic wound care, and a systematic approach to management is obligatory.

organisms and modify treatment in patients that do not respond to the original regimen.

The search for underlying osteomyelitis is important in persons with diabetes, who develop foot ulcers as a late manifestation of their long-term diabetes. An in-depth appreciation of the limitations of local and systemic host resistance in patients with chronic ulcers allows the care giver to systematically evaluate potentially correctable patient factors.

The presence of multiresistant microorganisms, such as MRSA, has major implications for infection control. The potential for wound infection with a more problematic pathogen increases the risks of systemic sepsis especially if the organism has gone unrecognized. More accurate diagnosis of infection, use of nonantibiotic treatment modalities, and rational antibiotic prescribing habits should reduce the risk of antimicrobial resistance in the future.

Self-Assessment Questions

1. The gold standard for the diagnosis of chronic wound deep tissue infection is best expressed as:
   A. The presence of the 4 classic signs of inflammation, along with dishwater pus
   B. A wound that resembles cooked rather than raw hamburger
   C. There is no gold standard
   D. The presence of delayed healing, foul odor, wound breakdown, local pain, serous drainage and friable granulation tissue

2. The best approach to the treatment of a suspected wound infection in an afebrile, ambulatory diabetic neuropathic ulcer would be:
   A. To admit the patient to hospital for short-term antimicrobial therapy using oral clindamycin and intravenous ceftriaxone
   B. To debride the wound, obtain cultures and start the patient on oral amoxicillin/clavulanate for 14 days, with follow-up in 3–5 days in clinic
   C. To apply a local antiseptic dressing, such as povidone-iodine
   D. To debride the wound, obtain cultures, apply a nanocrystalline silver dressing and begin oral clindamycin and a Quinalone antibiotic (ciprofloxacin or Moxifloxacin)

3. A patient with a sacral pressure ulcer that reveals the presence of MRSA colonization is best managed with:
   A. Contact isolation and daily applications of topical mupirocin (Bactroban®) to the wound bed for 7–10 days
   B. Notification of relevant health care staff, removal of unnecessary indwelling percutaneous lines or catheters, and screening of other body sites for MRSA, such as nares, axillae, and perineum
   C. Surgical wound closure to guarantee elimination of wound space
   D. Immediate institution of topical povidone-iodine to decontaminate the ulcer bed

Answers: 1-C, 2-D, 3-B

References

1. Howell-Jones RS, Wilson MJ, Hill KE, Howard AJ, Price PE, Thomas DW. A review of the microbiology, antibiotic usage and resistance in chronic skin wounds. *Journal of Antimicrobial Chemotherapy*. 2005;55(2):143-149.

2. Sibbald RG, Orsted H, Schultz GS, Coutts P, Keast D. Preparing the wound bed 2003: focus on infection and inflammation. *Ostomy Wound Manage*. 2003;49(11):24–51.

3. Schultz GS, Sibbald RG, Falanga V. Wound bed preparation: a systematic approach to wound management. *Wound Repair Regen*. 2003;11:1–28.

4. Bowler PG, Davies BJ, The microbiology of acute and chronic wounds. *WOUNDS*. 1999;11:72–99.

5. Hunt TK, Hopt HW. Wound healing and wound infection—what surgeons and anesthesiologists can do. *Surg Clin North Am*. 1997;77:587–606.

6. Carter S. Role of pressure measurements. In: Berstein E, ed. *Vascular Diagnosis*. 4th ed. St. Louis, Mo: Mosby; 1993:486–512.

7. Sorenson LT, Karlsmark T, Gottrup F. Abstinence from smoking reduces incisional wound infection: a randomized controlled trial. *Ann Surg*. 2003;238;1–5.

8. Dronge A, Perkal M, Kancir S, Concato J. Long-term glycemic control and post-operative infectious complications. *Arch Surg*. 2006;141:375–380.

9. Hansson C, Hoborn J, Moller A. The microbial flora in venous leg ulcers without clinical signs of infection. *Acta Dermatol Venereol*. 1995;75:24–30.

10. Edwards R, Harding KG. Skin and soft tissue infections. *Curr Opin Infect Diseases*. 2004;17(2):91–96.

11. Cutting K. Wound healing, bacteria and topical therapies. *EWMA J*. 2003;3(1):17–19.

12. Bowler P, Davies B. The microbiology of infected and non-infected leg ulcers. *Int J Dermatol*. 1999;38:573–578.

13. Bowler PG. The anaerobic and aerobic microbiology of wounds: a review. *WOUNDS*. 1998;10(6):170–178.

14. Bowler PG, Duerden BI, Armstrong DG. Wound microbiology and associated approaches to wound manage-

15. Cutting KF, Harding KG. Criteria for identifying wound infection. *J Wound Care*. 1994;3:198–201.

16. Neal G, Lindholm G, Lee M. Burn wound histological culture—a new technique for predicting burn wound sepsis. *J Burn Care Rehabil*. 1981;2:35–39.

17. Sibbald RG, Woo K, Ayello EA. Increased bacterial burden and infection: the story of NERDS and STONES. *Adv Skin Wound Care*. 2006;19(8):462–463.

18. Elek SD. Experimental staphylococcal infections in the skin of man. *Ann NY Acad Sci*. 1956;65(3):85–90.

19. Bendy R, Nuccio P, Wolfe, et al. Relationship of quantitative wound bacterial counts to healing decubiti: Effect of topical gentamicin. *Anticro Agents Chemother*. 1964;4:147–155.

20. Krizek TJ, Flagg SV, Wolfort FG, Jabaley ME. Delayed primary excision and skin grafting of the burned hand. *Plast Reconstr Surg*. 1973;51(5):524–529.

21. Noyes HE, Chi NH, Linh LT, Mo DH, Punyashthiti K, Pugh C Jr. Delayed topical antimicrobials as adjuncts to systemic antibiotic therapy of war wounds: bacteriologic studies. *Mil Med*. 1967;132(6):461–468.

22. Levine N, Lindberg R, Mason A. The quantitative swab culture and smear: a quick simple method for determining the number of viable aerobic bacteria on open wounds. *J Trauma*. 1976;16(2):89–94.

23. Thomson P, Taddonio T, Tait M. Correlation between swab and biopsy for the quantification of burn wound micro flora. *Proc In Cong Burn Inj*. 1990;8:381.

24. Gardner SE, Frantz RA, Doebbeling BN. The validity of the clinical signs and symptoms used to identify localized chronic wound infection. *Wound Repair Regen*. 2001;9:178–186.

25. Sheffield PJ. Tissue oxygen measurements. In: Davis JC, Hunt TK, eds. *Problem wounds, the role of oxygen*. New York, NY: Elsevier; 1988:17–51.

26. Grayson M, Gibbons G, Balogh K, Levin E. Probing to bone in infected pedal ulcers – a clinical sign of underlying osteomyelitis in diabetic patients. *JAMA*. 1995;273(9):721–723.

27. Caputo G, Cavanagh P, Ulbrecht J, Gibbons G, Karchmer A. Assessment and management of foot disease in patients with diabetes. *N Engl J Med*. 1994;331:854–860.

28. Wheat L, Allen S, Henry M, Diabetic foot infections bacteriologic analysis. *Arch Intern Med*. 1986;146:1935–1940.

29. Ehrenkranz NJ, Alfonso B, Nerenberg D. Irrigation-aspiration for culturing draining decubitus ulcers: correlation of bacteriological findings with a clinical inflammatory scoring index. *J Clin Microbiol*. 1990;28(11):2389–2393.

30. Heggers, JP, Robson MC, Frank DH, Ko F. Rapid slide technique with dextranomer beads for bacteriologic assessment of wounds in the elderly: comparison with quantitative biopsy method. *J Amer Ger Soc*. 1979;27(11):511–513.

31. Milner S. Acetic acid to treat pseudomonas aeruginosa in superficial wounds and burns. *Lancet*. 1992;340(8810):61.

32. George N, Faoagali J, Muller M. Silvazine (silver sulfadiazine and chlorhexidine) activity against 200 clinical isolates. *Burns*. 1997;23(6):493–495.

33. Burrell R, A scientific perspective on the use of topical silver preparations. *Ostomy Wound Manage*. 2003;49;(Suppl 5A):19–24.

34. Sibbald RG, Browne AC, Coutts P, Queen D. Screening evaluation of an ionized nanocrystalline silver dressing in chronic wound care. *Ostomy Wound Manage*. 2001;47(10):38–43.

35. Sibbald RG. The selective anti-inflammatory activity of prolonged release nanocrystalline silver dressing in the treatment of chronic venous leg ulcers Acticoat. Presented at the EWMA, Stuttgart, Germany, 2005.

36. Jorgensen B, Price P, Andersen KE, et al. The silver-releasing foam dressing, Contreet Foam, promotes faster healing of critically colonised venous leg ulcers: a randomised, controlled trial. *Int Wound J*. 2005;2(1):64–73.

37. Munter KC, Beele H, Russell L, et al. The CONTOP study: A large-scale, comparative, randomize study in patients treated with a sustained silver-releasing foam dressing. Presented at the EWMA, Stuttgart, Germany, 2005.

38. O'Meara SM, Cullen NA, Majid M. Systematic reviews of wound care management: (3) antimicrobial agents for chronic wounds; (4) diabetic foot ulceration. *Health Technol Assess*. 2000;4:1–237.

39. Grayson M, Gibbons G, Habershaw G. Use of ampicillin/sulbactam versus imipenem/cilastatin in the treatment of limb-threatening foot infections in diabetic patients. *Clin Infect Dis*. 1994;18:683–693.

40. Dow G, Thompson W, Brunham R. Duration of antimicrobial therapy for diabetic foot osteomyelitis. *Clin Invest Med*. 1994;(Suppl 17):B75.

41. Fridkin SK, Hageman JC, Morrison M. Methicillin-resistant Staphylococcus aureus disease in three communities. *N Engl J Med*. 2005;352(14):1436–1444.

42. Pittet D. Improving adherence to hand hygiene practice: a multidisciplinary approach. *Emerg Infect Dis*. 2001;7:234–242.

43. Vasquez JE, Walker ES, Franzus BW, Overbay BK, Reagan DR, Sarubbi FA. The epidemiology of mupirocin resistance among methicillin-resistant staphylococcus aureus at a Veterans' Affairs hospital. *Infect Control Hosp Epidemiol*. 2000;21(7);459–464.

44. Edwards-Jones V. Antimicrobial and barrier effects of silver against methicillin-resistant staphylococcus aureus. *J Wound Care*. 2006;15(7):285–290.

45. Mertz PM, Oliveira-Gandia MF, Davis SC. The evaluation of a cadexomer iodine wound dressing on methicillin resistant staphylococcus aureus (MRSA) in acute wounds. *Dermatol Surg*. 1999;25(2):89–93.

46. Frazee BW, Lynn J, Charlebois ED, Lambert L, Lowery D, Perdreau-Remington F. High prevalence of methicillin-resistant staphylococcus aureus on emergency department skin and soft tissue infections. *Ann Emerg Med*. 2005;45:311–320.

47. Loveday HP, Pellowe CM, Jones SR, Pratt RJ. A systematic review of the evidence for interventions for the prevention and control of methicillin-resistant staphylococcus aureus (1996–2004): report to the Joint MRSA Working Party (Subgroup A). *J Hosp Infect*. 2006;63(Suppl 1):S45–S70.

CHAPTER 9

Pain in People with Chronic Wounds: Clinical Strategies for Decreasing Pain and Improving Quality of Life

Kevin Y. Woo, PhD, RN, FAPWCA;
Diane L. Krasner, PhD, RN, CWCN, CWS, MAPWCA, FAAN;
R. Gary Sibbald, BSc, MD, MEd, FRCPC (Med, Derm), MACP, FAAD, MAPWCA

Objectives

The reader will be challenged to:

- Synthesize the complexity and pathophysiology of wound-associated pain
- Describe a systematized approach to address wound pain by examining the wound-related factors, procedure-related triggers, and modulating factors (cognitive, emotional, personal, sensory, and contextual)
- Identify methods to evaluate pain
- Appraise various pharmacological and non-pharmacological strategies to reduce pain.

Introduction

Pain is a common experience in people with chronic wounds. Pain impacts all aspects of everyday life, including physical activity, sleep, and social functioning, and erodes individuals' quality of life.[1-3] Even long after the ulcers are healed, some people continue to provide vivid descriptions of pain experiences.[4] While wound-associated pain often is caused by intrinsic wound pathology and exacerbated by local manipulation that is part of routine wound management, the intensity of pain is subjected to influences of many personal and social factors. The complexity of pain necessitates a systematized approach to obtain a thorough pain history, evaluate aggravating and alleviating factors, assess the wound and surrounding tissue, and monitor outcomes. Optimal pain management must be incorporated as an integral part of comprehensive wound care/caring in order to improve quality of life.

Prevalence of Pain in People with Chronic Wounds

Studies of patients with various chronic wound types validate the enormity and pervasiveness of pain. Szor and Bourguignon[5] reported that as many as 88% of people with pressure ulcers in their study expressed pressure ulcer pain at dressing change and 84% experienced pain even at rest. Of people with venous leg ulcers, the majority experienced moderate to severe levels of pain described as aching, stabbing, sharp, tender, and tiring.[6] Pain has been documented to persist up to at least 3 months after wound closure.[6,7]

Woo KY, Krasner DL, Sibbald RG. Pain in people with chronic wounds: clinical strategies for decreasing pain and improving quality of life. In: Krasner DL, ed. *Chronic Wound Care: The Essentials*. Malvern, PA: HMP Communications; 2014:111–122.

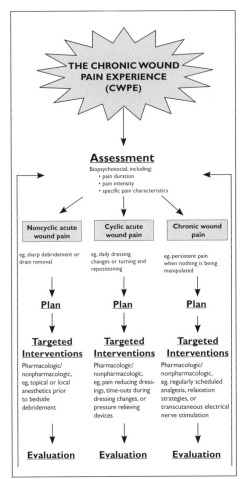

Figure 1. Proposed model of the chronic wound pain experience (CWPE). © 1995 Krasner.

Contrary to the commonly held belief that most patients with diabetic foot ulcers do not experience pain due to loss of protective sensation, up to 50% of patients experience varying degrees of predominantly neuropathic spontaneous painful symptoms at rest and approximately 40% experience moderate to extreme pain climbing stairs or walking on uneven surfaces, according to Evans and Pinzur.[8]

Consequences of Wound-Associated Pain

Pain has been described as the worst part of living with chronic wounds and constitutes a major stressor among people with chronic wounds.[3]

Stress-induced cytokine and neuroendocrine activity can activate sympathetic outflow, leading to vasoconstriction and subsequent compromised tissue oxygenation levels.[2] As part of the cascade of stress response, the overproduction of cortisol and catecholamines can have a significant impact, delaying wound healing due to alteration in the immune system.[9] Numerous studies have validated the deleterious impact of stress (and emotional distress) on wound healing.[9] Time to achieve complete wound closure is significantly prolonged for high-stress individuals. Woo and Sibbald[10] followed 111 home care clients with either leg or foot ulcers prospectively for 4 weeks to determine the effectiveness of comprehensive wound assessment and management. Wound-related pain was addressed by education, careful selection of wound dressings, application of topical analgesics during dressing changes, and use of systemic analgesics. The average pain intensity score was reduced from 6.3 at baseline to 2.8 at Week 4 ($P < .001$). To examine the relationship between pain and wound healing, pain intensity scores were compared among those who achieved wound closure by the end of data collection to those who did not. The mean pain intensity score was 1.67 for subjects who achieved wound closure as compared to an average score of 3.21 among those who did not achieve complete wound closure ($P < .041$). The result lends credence to the importance of pain management to promote wound healing.

Conceptualizations of Wound-Related Pain

According to a conceptual framework developed by Krasner,[11] wound-related pain is complex and dynamic, integrating the experience of noncyclic acute wound pain, cyclic acute wound pain, and chronic wound pain (Figure 1).

Chronic or persistent wound pain is described as the background symptom that is often associated with intrinsic wound-related factors often connected with the cause or aggravating factors of the wound. In contrast, acute wound pain (cyclic due to dressing change procedures and non-cyclic often associated with debridement) is conceptualized as episodic and triggered by wound-related procedures that are performed by healthcare providers (Figure 1).

Another conceptualization proposed by Woo

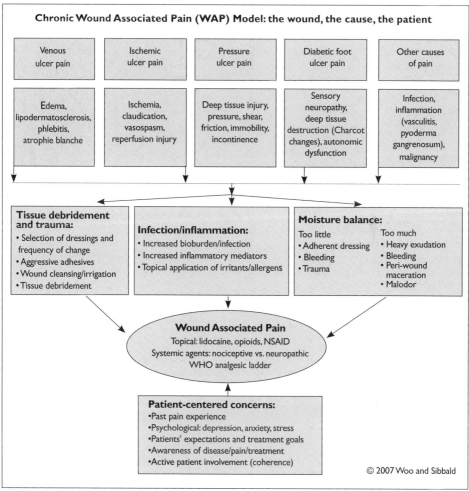

Chronic Wound Associated Pain (WAP) Model: the wound, the cause, the patient

Venous ulcer pain	Ischemic ulcer pain	Pressure ulcer pain	Diabetic foot ulcer pain	Other causes of pain
Edema, lipodermatosclerosis, phlebitis, atrophie blanche	Ischemia, claudication, vasospasm, reperfusion injury	Deep tissue injury, pressure, shear, friction, immobility, incontinence	Sensory neuropathy, deep tissue destruction (Charcot changes), autonomic dysfunction	Infection, inflammation (vasculitis, pyoderma gangrenosum), malignancy

Tissue debridement and trauma:
• Selection of dressings and frequency of change
• Aggressive adhesives
• Wound cleansing/irrigation
• Tissue debridement

Infection/inflammation:
• Increased bioburden/infection
• Increased inflammatory mediators
• Topical application of irritants/allergens

Moisture balance:
Too little
• Adherent dressing
• Bleeding
• Trauma

Too much
• Heavy exudation
• Bleeding
• Peri-wound maceration
• Malodor

Wound Associated Pain
Topical: lidocaine, opioids, NSAID
Systemic agents: nociceptive vs. neuropathic
WHO analgesic ladder

Patient-centered concerns:
•Past pain experience
•Psychological: depression, anxiety, stress
•Patients' expectations and treatment goals
•Awareness of disease/pain/treatment
•Active patient involvement (coherence)

© 2007 Woo and Sibbald

Figure 2. Chronic wound-associated pain model.

and Sibbald[12] provides further detail, linking various wound etiological causes, local wound factors, and patient-centered concerns to wound-associated pain (Figure 2).

Mechanisms of Wound-Related Pain

Wound-related triggers. Underlying mechanisms that lead to tissue breakdown also are implicated in the emergence of painful symptoms. According to Woo and Sibbald,[12] pressure ulcer pain stems from ischemic damages due to unrelieved pressure, shear, and friction. Pro-inflammatory mediators, such as bradykinin, histamine, serotonin, and prostaglandins, are released, rendering peripheral nociceptors to be hyperac-

tive. Venous ulcer pain is linked to venous abnormalities, including local leakage of fibrin that can become inflamed, precipitating acute lipodermatosclerosis; inflammation of the venous vessel wall and clotting, leading to thrombophlebitis; and venous hypertension with edema from leaky capillaries. Even in the absence of an ulcer, pain has been found in up to 43% of people with lipodermatosclerosis (due to acute inflammation of the dermal tissue).[13] Intermittent claudication (pain in the lower extremities that is precipitated by exercise) is a common yet extremely painful condition in people with peripheral arterial vascular disease. As arterial insufficiency progresses, ischemia rest pain may predominate.[14] Among persons with diabetes and coexisting neuropathy, spontaneous pain is thought to be caused by nerve damage (often accompanied with reddened and mottled skin, abnormal sensation to touch, and feelings of burning and electrical shocks) as a result of microvascular (vasa nervorum) and metabolic aberrations.[15]

Changes to the usual pattern of wound-associated pain can be a warning signal. The consensus among clinical experts is that the presence of unexpected pain/tenderness along with other criteria is indicative of infection in chronic wounds.[16,17] According to study results reported by Gardner et al,[18] pain as an indicator of infection has a specificity value of 100%; subjects did not experience any painful symptoms if wound infection was not detected based on bacteriology assessment. As a word of caution, there were only 31 subjects in this evaluation. The mechanism that explains how pain is connected to infection remains elusive. It may potentially involve *Toll-like receptors (TLRs)*, a family of pattern recognition receptors that mediate innate immune responses from pathogens or endogenous signals.[3] Following repeated insult, excessive and prolonged inflammation can lead to spontaneous "wind-up" pain or exaggerated or prolonged painful responses to normally painful stimuli (*hyperalgesia*) and even non-painful stimuli (*allodynia*).[19] The wind-up mechanism is complex, involving the remodelling of synaptic contacts between the neurons in the spinal dorsal horn circuitry (neuronal plasticity) and the increased activity of inflammatory substance P and glutamate on receptors for neurokinin 1 (NK1) and N-methyl-D-aspartic acid (NMDA).[20] Several types of exquisitely painful inflammatory skin lesions (eg, pyoderma gangrenosum, cutaneous vasculitis) are caused by sustained inflammatory response associated with autoimmune dysfunction. *Wound-associated pain may extend beyond the wound margins to periwound skin.* Unprotected skin in periwound regions is susceptible to irritation by enzyme-rich wound fluid. In a crossover, randomized, controlled trial,[21] patients with wound margin maceration and skin damage were prone to experience increased pain.

Practice tips to reduce wound-associated pain include the following:

• Identify and correct the wound cause
• Treat infection and inflammation
• Protect periwound skin from wound fluid.

Procedure-related triggers. Despite obvious therapeutic values and primary intentions to optimize wound healing, many wound management procedures are painful. Most obvious, debridement using a sharp surgical instrument can cause a considerable amount of pain.[22] A toolkit of various analgesic agents (topical or systemic), alternative debridement methods, and emerging technologies should be considered to minimize discomfort. Next to debridement, dressing removal has been documented to cause pain in several observational studies.[3] It has also been noticed that dressing materials often adhere to the fragile wound surface due to the glue-like nature of dehydrated or crusted exudate. Each time the dressing is removed, potential local trauma may evoke pain. In addition, the granulation tissue and capillary loops may grow into the product matrix — especially gauze dressings and with the use of negative pressure wound therapies — potentiating the likelihood of trauma and bleeding with dressing removal. According to a review of dressings and topical agents for secondary intention healing of post-surgical wounds, patients experienced significantly more pain with gauze than with other types of dressings.[23] *Wound care providers practicing evidence-based wound care should avoid the use of gauze products in painful wounds.* To ensure dressing securement, strong dressing adhesives or tapes are often used. However, repeated application and removal of adhesive tapes and dressings strip the stratum corneum from the skin epithelial cell surface, damaging the skin. In severe cases, contact irritant dermatitis results in local erythema, edema, and blistering of the wound margins.[24]

Next to dressing removal, *wound cleansing also is likely to cause pain* during dressing changes. In one study,[25] Woo asked 96 patients with chronic wounds to rate their levels of pain before dressing changes, at dressing removal, at wound cleansing, and after dressing reapplication. Wound cleansing was rated as most painful, indicating that *the routine practice of using abrasive materials and gauze to scrub the wound surface should be discouraged*. Clinicians must be mindful of the fact that pain can be caused by pressure-relieving equipment and treatment-related activities, such as repositioning, especially

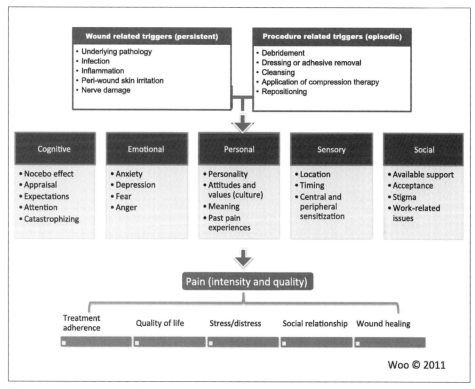

Figure 3. Integrated wound-associated pain model.

among patients who have significant contractures, increased muscle spasticity, and spasms. Some patients consider compression therapy treatment of venous stasis to be uncomfortable. Briggs and Closs[26] indicated that only 56% of patients in their study were able to tolerate full compression bandaging, with pain being the most common reason for nonadherence. *Elastic compression systems exert high pressure at rest and may not be tolerated until adequate pain control has been achieved.* Nonelastic systems exert their main effect with high pressure only with muscle contraction (during movement), and they may be tolerated at rest where there is a lower pressure against a fixed resistance.

Practical tips for procedural pain include the following:

• Use atraumatic dressings
• Avoid frequent removal or the use of strong adhesives (consider silicone adhesive alternatives)
• Avoid aggressive scrubbing of the wound base
• Provide information and support for patients and their circle of care.

Pain and its Dimensions

Pain is a complex biopsychosocial phenomenon. Melzack[27] introduced the term *neuromatrix* to connote the intricate interactions among a number of modulating factors. Despite seemingly comparable levels of pain intensity, persons with pain experience varying degrees of physical limitations, emotional distress, and suffering. The integrated wound-associated pain model in Figure 3 posits the multidimensionality of pain in response to wound- and procedure-related triggers. Understanding that emotions, cognitive process, social environment, and attitudes can influence how people feel, the various separate dimensions are created merely for heuristic purposes.

For instance, *nocebo effect* or *negative placebo effect* delineates pain amplification by expectation of pain and heightened anxiety. Colloca and

Benedetti[28] identified cholecystokinin (CCK) as a physiological mediator that augments nocebo hyperalgesia. Neuroimaging studies revealed that the link between anxiety and hyperalgesia may be located in the central nervous system (entorhinal area of the hippocampal formation, anterior cingulate cortex, amygdala, and insula).[29] The result is a vicious cycle of pain, stress/anxiety, and worsening of pain. In a study of 96 patients with chronic wounds, Woo[25] reported that patients who experienced high levels of anxiety also reported high levels of anticipatory pain, leading to high levels of pain at dressing change. Certain personalities may be more vulnerable to noxious stimuli in light of their propensity to experience anxiety and catastrophize their experience. ***Comprehensive wound pain management should incorporate an assessment of the person's anxiety level, stress, expectation, and social environment.***

How to Assess Pain

Pain assessments should be well documented to facilitate the continuity of patient care and to benchmark the effectiveness of management strategies. Many methods of pain assessment have been developed, ranging from subjective self-reports to objective behavioral checklists. Pain is a subjective experience. An individual's self-report of pain is the most reliable method to evaluate pain. Other assessment methodologies include physiological indicators, behavioral manifestations, functional assessments, and diagnostic tests. Categorical scales, numerical rating scales, pain thermometers, visual analogue scales, faces scales, and verbal categorical scales are one-dimensional tools commonly used to quantify pain in terms of intensity, quality (characteristics), pain unpleasantness, and pain relief.[30] To obtain a comprehensive assessment of pain, multidimensional measurements are available to evaluate the many facets of pain and its impact on daily functioning, mood, social functioning, and other aspects of quality of life. The key questions to ask about pain can be remembered by ***PQRSTU***:[31,32]

- **P — Provoking and palliating factors:** What makes your pain worse? What makes your pain better (eg, warm weather, walking, certain types of cleansing solutions or dressings)?
- **Q — Quality of pain:** What does your pain

feel like? Descriptors (eg, burning, electrical shocks, pricking, tingling pins) may help to differentiate the 2 types of pain: nociceptive and neuropathic.
- **R — Regions and radiation:** Where is the pain and does the pain move anywhere (eg, in and around the wound, the wound region, unrelated)?
- **S — Severity or intensity:** How much does it hurt on a scale of 0–10 with 0 representing no pain and 10 representing pain as bad as it could possibly be?
- **T — Timing or history:** When did the pain start? Is it present all the time? A pain diary may help to map out the temporal pattern of pain, eg, the pain worsens at night.
- **U — Understanding:** What is important to you for pain relief? How would you like to get better?

As an alternative, studies have shown that the observation of nonverbal indicators encompassing a wide range of vocalized signals and bodily movements may provide a means of assessing pain in patients (eg, neonates or cognitively impaired) who are not able to verbalize their pain. Several tools are available, including the following:
- Abbey Pain Scale Assessment of Discomfort in Dementia (ADD) Protocol
- Checklist of Nonverbal Pain Indicators (CNPI)
- Discomfort Scale-Dementia of the Alzheimer's Type (DS-DAT)
- Face, Legs, Activity, Cry, and Consolability (FLACC) Pain Assessment Tool
- Pain Assessment in Advanced Dementia (PAINAD) Scale
- Pain Assessment Scale for Seniors with Severe Dementia (PACSLAC)

Despite the robust psychometric properties of these measurement tools, it is important to remember behaviors (eg, facial expression, body movements, crying) that signal pain may vary significantly among individuals, and there is no evidence that any single behavior or number of behaviors is more reliable to measure the presence or intensity of pain.[30,33] Pain measurement tools may include word descriptors to qualify pain and allow clinicians to differentiate ***nociceptive*** from ***neuropathic pain.*** Nociceptive pain is incurred by tissue damage stimulating pain receptors in the

Table 1. Patient-oriented and multifaceted approach to pain management

Strategy	Objectives

Education	• Web-based learning
	• Face-to-face education:
	  o Explain mechanism of pain
	  o Dispel misconceptions about pain
	  o Address concerns about addiction
	  o Emphasize the availability of multiple strategies

Pharmacological	• Topical:
	  o Topical ibuprofen (dressing not available in the United States)
	  o Morphine
	  o Topical lidocaine
	• Systemic:
	  o Nociceptive pain: ASA, NSAIDs, acetaminophen for mild to moderate pain
	  o Opioids for moderate to intense pain
	  o Neuropathic pain: SNRI, anticonvulsants

Local Wound Care	• Atraumatic interface (silicone) • Sequester: remove inflammatory mediators • Protect periwound skin • Treat infections
Physical Therapies	• Heat/cold compress • Massage • Exercise
Anxiety Reduction	• Relaxation • Imagery • Distractions • Education • Music therapy • Support groups
Cognitive Therapy	• Cognitive behavior therapy • Problem-solving skills • Positive thinking
Therapeutic Alliance	• Communication techniques, eg, reflective listening • Goal setting • Align expectations • Demonstrate sympathy
Empowerment	• Allow individual to call "time out" • Respect individual's choices • Maximize autonomy: active participation • Functional focused therapy

© Woo 2011

muscle, bone, joints, and ligaments (somatic pain) or in the viscera and peritoneum (visceral pain). Nociceptive pain is often described as sharp, dull, aching, throbbing, or gnawing. In contrast, neuropathic pain is caused by injury and sensitization of the peripheral or central nervous system. Neuropathic pain is mostly described as burning, electrical shocks, pricking, tingling pins, and increased sensitivity to touch. Specific assessment protocols are developed to evaluate neuropathic pain.[34] All in all, no one tool has been deemed universal and useful for all patients. The selection of a specific pain scale must take into account the patient's age, language, educational level, sensory impairment, developmental stage, and cognitive status. *Once chosen, the same measurement scale should be used for subsequent assessments for ongoing comparison.* Changes in pain levels may

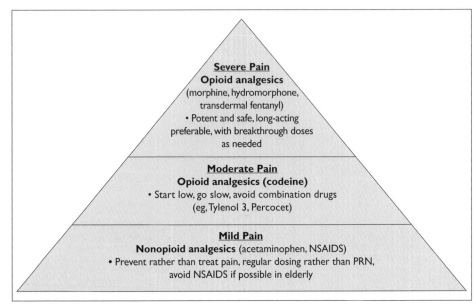

Figure 4. The World Health Organization (WHO) Analgesic Ladder.

Table 2. Neuropathic pain		
Type	**Symptom**	**Treatment**
Nerve irritation	Burning/stinging	Tricyclics — amitriptyline, nortriptyline, etc
Nerve damage	Shooting/stabbing	Anti-epileptics — gabapentin, carbamazepine

indicate a need to reassess the choice and timing of analgesics and/or other interventions used in pain management.

How to Manage Wound-Associated Pain

A patient-oriented and multifaceted approach (Table 1) is recommended for the management of wound-associated pain with the objectives to address pain relief, increase function, and restore overall quality of life. Pharmacotherapy continues to be the mainstay for pain management. Appropriate agents are selected based on severity and specific types of pain. The World Health Organization's analgesic ladder[35] proposes that treatment of mild (1–4 out of 10) to moderate (5–6 out of 10) nociceptive pain should begin with a non-opioid medication, such as acetaminophen and nonsteroidal anti-inflammatory drugs (Figure 4 and Table 2).

For controlling more severe (7–10 out of 10)

and refractory pain, opioid analgesics should be considered. Management of neuropathic pain or associated symptoms (eg, anxiety and depression) may include the possibility of adding adjuvant treatments. Three classes of medications are recommended as first-line treatments for neuropathic pain (Table 3): antidepressants with both norepinephrine and serotonin reuptake inhibition (TCAs and selective serotonin and norepinephrine reuptake inhibitors [SSNRIs]), calcium channel $\alpha_2\delta$ ligands (gabapentin and pregabalin), and topical lidocaine (lidocaine patch 5%).[19] In addition to the severity and pain types, selection of appropriate pharmaceuticals should always take into account the characteristics of the drug (onset, duration, available routes of administration, dosing intervals, side effects) (Table 3) and individual factors (age, coexisting diseases, and other over-the-counter or herbal medications).[19]

Table 3. Analgesics: mode of action, dosage, and side effects

Medication	Mode of Action	Dosage	Side Effects
Non-Opioid			
Acetaminophen	Affects nitric oxide cycle, antipyretic property	325–650 mg q 4 h up to a maximum of 4 g/d in healthy people	Do not exceed 4 g/d to avoid liver toxicity
Acetylsalicylic acid (ASA)	Inhibits the enzyme cyclooxygenase (COX)	325–650 mg q 4–6 h up to 4 g/d	Gastritis, gastrointestinal bleeding, acute renal failure, may interact with anticoagulants
NSAIDs and COX-2 selective NSAIDs	Inhibit COX	Common NSAIDs: Ibuprofen 200–400 mg q 4–6 h Ketoprofen 25–50 mg q 6–8 h Naproxen 250 mg q 6 h Common COX-2 NSAIDs: Celecoxib 200–400 mg od Rofecoxib 25–50 mg od Meloxicam 7.5–15 mg od	Similar as ASA, less side effects with COX-2 NSAIDs
Co-analgesic (Adjuvant)			
Tricyclic antidepressant (TCA)	Inhibit serotonin and NE reuptake; block sodium channels	Common TCAs: Amitriptyline, doxepin, nortriptyline 10–25 mg q hs titrate up to 150–200 mg/d	Dry mouth, drowsiness, orthostatic hypotension
Anticonvulsants	Most agents block sodium channels; unknown for gabapentin	Common anticonvulsants: Carbamazepine 100 mg od to maximum dose 1200 mg/d, gabapentin 100 mg TID titrate up to 3000 mg/d	Drowsiness, dizziness, fatigue
Opioids (CR/SR)			
Morphine	Gold standard mu agonist	For patients who are opioid naive, start on morphine 2.5–10 mg po q 4 h with 10% of total daily dose (TDD) q 1 h as needed	
Codeine	Weak mu agonist; 0.125 as potent as morphine; convert to active analgesic by enzyme CYP2D6	Codeine 100 mg = morphine 10 mg (~10:1)	Constipation, delirium, sedation, nausea, vomiting, urinary retention
Oxycodone (may be combined with ASA or acetaminophen)	Mu and kappa agonist; 2x as potent as morphine	Oxycodone 5 mg or Percocet 1 tab (5/325) = morphine 10 mg (1:2)	
Hydromorphone	5–7.5x as potent as morphine	Hydromorphone 2 mg = morphine 10 mg (1:5)	
Methadone	Mu and delta agonist; blocks NMDA; 10x more potent than morphine	Variable	

© Woo 2011

Legend: h = hour; d = day; q = every; od = daily; hs = evening; TID = 3 times a day; NSAID = nonsteroidal anti-inflammatory drug; NE = norepinephrine; po = by mouth

How to Use Analgesics

As a general rule of thumb, analgesics should be taken at regular intervals until pain is adequately relieved. Whenever possible, the oral route of medication administration is preferred. After a titration period with short-acting preparations (it takes 5 half-lives of an analgesic agent to reach a steady state) to estimate the required dosing for managing continuous stable pain, controlled release medications should be considered to facilitate around-the-clock dosing, especially at night. Nonetheless, short-acting medications should still be made available for occasional breakthrough pain. In some cases, it may be necessary to consider the use of 2 or more drugs from different classes. Their complementary mechanisms of action may provide greater pain relief with less toxicity and lower doses of each drug. *For the elderly population, it is advisable to "start low and go slow"[36] in order to circumvent untoward adverse effects* (see common side effects of analgesics in Table 3). Common side effects, such as constipation, nausea, confusion, and drowsiness, should be monitored and managed appropriately. However, if the pain is (anticipated to be) severe pain, conscious sedation, combining sedatives and potent narcotic analgesics, such as sublingual fentanyl or sufentanil (approximately 100 times more potent than morphine) and ketamine, can be used with success.[19] In resistant cases, options may include general anesthesia, local neural blockade, spinal analgesia, or the use of mixed nitrous oxide and oxygen.

Topical agents play a critical role in alleviating wound-related pain. Slow-release ibuprofen foam dressings (available in Canada and Europe but not in the United States) have demonstrated reduction in persistent wound pain between dressing changes and temporary pain on dressing removal.[37] The topical use of morphine, tricyclic, nonsteroidal anti-inflammatory drugs (NSAIDs), capsaicin, and lidocaine/prilocaine (EMLA® or Eutectic Mixture of Local Anesthetics including lidocaine and prilocaine, AstraZeneca, Wilmington, Delaware) has demonstrated effectiveness for pain relief.[3,12,38] However, the lack of pharmacokinetic data precludes the routine clinical use of these compounds at this time. There are many advantages to using local rather than systemic treatment. Any active agent is delivered directly to the affected area, bypassing the systemic circulation, and the dose needed for pain reduction is lower, minimizing the risk of side effects.

How to Reduce Procedural Pain

In addition to pharmacotherapy, careful selection of *dressings with atraumatic and nonadherent interfaces, such as silicone, has been documented to limit skin damage/trauma with dressing removal and to minimize pain at dressing changes.*[39] Silicone coatings do not adhere to moist wound beds and have a low surface tension due to their unique structure, which consists of chains of hydrophobic polymers with alternate molecules of silicone and oxygen.

Numerous sealants, barriers, and protectants, such as wipes, sprays, gels, and liquid roll-ons, are designed to protect the periwound skin from trauma induced by adhesives.[40] Wound cleansing should involve less abrasive techniques, such as compressing and irrigating usually with normal saline or water. Topical antimicrobial dressings and related products should be considered when surface compartment critical colonization is indicated by increased pain.

Education is a key strategy to empower patients with wounds and individuals within their circle of care and to improve wound-related pain control. Patients and individuals within their circle of care should be informed of various treatment options and be empowered to be active participants in care. Being an active participant involves taking part in the decision-making for the most appropriate treatment, monitoring response to treatment, and communicating concerns to healthcare providers. Common misconceptions about pain management should be addressed.[2]

Fear of addiction and adverse effects has prevented patients from taking regular analgesics. In a pilot study,[41] chronic wound patients described dressing change pain as being more manageable after receiving educational information. Pain-related education is a necessary step in effecting change in pain management by debunking common misconceptions and myths that may obstruct effective pain management. *Cognitive therapy that aims at altering anxiety by modify-*

ing attitudes, beliefs, and expectations by exploring the meaning and interpretation of pain concerns has been successful in the management of pain.[25] This may involve distraction techniques, imagery, relaxation, or altering the significance of the pain to an individual. Patients can learn to envision pain as less threatening and unpleasant through positive imagery by imagining pain disappearing or by conjuring a mental picture of a place that evokes feelings and memories of comfort, safety, and relaxation. In addition to pain, clinicians should pay attention to other sources of anxiety that may be associated with stalled wound healing, fear of amputation, body disfigurement, repulsive odor, social isolation, debility, and disruption of daily activities.[2]

Relaxation exercises can help to reduce anxiety-related tension in the muscle that contributes to pain.

Conclusion

Pain is a common concern and affects quality of life in people with chronic wounds. It is imperative to approach wound-associated pain by first identifying the triggers (related to wound pathologies or procedures), followed by evaluating the number of neurobiopsychosocial factors that may affect the pain experience. A variety of approaches drawing on expertise from interprofessional teams is crucial to optimize pain management.

Take Home Messages for Practice

• Wound-associated pain is complex: comprehensive assessment should entail how pain is affected by wound etiologies, procedure-related triggers, and biopsychosocial factors.

• Wound-associated pain assessment should be comprehensive. Remember PQRSTU.

• Selected pharmacological agents for the treatment of wound-associated pain should be based on the WHO recommendations, taking into account pain severity and types of pain (nociceptive versus neuropathic pain).

• A non-pharmacological approach to pain management should include the use of atraumatic dressings, education, empowerment, and anxiety reduction.

Self-Assessment Questions

1. Mrs. Lebert experiences severe pain due to her leg ulcers. The wound care clinician should assess for which of the following?
   A. Lipodermatosclerosis
   B. Other signs of infection
   C. Anxiety due to cleansing of the wound
   D. All of the above

2. Mrs. Lebert rated her pain as 10 out of 10 on a numerical rating scale. Which of the following pain management strategies is most appropriate for Mrs. Lebert?
   A. Give short-acting morphine 5 mg once daily
   B. Give acetaminophen every 6 hours
   C. Consider changing gauze dressings to silicone dressings
   D. Inform Mrs. Lebert that pain is a good indicator of healing

Answers: 1–D, 2–C

References

1. Krasner D. *Carrying on Despite the Pain: Living with Painful Venous Ulcers. A Heideggerian Hermeneutic Analysis* [dissertation]. Ann Arbor, MI: UMI; 1997.

2. Woo KY. Meeting the challenges of wound-associated pain: anticipatory pain, anxiety, stress, and wound healing. *Ostomy Wound Manage.* 2008;54(9):10–12.

3. Woo K, Sibbald G, Fogh K, et al. Assessment and management of persistent (chronic) and total wound pain. *Int Wound J.* 2008;5(2):205–215.

4. Flaherty E. The views of patients living with healed venous leg ulcers. *Nurs Stand.* 2005;19(45):78,80,82–83.

5. Szor JK, Bourguignon C. Description of pressure ulcer pain at rest and at dressing change. *J Wound Ostomy Continence Nurs.* 1999;26(3):115–120.

6. Nemeth KA, Harrison MB, Graham ID, Burke S. Understanding venous leg ulcer pain: results of a longitudinal study. *Ostomy Wound Manage.* 2004;50(1):34–36.

7. Pieper B, Szczepaniak K, Templin T. Psychosocial adjustment, coping, and quality of life in persons with venous ulcers and a history of intravenous drug use. *J Wound Ostomy Continence Nurs.* 2000;27(4):227–237.

8. Evans AR, Pinzur MS. Health-related quality of life of patients with diabetes and foot ulcers. *Foot Ankle Int.* 2005;26(1):32–37.

9. Kiecolt-Glaser JK, Marucha PT, Malarkey WB, Mercado AM, Glaser R. Slowing of wound healing by psychological stress. *Lancet.* 1995;346(8984):1194–1196.

10. Woo KY, Sibbald RG. The improvement of wound-associated pain and healing trajectory with a comprehensive foot and leg ulcer care model. *J Wound Ostomy Continence Nurs.* 2009;36(2):184–191.

11. Krasner D. The chronic wound pain experience: a con-

ceptual model. *Ostomy Wound Manage.* 1995;41(3):20–25.

12. Woo KY, Sibbald RG. Chronic wound pain: a conceptual model. *Adv Skin Wound Care.* 2008;21(4):175–190.

13. Bruce AJ, Bennett DD, Lohse CM, Rooke TW, Davis MD. Lipodermatosclerosis: review of cases evaluated at Mayo Clinic. *J Am Acad Dermatol.* 2002;46(2):187–192.

14. Aquino R, Johnnides C, Makaroun M, et al. Natural history of claudication: long-term serial follow-up study of 1244 claudicants. *J Vasc Surg.* 2001;34(6):962–970.

15. Grey JE, Harding KG, Enoch S. Venous and arterial leg ulcers. *BMJ.* 2006;332(7537):347–350.

16. Cutting KF, White RJ. Criteria for identifying wound infection--revisited. *Ostomy Wound Manage.* 2005;51(1):28–34.

17. Moore Z, Cowman S. Effective wound management: identifying criteria for infection. *Nurs Stand.* 2007;21(24):68,70,72.

18. Gardner SE, Frantz RA, Doebbeling BN. The validity of the clinical signs and symptoms used to identify localized chronic wound infection. *Wound Repair Regen.* 2001;9(3):178–186.

19. Jovey RD, ed. *Managing Pain: The Canadian Healthcare Professional's Reference.* Toronto, Ontario, Canada: Healthcare & Financial Publishing, Rogers Media; 2002.

20. Ji RR, Woolf CJ. Neuronal plasticity and signal transduction in nociceptive neurons: implications for the initiation and maintenance of pathological pain. *Neurobiol Dis.* 2001;8(1):1–10.

21. Woo KY, Coutts PM, Price P, Harding K, Sibbald RG. A randomized crossover investigation of pain at dressing change comparing 2 foam dressings. *Adv Skin Wound Care.* 2009;22(7):304–310.

22. Sibbald RG, Goodman L, Woo KY, et al. Special considerations in wound bed preparation 2011: an update©. *Adv Skin Wound Care.* 2011;24(9):415–436.

23. Ubbink DT, Vermeulen H, Goossens A, Kelner RB, Schreuder SM, Lubbers MJ. Occlusive vs gauze dressings for local wound care in surgical patients: a randomized clinical trial. *Arch Surg.* 2008;143(10):950–955.

24. Thomas S. Atraumatic dressings. Available at: www.worldwidewounds.com/2003/january/Thomas/Atraumatic-Dressings.html. Accessed February 7, 2008.

25. Woo KY. *Wound Related Pain and Attachment in the Older Adults.* LAP Lambert Academic Publishing; 2011.

26. Briggs M, Closs SJ. Patients' perceptions of the impact of treatments and products on their experience of leg ulcer pain. *J Wound Care.* 2006;15(8):333–337.

27. Melzack R. From the gate to the neuromatrix. *Pain.* 1999;Suppl 6:S121–S126.

28. Colloca L, Benedetti F. Nocebo hyperalgesia: how anxiety is turned into pain. *Curr Opin Anaesthesiol.* 2007;20(5):435–439.

29. Tracey I. Neuroimaging of pain mechanisms. *Curr Opin Support Palliat Care.* 2007;1(2):109–116.

30. Powell RA, Downing J, Ddungu H, Mwangi-Powell FN. Pain history and pain assessment. Available at: http://www.iasp-pain.org/AM/Template.cfm?Section=Home&Template=/CM/ContentDisplay.cfm&ContentID=12173. Accessed January 14, 2012.

31. RNAO. Assessment of pain: questions to consider during assessment of pain (PQRST). Available at: http://pda.rnao.ca/content/assessment-pain-questions-consider-during-assessment-pain-pqrst. Accessed December 28, 2011.

32. Herr K, Coyne PJ, McCaffery M, Manworren R, Merkel S. Pain assessment in the patient unable to self-report: position statement with clinical practice recommendations. *Pain Manag Nurs.* 2011;12(4):230–250.

33. City of Hope Pain & Palliative Care Resource Center. Pain and symptom management. Available at: http://prc.coh.org/pain_assessment.asp. Accessed December 28, 2011.

34. Arnstein P. Assessment of nociceptive versus neuropathic pain in older adults. Available at: http://consultgerirn.org/uploads/File/trythis/try_this_sp1.pdf. Accessed December 28, 2011.

35. World Health Organization. WHO's pain ladder. Available at: http://www.who.int/cancer/palliative/painladder/en/. Accessed December 28, 2011.

36. The AGS Foundation for Health in Aging. *Medications for Persistent Pain. An Older Adult's Guide to Safe Use of Pain Medications.* Available at: http://www.healthinaging.org/public_education/pain/know_your_pain_medications.pdf. Accessed December 28, 2011.

37. Romanelli M, Dini V, Polignano R, Bonadeo P, Maggio G. Ibuprofen slow-release foam dressing reduces wound pain in painful exuding wounds: preliminary findings from an international real-life study. *J Dermatolog Treat.* 2009;20(1):19–26.

38. Briggs M, Nelson EA. Topical agents or dressings for pain in venous leg ulcers. *Cochrane Database Syst Rev.* 2010;(4):CD001177.

39. Woo KY, Harding K, Price P, Sibbald G. Minimising wound-related pain at dressing change: evidence-informed practice. *Int Wound J.* 2008;5(2):144–157.

40. Woo KY, Sibbald RG. The ABCs of skin care for wound care clinicians: dermatitis and eczema. *Adv Skin Wound Care.* 2009;22(5):230–238.

41. Gibson MC, Keast D, Woodbury MG, et al. Educational intervention in the management of acute procedure-related wound pain: a pilot study. *J Wound Care.* 2004;13(5):187–190.

Health-Related Quality of Life and Chronic Wounds: Evidence and Implications for Practice

Patricia Price, BA (Hons), PhD, AFBPsS, CPsychol, FHEA;
Diane L. Krasner, PhD, RN, CWCN, CWS, MAPWCA, FAAN

Objectives

The reader will be challenged to:

- Distinguish between the concepts of health-related quality of life (HRQoL) and life quality
- Discuss the benefits of HRQoL for clinical practice, research, and audit/quality improvement
- Identify the limitations associated with measuring HRQoL using generic and condition-specific tools, such as pain and wound assessment tools
- Value quality-of-life issues for people with wounds and incorporate this assessment into clinical practice.

Introduction

There is growing awareness that an individual's perspective on health and illness represents an important aspect of total healthcare. Increasingly, the person's experience plays a significant role in helping professionals adapt their care to the needs of the individual. Healthcare providers are increasingly formalizing the way in which this information is reported using *patient-reported outcome measures (PROMs).*[1] These measures provide a way in which professionals can gain insight into how patients perceive their conditions and the impact their conditions have on the quality of their lives, as well as monitor the impact of different treatments on life quality. This information will help the clinicians of the future deliver individualized care that focuses not only on healing the wound, but also on optimizing the quality of life of the person with a wound and his or her circle of care.

There have been substantial changes in this field over the past 10–15 years as researchers and clinicians have worked together to build on earlier work that described patient experiences while living with acute or chronic wounds. This fundamental work has led to the increased availability of tools for use in research and clinical contexts that allow us to measure improvements in this area. For example, in the United States, the Centers for Medicare & Medicaid Services (CMS) now require that residents in long-term care facilities be interviewed about their quality of life as part of the Minimum Data Set (MDS) 3.0 regulatory process. Every facility is required to capture person-centered concerns on an ongoing basis and to connect them to the care planning process. Few clinicians

Price P, Krasner DL. Health-related quality of life and chronic wounds: evidence and implications for practice. In: Krasner DL, ed. *Chronic Wound Care: The Essentials.* Malvern, PA: HMP Communications; 2014:123–130.

would disagree that the presence of a wound has a great impact on the individual. This chapter will outline key considerations in defining **health-related quality of life** and using robust tools to measure this outcome and outline the importance of qualitative work in reviewing the life quality of patients with nonhealing wounds. We will provide examples of ways in which consideration for quality-of-life issues for the person with a wound and his or her circle of care can be built into routine clinical care.

What is Quality of Life?

The term *quality of life* first appeared in the United States in the 1950s as a slogan to represent "the good life" and was featured during the next decade in European political discussions. More recently, however, it has become part of a holistic view of the individual within healthcare systems. Quality of life is a broad concept that reflects an individual's perspective on the level of life satisfaction experienced in a variety of situations, including housing, recreation, and environmental conditions. In this way, it is a subjective measure that is affected by factors well beyond health status.

Consequently, most authors since the 1980s have restricted their definitions to **health-related quality of life (HRQoL)** outcomes, referring to the impact of health and illness on physical and social functioning and psychological well-being. In the 1990s, HRQoL assessments were further refined and aimed to capture data on both objective functioning and subjective well-being. This approach tackles the controversy over the relative importance of these two aspects of this concept while acknowledging the patient's experience of disease and treatment as a central component of healthcare and healthcare research.[2,3]

HRQoL is a complex multidimensional concept that reflects the total impact of health and illness on the individual. However, many studies infer improvements in HRQoL from change in a single clinical parameter, usually pain. While all those involved in wound care would acknowledge the profound impact pain can have on an individual, it is important to note that pain and HRQoL are not equivalent concepts. Just as a clinician will require information on a range of physiological parameters before making a diagnosis, so, too, is information on a range of dimensions needed before statements can be made about the HRQoL status of an individual.[4]

PROMs include a range of validated tools that are designed to measure either a person's perception of his or her general health or in relation to a specific disease or conditions (eg, pain, chronic wound). HRQoL tools come into this category: HRQoL is measured using robust, validated questionnaires where people rate their health in response to individual items. These tools may be a *generic measure* of HRQoL when the questions are related to general health, allowing for HRQoL comparisons to be made across a range of health states, or *condition-specific measures*, where tools have been developed to assess the impact of a particular condition or illness. Condition-specific tools are often more sensitive to change in a person's condition over time (eg, improvement toward healing) as the individual items included in the questionnaire have been developed from the experiences of people who have lived with that particular condition. However, *generic HRQoL tools* allow the health state of a person with a chronic wound to be compared with any other health state, for example, a person with a fractured femur — such comparative data can be important when planning resource allocation and the provision of services.

However, important qualitative approaches also are used to ensure that the rich data that emerges from this approach can capture the detail of the everyday life experiences of people with chronic wounds, such as the social stigma, guilt, and shame associated with living with a malignant wound.[5,6] Work in this area has shown that an improvement in daily life quality is an important health outcome that may, in the short term, affect a person's motivation to continue with treatment in the long term and so improve clinical outcomes.[7] Research into the life quality of people with wounds using qualitative approaches is just as important as quantitative research in informing our clinical practice so that wound care outcomes can be optimized.

Why Measure HRQoL?

Improved HRQoL for people has become increasingly recognized as an important outcome measure for a range of interventions and particularly important for people with chronic conditions or those receiving palliative care. The importance of the measure can be grouped under 3 headings: *clinical practice, research,* and *audit/quality improvement-quality assurance.*

Clinical practice. During routine clinical practice, healthcare professionals intuitively take into account life quality issues when making clinical decisions. Robust quality data in this area will help formalize some of these decisions. HRQoL data may be particularly relevant when expensive or hazardous options need to be considered for those patients not healing using conventional treatment. With the increasing costs associated with patient care, HRQoL may be a useful measure for allocating finances to patient care. There is, as yet, no "gold standard" to measure cost effectiveness or to analyze costs, but at some point in the development of appropriate formulae, the "human" cost needs to be considered. On the individual level, considerations about treatment options may be influenced by those aspects of living with a wound that have the greatest impact on the person, while at the population level, HRQoL data are generally considered as valid indicators of service needs and intervention outcomes.

Research. HRQoL data may prove to be useful as an additional outcome measure for research in wound care, as an alternative to "days to healing" (particularly for those patients where healing is not a realistic option), or as an additional measure of efficacy of the clinical treatment plan. In some areas, HRQoL has become an accepted endpoint in clinical trials, particularly when comparing treatments with similar or no impact on disease progression or survival.[8] The development of new therapies, particularly those using new technologies, should include HRQoL data: enormous amounts of time could be devoted to the development of a new technique only to find that it is not acceptable to patients (eg, because of side effects like burning or stinging).

Audit/quality improvement-quality assurance. HRQoL data may be extremely useful within audits or quality improvement or quality assurance programs to demonstrate effectiveness and as a means of measuring change. Certainly, the work within this area could eventually allow us to provide a patient-based view of the service and treatment provided. Measuring HRQoL can help identify the burden of disease and disabilities and help countries monitor health objectives (eg, identify subgroups with poor perceived health in order to guide service interventions).[9] HRQoL data may be particularly important for planning services for the elderly in an era when life expectancy is increasing, given the expectation for improving both the number and quality of life years despite the consequences of the normal aging process.[9]

Quality of Life and Pressure Ulcers

Compared to other wound types, there is limited empirical evidence for the impact of pressure ulcers on HRQoL, although a systematic review[10] in 2009 included 31 studies with 2,463 patients. These studies included 10 qualitative studies (described as "good quality" studies) on life quality and 21 quantitative studies (described as "poor quality" studies) across a range of patients, including frail elderly and those with spinal-cord injury. Collectively, these studies cover 11 key themes that cover a range of issues from physical restrictions, social isolation, the impact of wound symptoms, body image, and self-concept, as well as the importance of the relationship between the patient and the healthcare provider. The major issues raised related to *severe wound pain* and the concern that healthcare providers did not listen to patient concerns, particularly in relation to responding to early warning symptoms of deterioration.

The age range of patients included in this review and the range of conditions included make it difficult to assess whether the issues raised by those with spinal-cord injury are the same as those who are elderly. Many of those who develop pressure ulcers are elderly and frail with profound mobility problems and a wide range of additional concomitant disorders. Such patients are often unable to complete self-ratings of HRQoL due to impairment in cognitive functioning, so qualitative studies are more likely to capture the extent of their experiences, while high-quality, large scale studies using validated tools are still urgently needed.

While the sociological and psychological histories of the patient are deemed important aspects of patients' assessment, it is clear that the majority of work in this area focuses on symptom control (eg, pain at dressing change) or overall patient discomfort.[11,12] The need for detailed research work in this area is paramount, and clinicians and researchers must tackle and address the methodological difficulties inherent in conducting research in this area.

Clinical Application

Using HRQoL measures to drive the wound care plan of care. Many of the issues raised by those with pressure ulcers can be approached with good communication between the patient and healthcare provider. Activities, such as attentive listening, responding to the patient's needs for information, and reacting proactively to patient concerns, can help to build a strong relationship around managing wound symptoms in a way that the patient feels supported and a partner in his or her own care.

HRQoL measures that can drive the pressure ulcer plan of care include:

- *Attention to the person's pressure ulcer-related concerns/complaints, especially wound pain*
- *Timely assessment of changes in pressure ulcer status/deterioration*
- *Appreciation for the person's psychosocial concerns*
- *Attention to the individual's mobility problems and other comorbidities.*

Quality of Life and Diabetic Foot Ulceration

While the literature contains many references to the devastating effects of diabetic foot wounds for the person with diabetes, the literature specifically on HRQoL has taken longer to emerge. However, recent studies have shown that the emotional status of the person at the time when the first diabetic ulcer appears can have long-term consequences for the individual, as a 5-year follow-up study has shown a 2-fold increase in mortality for those with depressive symptoms at initial presentation.[13]

Research work using generic questionnaires to measure HRQoL have indicated that **people with diabetic foot ulcers have a significantly poorer quality of life** than those with diabetes but no foot ulcers. For example, in a cross-sectional study in Norway[14] with 127 adults with diabetic foot ulcers compared with 221 patients with diabetes but no ulcers and 5,903 controls from the general population, Ribu and colleagues demonstrated that those with foot ulcers had statistically significantly poorer HRQoL when measured using the Short Form 36 (SF-36) — with particular restrictions in physical functioning that limited their abilities in activities of daily living. These findings were confirmed in a longitudinal study from the same group who followed these patients for 1 year. HRQoL scores improved significantly for those patients whose ulcers went on to heal.[15] Data from Spain[16] also

support the finding that having a diabetic foot ulcer reduces HRQoL; a study of 258 people with diabetes but no foot ulceration compared with 163 people with diabetes-related foot ulcers indicated a statistically poorer HRQoL when an ulcer is present using the SF-36. The study also showed that **neuropathy, amputation history, and poor metabolic control were all associated with poorer quality of life**. Data from Brazil also indicate this pattern of poorer HRQoL in those with active ulceration, although the study showed no difference in self-esteem scores.[17]

The impact of wound healing on quality of life was confirmed by an American study (N = 253) that showed a 5- to 6-point deterioration in the mental component of the SF-36 for those whose diabetic foot ulcers did not heal over an 18-month period.[18] Similar patterns were observed in a Swedish study (N = 75) that showed mental health summary scores, social functioning, and limits on daily living through physical and emotional limitations were significantly higher in those who went on to heal over a 12-month period, again using SF-36.[19] However, a British multicenter study of 317 patients[20] with diabetic foot ulcers found no statistical differences between those who had healed ulcers and those with ongoing ulceration/withdrawn at either 12 or 24 weeks using the SF-36. The researchers were able to demonstrate a statistically significant difference in physical functioning and well-being in those who were healed at both 12 and 24 weeks and a difference also in social functioning at 24 weeks alone when a condition-specific tool, the ***Cardiff Wound Impact Schedule*** or ***CWIS***, was used.

The CWIS has been shown to be a valid and reliable condition-specific tool for chronic wounds on the lower limb. This tool has been recommended as a research outcome measure when evaluated for use in people with diabetic foot ulcers.[21] This is just one of a number of condition-specific tools that can be used to assess HRQoL in this group. A review of all the available tools is outside the scope of this chapter, but those interested in finding out more about the range of tools available should refer to a systematic review by Hogg et al.[22]

Studies on the life quality of people with diabetic foot ulceration have emphasized that this is a life of fear, mainly of amputation but also infection, with wound pain being an underestimated problem in this group.[23,24] Qualitative studies have shown that the presence of a diabetic foot ulcer is "inconvenient" and "burdensome," with the fear of amputation precipitating anxiety and stress.[25] For people with diabetes, ongoing experiences of pain affected the ability to sleep and impacted mobility and social life. These people also described feelings of depression, isolation, and loss of independence.[26] Patients with unhealed ulcers were frustrated with healing and had anxiety about the wound, reported problems with a range of activities of daily living, had problems with footwear, and complained of a limited social life.[27] One qualitative study indicated that both the ulcer and the treatment for the ulcer restricted mobility and independence, leading to feelings of anger, fear, depression, helplessness, and boredom, and also showed that podiatrists were aware of the negative impact of ulceration on their patients' lives but felt they lacked the skills necessary to deal with their patients' emotional needs.[28]

Nearly 20 years ago, Williams[29] noted the severity of a situation in which we did not have quantitative information on the impact of foot disorders on quality-of-life dimensions and stated, "The lack of such information must rank as the most serious deficiency in our current knowledge of the impact of these disorders." Considerable steps were taken during that time to address the situation, with both qualitative data on life quality and quantitative data on HRQoL collected from a range of countries using a range of methods, all indicating the profound impact that diabetic foot ulceration has on patients. A greater understanding of these issues should help us tailor clinical practice to assist patients while they live with ulceration and work to adopt positive foot self-care as a preventive measure against further deterioration.

Clinical Application

Be aware of the potential for unrecognized pain in this group and consider the frustrations that patients may experience during the long road to healing and the lifetime of changes that will be needed to prevent recurrence. Using an holistic approach will help to pick up on the anxieties and stress that patients may feel and consider approaches, such as motivational interviewing, to assist in behavior change.[30]

HRQoL measures that can drive the diabetic foot ulcer plan of care include:

- *Attention to the person's diabetic foot ulcer-related concerns, including pain*
- *Empathy for the person's change in mobility and functioning (activities of daily living), sleep, and social functioning*
- *Appreciation of any signs and symptoms of anxiety, stress, or depression*
- *Assessment of concerns related to amputation and infection.*

Quality of Life and Chronic Leg Ulceration

There is probably more data on quality-of-life issues and patients with leg ulceration than any other wound type due to the qualitative and quantitative work undertaken in the early 1990s. A synthesis analysis[31] in 2007 included 12 qualitative studies from the United States, Australia, Sweden, and the United Kingdom that identified *5 common themes: physical effects of leg ulceration, describing the leg ulcer journey, patient-professional relationships, cost of a leg ulcer, and psychological impact.* Using software designed for the synthesis of qualitative research by the Joanna Briggs Institute,[32] the synthesis[31] clearly demonstrated that living with the physical symptoms associated with an open, chronic wound dominated the data from all 12 studies. These physical symptoms included pain, odor, itch, leakage, and infection. The synthesis also demonstrated how many patients had initially been guided by their own health beliefs and aided by family members before accepting that the wound was not a "simple scratch" and that professional help was needed. The relationship with the professional was described in both positive and negative ways. Positive themes associated with the relationship focused on therapeutic value, providing continuity of care, providing strategies to cope with a chronic condition, and — whenever possible — aiding patients in regaining control of their lives. The negative comments from the data included disputes between patients and their health professionals and patients being given conflicting advice. Across a number of studies (n = 8), patients perceived a lack of time, trust, empathy, and understanding — *patients felt they were not listened to, and dissatisfaction with treatment was highlighted.*

Although not all studies included in the synthesis[31] focused on psychological problems, many patients reported feelings of embarrassment associated with the leg ulcer, the negative impact on body image, fear of amputation, negative self-esteem, anger, depression (in some cases linked to suicidal thoughts), and a general sense of identity loss (as the wound dominated their lives).

The authors concluded that many professionals work to a code of practice whereby the **emphasis is on the route to healing**, with the assumption that a healed wound will improve quality of life. However, they also noted that aiming for healing may not be the most appropriate route for those with large, hard-to-heal wounds or those whose wound duration is extensive, as this may "initiate a spiral of hopelessness."

A more recent review that only included 8 qualitative studies[33] (focusing on venous leg ulceration) confirmed that **physical symptoms, especially pain, dominate everyday living with mobility, sleep disruption, exudate, and odor all causing significant problems.** The authors also commended qualitative studies for their ability to provide insight into the lives of people with chronic wounds.

Integrative reviews that included both qualitative and quantitative studies[34,35] looking at quality-of-life issues for people with venous leg ulceration also have concluded that the impact of living with a chronic ulcer is profound, with individuals reporting more pain, more restrictions on their physical and social lives, and poorer sense of well-being compared to controls. Together, these data suggest that regardless of methodology, theoretical philosophy, or study location, the findings are increasingly confirmative that the impact on people is extensive, and we, as health professionals, now have to investigate ways in which we can deliver care that addresses these concerns.

Two recent reviews focused on the different tools that have been used to conduct quantitative studies of HRQoL,[35,36] including both generic and condition-specific questionnaires. The reviews demonstrated that many researchers still question the relevance of using generic tools (those designed to be used with any health condition), as the resulting data make it difficult to attribute HRQoL scores to leg ulceration rather than any other comorbidity that may be present. Both reviews also described the growing number of condition-specific tools that are available and have been developed based on the experiences of

people with chronic wounds. These reviews concluded that many tools have been able to demonstrate acceptable levels of reliability, validity, and discrimination between healed and active ulceration. Some are available in several languages, and some are still in the early stages of development. Researchers have concluded that at this stage in the development of these relatively new tools, it may be wise to use both a generic and condition-specific tool in clinical trials.[37] HRQoL work with condition-specific tools may still be in its infancy, but we must endeavor to investigate the specific impact of wounds on the individual if we are to truly understand the condition from the perspective of the person. Those interested in finding out more about specific tools will find relevant details in these reviews.[35,36]

Clinical Application

The data strongly suggest that patients' experiences of living with wounds are dominated by symptom management, with all studies showing that the wound and its treatment have a profound effect on quality of life. Nurses predominate in the care of these patients, and where that relationship works well, the benefits to the patients are substantial. Unfortunately, not all relationships work so well, indicating a need for more training and education around quality-of-life issues as the patient's needs go far beyond the routine treatment of wounds. The data suggest that a holistic approach to assessment is important and that patients and professionals need to build relationships based on mutual trust and respect if the patient's overall experience is to improve.

HRQoL measures that can drive the venous ulcer plan of care include:

- *Attention to the person's venous ulcer-related concerns, including symptoms, body image changes, and other psychosocial concerns*
- *Appreciation for the person's change in mobility and functioning (activities of daily living), sleep, and social functioning*
- *Regular review of patient concerns through active listening.*

Conclusion

Formal HRQoL assessment in patients with chronic wounds is relatively new, with investigators using a range of methodologies and measures with this patient population. Many of the studies are cross-sectional in design and descriptive in nature, indicating that there is still a large amount of basic theoretical and empirical work yet to be completed despite the huge progress that has been made in recent years. Compared to trials in other patient populations (eg, cancers, AIDS, asthma), relatively few randomized, controlled, chronic wound trials have included HRQoL data, although some studies are now including such measures as secondary outcomes.[8] Yet, anyone who spends even a short amount of time with a frail elderly patient who is house-bound with large wounds on both legs cannot help but be moved to appreciate the impact of living with that condition on everyday life. Attention to and appreciation for a person's HRQoL concerns should drive the individual's wound care plan of care.

The challenge for the future is to ensure that we pay as much attention to HRQoL and life quality as we do to other important clinical parameters and start to build new ways of delivering care that ensure that we keep patients' well-being as our central focus. The data are now consistently showing us that the quality of life of patients with chronic wounds is very poor — regardless of where the study has been conducted, whether qualitative or quantitative approaches have been used, or the sector within which the healthcare was provided. We now need to go beyond describing the situation and consider ways in which we can work in partnership to ensure we provide optimal care and work for the best possible outcomes for people with wounds, including an improvement in their sense of well-being.[38]

Self-Assessment Questions

1. Why is assessing HRQoL important?
   A. Patients like to talk to us about their lives
   B. Government tells us to assess everything
   C. Clinical, research, audit/quality reasons exist that can lead to improved outcomes
   D. Clinicians do it routinely, so there is no need to assess HRQoL

2. What sort of tool would you use to assess HRQoL in a way that you could compare it for different groups of patients?
   A. Condition-specific tools
   B. Generic tools
   C. Qualitative methods
   D. Ask the clinician

3. If you wanted to find out more about the life quality of your patients, which approach would you take?
   A. Condition-specific tools
   B. Generic tools
   C. Qualitative methods
   D. Ask the clinician

Answers: 1–C, 2–B, 3–C

Take Home Messages for Practice

- HRQoL measures will help the clinicians of the future deliver individualized care that focuses not only on healing the wound but also on optimizing the quality of life of the person with a wound and his or her circle of care.
- HRQoL is a complex multidimensional concept that reflects the total impact of health and illness on the individual.
- HRQoL measures should help guide clinical practice, research, and audit/quality improvement-quality assurance initiatives.
- HRQoL data suggest that a holistic approach to assessment is important and that patients and professionals need to build relationships based on mutual trust and respect if the patient's overall experience is to improve.

References

1. Dawson J, Doll H, Fitzpatrick R, Jenkinson C, Carr AJ. The routine use of patient reported outcome measures in healthcare settings. *BMJ*. 2010;340:c186.
2. Muldoon MF, Barger SD, Flory JD, Manuck SB. What are quality of life measurements measuring? *BMJ*. 1998;316(7130):542–545.
3. Gandek B, Sinclair SJ, Kosinski M, Ware JE Jr. Psychometric evaluation of the SF-36 health survey in Medicare managed care. *Health Care Financ Rev*. 2004;25(4):5–25.
4. Price P. An holistic approach to wound pain in patients with chronic wounds. *WOUNDS*. 2005;17(3):55–57.
5. Dolbeault S, Flahault C, Baffie A, Fromantin I. Psychological profile of patients with neglected malignant wounds: a qualitative exploratory study. *J Wound Care*. 2010;19(12):513–521.
6. Piggin C, Jones V. Malignant fungating wounds: an analysis of the lived experience. *J Wound Care*. 2009;18(2):57–64.
7. Speight J, Reaney MD, Barnard KD. Not all roads lead to Rome — a review of quality of life measurement in adults with diabetes. *Diabet Med*. 2009;26(4):315–327.
8. Gottrup F, Apelqvist J, Price P; European Wound Man-

agement Association Patient Outcome Group. Outcomes in controlled and comparative studies on non-healing wounds: recommendations to improve the quality of evidence in wound management. *J Wound Care*. 2010;19(6):237–268.

9.   Centers for Disease Control and Prevention. Health-Related Quality of Life (HRQOL). Available at: http://www.cdc.gov/hrqol/concept.htm. Accessed January 3, 2012.

10. Gorecki C, Brown JM, Nelson EA, et al; European Quality of Life Pressure Ulcer Project group. Impact of pressure ulcers on quality of life in older patients: a systematic review. *J Am Geriatr Soc*. 2009;57(7):1175–1183.

11. Benbow M. Quality of life and pressure ulcers. *J Community Nursing*. 2009;23(12):14–18.

12. Rastinehad D. Pressure ulcer pain. *J Wound Ostomy Continence Nurs*. 2006;33(3):252–257.

13. Winkley K, Sallis H, Kariyawasam D, et al. Five-year follow-up of a cohort of people with their first diabetic foot ulcer: the persistent effect of depression on mortality. *Diabetologia*. 2012;55(2):303–310.

14. Ribu L, Hanestad BR, Moum T, Birkeland K, Rustoen T. A comparison of the health-related quality of life in patients with diabetic foot ulcers, with a diabetes group and a nondiabetes group from the general population. *Qual Life Res*. 2007;16(2):179–189.

15. Ribu L, Birkeland K, Hanestad BR, Moum T, Rustoen T. A longitudinal study of patients with diabetes and foot ulcers and their health-related quality of life: wound healing and quality-of-life changes. *J Diabetes Complications*. 2008;22(6):400–407.

16. Garcia-Morales E, Lázaro-Martínez JL, Martínez-Hernández D, Aragón-Sánchez J, Beneit-Montesinos JV, Gonzàlez-Jurado MA. Impact of diabetic foot related complications on the Health Related Quality of life (HRQol) of patients — a regional study in Spain. *Int J Low Extrem Wounds*. 2011;10(1):6–11.

17. de Meneses LC, Blanes L, Francescato Veiga D, Carvalho Gomes H, Masako Ferreira L. Health-related quality of life and self-esteem in patients with diabetic foot ulcers: results of a cross-sectional comparative study. *Ostomy Wound Manage*. 2011;57(3):36–43.

18. Winkley K, Stahl D, Chalder T, Edmonds ME, Ismail K. Quality of life in people with their first diabetic foot ulcer: a prospective cohort study. *J Am Podiatr Med Assoc*. 2009;99(5):406–414.

19. Löndahl M, Landin-Olsson M, Katzman P. Hyperbaric oxygen therapy improves health-related quality of life in patients with diabetes and chronic foot ulcer. *Diabet Med*. 2011;28(2):186–190.

20. Jeffcoate WJ, Price PE, Phillips CJ, et al. Randomised controlled trial of the use of three dressing preparations in the management of chronic ulceration of the foot in diabetes. *Health Technol Assess*. 2009;13(54):1–86.

21. Jaksa PJ, Mahoney JL. Quality of life in patients with diabetic foot ulcers: validation of the Cardiff Wound Impact Schedule in a Canadian population. *Int Wound J*. 2010;7(6):502–507.

22. Hogg FRA, Peach G, Price P, Thompson MM, Hinchliffe RJ. Measures of health-related quality of life in diabetes-related foot disease: a systematic review. *Diabetologica*. 2012;55(3):552–565.

23. Ribu L, Rustoen T, Birkeland K, Hanestad BR, Paul SM, Miaskowski C. The prevalence and occurrence of diabetic foot ulcer pain and its impact on health-related quality of life. *J Pain*. 2006;7(4):290–299.

24. Bengtsson L, Jonsson M, Apelqvist J. Wound-related pain is underestimated in patients with diabetic foot ulcers. *J Wound Care*. 2008;17(10):433–435.

25. Watson-Miller S. Living with a diabetic foot ulcer: a phenomenological study. *J Clin Nurs*. 2006;15(10):1336–1337.

26. Bradbury S, Price PE. Diabetic foot ulcer pain (part 2): the hidden burden. *EWMA J*. 2011;11(2):25–37.

27. Goodridge D, Trepman E, Sloan J, et al. Quality of life of adults with unhealed and healed diabetic foot ulcers. *Foot Ankle Int*. 2004;27(4):274–280.

28. Searle A, Campbell R, Tallon D, Fitzgerald A, Vedhera K. A qualitative approach to understanding the experience of ulceration and healing in the diabetic foot: patient and podiatrist perspectives. *WOUNDS*. 2005;17(1):16–26.

29. Williams DRR. The size of the problem: epidemiological and economic aspects of foot problems in diabetes. In: Boulton AJ, Connor H, eds. *The Foot in Diabetes*. 2nd ed. Chichester, UK: Wiley & Sons; 1994.

30. Gabbay RA, Kaul S, Ulbrecht J, Scheffler NM, Armstrong DG. Motivational interviewing by podiatric physicians: a method for improving patient self-care of the diabetic foot. *J Am Podiatr Med Assoc*. 2011;101(1):78–84.

31. Briggs M, Flemming K. Living with leg ulceration: a synthesis of qualitative research. *J Adv Nurs*. 2007;59(4):319–328.

32. Pearson A. Balancing the evidence: incorporating the synthesis of qualitative data into systematic reviews. *JBI Reports*. 2004;2(2):45–64.

33. Green J, Jester R. Health-related quality of life and chronic venous leg ulceration: part 1. *Br J Community Nurs*. 2009;14(12):S12–S17.

34. Herber OR, Schnepp W, Rieger MA. A systematic review on the impact of leg ulceration on patients' quality of life. *Health Qual Life Outcomes*. 2007;5:44.

35. González-Consuegra RV, Verdú J. Quality of life in people with venous leg ulcers: an integrative review. *J Adv Nurs*. 2011;67(5):926–944.

36. Green J, Jester R. Health-related quality of life and chronic venous leg ulceration: part 2. *Br J Community Nurs*. 2010;15(3):S4–S14.

37. Palfreyman S. Assessing the impact of venous ulceration on quality of life. *Nurs Times*. 2008;104(41):34–37.

38. Gray D, Boyd J, Carville K, et al. Effective wound management and wellbeing: guidance for clinicians, organizations and industry. *Wounds UK*. 2011;7(1):86–90.

CHAPTER 11

Nutritional Strategies for Wound and Pressure Ulcer Management

Mary Ellen Posthauer, RDN, CD, LD;
Jos M.G.A. Schols, MD, PhD

Objectives

The reader will be challenged to:

• Define the direct and indirect roles of nutrients in the wound healing process

• Analyze the role of nutrition in pressure ulcer prevention and healing

• Establish an interprofessional approach to wound care, including nutrition.

Introduction

No one will argue the importance of adequate nutrition for preserving skin and tissue viability and promoting tissue repair processes like wound healing. Good nutritional status generally reflects a healthy condition and adequate body power. However, despite this assumption, little scientific evidence about the relationship between nutrition or nutrition intervention and wound healing is available. Most studies that have been performed are related to the problem of pressure ulcers. Hence, this chapter focuses on nutritional strategies for pressure ulcer management.

Prevalence of Pressure Ulcers

Pressure ulcers are common across all healthcare sectors throughout the world and have been described as one of the most costly and physically debilitating care problems. A survey by the European Pressure Ulcer Advisory Panel (EPUAP) found an overall prevalence of 18.1% in 5 different European countries, and a study of the National Pressure Ulcer Advisory Panel (NPUAP) found a similar prevalence of 15% together with an incidence of 7% in American hospitals.[1,2] The Agency for Healthcare Research and Quality (AHRQ) in the United States noted that pressure ulcer-related hospitalizations increased by 80% from 1993 to 2006. Specifically, the prevalence figures are highest among vulnerable populations, such as frail and disabled residents in long-term care facilities, individuals receiving palliative care, and medically complex patients in intensive care units.[3]

Posthauer ME, Schols J. Nutritional strategies for pressure ulcer management. In: Krasner DL, ed. *Chronic Wound Care: The Essentials.* Malvern, PA: HMP Communications; 2014:131–144.

The impact of pressure ulcers is significant to individuals and the healthcare system.[4] Individuals with pressure ulcers have increased awareness about their pain, reduced quality of life, and limited abilities to participate in activities and rehabilitation. The amount of healthcare resources to manage the care of individuals with pressure ulcers in addition to frequent hospital stays is staggering.[5] The **pressure ulcer cost-of-illness** has been calculated to be at least 1% of the total Dutch healthcare budget and 4% of the United Kingdom healthcare budget.[6,7] In the United States, the Centers for Medicare & Medicaid Services (CMS) reported that the cost of treating a pressure ulcer in acute care, as a secondary diagnosis, in 2008 was $43,180.00 per hospital stay.[8-10] In the United States, the cost of litigation adds to the burden of healthcare costs, especially in long-term care, where 87% of settlements against facilities are awarded to the plaintiffs.[11] Therefore, addressing the overall management of pressure ulcers is now a prominent national healthcare issue in many western countries. Despite advances in healthcare, pressure ulcers remain a major cause of morbidity and mortality.

Both **poor nutritional intake** and **poor nutritional status** have been identified as the key risk factors for pressure ulcer development and protracted wound healing. Notwithstanding methodological shortcomings, cross-sectional and prospective studies suggest a fairly strong correlation between malnutrition and pressure ulcer development.[12-15] Malnutrition is a status of nutrition in which a deficiency, excess, or imbalance of energy, protein, and other nutrients causes measurable adverse effects on tissue, body structure, body function, and clinical outcome. The studies related to pressure ulcers have mostly focused on the relationship between pressure ulcers and undernutrition. Multivariate analysis of epidemiological data indicates that poor nutritional status and related factors, such as low body weight and poor oral food intake, are independent risk factors for pressure ulcer development.[16-18] Moreover, it appears that many acute and chronically ill as well as elderly individuals at risk for pressure ulcer development or with established pressure ulcers suffer from undesired weight loss.[17-20] A recent study from Shahin et al on the relationship between malnutrition parameters and pressure ulcers

in German hospitals and nursing homes clearly established a significant relationship between the presence of pressure ulcers and undesired weight loss (5%–10%). Inadequate and poor nutritional intake was strongly related to the presence of pressure ulcers in both healthcare settings as well.[21]

These findings confirm the importance of adequate nutritional care in individuals prone to pressure ulcer development, especially since malnutrition is a reversible risk factor for wounds (including pressure ulcers), unless the individual has a terminal illness.

Pathophysiology

In the NPUAP and EPUAP clinical practice guideline on pressure ulcer prevention and treatment, a pressure ulcer is defined as a localized injury to the skin and/or underlying tissue, usually over a bony prominence, as a result of pressure or pressure in combination with shear.[22] The external mechanical loading of the skin can be a force perpendicular to the skin surface (direct pressure), a force parallel to the skin surface (shear), or a combination of both. Depending on the magnitude, time duration, and type of the mechanical load, the mechanical and geometrical properties of the tissues, as well as the susceptibility of the individual, ischemia as a result of the deformation of the tissues will lead to hypoxia. In addition, blocking of the nutrient supply and blocking of waste product removal combined with a subsequent change in pH will eventually lead to tissue damage. Finally, reperfusion after a period of ischemia may increase the ultimate cell death damage. The resultant tissue necrosis may cause local injured tissue alterations and even further exacerbate the damage.[22]

The development of pressure ulcers depends on extrinsic and intrinsic risk factors. The most important extrinsic risk factors are pressure, shear, and friction, which lead to mechanical loading and secondary damage to the skin and soft tissue. Intrinsic factors have an effect on tissue viability and consequently influence the pathophysiological response to mechanical loading. Studies have found significant associations with age, sex, limited activity, care dependency, incontinence (bowel and bladder), acute disease (eg, infection), and nutritional status. The relative influence of each of these intrinsic risk factors is still unclear.[22]

Pressure Ulcer Risk Assessment, Prevention, and Treatment

Pressure ulcer risk assessment. Based on targeted parameters, risk assessment aimed at identifying susceptible individuals is of utmost importance in daily clinical practice. Next to the overall clinical assessment of general health status and, related to this, the possible diseases affecting tissue perfusion and sensory perception (eg, cardiovascular diseases, diabetes, and neurological diseases), pressure ulcer risk assessment should be performed in a structured, interprofessional way and should include activity, mobility, the skin's viability and moisture, and nutritional status.

Pressure ulcer risk assessment scales can be used to support risk assessment. Several widely used risk assessment scales include the Waterlow pressure sore risk scale and the Braden scale, which consists of 6 items referring to sensory perception, skin moisture, activity, mobility, nutritional status, and the extent of friction and shear forces.[23,24] In scientific research, risk assessment scales in general appear to have a poor predictive value, yet the advice is to incorporate them in the daily care process because they can be regarded as a means of alerting healthcare professionals to the possibility of pressure ulcers. Their use indeed may lead to structural systematic assessment and a stimulus for treatment of pressure ulcer risk within the healthcare organization.

Pressure ulcer prevention.[22] After establishing pressure ulcer risk or pressure ulcer diagnosis, preventive measures should be initiated. Relevant preventive measures include:

- Regular inspection of the skin for signs of redness in individuals identified as being at risk of pressure ulceration together with the use of skin emollients to hydrate dry skin
- Reduction of the duration and magnitude of pressure on vulnerable areas of the body by repositioning at-risk individuals in combination with using pressure redistribution surfaces, such as mattresses, beds, seats, and cushions
- Optimization of the individual's general health condition, including improvement of mobility and nutritional status.

Pressure ulcer treatment.[22] In the case of a confirmed pressure ulcer, therapeutic measures must be taken directly and in agreement with an additional comprehensive assessment of the individual involved. During the course of the treatment, the aforementioned preventive measures remain in force.

Curative intervention consists primarily of appropriate wound care to encourage tissue repair as much as possible. This process includes cleaning the wound (removal of any necrosis, disinfection, and cleansing of the wound) and application of appropriate wound dressings. Sometimes surgical interventions may be indicated.

In addition, attention must be paid to the individual's general health status, the management of secondary infection, pain, and psychosocial suffering, and, last but not least, adequate nutritional care.

Basic Aspects of Wound Healing

Healing wounds is a complex process directly influenced by the status of the local wound environment and also by the overall physical condition of the individual. The wound healing process involves the overlapping sequential stages of blood coagulation, inflammation, migration and proliferation of defense and repair cells (eg, neutrophils, macrophages, lymphocytes, endothelial cells, fibroblasts, and keratinocytes), remodelling of tissue structure, scar formation, and maturation. To promote wound healing, several endogenous factors are crucial. One such factor is the body's ability to generate an adequate inflammatory and defense response to manage the bacterial burden of the wound and to create the required enzymatic environment needed for the various wound repair tasks. These tasks include prevention of ischemia-reperfusion damage and counteracting of oxidative damage; removal of devitalized tissue; prevention of cell migration; epidermal-mesenchymal interactions during keratinocyte migration; angiogenesis; remodelling of newly synthesized connective tissue during maturation; and regulation of growth factor activities. In the total process of wound repair, nutrients also play an important role.

Role of Nutrients in Wound Healing

Carbohydrates, fats, and proteins supply the energy source (kilocalories) for the body. Consumption of adequate kilocalories supports collagen and nitrogen synthesis for healing. External consumption also promotes anabolism by sparing the body's endogenous protein from being used as an energy source.[25] When the energy from carbohydrates and fats fails to meet the body's requirements, glucose is synthesized by the liver and kidney from non-carbohydrate sources, such as protein or amino acids. Gluconeogenesis occurs when the nitrogen is removed from the amino acid that is part of the protein structure leaving the carbon skeleton that can be used as an energy source by the body. When visceral protein stores in the muscle are converted to glucose, the caloric requirement needed to promote anabolism and reverse catabolism (a breakdown of protein and other body energy sources) is increased. The decline in lean body mass can lead to muscle wasting, loss of subcutaneous tissue, and poor wound healing.

Fat. Fat, the most concentrated source of kilocalories, transports the fat-soluble vitamins (A, D, E, and K) and provides insulation under the skin and padding to bony prominences. Meats, eggs, dairy products, and vegetable oils contain fat.

Protein and amino acids. Protein is the only nutrient containing nitrogen and is composed of amino acids that form the building blocks of protein. Protein is important for tissue perfusion, preservation of immune function, repair and synthesis of enzymes involved in wound healing, cell multiplication, and collagen and connective tissue synthesis. Protein is required to compensate for the nitrogen lost through pressure ulcer skin breakdown and exudate.[26]

Foods that provide all 9 essential amino acids, such as meat, poultry, fish, eggs, milk products, and soybeans, are considered complete proteins. Essential or indispensable amino acids must be obtained from the diet. The body requires an adequate supply of the essential amino acids plus enough nitrogen and energy to synthesize the 11 other amino acids. Legumes, grains, and vegetables contain incomplete proteins, meaning they are lacking or low in one or more of the essential amino acids.

During periods of stress or trauma, such as injury, wound healing, or sepsis, certain amino acids, such as arginine and glutamine, become conditionally essential. *L-arginine*, which is 32% nitrogen, has been shown in some studies to increase concentrations of hydroxyproline, which is an amino acid that is a constituent of collagen and an indicator of collagen deposition and protein in the wound site.[27,28] Desneves et al conducted a randomized controlled trial to measure pressure ulcer healing for 3 groups of subjects using the Pressure Ulcer Scale for Healing (PUSH) scores. One group received a standard hospital diet. A second group received the standard hospital diet plus 2 high-calorie supplements totalling 500 Kcalories, 18 g of protein, 72 mg of vitamin C, and 7.5 mg of zinc. The third group received the standard diet plus 2 high-calorie supplements totalling 500 Kcalories, 21 g of protein, 9 g of added arginine, 500 mg of vitamin C, and 50 mg of zinc. The third group noted a reduction in the PUSH score (indicating clinical improvement) when they consumed the oral nutritional supplement containing arginine.[29] This was a small study of 16 people. In a randomized controlled trial, van Anholt et al discovered significantly reduced PUSH scores and significantly faster wound healing in non-malnourished individuals aged 18 to 90 years with normal body mass indices (BMIs), no undesired weight loss, and stage III or stage IV pressure ulcers who received an oral nutritional supplement with arginine, protein, zinc, ascorbic acid, and vitamin E.[30] Additional research is needed to determine the impact of using arginine alone or combined with other nutrients.[31]

While it has been shown that inflammatory cells within the wound use *glutamine* for proliferation and as a source of energy, studies on the effectiveness of consuming supplements containing glutamine are inconclusive.[32]

Water. Water is distributed throughout the body in our intracellular, interstitial, and intravascular compartments and serves as the transport medium for moving nutrients to the cells and removing waste products. Fluids are the solvent for minerals, vitamins, amino acids, glucose, and other small molecules, thus enabling them to diffuse into and out of cells.

Individuals with draining wounds, emesis, diarrhea, increased insensible loss due to elevated temperature, or increased perspiration require additional fluids to replace lost fluid.[33] Water constitutes 60% of an adult's body. The elderly individual generally has increased body fat and decreased lean body mass, resulting in a decreased percentage of water stored. The decrease in water stored coupled with a declined sense of thirst places the elderly at risk for dehydration. Schols et al noted that illness and warm weather are contributing factors to dehydration in the elderly.[34] Hydration needs are met with liquids plus the water content of food, which accounts for 19% to 27% of the total fluid intake of healthy adults.[35] Adequate intake of fluids for healthy adults is 2.7 L/day for women and 3.7 L/day for men. This includes all beverages as well as the moisture content of food.

Vitamins and minerals. The role of micronutrients that are assumed to promote wound healing is debatable. Ascorbic acid (vitamin C), a water-soluble vitamin, is a cofactor with iron during the oxidation of proline and lysine in the production of collagen. Hence, a deficiency of vitamin C prolongs the healing time and contributes to reduced resistance to infection.[36] The Dietary Reference Intake (DRI) of 70–90 mg/day of vitamin C is achieved with the consumption of fruits and vegetables, such as citrus fruits, tomatoes, potatoes, and broccoli. Most oral nutritional supplements provide ascorbic acid along with calories, protein, and other vitamins and minerals. Mega doses of ascorbic acid have not resulted in accelerated pressure ulcer healing.[37]

Vitamin A and vitamin E are fat-soluble vitamins, and the dietary intake of these vitamins comes from a variety of foods. Vitamin A acts as a stimulant during the wound healing process to increase collagen formation and promote epithelization. Mega doses of vitamin A above 3,000 ug of the DRI's Tolerable Upper Limit (UL), the maximum level of daily nutrient intake that is likely not to pose concern, should not be recommended without consultation with the physician. Vitamin E acts as an antioxidant, and the DRI can easily be met with food and/or a multivitamin, unless a deficiency is confirmed.

Zinc, a cofactor for collagen formation, also metabolizes protein, liberates vitamin A from storage in the liver, and assists in immune function. Individuals who have large draining wounds, poor dietary intake over an extended time, or excessive gastrointestinal losses may trigger a zinc deficiency. Unless a deficiency is confirmed, elemental zinc supplementation, above the UL of 40 mg/day, is not recommended for individuals with pressure ulcers.[38,39] *Copper* is an essential mineral for collagen cross-linking. Zinc and copper compete for the same binding site on the albumin molecule, thus high serum zinc levels interfere with copper metabolism, inducing a copper deficiency.[40,41] If deficiencies are suspected, a multivitamin with minerals may be appropriate. Check the nutrient analysis of oral nutritional supplements or enteral formulas recommended to individuals with pressure ulcers, since they usually contain additional micronutrients.

Nutritional Screening and Assessment

Screening and assessment of nutritional status should be part of the prevention and treatment plan for individuals at risk for pressure ulcer development and those with pressure ulcers.

Nutritional screening. Unless the individual has a terminal illness, under-nutrition is a reversible risk factor for pressure ulcer development, making early identification and management critical. Individuals at risk for pressure ulcer development may also be in danger of under-nutrition, so nutritional screening should be completed.[17-20,26,42] Healthcare organizations should have a policy on nutritional screening and its frequency. Screening should be completed upon admission to a healthcare setting and with each condition change. Since individuals frequently move from one healthcare setting to another, the screening results must be documented and communicated from one care setting to another.[26,43] Screening tools should be quick and easy to use, validated, and reliable for the patient population served.[44] Any qualified healthcare professional may complete a screening. Validated screening tools are more widely used in Europe than in the United States. In a cross-sectional study, Langkamp-Henken et al noted an advantage to using the *Mini-Nutritional Assessment (MNA)* and the *MNA short form (MNA-SF)* over using visceral protein when screening and assessing nutritional status.[45,46] The MNA-SF was revised to 6 questions and revalidated for adults age 65 and older and has an 80% sensitivity and specificity and a 97% positive predictive value according to clinical status.[47] The *Malnutrition Universal Screening Tool (MUST)* was validated in acute care, long-term care, and the community and identifies those individuals who are underweight or at risk for under-nutrition.[48] The MUST tool uses

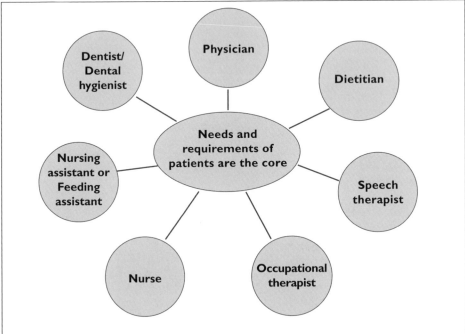

Physician:
- Diagnoses medical reasons for altered/disturbed nutritional status
- Responsible for ordering all medications and treatments

Dietitian:
- Completes nutrition assessment and estimates nutrition/hydration requirements
- Provides dietary recommendations and monitors nutritional status

Speech Therapist:
- Screens and evaluates chewing and swallowing ability
- Determines training compensation and recommends food/fluid consistency

Occupational Therapist:
- Assesses feeding skills and/or recommends techniques to improve motor skills
- Recommends appropriate position for eating and/or self-help feeding devices, ie, special utensils

Nurse:
- Monitors acceptance and tolerance of oral and/or enteral nutrition
- Alerts physician, dietitian, and patient of changes in nutritional status, such as meal refusal, and changes in weight or hydration status

Nursing Assistant or Feeding Assistant:
- Delivers food (trays) and provides feeding assistance, if needed
- Alerts nurse and/or other team members of refusal of or decline in oral intake

Dentist/Dental Hygienist:
- Assesses oral/dental status (eg, inflamed gums, oral lesions, denture problems)
- Offers oral healthcare

Figure 1. Nutrition for pressure ulcer prevention and treatment is interprofessional care.

5 steps to establish nutritional risk and determine a plan of care. First, the height and weight are recorded to determine BMI. In step 2, percentage of unplanned weight loss is recorded. In step 3, established acute disease effect is scored. In step 4, the previous 3 scores are added to obtain the overall risk of malnutrition, and step 5 uses either the management guide or local policy to develop

a plan of care.

When the screening tool triggers a nutrition assessment, timely referral to the appropriate professionals is critical. Conditions requiring immediate assessment and intervention include unplanned weight loss, dysphagia, poor appetite or the inability to consume adequate food or fluid, and pressure ulcers or other wounds. The registered dietitian (RD) completes the nutrition assessment and collaborates and communicates with the other healthcare team members. In addition to the RD, the members of the nutritional team include the speech therapist who is responsible for screening, evaluating, and treating swallowing problems; the occupational therapist who works to strengthen the individual's ability to feed him or herself; and the nursing staff whose responsibilities include monitoring factors, such as mood, pain, and dentition, which can affect oral intake. The physician is responsible for the overall care of the individual and ordering any treatments recommended by the team (Figure 1).

Nutrition assessment. Nutrition assessment is a methodical process of obtaining, verifying, and interpreting data in order to make decisions about the basis of nutrition-related problems. The American Dietetic Association (ADA) Nutrition Care Process includes 4 steps:
- Nutrition assessment
- Nutrition diagnosis
- Nutrition intervention
- Nutrition monitoring and evaluation.[49]

The assessment includes obtaining anthropometric measurements; evaluating visual signs of poor nutrition, oral status, chewing/swallowing ability, and/or diminished ability to eat independently; and interpreting and analyzing medical, nutritional, and biochemical data along with food-medication interactions.

Anthropometrics. Anthropometric measurements include height, weight, and BMI. Obtaining accurate height and weight is important, since these values are the basis for calculating BMI and caloric requirements. Individuals should be weighed on a calibrated scale at the same time of the day and wearing the same amount of clothing. Specialty beds often are equipped with a device to weigh an immobile individual. The RD evaluates the severity of the weight loss, considering the effect of recent surgery, diuretic therapy, and other traumatic events. Significant weight loss places an individual at increased nutritional risk and has a negative effect on wound healing. Several studies support the theory that *unintentional weight loss of 5% in 30 days or 10% in 180 days is a predictor of mortality in the elderly.*[50–53] During the interview with the individual or care-giver, the RD/clinician asks what the usual body weight has been over the past few months. Usual body weight is used to calculate the percentage of weight lost or gained over time thus determining the significance of any weight change.

BMI, an index of an individual's weight in relationship to his or her height, is calculated as weight (kg)/height (m^2), or weight (lb)/height (in^2) x 705. BMI is highly correlated with body fat, but increased lean body mass or a large body frame can also increase the BMI. It is generally agreed that a normally hydrated individual with a BMI $\geq$ 30 is obese and an individual with a BMI less than 20 is considered underweight. The National Pressure Ulcer Long Term Care Study (NPULS) of residents in nursing homes who were at risk for developing a pressure ulcer reported that more than 50% of the residents had a 5% weight loss during a 12-week study, and 45.6% were considered underweight (defined by a BMI of 22 or less). Residents with the highest percentage of weight loss more often had a recent pressure ulcer.[54] Under-nutrition has been defined in the literature as protein and energy deficiency often associated with coexisting deficiencies of micronutrients, which is reversed solely by nutrients.[55] Unintentional weight loss, poor food intake, and the inability to eat independently impact the healing process.[56]

The obese individual is also at risk for pressure ulcer development, and healing may be delayed when the diet consumed is inadequate in nutrients, including protein. When pressure ulcer healing is the goal, the interprofessional team should evaluate the risks versus the benefits of recommending a low-calorie diet.

Nutrition-focused clinical examination. The interprofessional team, including the RD, should examine the individual for physical signs of under-nutrition and protein depletion as evidenced by changes in the hair, skin, or nails, such as thin, dry hair; brittle nails; or cracked lips. Individuals with missing or decayed teeth or ill-fitting dentures often reduce their intake of difficult-to-chew protein foods, thus restricting their caloric intake and increasing the chance for weight loss. If untreated, individuals with swallowing problems or dysphagia may become dehydrated, lose weight, and develop pressure ulcers. Loss of dexterity and/or the ability to self-feed is a risk factor

Table 1. Recommendations of the NPUAP/EPUAP Guideline[22]

Adapted with permission of the European Pressure Ulcer Advisory Panel and the National Pressure Ulcer Advisory Panel. Prevention and treatment of pressure ulcers: quick reference guide. Washington, DC: National Pressure Ulcer Advisory Panel; 2009.

Nutrition for Pressure Ulcer Prevention

General Recommendations

1. Screen and assess the nutritional status of every individual at risk for pressure ulcer development in each healthcare setting.
    1.1. Use a valid, reliable, and practical tool for nutritional screening that is quick and easy to use and acceptable to both the individual and the healthcare worker.
    1.2. Establish and implement a nutritional screening policy in all healthcare settings, along with recommended frequency of screening.
2. Refer each individual with nutritional risk and pressure ulcer risk to a registered dietitian and also, if needed, to a multidisciplinary nutritional team that includes a registered dietitian, a nurse specializing in nutrition, a physician, a speech and language therapist, an occupational therapist, and, when necessary, a dentist.
    2.1. Provide nutritional support to each individual with nutritional risk and pressure ulcer risk, following the nutrition cycle. This support should include:
        • Nutritional assessment
        • Estimation of nutritional requirements
        • Comparison of nutrient intake with estimated requirements
        • Provision of appropriate nutritional intervention, based on appropriate feeding route
        • Monitoring and evaluation of nutritional outcome, with reassessment of nutritional status at frequent intervals while the individual is at risk.
    2.2. Follow relevant and evidence-based guidelines on enteral nutrition and hydration for individuals at risk for pressure ulcer development who show nutritional risk or nutritional problems.
    2.3. Offer each individual with nutritional risk and pressure ulcer risk a minimum of 30–35 kcal/kg/day, with 1.25–1.5 g/kg/day protein and 1 mL of liquid intake per kcal per day

Specific Recommendations: Nutrition Prevention

1. Offer high-protein mixed oral nutritional supplements and/or tube feeding, in addition to the usual diet, to individuals with nutritional risk and pressure ulcer risk because of acute or chronic diseases or following surgical intervention (strength of evidence = A).
    1.1. Administer oral nutritional supplements and/or tube feeding in between the regular meals to avoid reduction of normal food and fluid intake during regular mealtimes (strength of evidence = C).

often resulting in poor oral intake. All of these conditions are roadblocks to wound healing.

Biochemical data. Analysis of current laboratory values is one component of the nutrition assessment. Biochemical assessment data must be used with caution because values can be altered by hydration, medication, and changes in metabolism. There is not one specific laboratory test that can expressly determine an individual's nutritional status. Serum hepatic proteins including albumin, prealbumin (transthyretin), and transferrin may not correlate with the clinical observa-

tion of nutritional status.[57] Serum albumin has a long half-life (12–21 days), and multiple factors, such as infection, acute stress, hydration, and excess cortisone, decrease the albumin level, making it a poor indicator of visceral protein status. Edema depresses albumin levels and dehydration falsely elevates both prealbumin and albumin levels. Low albumin levels may manifest the presence of inflammatory cytokine production or other comorbidities rather than poor nutritional status (eg, from the local wound bed or a systemic inflammatory process).[58] Prealbumin also decreases

Table 1. Recommendations of the NPUAP/EPUAP Guideline[22] *continued*

Adapted with permission of the European Pressure Ulcer Advisory Panel and the National Pressure Ulcer Advisory Panel. Prevention and treatment of pressure ulcers: quick reference guide. Washington, DC: National Pressure Ulcer Advisory Panel; 2009.

Nutrition for Pressure Ulcer Healing

Role of Nutrition in Pressure Ulcer Healing

1. Screen and assess nutritional status for each individual with a pressure ulcer at admission and with each condition change and/or when progress toward pressure ulcer closure is not observed (strength of evidence = C).

    1.1. Refer all individuals with pressure ulcers to the dietitian for early assessment and intervention for nutritional problems (strength of evidence = C).

    1.2. Assess weight status for each individual to determine weight history and significant weight loss from usual body weight (≥ 5% change in 30 days or ≥ 10% in 180 days) (strength of evidence = C).

    1.3. Assess the individual's ability to eat independently (strength of evidence = C).

    1.4. Assess the adequacy of total nutrient intake (food, fluid, oral supplements, enteral/parenteral feedings) (strength of evidence = C).

2. Provide sufficient calories (strength of evidence = B).

    2.1. Provide 30–35 kcal/kg for individuals with a pressure ulcer under stress. Adjust formula based on weight loss, weight gain, or level of obesity. Individuals who are underweight or who have had significant unintentional weight loss may need additional kilocalories to cease weight loss and/or regain lost weight (strength of evidence = C).

    2.2. Revise and modify (liberalize) dietary restrictions when limitations result in decreased food and fluid intake. These adjustments are to be managed by a dietitian or medical professional (strength of evidence = C).

    2.3. Provide enhanced foods and/or oral supplements between meals if needed (strength of evidence = B).

    2.4. Consider nutritional support (enteral or parenteral nutrition) when oral intake is inadequate. This must be consistent with the individual's goals (strength of evidence = C).

3. Provide adequate protein for positive nitrogen balance for an individual with a pressure ulcer (strength of evidence = B).

    3.1. Offer 1.25–1.5 g/kg/day protein for an individual with a pressure ulcer when compatible with the goals of care and reassess as condition changes (strength of evidence = C).

    3.2. Assess renal function to ensure that high levels of protein are appropriate for the individual (strength of evidence = C).

4. Provide and encourage adequate daily fluid intake for hydration (level of evidence = C).

    4.1. Monitor individuals for signs and symptoms of dehydration: changes in weight, skin turgor, urine output, elevated serum sodium, or calculated serum osmolality (strength of evidence = C).

    4.2. Provide additional fluid for individuals with dehydration, elevated temperature, vomiting, profuse sweating, diarrhea, or heavily draining wounds (strength of evidence = C).

5. Provide adequate vitamins and minerals (strength of evidence = B).

    5.1. Encourage consumption of a balanced diet that includes good sources of vitamins and minerals (strength of evidence = B).

    5.2. Offer vitamin and mineral supplements when dietary intake is poor or deficiencies are confirmed or suspected (strength of evidence = B).

with metabolic stress, inflammation, infection, and surgical trauma. Studies indicate that hepatic proteins may correlate with the severity of illness rather than with nutritional status.[58-65]

Since the blood carries oxygen to the wound bed, anemia may have an adverse effect on wound healing. Blood loss, poor dietary intake, malabsorption, and increased iron needs are causes of anemia. Biochemical data used to diagnose iron-deficiency anemia include low hemoglobin and hematocrit, low mean corpuscular volume (MCV), low serum iron, low ferritin, and elevated total iron-binding capacity (TIBC). Treatment for iron-deficiency anemia is oral iron therapy.

Older adults often have pernicious anemia or *vitamin B12 deficiency* that is caused by inadequate intrinsic factor. The prevalence of anemia[66] increases with each decade of life after age 70. Without adequate intrinsic factor, vitamin B12 cannot be properly absorbed. Laboratory results include low hemoglobin, hematocrit, and serum B12; normal or elevated MCV; and elevated serum iron, ferritin, folate, and homocysteine. There are several ways to supply vitamin B12, but the monthly injection is most effective. Some individuals with low B12 levels respond to daily intake of oral B12 with the suggested dose of 1000 IU or to the use of nasal sprays or patches.

Diet history. The *diet history* includes consultation with the individual and/or caregivers to determine the type, quantity, and frequency of food usually consumed by the individual. Questions about any vitamin, mineral, or herbal supplements taken by the individual should also be noted. The healthcare team should consider any factors that may influence the individual's decision about nutrition, such as culture, tradition, religion, and belief systems of ethnic and minority groups. Often, culture or religion strongly influence food intake and may affect nutritional status. Since the individual is the center of the wound care model, recommendations for nutritional interventions should incorporate the values and beliefs of the individual.

Nutrition Intervention

Ultimately, the nutrition assessment will lead to a nutrition diagnosis and nutritional support.

The cycle for both prevention and treatment should include:
- Nutrition assessment
- Estimation of nutritional requirements
- Comparisons of intake with estimated requirements
- Provision of appropriate nutrition intervention, based on appropriate feeding route
- Monitoring and evaluation of nutritional outcome, with reassessment of nutritional status at frequent intervals.

Early nutrition intervention and subsequent monitoring of the nutritional plan can reverse poor outcomes associated with under-nutrition and promote healing. Caloric, protein, and fluid requirements should be individualized and increased or decreased, depending on the assessed requirement of the individual. Hypermetabolic conditions, such as infection, stress, and trauma, require calories above the baseline requirements. *Renal function should be assessed routinely to ensure that high levels of protein are appropriate.*[67] The interprofessional team should frequently review the type and amount of food and fluid consumed by the individual to determine when fortified foods and/or oral nutritional supplements should be incorporated into the treatment plan. Fortified foods include commercial products, such as cereal, soup, cookies, or dairy products enriched with additional calories and protein, or enriched menu items prepared by the staff of a care facility.

Research supports the theory of providing oral nutritional supplements to reverse under-nutrition, prevent pressure ulcer occurrence, and promote pressure ulcer healing.[68-70] As previously noted, *oral nutritional supplements* provided in addition to the diet for non-malnourished individuals also decreased the healing time.[30] One study noted that individuals who consume oral nutritional supplements between meals, in addition to the usual diet, experience better absorption of nutrients.[71]

Therapeutic or restricted diets often result in unappealing meals that are refused, thus delaying wound healing. The American Dietetic Association's 2010 position statement noted that "the quality of life and nutritional status of older adults residing in healthcare communities can be enhanced by individualization to the least restrictive diet appropriate."[72]

When normal oral intake is inadequate to promote healing, *enteral or parenteral nutrition* is considered if it is consistent with the individual's goal of overall treatment. The interprofessional team should discuss the risks and benefits with the individual or his or her caregiver. When the gut is functioning, enteral feeding via oral nutritional supplements in addition to the diet or total tube feeding is the preferred route. Provision of an adequate nutrient supply can lower the incidence of metabolic abnormalities, reduce septic morbidity, and improve survival rates. However, research fails to show the benefit of initiating enteral tube feeding to improve pressure ulcer healing rates.[73,74]

The *NPUAP/EPUAP guideline* on prevention and treatment of pressure ulcers is the most recently published international guideline on pressure ulcer care.[22] The guideline was developed following a systematic, comprehensive review of peer-reviewed, published research on pressure ulcers from January 1998 to January 2008 and will be updated routinely as new research becomes available. This guideline also gives the most relevant recommendations regarding nutritional care for individuals prone to pressure ulcer development (Table 1).

Conclusion

Nutrition is a key element in pressure ulcer prevention and the treatment of individuals with pressure ulcers. The early identification of under-nutrition and the correction of nutritional deficits prevent pressure ulcer occurrence, promote pressure ulcer healing, and improve the individual's quality of life. Nutritional care has to be incorporated into integrated and multidisciplinary pressure ulcer care, performed by a dedicated interprofessional team. In order to achieve optimal nutrition for each individual prone to pressure ulcer development, goals should be evaluated frequently and revised with each condition change or when progress toward healing is not occurring. The amount and type of nutritional support should be consistent with medical goals and the individual's wishes. While each member of the interprofessional team has a distinct role in the care and treatment of the individual prone to pressure ulcer development, collaboration, communication, complementariness, and continuity are fundamental to benefit the individuals involved.

Take-Home Messages for Practice
- Screen and assess the nutritional status of individuals at risk for or with pressure ulcers and determine appropriate interventions.
- Encourage consumption of a balanced diet, which includes good sources of calories, protein, vitamins, and minerals.
- Provide enriched food and/or oral nutritional supplements between meals, if appropriate and consistent with the person's overall plan of care.

Self-Assessment Questions

1. The appropriate daily kilocalories for an individual with a category/stage IV pressure ulcer weighing 120 pounds (54.5 kg) is:
   A. 1,100 kilocalories
   B. 1,650 kilocalories
   C. 1,909 kilocalories
   D. 1,275 kilocalories

2. The non-malnourished individual with a category/stage III pressure ulcer may benefit from:
   A. An oral nutritional supplement with calories, protein, vitamin A, and copper
   B. A balanced 2,200 kilocalorie diet plus a vitamin supplement
   C. A 1,200 kilocalorie diet plus 1,000 mg of ascorbic acid and 220 mg of zinc sulfate
   D. An oral nutritional supplement with added protein, arginine, zinc, vitamin C, and vitamin E

3. Mr. B has a wound infection, a draining pressure ulcer, and a fever. Wound healing can be facilitated by increasing:
   A. Fluid
   B. Vitamin C
   C. Iron
   D. Protein

Answers: 1-C, 2-D, 3-A

References

1. Vanderwee K, Clark M, Dealey C, Gunningberg L, Defloor T. Pressure ulcer prevalence in Europe: a pilot study. *J Eval Clin Pract*. 2007;13(2):227–235.
2. National Pressure Ulcer Advisory Panel. Cuddigan J, Ayello EA, Sussman C, eds. *Pressure Ulcers in America:*

Prevalence, Incidence, and Implications for the Future. Reston, VA: NPUAP; 2001.

3. Russo CA, Steiner C, Spector W. Hospitalizations related to pressure ulcers among adults 18 years and older, 2006. Available at: http://www.hcup-us.ahrq.gov/reports/statbriefs/sb64.jsp. Accessed December 22, 2008.

4. Hopkins A, Dealey C, Bale S, Defloor T, Worboys F. Patient stories of living with a pressure ulcer. *J Adv Nurs.* 2006;56(4):345–353.

5. Allman RM, Goode PS, Burst N, Bartolucci AA, Thomas DR. Pressure ulcers, hospital complications, and disease severity: impact on hospital costs and length of stay. *Adv Wound Care.* 1999;12(1):22–30.

6. Severens JL, Habraken JM, Duivenvoorden S, Frederiks CM. The cost of illness of pressure ulcers in The Netherlands. *Adv Skin Wound Care.* 2005;15(2):72–77.

7. Bennet G, Dealey C, Posnett J. The cost of pressure ulcers in the UK. *Age Ageing.* 2004;33(3):230–235.

8. Centers for Medicare & Medicaid Services. Proposed fiscal year 2009 payment, policy changes for inpatient stays in general acute care hospitals. Available at: http://www.cms.hhs.gov/apps/media/press/factsheet.asp?Counter=3045&intNumPerPage=10&checkDate=&checkKey=&srchType=1&numDays=3500&srchOpt=0&srchData=&keywordType=All&chkNewsType=6&intPage=&showAll=&pYear=&year=&desc=&cboOrder=date. Accessed December 3, 2008.

9. Centers for Medicare & Medicaid Services. Medicare program; proposed changes to the hospital inpatient prospective payment systems and fiscal year 2009 rates; proposed changes to disclosure of physician ownership in hospitals and physician self-referral rules; proposed collection of information regarding financial relationships between hospitals and physicians; proposed rule. Federal Register. 2008;73(84):23550. Available at: http://edocket.access.gpo.gov/2008/pdf/08-1135.pdf. Accessed December 3, 2008.

10. Dorner B, Posthauer ME, Thomas D; National Pressure Ulcer Advisory Panel. The role of nutrition in pressure ulcer prevention and treatment: National Pressure Ulcer Advisory Panel white paper. *Adv Skin Wound Care.* 2009;22(5):212–221.

11. Voss AC, Bender SA, Ferguson ML, Sauer AC, Bennett RG, Hahn PW. Long-term care liability for pressure ulcers. *J Am Geriatr Soc.* 2005;53(9):1587–1592.

12. Pinchcofsky-Devin GD, Kaminski MV Jr. Correlation of pressure sores and nutritional status. *J Am Geriatr Soc.* 1986;34(6):435–440.

13. Thomas DR. The role of nutrition in prevention and healing of pressure ulcers. *Clin Geriatr Med.* 1997;13(3):497–511.

14. Berlowitz DR, Wilking SV. Risk factors for pressure sores. A comparison of cross-sectional and cohort-derived data. *J Am Geriatr Soc.* 1989;37(11):1043–1050.

15. Green SM, Winterberg H, Franks PJ, Moffatt CJ, Eberhardie C, McLaren S. Nutritional intake in community patients with pressure ulcers. *J Wound Care.* 1999;8(7):325–330.

16. Guenter P, Malyszek R, Bliss DZ, et al. Survey of nutritional status in newly hospitalized patients with stage III or stage IV pressure ulcers. *Adv Skin Wound Care.*

2000;13(4 Pt 1):164–168.

17. Thomas DR, Verdery RB, Gardner L, Kant A, Lindsay J. A prospective study of outcome from protein-energy malnutrition in nursing home residents. *JPEN J Parenter Enteral Nutr.* 1991;15(4):400–404.

18. Mathus-Vliegen EMH. Clinical observations: nutritional status, nutrition, and pressure ulcers. *Nutr Clin Pract.* 2001;16:286–291.

19. Ek AC, Unosson M, Larsson J, Von Schenck H, Bjurulf P. The development and healing of pressure sores related to the nutritional state. *Clin Nutr.* 1991;10(5):245–250.

20. Kerstetter JE, Holthausen BA, Fitz PA. Malnutrition in the institutionalized older adult. *J Am Diet Assoc.* 1992;92(9):1109–1116.

21. Shahin ES, Meijers JM, Schols JM, Tannen A, Halfens RJ, Dassen T. The relationship between malnutrition parameters and pressure ulcers in hospitals and nursing homes. *Nutrition.* 2010;26(9):886–889.

22. National Pressure Ulcer Advisory Panel and European Pressure Ulcer Advisory Panel. Prevention and treatment of pressure ulcers: clinical practice guideline. Washington, DC: NPUAP; 2009.

23. Bergstrom N, Braden BJ, Laguzza A, Holman V. The Braden Scale for Predicting Pressure Sore Risk. *Nurs Res.* 1987;36(4):205–210.

24. Jalali R, Rezaie M. Predicting pressure ulcer risk: comparing the predictive validity of 4 scales. *Adv Skin Wound Care.* 2005;18(2):92–97.

25. Clark M, Schols JM, Benati G, et al; European Pressure Ulcer Advisory Panel. Pressure ulcers and nutrition: a new European guideline. *J Wound Care.* 2004;13(7):267–272.

26. Stratton RJ, Green CJ, Elia M. *Disease-Related Malnutrition: An Evidence-Based Approach to Treatment.* Oxon, UK: CABI Publishing; 2003.

27. Kirk SJ, Hurson M, Regan MC, Holt DR, Wasserkrug HL, Barbul A. Arginine stimulates wound healing and immune function in elderly human beings. *Surgery.* 1993;114(2):155–160.

28. Barbul A, Lazarou SA, Efron DT, Wasserkrug HL, Efron G. Arginine enhances wound healing and lymphocyte immune responses in humans. *Surgery.* 1990;108(2):331–337.

29. Desneves KJ, Todorovic BE, Cassar A, Crowe TC. Treatment with supplementary arginine, vitamin C and zinc in patients with pressure ulcers: a randomised controlled trial. *Clin Nutr.* 2005;24(6):979–987.

30. van Anholt RD, Sobotka L, Meijer EP, et al. Specific nutritional support accelerates pressure ulcer healing and reduces wound care intensity in non-malnourished patients. *Nutrition.* 2010;26(9):867–872.

31. Langer G, Schloemer G, Knerr A, Kuss O, Behrens J. Nutritional interventions for preventing and treating pressure ulcers. *Cochrane Database Syst Rev.* 2003;(4):CD003216.

32. Ziegler TR, Benfell K, Smith RJ, et al. Safety and metabolic effects of L-glutamine administration in humans. *JPEN J Parenter Enteral Nutr.* 1990;14(4 Suppl):137S–146S.

33. Thomas DR, Cote TR, Lawhorne L, et al; Dehydra-

tion Council. Understanding clinical dehydration and its treatment. *J Am Med Dir Assoc.* 2008;9(5):292–301.

34. Schols JM, De Groot CP, van der Cammen TJ, Olde Rikkert MG. Preventing and treating dehydration in the elderly during periods of illness and warm weather. *J Nutr Health Aging.* 2009;13(2):150–157.

35. Institute of Medicine of the National Academies. Dietary Reference Intakes: Water, Potassium, Sodium, Chloride, and Sulfate. Available at: http://iom.edu/Reports/2004/Dietary-Reference-Intakes-Water-Potassium-Sodium-Chloride-and-Sulfate.aspx. Accessed June 5, 2010.

36. Ronchetti IP, Quaglino D Jr, Bergamini G. Ascorbic acid and connective tissue. In: Harris JR, ed. *Subcellular Biochemistry Volume 25 Ascorbic Acid: Biochemistry and Biomedical Cell Biology.* New York: Plenum Press; 1996:249–264.

37. Ter Riet G, Kessels AG, Knipschild PG. Randomized clinical trial of ascorbic acid in the treatment of pressure ulcers. *J Clin Epidemiol.* 1195;48(12):1453–1460.

38. Institute of Medicine of the National Academies. *Dietary Reference Intakes: The Essential Guide to Nutrient Requirements.* Washington, DC: The National Academies; 2006.

39. Cataldo CB, DeBruyne LK, Whitney EN. *Nutrition and Diet Therapy, Principles and Practice.* Belmonth, CA: Wadsworth; 2003.

40. Reed BR, Clark RA. Cutaneous tissue repair: practical implications of current knowledge. II. *J Am Acad Dermatol.* 1985;13(6):919–941.

41. Goode HF, Burns E, Walker BE. Vitamin C depletion and pressure sores in elderly patients with femoral neck fracture. *BMJ.* 1992;305(6859):925–927.

42. Elia M, Zellipour L, Stratton RJ. To screen or not to screen for adult malnutrition? *Clin Nutr.* 2005;24(6):867–884.

43. Kondrup J, Allison SP, Elia M, Vellas B, Plauth M; Educational and Clinical Practice Committee, European Society of Parenteral and Enteral Nutrition (ESPEN). ESPEN guidelines for nutrition screening 2002. *Clin Nutr.* 2003;22(4):415–421.

44. Ferguson M, Capra S, Bauer J, Banks M. Development of a valid and reliable malnutrition screening tool for adult acute hospital patients. *Nutrition.* 1999;15(6):458–464.

45. Langkamp-Henken B, Hudgens J, Stechmiller JK, Herrlinger-Garcia KA. Mini nutritional assessment and screening scores are associated with nutritional indicators in elderly people with pressure ulcers. *J Am Diet Assoc.* 2005;105(10):1590–1596.

46. Hudgens J, Langkamp-Henken B, Stechmiller JK, Herrlinger-Garcia KA, Nieves C. Immune function is impaired with a mini nutritional assessment score indicative of malnutrition in nursing home elders with pressure ulcers. *JPEN J Parenter Enteral Nutr.* 2004;28(6):416–422.

47. Kaiser MJ, Bauer JM, Ramsch C, et al; MNA-International Group. Validation of the Mini Nutritional Assessment short-form (MNA-SF): a practical tool for identification of nutritional status. *J Nutr Health Aging.* 2009;13(9):782–788.

48. BAPEN (British Association of Parenteral and Enteral Nutrition) Malnutrition Advisory Group, The MUST Report, Nutritional screening of adults: a multidisciplinary responsibility. Available at: http://www.bapen.org.uk/must_tool.html. Accessed June 3, 2011.

49. American Dietetic Association. *International Dietetics & Nutrition Terminology (IDNT) Reference Manual: Standardized Language for the Nutrition Care Process.* 3rd ed. Chicago, IL: The American Dietetic Association; 2011.

50. Landi F, Onder G, Gambassi G, Pedone C, Carbonin P, Bernabei R. Body mass index and mortality among hospitalized patients. *Arch Intern Med.* 2000;160(17):2641–2644.

51. Ryan C, Bryant E, Eleazer P, Rhodes A, Guest K. Unintentional weight loss in long-term care: predictor of mortality in the elderly. *South Med J.* 1995;88(7):721–724.

52. Sullivan DH, Johnson LE, Bopp MM, Roberson PK. Prognostic significance of monthly weight fluctuations among older nursing home residents. *J Gerontol A Biol Sci Med Sci.* 2004;59(6):M633–M639.

53. Murden RA, Ainslie NK. Recent weight loss is related to short-term mortality in nursing homes. *J Gen Intern Med.* 1994;9(11):648–650.

54. Horn SD, Bender SA, Bergstrom N, et al. Description of the National Pressure Ulcer Long-Term Care Study. *J Am Geriatr Soc.* 2002;50(11):1816–1825.

55. ASPEN Board of Directors and the Clinical Guidelines Task Force. Guidelines for the use of parenteral and enteral nutrition in adult and pediatric patients. *JPEN J Parenter Enteral Nutr.* 2002;26(1 Suppl):1SA–138SA.

56. Gilmore SA, Robinson G, Posthauer ME, Raymond J. Clinical indicators associated with unintentional weight loss and pressure ulcers in elderly residents of nursing facilities. *J Am Diet Assoc.* 1995;95(9):984–992.

57. Myron Johnson A, Merlini G, Sheldon J, Ichihara K; Scientific Division Committee on Plasma Proteins (C-PP), International Federation of Clinical Chemistry and Laboratory Medicine (IFCC). Clinical indications for plasma protein assays: transthyretin (prealbumin) in inflammation and malnutrition. *Clin Chem Lab Med.* 2007;45(3):419–426.

58. Mahan LK, Escott-Stump S, eds. *Krause's Food, Nutrition, & Diet Therapy.* St Louis, MO: WB Saunders (Elsevier); 2008.

59. Shenkin A. Serum prealbumin: Is it a marker of nutritional status or of risk of malnutrition? *Clin Chem.* 2006;52(12):2177–2179.

60. Lim SH, Lee JS, Chae SH, Ahn BS, Chang DJ, Shin CS. Prealbumin is not a sensitive indicator of nutrition and prognosis in critical ill patients. *Yonsei Med J.* 2005;46(1):21–26.

61. Robinson MK, Trujillo EB, Mogensen KM, Rounds J, McManus K, Jacobs DO. Improving nutritional screening of hospitalized patients: the role of prealbumin. *JPEN J Parenter Enteral Nutr.* 2003;27(6):389–395.

62. Bachrach-Lindstrom M, Unosson M, Ek AC, Arnqvist HJ. Assessment of nutritional status using biochemical and anthropometric variables in a nutritional intervention study of women with hip fracture. *Clin Nutr.* 2001;20(3):217–223.

63. Fuhrman MP, Charney P, Mueller CM. Hepatic proteins and nutrition assessment. *J Am Diet Assoc.* 2004;104(8):1258–1264.

64. Steinman TI. Serum albumin: its significance in patients with ESRD. *Semin Dial.* 2000;13(6):404–408.

65. Dutton J, Campbell H, Tanner J, Richards N. Pre-dialysis serum albumin is a poor indicator of nutritional status in stable chronic hemodialysis patients. *EDTNA ERCA J.* 1999;25(1):36–37.

66. American Medical Directors Association (AMDA). *Anemia in the Long-Term Care Setting.* Columbia, MD: American Medical Directors Association; 2007.

67. Clinical practice guidelines for nutrition in chronic renal failure. K/DOQI, National Kidney Foundation. *Am J Kidney Dis.* 2000;35(6 Suppl 2):S1–S140.

68. Horn SD, Bender SA, Ferguson ML, et al. The National Pressure Ulcer Long-Term Care Study: pressure ulcer development in long-term care residents. *J Am Geriatr Soc.* 2004;52(3):359–367.

69. Bergstrom N, Horn SD, Smout RJ, et al. The National Pressure Ulcer Long-Term Care Study: outcomes of pressure ulcer treatments in long-term care. *J Am Geri-atr Soc.* 2005;53(10):1721–1729.

70. Bourdel-Marchasson I, Barateau M, Rondeau V, et al. A multi-center trial of the effects of oral nutritional supplementation in critically ill older inpatients. *Nutrition.* 2000;16(1):1–5.

71. Wilson MM, Purushothaman R, Morley JE. Effect of liquid dietary supplements on energy intake in the elderly. *Am J Clin Nutr.* 2002;75(5):944–947.

72. Dorner B, Friedrich EK, Posthauer ME; American Dietetic Association. Position of the American Dietetic Association: individualized nutrition approaches for older adults in health care communities. *J Am Diet Assoc.* 2010;110(10):1549–1553.

73. Henderson CT, Trumbore LS, Mobarhan S, Benya R, Miles TP. Prolonged tube feeding in long-term care: nutritional status and clinical outcomes. *J Am Coll Nutr.* 1992;11(3):309–325.

74. Mitchell SL, Kiely DK, Lipsitz LA. The risk factors and impact on survival of feeding tube placement in nursing home residents with severe cognitive impairment. *Arch Intern Med.* 1997;157(3):327–332.

CHAPTER 12

The Development of Wound Management Products

Sarah M.E. Cockbill, PhD, LL.M, B.Pharm, M.Pharm, DAgVetPharm, MIPharmM, FCPP, FRPharmS; **Terence D. Turner**, OBE, FRPharmS, MPharm

Objectives

The reader will be challenged to:

- Distinguish between passive, interactive, and bioactive products
- Analyze the characteristics of an ideal wound dressing
- Review the development of products for wound management.

Introduction

Throughout history, many diverse materials of animal, vegetable, and mineral origin have been used to treat wounds. They range from the hot oils and waxes reported in the Ebers papyrus[1] to the animal membranes and feces of the Middle Ages to the picked oakum of the 19th century. Some of these products have survived; both absorbent cotton and Gamgee tissue were as familiar to the surgeon of 1880 as they are to the physician of today. The first monographs related to wound dressing materials appeared in early London and Edinburgh hospital dispensatories followed later by the British Pharmaceutical Codices and the British Pharmacopoeia.[2] Information relating to the development of wound management products is reflected in similar publications in the United States Pharmacopoeia and in other national standards.

Until 1960, advances in the design and efficacy of wound management products had been spasmodic and limited to the adaptation of available materials that were being used for other purposes. The older products (eg, absorbent cotton, lint, and gauze) were primarily of the plug-and-conceal variety and could be considered *passive* products that took no part in the healing process. Little attention was paid to the functional performance of a product, and minimal consideration was given to the healing environments required for different wound types.

A new generation of products was potentiated by the advances in knowledge of the humoral and cellular factors associated with the healing process and the realization that a

Cockbill SME, Turner TD. The development of wound management products. In: Krasner DL, ed. *Chronic Wound Care: The Essentials.* Malvern, Pa: HMP Communications, 2014:145–164.

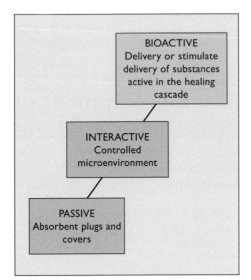

Figure 1. Classification of wound management product activity.

controlled microenvironment at the wound surface was needed if wound healing was to progress at the optimal level. These environmental control dressings are classified as *interactive* dressings; current developments are directed at bioactive products (Figure 1), which will directly or indirectly stimulate some part of the healing cascade (Figure 2) and optimize the wound microenvironment to allow the free movement of cells, cytokines, and growth factors involved in the healing process.

This chapter surveys the progressive development of wound management products and offers performance profiles for different product groups with their possible clinical usage. The ever-increasing new product appearance in the medical market, many of which are "me-too" duplicates of other products, precludes the use of brand names and allows a broader perspective of the advances in real-term formulations.

Linteum and Oakum

Linteum was the first woven fabric to be recognized as a surgical material. In 1816, William Cade King, Governor of St. Bartholomew's Hospital, London, presented a sample of patent lint to the House Committee to consider its adoption within the hospital.[3] It consisted of a cloth that had its nap raised on one side by scraping with

a knife to produce a soft pile. With the advent of the Crimean War came power-driven machines, which stimulated William Bradbury Robinson of Chesterfield, England to produce a lint machine that could produce an amount of woven material equal to 6 people working on hand machines. The lint was also bleached and purified. It was often formed into dossils (cylindrical pieces), pledgets (oval shaped), and boulsters or tents (conical compresses).

In 1819, Abraham Rees summarized the uses as follows:[4]

1. To stop blood in fresh wounds by filling with dry lint—in large hemorrhages, dip lint into alcohol or oil of turpentine
2. To agglutinate and heal wounds when spread with ointments
3. To dry wounds and ulcers, thus forwarding the formulation of a cicatrix
4. To keep the tops of wounds at proper distance so that they do not hastily unite before the bottom is well digested and healed
5. To prevent the access of air.

He added, "that when used to dress deep wounds a thread should be tied to each portion before insertion to assist in its removal." This product was used with minimal modification for more than 100 years.

A similar development on fibrous materials was to be initiated by another war stimulus (Table 1). Dr. Lewis A. Sayre of New York wrote enthusiastically about the use of oakum in the American Civil War.[1] This was a fibrous mass produced by shredding tarred or untarred rope, the former sometimes being referred to as marine lint (a name also retained for tow impregnated with fresh Stockholm tar). An edition of *The Lancet*[5] in 1870 reported that it "absorbs discharges, destroys bad odors, and supersedes the use of lint, ointments, and linseed meal or bread poultices." Picking oakum was often considered good occupational therapy for prisoners, with obvious difficulties in producing good and reproducible quality. In 1871, Southall Son and Dymond, manufacturing chemists of Birmingham, England, reduced selected quality rope to oakum. Joseph Samson Gamgee[6] referred to this material in his clinical lectures at Queen's Hospital, Birmingham, in 1876. He told of his extensive use of oakum as an absorbent dressing either by itself

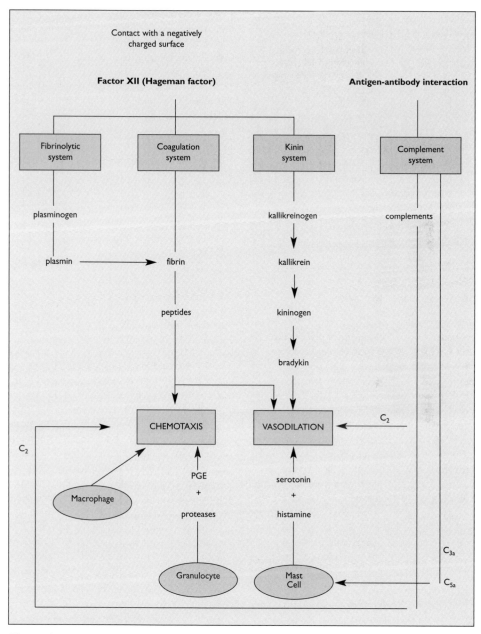

Figure 2. Healing cascade, cellular and humoral factors.

or over a thin layer of fine cotton or stitched into gauze bags to make absorbent pads.

Gamgee also noted that in 1870, M. Alphonso Guerin of Paris had reported a method of dressing amputation stumps using cotton wool. This was raw cotton that, although nonabsorbent, had been washed and carded. Gamgee, wishing to emulate Guerin, obtained the best quality cotton available, a material prepared as packing for jewelers' goods, and rejected all lesser grades as

Table 1. Nineteenth century products
Lewis A Sayre • oakum fiber
Joseph Samson Gamgee • oakum on cotton pads
M. Alphonso Guerin • washed and carded cotton
Joseph Samson Gamgee • jewelers cotton and tiffany
Robinson's & Son, Chesterfield • gauze and cotton tissue

Table 2. Surgical Materials, British Pharmaceutical Codex, 1923	
Cotton wools	15
Gauzes	13
Tows	4
Gauze and cotton tissue	2
Bandages	9
Protectives (Jaconet etc.)	4
Emplastrums	32
Lints	8

Table 3. Surgical Materials British Pharmacopoeia 1988	
Gauze products	9
Ribbon gauze	3
Dressing pads	5
Fibrous absorbents	3
Surgical felts	3
Bandages	20
Surgical tapes	7
Impregnated gauze	3
Stockinette	8
Adhesive dressings	4
Film dressings	1
Foam dressings	3

unsuitable. His interest encouraged the production of better grades in which the fibers were treated to remove traces of grease and thus were not only rendered absorbent but had a markedly reduced level of bacterial contamination. In 1880, Gamgee wrote a paper describing experiments in which he had used the cotton pads covered with tiffany, a fine bleached gauze used by nurserymen to stretch under the roofs of their conservatories to protect their plants from invading birds. Working in collaboration with Robinson and his son of Chesterfield, England, Gamgee showed that the gauze could be made more absorbent by bleaching, thus formulating the Gamgee tissue, which was the forerunner for today's gauze and cotton tissue. It was the first-named pad to be designed using a woven fabric and a fibrous mass with the criterion of function as the basis of the design.

The 1923 British Pharmaceutical Codex,[7] then the only accepted source of quality standards for pharmaceutical products, gave monographs for gauze and cotton tissue: 8 lints, 13 gauzes, and 15 cotton wools (Table 2). The 1988 British Pharmacopoeia[2] still contained 12 gauze products and 3 fibrous absorbents but excluded lint and Gamgee tissue (Table 3). Gauze, the survivor of those early fabrics, although currently contraindicated as a wound contact dressing, is used widely in surgery. The 2007 British Pharmacopoeia, however, contains monographs for absorbent cotton and absorbent viscose wadding only, and the current European Pharmacopoeia[8] has a monograph for absorbent cotton only. This diminution of formal standards for the materials used to formulate wound management products can only mean that the patient has fewer safeguards against exaggerated claims made by product manufacturers.

Absorbents[9]

The overall function of clinical absorbents is self-explanatory, and they have demonstrated minimal development in the past decades. Absorbents are required to absorb and retain a wide range of fluids from the blood and serous exudate of damaged tissue to the variable gut content met during surgical intervention.[6,7] They are found in a number of forms: fibrous (staple), fabric, and fiber plus fabric.

Fibrous absorbents. These absorbents are made from cotton staple or from the fibers of viscose or cellulose; viscose and cotton and viscose or cotton and acrylic fibers may be combined.

Absorbent cotton is available in different qualities varying with the length and diameter of the cotton staple. It is available in the form of rolls and balls and is used for cleansing and swabbing wounds, preoperative skin preparation, and the application of topical medicaments to the skin.

The absorption, performance, and physical character of absorbent viscose vary markedly with the manufacturing process. Viscose is available in the bright or dull form, the latter containing a particulate material, such as titanium dioxide, within the fiber. The fibers are, in general, a continuous staple with a crenate transsectional profile, but smooth and laminated forms are available, which show different degrees of absorptive capacity and wet tensile strength.

Some fibrous absorbents were developed containing a proportion of acrylamide or other synthetic polymeric fiber. These frequently enhance the absorptive performance and give body to the fleece, thus improving fluid retention and avoiding fluid squeeze out, which is caused by fleece collapse after wetting.

Cellulose wadding is produced from delignified wood pulp and manufactured in a multiple laminate material form. It is used in large pieces to absorb large volumes of fluid in incontinence, but is not used in contact with a wound unless enclosed in an outer fabric sleeve to prevent fiber loss to the wound.

Fabric absorbents. Absorbent lint is a close-weave cotton cloth with a raised nap on one side, which offers a large surface area for evaporation when placed with the nap upward on an exuding wound. It is generally unacceptable for modern wound management.

Absorbent gauze is the most widely used absorbent and consists of a cotton cloth of plain weave that is bleached and made reasonably free from weaving defects, cotton leaf, and shell. It may be slightly off white if sterilized. It absorbs water readily, but its performance may be reduced by prolonged storage or exposure to heat.

Surgical usage of absorbent gauze. Gauze products are primarily absorbents when used preoperatively, perioperatively, and postoperatively. Perioperatively, they may protect tissue and organs by occluding areas not involved in the

procedure, which may establish tissue viability.[8] To contribute to hemostasis, the gauze fabric may contain a proportion of viscose incorporated with the cotton either in the warp and the weft or exclusively in the weft. A maximum level of 45% of viscose is widely accepted.

Gauze products fall into 2 broad categories— the swab or sponge type (produced by folding and stitching the cloth) and the plain cloth. The swab type includes swabs, strips, pads, and pledgets. The plain type includes packs and ribbon. They are available with and without a radio opaque (X-ray detectable) element, and some are colored with a suitable nontoxic dye for recognition and use by the anesthetist.

Nonwoven fabrics include a wide range of products manufactured from synthetic and semi-synthetic fibers. Nonwoven viscose fabric swabs are available in folded pieces of various dimensions. They are occasionally used in error as a single wound dressing. They have a lower total absorptive capacity than gauze, but absorb more quickly because of the random orientation of the viscose fibers. They can replace the more sophisticated cotton swab for general purpose swabbing and cleansing procedures. As fabrics, they constitute the outer layer on a number of wound dressing pads: sometimes suitably coated with a polymer to reduce adherence at dressing change.

A cellulose sponge is a cavity foam cellulose-based sponge available in sheets and thin bands. It is for absorption at small sites in surgery.

Neuropatties are small squares or strips of non-woven absorbent viscose with thread stitched through the nonwoven fabric and left long. They are used as spot absorbents, particularly in neurosurgery. They are frequently moistened in saline before application. The threads are left outside the surgical area. On completion of surgery, the recovery of each pattie is facilitated by lifting each thread. Products vary in size and shape, and there is also a device for attaching the ends of all the threads, thus producing a mini count rack.

Fiber plus fabric absorbents. Gauze and cellulose wadding consists of a thick layer of cellulose wadding enclosed in a tubular-form gauze. The properties of the 2 separate materials have already been described. Combined, gauze and cellulose wadding tissue are used as an absorbent and protective pad. Together, they should only be used as a wound dressing with a nonadherent layer placed between the pad and the wound. This combination has a high absorbency and, because of its thickness, the additional property of insulation, which results in raising the temperature at the skin surface. This increase in temperature has been shown to accelerate the wound-healing rate. On a highly exuding surface, there is a tendency for the cellulose wadding element to collapse when wet and become a semisolid wet mass, which may cause difficulty in practice. In such fluid-loss situations, gauze and cotton tissue are preferred.

Gamgee tissue is a thick layer of absorbent cotton enclosed in a tubular form gauze. It has the same uses as gauze and cellulose wadding tissue but has the advantage of a higher absorbent capacity and less wet collapse. It is also softer in use and thus conforms more easily to the wound surface. It should be used in place of gauze and cellulose wadding tissue on highly exuding surfaces, such as burns, but, as previously stated, it should not be used in direct contact with the wound surface but rather placed upon a nonadherent dressing.

Ideal Wound Dressing

In the 1960s, the recognition that gauze was a passive product that plugged and concealed but did little to encourage wound healing resulted in the creation of a minimal set of criteria for an ideal wound dressing. Such a dressing would allow a wound to heal at the optimum rate concomitant with the physiological state of the patient. Gauze and similar materials did not meet these requirements and their uses have diminished relative to the development of new products, which meet some, but not all, of the stated criteria.

The performance parameters of an ideal wound dressing[9] specified in 1979 were the result of observations in clinical situations of failures of the then contemporary dressings to optimize wound healing. The dressing criteria are as follows:

- To remove excess exudate and toxic components
- To maintain a high humidity at wound/ dressing interface
- To allow gaseous exchange
- To provide thermal insulation
- To afford protection from secondary infection

- To be free from particulate or toxic contaminants
- To allow removal without trauma at dressing change.

Acceptable handling characteristics were also specified to include variability of size, resistance to tear and disintegration when wet or dry, conformability, sterilizability, and disposability.

These parameters were the initial stimuli for the development of functionally designed *interactive* products using the advances in the technology of materials. They have since been expanded to incorporate our increased knowledge of the humoral and cellular factors associated with the healing process. They mark the progression toward the production of an ideal wound dressing. *However, it should be emphasized that no single dressing will produce the optimum microenvironment for all wounds or for all of the healing stages of one wound. The spectrum of performance requires that following wound diagnosis, treatment progresses by prescribing the most suitable dressing.*

The first progression toward interactive products was the development of wound dressing pads with high-absorptive capacity, slow strike through, and a low-adherence wound contact surface. These were initially available in simple-sleeved pads containing cotton, viscose, or cellulose fibers with an outer sleeve of gauze or nonwoven fabric. They were reformulated as laminate pads with multiple layer cores, having outer sleeves of cotton, which were viscose or nonwoven fabric that may have been treated with a polymer (polypropylene) to reduce adherence. The multilayer core is designed to increase absorptive capacity and to prolong usage by delaying strike through to the outer surface. This delay is facilitated by using a fluid-retardant layer within the upper and outer sleeve, which encourages lateral rather than vertical movement of fluid within the pad. *Strike through is undesirable because it provides a band of wet dressing that may allow transmission of airborne organisms to a clean wound, or bacteria from an infected wound to the outer dressing surface, thus acting as a possible vector in infection transmission.*

Pads with wound-contact surfaces designed to be of low adherence were produced for low exudate and drying wounds where high adherence can be expected and high absorptive capacity becomes irrelevant. They vary from aluminum-coated fabrics to perforated polymeric films or heat-bonded polyethylene films. The wound contact film is attached to an absorbent fibrous mat and an outer woven or nonwoven fabric. In some products, the polymeric film forms a continuous sleeve on both dressing surfaces. These low-adherence, low-absorptive capacity dressings are sometimes centered on adhesive backing to produce an island dressing, which may be used as a postoperative adhesive dressing or in the more familiar form of a first-aid island or strip dressing for superficial injuries.

Low-adherence primary dressing manufacturers found difficulties in producing wound-dressing pads that would meet all the ideal parameters—in particular, that of low adherence. They produced low-adherence wound contact products that consisted of partially open-cell structured nylon or viscose fabric, which may be finished with a silicone coating. The open-cell structure allows fluid transmission to a secondary, superimposed absorbent dressing, which can be changed when necessary without disturbing the primary, low-adherent contact layer.

The 2-layer system heralded the concept of a primary and secondary wound management regime where the primary dressing would meet the requirements of permeability, nonadherence, and bacterial impermeability and the secondary dressing would meet the need for absorption, protection, and insulation. This concept resulted in a number of products being specified as primary dressings and their associated secondary pads as low- or high-exudate absorption performers.

Impregnated Dressings

Close-weave gauze and open-weave tulles are used as carriers of medicated and unmedicated ointments to the wound surface and were developed initially to lower adherence and, subsequently, release systems for antibacterials and antibiotics.

Paraffin gauze (tulle dressing). Paraffin gauze was developed during World War I. It is bleached cotton or combined cotton and viscose cloth impregnated with yellow or white soft paraffin. It is available as sterile, individually wrapped, single pieces. The paraffin is present to prevent

the dressing from adhering to a wound. The gauze, which may be leno in nature, is coated so all the threads of the fabric are impregnated, but the spaces between the threads are free of paraffin. The material is used primarily in the treatment of wounds, such as burns and scalds, where the protective function of the stratum corneum is lost and water vapor can escape. Paraffin-gauze dressing functions by reducing the fluid loss while the water barrier layer is reforming. The 2 properties of the paraffin gauze that are most useful are those of nonadherence and semi-occlusiveness.

In addition to burns and scalds, the dressing is used as a wound contact layer in lacerations, abrasions, and ulcers as a packing material to promote granulation. Postoperatively, it is used as a vaginal or perineal dressing and for sinus packing. A recent development has been the substitution of cotton gauze with cellulose acetate and a paraffin emulsion impregnation.

Examples of available impregnations that are recommended for the reduction of infection are povidone iodine 10%, chlorhexidine 0.5% w/w, and cod liver oil with honey. Diffusion of the antibacterial agent into or onto an infected and exuding wound has been shown to be minimal. The possibility of development of resistant strains of infective organisms together with an increased incidence of sensitivity reactions has reduced the usage of these products and has led to the development of antibacterial products containing silver ions. One such material uses a vapor-permeable film as a base with a coating of a controlled-release polymer that dissolves in either water or water vapor to release silver ions to the wound. The sustained release is said to continue over a period of 5–7 days. A similar product contains activated carbon, which may be used as a deodorizing dressing. Silicone dressings have been used clinically as an alternative to paraffin gauze for the fixation of pediatric skin grafts where it was found that changing the outer absorbent dressing was painless as was the removal of the silicone dressing itself so that no analgesia or anesthesia was required. Generally, silicone dressings have a porous, semitransparent wound contact layer consisting of a flexible, polyamide net coated with silicone. The dressing is nonabsorbent, but the pores within its matrix allow the passage of exudate from the wound to a secondary dressing.

Its use is limited to minor skin grafts because the dressing requires a margin of healthy skin for application of at least 2 cm surrounding the wound. Reports have indicated that use of silicone dressings leads to improvements in the appearance (eg, scar size, erythema, elasticity) and symptoms (eg, pruritis, burning pain) after application to hypertrophic scars and keloids.[10] Silicone dressings are thought to effect this by promoting hydration of the scar and applying pressure, thereby flattening scar tissue, increasing wound elasticity, and reducing discoloration.

Other impregnations now available include gauze pads saturated with zinc sulfate, zinc oxide, or hypertonic saline, coated with a partially hydrated hydrogel or hydrogel acemannan derived from *aloe vera*.

Deodorizing Dressings

These dressings were developed as functionally specific primary dressings. Infected wounds frequently produce obnoxious odors that are embarrassing to the patient and may have a detrimental effect upon the wound-management procedure. Fungating carcinomas and venous ulcers are but 2 of the conditions that would be advantaged by the use of a deodorizing dressing.

Deodorizing dressings have been formulated from the high gaseous sorptive material, activated carbon, incorporated into a woven fabric or a fibrous mat backed by a nylon sleeve, a vapor-permeable film, or a polyurethane foam. In each formulation, the objective is to reduce odor. Therefore, the dressings must be large enough to cover the entire malodorous area. One product encourages direct contact of the carbon layer with wound exudate. This dressing adsorbs polarized bacteria onto the surface of the charcoal cloth used in the formulation. The silver present in the dressing exerts a bactericidal effect, which gradually diminishes as wound exudate saturates the material. It follows that once the activated carbon has absorbed serum plus bacteria it will cease to act specifically as a deodorizer.

Polymeric Dressings

Despite the advances in fiber technology and better understanding of the physiological parameters associated with wound healing, the fabric dressing development process has failed to pro-

vide the optimum microenvironment for wound healing, in particular, by the controlled absorption of wound exudate to allow a moist environment without tissue maceration due to excess moisture. The incorporation of new technology fibers, such as acrylics and viscose variants, and the production of nonwoven fabrics in swab and pad formulations were the precursors to the use of synthetic and semisynthetic polymers with prespecified performance parameters that would produce the required microenvironment for differing wound types at various stages of healing. The first of these interactive polymeric products appeared in the 1960s, and ongoing development has resulted in polymeric films, polymeric foams, particulate and fibrous polymers, hydrogels, xerogels, and hydrocolloids. The polymers range from polyurethane to naturally occurring polysaccharides and collagens.

Polymeric films.[11] Studies of superficial wounds emphasized the importance of avoiding dehydration and maceration of a wound surface while maintaining a moist wound interface and a gaseous exchange system similar to healthy skin.[11-13] These requirements potentiated the development of a material that would, in part, mimic the performance of skin. The resultant products were transparent, synthetic, adhesive films generically described as vapor-permeable adhesive membranes or synonymously as vapor-permeable films. They consist of transparent polyurethane or other synthetic film of low reflectance, evenly coated on one side with a synthetic adhesive mass.

The films are adhesive and cohesive, producing intimate adhesion to a dry skin surface and nonadhesion to a wet surface. They have highly elastomeric and extensible properties that contribute to both their conformability and their resistance to shear and tear. The products are sterile and particle free.

The films also possess permeability functions that are essential to their efficacy as wound management materials. It should be noted that the removal of the stratum corneum results in a water vapor loss from tissues between 3,000 g/m^2 and 5,000 g/m^2 over 24 hours. This loss will result in progressive dehydration, which could be of great significance, particularly in a full-thickness burn. The loss through a positioned vapor-permeable membrane is reduced to 2,500 g/m^2 over 24 hours or less, depending upon the structure of the membrane. This reduction allows excess fluid to be lost by water-vapor transmission through the membrane, but prevents dehydration and maintains a moist wound interface. Where the volume of exudate produced is significantly greater than the volume removed as vapor, the water impermeability will result in serous effusion accumulating below the film. Obtrusive exudate can be aspirated using aseptic technique, or preferably, the entire dressing can be changed or upgraded to one with greater vapor permeability. Impermeability to water prevents wetting from external sources.

The importance of a moist interface to wound healing is now well recognized. It allows the rapid migration of keratinocytes across the wound surface, precludes trauma due to adherence at dressing change, and contributes to gaseous diffusion in the damaged tissue. Oxygen and carbon dioxide transfer are accomplished by intramolecular diffusion through the membrane and by solution in the wound-surface moisture. The oxygen permeability of the films is variously described as 4,000 to 10,000 cm^3 m^2 24 hours at ambient atmospheric pressure. The pO_2 and pH levels of the wound surface are directly related to gaseous permeability and contribute to cellular activity. The wound is protected against secondary infection by the bacterial impermeability of the film to organisms, such as *Pseudomonas aeruginosa*, *Staphylococcus aureus*, and *Escherichia coli*.

The physical performance is applicable to the management of superficial tangential wounds, such as dermabrasions, split-skin graft donor sites, and burns. In a dermabrasion, hemostasis must first be obtained and the margin of the wound dried before the film is applied. Correctly positioned film may be left *in situ* until epithelization is complete. In its application for the treatment of burns, careful disinfection must precede the positioning of the film. It is only recommended for superficial and clinically clean burns and contraindicated for deep burns where it retards the separation of necrotic tissue.

Pressure ulcers can be covered with a vapor-permeable film with the added advantage of film resistance to shear and low frictional surface properties, which protect the dermal layers from additional physical abrasion while producing the minimal barrier to normal skin function. This performance allows the film to be used as a prophylactic in areas that are traumatized by pressure but not ulcerated.

Film dressings can also be used for the retention of cannulae and tubes in operating rooms and patient care units. Specific products have now been produced with a variable water-vapor permeability to reduce the build up of moisture beneath the film and the resultant infective hazard.

Technological development has resulted in several new intelligent vapor-permeable films that allow high permeability in high-exudate conditions, but respond to low exudate by a reduction in the moisture vapor transmission rate, thus maintaining the moist environment conducive to the optimization of the microenvironment. Recently, film dressings impregnated with an antibacterial (silver) for the management of infected wounds or a deodorizer (charcoal) for malodorous wounds have been developed.

Polymeric Foams

Foam dressings were developed alongside film dressings and have certain properties in common, but differences in their structure and composition have important implications for their performance in the clinical situation. The dressings are available as sheet dressings and foams formed *in situ*.

The sheet dressings are mainly polyurethane foams where the absorbency and water-vapor permeability are varied either by a physical modification to the foam or by combining the foam with an additional sheet component. They have many of the attributes of an ideal dressing with the added advantage of the ability to be tailored for particular applications, such as that of a tracheostomy dressing, without particle loss to the wound or loss of conformable characteristics.

Partially expanded, modified polyurethane foam was developed by Lock.[12] It comprised a lower layer of open cells and an upper hydrophilic surface with closed impermeable layers, which reduced the loss of water vapor and prevented strike through of absorbed fluid. This primary dressing expands when it becomes wet and conforms to the contours of the wound producing an environmental chamber with entrapped solutes and cell debris. It is claimed this function enhances the inflammatory response of the wound and subsequently stimulates the production of granulation tissue and revascularization. These polyurethane foam dressings are recommended specifically for the management of stasis ulcers with a superimposed absorbent pad and graduated pressure applied either by stretch bandages or elasticized stockings.

A foam dressing with the prime function of absorbency has been designed for the management of burns. It consists of a highly absorbent hydrophilic polyurethane foam, backed with a moisture permeable polyurethane membrane and bonded to an apertured polyurethane net on the wound contact face. It is capable of absorbing and retaining large volumes of fluid even under pressure. The backing, while permeable to water vapor, is impermeable to water thus avoiding strike through. As the exudate level decreases, the membrane retains moisture and prevents the drying of the wound. The apertured polyurethane net interface reduces adherence to the wound surface. While recommended for burns, these dressings have been used successfully on other exuding lesions.

Low-absorptive capacity primary foam dressings have been produced from a carboxylated styrene butadiene rubber latex foam. The foam is bonded to a nonwoven fabric coated with a polyethylene film, which has been vacuum ruptured. The basic foam is naturally hydrophobic, and a surface-active agent is incorporated to facilitate the uptake of wound exudate. The polyethylene film layer is particularly effective in preventing adherence, and the dressing is recommended for minor wounds and abrasions where exudate levels are low and adherence is a prominent hazard at dressing change.

Foam Cavity Wound Dressings

One major problem in wound management is the treatment of large cavity wounds produced either perioperatively (eg, pilonidal sinus) or by trauma (eg, pressure ulceration). *It is necessary to occlude the cavity by packing to absorb excess exudate, prevent fistula formation, and stimulate the production of granulation tissue, neovascularization, and collagen deposition.*

The traditional procedure is to pack the cavity with ribbon gauze (see cellulosic absorbents) variously impregnated. The subsequent removal of such a dressing is difficult, and the pain and stress associated with the dressing change may require low-level anesthesia and the use of a special procedures or operating room.

A foam that could be formed *in situ* was developed by Dow Corning[13] and found to be clinically superior to ribbon gauze. Its status in cytotoxic terms was open to question, and it was taken off the market, but a similar product has now been developed and is used with comparable clinical success. This material consists of a 2-component foam, mixed prior to use and poured directly into the wound where the dressing expands to 4 times its original volume. It then sets to a soft spongy foam that accurately conforms to the contours of the wound cavity. The resulting stent may be removed twice daily, soaked in a mild antiseptic, rinsed in saline, and replaced. A new dressing is formed when required, usually after 7 to 10 days, to match the reduction in size of the cavity. It does not adhere to tissue, and the slight pressure produced on the cavity surfaces contributes to the production of granulation tissue. It is indicated for the management of pilonidal sinus, hydradenitis suppurativa, perianal and perineal wounds, and dehisced abdominal wounds.

Other cavity wound dressing developments have been based upon the tailoring of prepacked absorption foam fragments into nonwoven outer layers of various dimensions. These foam pillows are positioned directly in the wound and, unlike the *in situ* foams, have high absorbency and can be removed and replaced with ease at predetermined intervals.

A polyurethane/polyacrylic polymer sheet described as a hydroactive dressing is also available. It has an island configuration with a unique adhesive portion. It is nonadhesive to the wound surface and, due to its high absorptive capacity when positioned on a wound, such as a pressure or venous ulcer, expands and conforms to the wound cavity. It has the ability to re-adhere once lifted, enabling manipulation of the product for fit or assessment of the wound without dressing change. The polymer wicks fluid into the upper layers of the dressing where it escapes through the backing.

Along with the vapor-permeable films, the foams continue to evolve toward a more precise control of the wound microenvironment.

Hydrogels[14]

Hydrogels, or water polymer gels, are 3-dimensional networks of hydrophilic polymers prepared from materials, such as gelatin, polysaccharides, cross-linked polyacrylamide polymers, polyelectrolyte complexes, and polymers or copolymers derived from methacrylate esters. They interact with aqueous solutions by swelling to an equilibrium value and retain a significant proportion of water within their structure. They are insoluble in water and are available as dry or hydrated sheets or a hydrated gel in an individual delivery system. The tissue-like structure of most hydrogels will contribute to their biocompatibility by minimizing mechanical irritation to surrounding cells and tissues. Sheet hydrogels currently used as wound dressings possess most of the properties of an ideal dressing. Their high moisture content maintains a desirable moist interface with the surface of the wound, which facilitates cell migration and prevents dressing adherence. The gels are able to absorb fluid into the polymer matrix and swell in a 3-dimensional manner, and they maintain a sheet form without intruding into the wound cavity. Water can be transmitted through the saturated gel while the unsaturated gel has a water-vapor permeability comparable to that of vapor-permeable membranes.

The first wound management hydrogel product developed was a cross-linked polymer of polyacrylamide and agarose. The mesh size allowed the absorption and desorption of both high molecular-weight proteins and low molecular-weight solutes. While this performance parameter is essential in its function as an environmental dressing, it could also be utilized to transport compounds to the wound and thus act as the release component in a sustained-release system. Some success has been evident in using topical antibacterials in this way, but it would seem that there may be a greater potential still to be exploited. The ability to sustain release can be seen from the results of the growth curves of L929 and epithelial cells growing *in vitro* beneath a nutrient-saturated hydrogel.[15] Growth is maintained at a higher level than that observed with the control where the cells are surrounded by media. The cells become a confluent layer adhering to the lower surface of the gel. This property can be utilized to transfer epithelial seed cultures

to large partial-thickness wound areas and thus supplement the current practice of skin grafting. If the epithelial layer is derived from the patient's own tissue, this may avoid problems associated with graft rejection.

Diffusion rates from the hydrogel can also be controlled by the degree of cross linkage. For example, initial cross linking of aqueous solutions of sodium alginate and calcium chloride followed by external cross linking of the produced suspension using poly-L-lysine or poly-ethylene-imine will result in a predetermination of the mesh size and thus control the release rate of sorbed compounds, such as polypeptides or growth factors.

Other hydrogel properties could also be utilized as release mechanisms. Gel synapsis at the Theta, Ø, critical temperature of temperature-sensitive hydrogels results in expansion or collapse of the hydrophilic networks. This process could be used to design a release system for wound management where a drug could be incorporated into the hydrogel structures at one temperature and the active component released abruptly as the critical temperature approaches 32°C when phase separation occurs. pH-sensitive hydrogels may be polybasic or polyacidic and will preferentially release compounds in a pH-changed environment. This property is being developed for periodontal medication using glassy hydrophobic hydrogels, which become highly hydrated from pH2 to pH6. The pH changes in infected wounds might well be used to initiate the release of topical antibacterials until the pH reverts to normal and the sustained-release system ceases to operate. All of these properties have been the subject of investigation with the objective of developing new products.

It has been observed that the use of a hydrogel frequently results in a marked reduction in pain response in patients. It is suggested that the high humidity protects the exposed neurons from dehydration and also produces acceptable changes in pH. A secondary effect, which may contribute to this response, is the property of the gels to immediately cool the wound surface and maintain a lower temperature for up to 6 hours. In a wound, this lowering of temperature results in a reduction of the inflammatory response.

Hydrogel sheets or gels of similar composition have been developed to allow continuity of formulation and function in, for example, cavity wounds. The wound volume is filled with the amorphous hydrogel, and the hydrogel sheet is superimposed over the wound. Hydrogels are nonadherent, so a secondary dressing, such as a vapor-permeable film, will be required.

Hydrogels have been developed to produce a moisture "donor" effect for necrotic wounds that require debriding. They are at present available only in the amorphous hydrogel form. Some manufacturers have produced gauze pads presaturated and impregnated with a hydrogel. Recent developments have been directed at producing hydrogel sheets bonded onto a vapor-permeable film to control water-vapor transmission and to prevent the possible hazard of wet hydrogels becoming dry sheets, which would be incompatible with a healing surface.

The recommendation for use of these products includes the management of donor sites and superficial operation sites and also the treatment of chronically damaged epithelium. In chronic ulcers, they are used to promote autolytic debridement and to encourage granulation and the formation of a cellular matrix.

Particulate and Fibrous Polymers[16]

The group of xerogel dressings includes synthetic, semisynthetic, and naturally occurring products embracing a range of polysaccharide materials, such as alginates and dextranomers. They are in an ongoing state of development with new and "me-too" products appearing at frequent intervals.

The xerogel dressings may be regarded as a subgroup of products within the larger group of polysaccharide dressings. The latter contains the well known cellulosic dressing products, such as gauze and absorbent cotton (these have been dealt with earlier in this chapter under Absorbents). However, the products that consist of dextranomer beads, dehydrated hydrogels of the agar/acrylamide group, calcium alginate fibers, and dehydrated granulated Graft T starch polymers are identified specifically as xerogels,[16] the material remaining after the removal of most or all of the water from a hydrogel (or the disperse phase from any type of simple gel).

Particulate dextranomer. Dextranomer is prepared from dextran, a naturally derived poly-

mer of glucose produced by cultures of a microorganism, *Leuconostoc mesenteroides*. The gel is formed when the dextran molecules comprising the disperse phase of the hydrogel are crosslinked by a chemical process utilizing epichlorhydrin and sodium hydroxide.

The dextranomer is supplied in beads of 100 μm to 300 μm diameter containing poloxamer 187, polyethylene glycol 300 (PEG 300), and some water. A paste formulation is also available, which is the dextranomer in polyethylene glycol 600 (PEG 600). The beads are offered as discrete particles or enclosed in a low-adherence pouch for insertion into a cavity wound. One company (Pharmacia AB, Sweden) offers a polymeric net that can be placed into a cavity wound before the addition of either granules or paste, facilitating removal of the product. A vapor-permeable film is superimposed on the dextranomer dressing in a low exuding wound to control evaporation and retard drying of the dressing. The dextranomer acts as a selective sorbent, as the hydrophilic beads will absorb the aqueous component of wound exudate and dissolved materials ranging from inorganic salts to low molecular-weight proteins. Dextranomer has a pore size that produces an exclusion limit of 1,000 to 8,000 Daltons, precluding the sorption of viruses and bacteria. Microorganisms are removed from the wound by a capillary action between the beads, a function that is absent from the paste formulation. This function, however, demonstrates a marked increase in absorbing capacity for malodorous elements and pain-producing compounds released during the inflammatory response.

It may be used as a debriding agent on sloughy and exuding wounds where the objective is to produce a clean tissue bed for the production of a granulating tissue. It is not a product that should be used beyond this phase of the wound-healing process, as its continued application will impair epithelization. Dextranomer is not biodegradable and both granules and paste must be carefully removed with saline to avoid particulate residues and the subsequent development of granulomas.

Fibrous polymers. Alginate fibers are derived from alginic acid, which is a polyuronic acid composed of residues of D-mannuronic acid and L-guluronic acid. Alginic acid is obtained chiefly from algae belonging to the Phaeophyceae, a species of *Laminaria*.

The isomeric acids are present in varying proportions dependent upon the seaweed source. Calcium alginate is capable of gel formation. The guluronic acid forms an association with calcium, providing the stimulus to produce the continuous disperse phase of a hydrogel. Ca^{2+} ion and a phospholipid surface promote the activation of prothrombin in the clotting cascade. *Calcium alginate products are used as the source of these ions to arrest bleeding, both in superficial injuries and as an absorbable hemostat in surgery. The rate of biodegradation is related to the sodium/calcium balance in the preparation.*

The alginates are produced in fiber form and have been developed as a fleece or layered needled fabric. When applied to a bleeding surface, the availability of the Ca^{2+} ions and the fibrous matrix contribute to coagulation, and serum absorption produces a gel-like mass. The dressings may be removed either with sterile 3% sodium citrate solution followed by washing with sterile water or with sterile normal saline.

The wet integrity of the dressing, which facilitates removal from the wound, may be improved by incorporating fibers of greater strength, such as viscose (rayon) staple fiber, or fibers that interact with the alginate fibers when wet, such as chitosan staple fibers.

Alginate gauze and staple products are applied using normal sterile dressing procedures. The frequency of change will be a matter for clinical assessment of the injury and depend on the type of wound and the degree of exudation.

The primary hemostatic usage of calcium alginate is in the packing of sinuses, fistulae, and bleeding tooth sockets. The use of calcium alginate as a hemostatic agent dates back to the 1950s. Its subsequent development as a xerogel, which is converted to a hydrogel in the presence of wound exudate, came in the late 1970s. It was at this stage that the significance of the Ca^{2+} and Na^+ ion ratios became apparent in physical differences between the gel strength of products containing high or low Na^+ ion levels. This discovery has led to a range of Ca/Na alginate dressings in the form of fibrous and fabric preparations, which have different absorptive capacities and gelling properties. The alginates also have been

cross formulated with a collagen type 1 and chitosan to increase the possible bioactivity.

Recent studies have indicated an auto oxidation property of alginates, which stimulates the production of hydrogen peroxide. In addition to containing Ca^{2+} ions, alginates have been identified as contributing to the initial inflammatory response required to kick start the healing cascade by causing lysis of mast cells with the subsequent release of histamine and 5HT.

Alginate dressings have been used successfully as hemostats for lacerations and abrasions and are effective in the management of hypergranulation (proud flesh), interdigital maceration, and heloma molle. They are used in hospitals and communities to accelerate healing in intractable skin and pressure ulcers and in the successful management of diabetic ulcers, venous ulcers, and burns.

Alginates have also proven to be useful autolytic debriding agents. When applied to these injury types, the alginate must be covered by a secondary dressing of foam or film.

Hydrocolloids[17]

Hydrocolloid dressings have developed from the adhesive flanges used for long-term protection of skin surrounding a stoma. The barrier produced prevented the excretions from eroding or denuding the skin, and the flange acted as a base for the adhesive attachment of ostomy collection devices. The development of the hydrocolloid as a wound management product has resulted in new formulations and a range of technologically superior products available in adhesive sheet, granular, and paste forms.

The early hydrocolloid dressings consisted of composite agents based on naturally occurring hydrophilic polymers. In general, they have a pressure-sensitive adhesive layer composed of a so-called hydrocolloid, dispersed with the aid of a tackifier in an elastomer and, secondly, a film coating composed of a variable vapor-permeable but water-impermeable, flexible, elastomeric material. One of the first hydrocolloid dressings described had a pressure-sensitive adhesive hydrocolloid layer, which consisted of a mixture of gelatine and sodium carboxymethylcellulose, 40%–50% by weight, dispersed in polyisobutylene with an antioxidant and a tackifier (mineral oil and terpene resin). This mixture was then laminated with a semi-open–cell, flexible polyurethane foam previously laminated with a closed-cell, flexible polyurethane film. A currently available hydrocolloid dressing is a flexible mass with an adherent inner face and an outer vapor-permeable polyurethane foam. The modified formulation is as follows: sodium carboxymethylcellulose 20%; polysiobutylene 40%; gelatine 20%; pectin 20%. This product is also available as a paste of similar formulation allowing a continuous fill for cavity wounds.

Other hydrocolloid dressings with formulations consisting of sodium carboxymethylcellulose combined with karaya gum or sodium carboxymethylcellulose alone are also available.

The adhesive formulation of hydrocolloids gives an initial adhesion higher than some surgical adhesive tapes. After application, the absorption of transepidermal water vapor modifies the adhesive flow to maintain a high-tack performance throughout the period of use. *In situ*, the dressings provide a gaseous and moisture-proof environmental chamber strongly adhered to the area surrounding the wound and offering protection against contamination from incontinence or other sources. In the wound contact area, the exudate is absorbed to form a gel that swells in a linear fashion with a higher moisture retention at the contact surface. This higher moisture retention results in an expansion of the gel into the wound cavity with the continued support and increasing pressure from the remainder of the elastomeric dressing. The larger the volume of exudate, the greater the expansion into the cavity, up to the limitation imposed by the availability of the gel. *The advantage of this system is that it applies a firm pressure to the floor of a deep ulcer, a basic surgical maxim for the production of healthy granulating tissue. It is this function that contributes to its recommended usage for venous ulcers.*

The formed colloidal gel will also produce a sorption gradient for soluble components within the serous exudate and thereby allowing the removal of toxic compounds arising from bacterial or cellular destruction. The moist gel is soft and conforms to the wound contours. When the dressing is removed, the gel remains in the wound and can be washed away with normal saline. No damage to the wound results from this procedure. During use, the dressing in contact with

the wound liquifies to produce a pus-like liquid with a somewhat strong odor. The hydrocolloids are suitable for de-sloughing and for light-to-medium exuding wounds but are contraindicated if an anaerobic infection is present. They have been used successfully in the treatment of chronic leg ulcers, pressure ulcers, and skin barriers in the management of stomas.

As with hydrogels, hydrocolloids are available in both powder and paste form where the powders and pastes have similar formulations to that of the hydrocolloid mass in the sheet dressing. This versatility will allow larger cavity wounds to be treated with a continuous hydrocolloid system.

A recent development for deep exuding pressure ulcer management is a hydrocolloid dressing with a formulation including sodium alginate in a spiral form rolled into a round disc, which can be positioned in the cavity and covered with a hydrocolloid sheet dressing. A further advance has been the development of thin hydrocolloid sheets with improved conformability and a degree of transparency that allows the wound to be observed without removal of the dressing. This latter product is comparable in performance with a vapor-permeable film. *It should be noted that although the hydrocolloids are primarily considered to be interactive dressings, incorporating silver into their formulation, as has been done by several manufacturers, must contribute a bioactive function to the material.*

Superabsorbents

Superabsorbent hydrocolloid dressings are highly absorbent and entrap exudate so that it cannot be squeezed out once absorbed. One product incorporates the highly absorbent material into an island pad covered by a nonwoven absorbent and surrounded by an extra thin hydrocolloid as the adhesive portion. The covering acts as a transfer layer while its surface stays dry.[18]

Hydrofibers

Hydrofibers are fibers of carboxymethylcellulose formed into flat, nonwoven pads for application to large, open wounds. They appear as a textile fiber and are presented in the form of a fleece held together by a needle-bonding process. Hydrofibers are also available as a "ribbon" for packing cavities. The dressing absorbs and interacts with wound exudate to form a soft, hydrophilic, gas-permeable gel that traps bacteria and conforms to the contours of the wound while providing a microenvironment that is believed to facilitate healing. The resultant gel is similar to a sheet hydrogel, but it does not dry out or wick laterally, which ensures that there is no maceration of the skin surrounding the wound. The high absorbent capacity reduces the frequency of dressing changes.

Hydrofiber dressings are easy to remove without causing pain or trauma and leave minimal residue on the surface of the wound. They may be applied to exuding lesions, including leg ulcers, pressure areas, donor sites, and most other granulating wounds, but for deeper cavity wounds and sinuses, the ribbon packing is generally preferred.[18]

Bioactive Products

When developing interactive products, the environment sought was obtained, but some chronic injuries still refused to respond adequately. Since most wounds, when not infected, heal spontaneously in endocrinologically and nutritionally normal mammals, it had always been considered axiomatic that the rate of healing represents a biologic maximum and therefore could not be accelerated beyond the available capacity of the tissues. However, the experimental use of processed cartilage and cartilage extracts showed the potential to stimulate through topical application the normal or enhanced activity of the acellular and cellular mechanisms involved in tissue repair. Such products may be considered to produce a localized systemic intervention and can be defined as bioactive.

A brief reexamination of the healing cascade (Figure 2) is sufficient to identify those parts of the cycle that could be influenced by such materials either by correcting some deficiency in the biochemical pathway or by stimulating the involved cellular elements to increase their activity and accelerate their biofunction.

The initial inflammatory response is predominantly acellular by comparison with the regeneration and repair processes. It is in these 2 latter processes that the designated bioactive compounds need to perform as the biologic primers for cell proliferation and tissue reconstruction.

Naturally occurring polysaccharides, such as hyaluronic acid and chondroitin sulphate, are glycosaminoglycans (GAGs), which have been shown to be involved in diverse structural and organization functions in tissues. They and other GAGs, such as heparin and dermatan sulphate, show a partial specification for cell surface interactions, cell/cell interactions, cell substrate interactions, or cell proliferation. They have an important bioactive influence on the microenvironment and, therefore, on tissue regeneration. Noncollagenic proteins, such as fibronectin (C1g) laminin and chondronectin, are still to be fully characterized, but their *in vitro* effects on cell division are well documented. Fibronectin demonstrates chemokinesis on fibroblasts (general stimulation of movement) and, in the presence of a concentration gradient, chemotaxis (directional movement stimulated by a gradient of diffusable substance) and hapotaxis (directional movement stimulated by a gradient of substrate adhesiveness). These proactive materials are now becoming available after being challenged for their levels of quality, safety, and efficacy.

Polymeric materials, such as pectins, alginates, and chitosan, which act as pro-oxidants are important. In other words, in the presence of traces of transition metal catalysts, such as iron and copper ions, they interact with dissolved molecular oxygen to form superoxide, which dismutases spontaneously to form hydrogen peroxide.[15] This reactive oxygen species initiates oxidative processes and has been shown at concentrations of 10^{-6} M to 10^{-9} M to stimulate both the proliferation of fibroblasts and the macrophage respiratory burst. The Superoxide Assisted Fenton Reaction is as follows:

$$Fe^{3}+ + O_2 \downarrow Fe^{2}+ + O_2$$

$$Fe^{2} + H_2O_2 \downarrow Fe^{3} + \bullet OH^- + -OH$$

The use of hydrogen peroxide has been discouraged in wound management. Its toxicity in fibroblast cultures and its tissue destruction properties in vivo have been reported at higher concentrations than those quoted here. At these low concentrations, there is a 20% increase in murine fibroblast proliferation over a period of 3–6 days. Work involving the use of low passage number human fibroblasts has also shown substantially higher increases.[19]

The generation of superoxide also contributes to leukotaxin formation, which could reinitiate the inflammatory response in recalcitrant wounds. The resultant influx of monocytes/macrophages would contribute further superoxide and hydrogen peroxide to the wound environment. Following NADPH oxidase activity, the higher concentrations of hydrogen peroxide would initially inhibit the proliferation of fibroblasts, but as its concentration falls, the rate of cell division is enhanced leading to collagen synthesis.

Further investigations completed and in progress have identified similar antioxidant activity in other hydrogel and hydrocolloid products.[19]

It would appear that the application of antioxidant wound contact materials to soft tissue lesions in patients whose intrinsic antioxidant defenses are compromised by age, dietary deficiency, or physiological deficiency, such as diabetes, would contribute to an improved antioxidant status in the wound locality and thus establish and maintain the reducing environment necessary for energy production and hence cell division.[20] This process, plus the maintenance of moist wound healing, could contribute to the rate of healing and repair of the soft tissue injury by normalizing the complete bioenvironment.

Growth Factors

The year 1986 was a landmark in wound healing. This was the year that Cohen and Levi-Montaleini shared a Nobel prize for their work on epidermal and nerve growth factors. This research stimulated many other workers to investigate the potential of other growth factors.

Growth factors and cytokines are polypeptides transiently produced by cells that exert their hormone-like function on other cells via specific cell-surface receptors and thereby increase the mitotic index of proliferating cells. They have been broadly classified as paracrine when they act upon neighboring cells and autocrine when they act upon producing cells. Their activities overlap, and the effect of most of them depends on the group and pattern of regulatory molecules to which the cell is exposed.[21] Growth factors are so named because of their stimulatory effect on cell proliferation. They display both stimulatory and inhibitory activities even with the same cells

depending on the state of activation and differentiation of the cells and the presence of other stimulating factors. Several growth factors have been identified in wounds, but their precise functions are still a matter of debate.

Three types of growth factor are recognized based upon the apparent cellular response: proliferative, migratory, or producing an alteration in the phenotypic state.

The proliferative response can be stimulated by the following:

1) The cell moves from the resting state, inducing DNA replication and proving the competence of the cell; the cell is then sensitive to the progressive factor that leads to cell replication

2) Chemoattractants stimulate migration or movement of cells

3) The transforming growth factors produce a phenotypic alteration. There are 5 families of peptide growth factors that are thought to be involved in wound healing: epidermal growth factor (EGF), transforming growth factor-ß (TGF-ß), platelet-derived growth factor (PDGF), insulin-like growth factor (IGF), and fibroblast growth factor (FGF).

Macrophages are the cells pivotal in bringing about the first stages of healing after which they then control and direct it before finally stopping it when the repair is complete. The cells modulate the immune response by induction of lipoxygenase products through stimulation of the arachidonic acid cascade.[22] In addition to aiding debridement at the wound site, they are involved in the secretion and synthesis of the collagenases neutrophil elastase and matrix metalloproteinase 8 (MMP 8) preparatory to laying down new extracellular matrix (connective tissue). They are a source of the growth factors PDGF and TGF-ß and regulate fibroblast migration and proliferation by production of the cytokine interleukin-1ß (IL-1ß).[23,24]

The possible bioactivity of platelet-derived angiogenesis factor (PDAF), of platelet-derived growth factor (PDGF), and their interrelationship with the healing cascade is summarized in Figure 3.

A commentary in *The Lancet*[25] emphasized the clinical potential of the cytokine TGF-ß, which exhibits autocrine, paracrine, and endocrine ef-

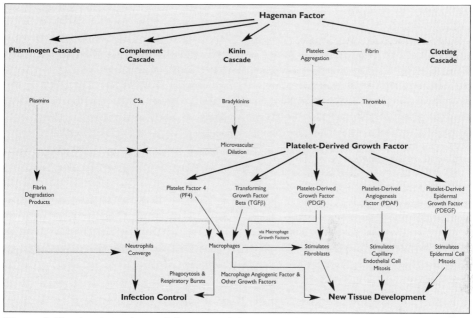

Figure 3. Platelet-derived growth factors and their interrelationship with the healing cascade.

fects. TGF-ß acts through the heteromultimers of receptors on the cell surface. Clinical interest has been focused on this growth factor's role in extracellular matrix deposition and leukocyte infiltration, which are important factors in wound healing. The chemotactic effect of TGF-ß on fibroblasts stimulates the deposition of collagen and other components of the extracellular matrix. Dermal wounds in rats are reported to heal with reduced scarring, and a clinical trial on venous ulcers showed a marked promotion of healing.[25]

The ongoing development of these products and their introduction as pharmacological agents in wound management are dependent upon a number of factors, not the least of which is the level at which the increase in cell replication is considered to be therapeutically significant and is further complicated by the difficulty of determining the rate in connective tissue.

The quantitative and qualitative effects must be the subject of new laboratory and clinical assessment procedures. The use of reproducible models, such as skin graft donor sites or implanted wound tissue sampling devices and bioassay techniques using cell cultures, will contribute to our characterization and ultimate usage of these factors.

The clinical expectation of application is wide, and the number of organizations involved internationally in research development and production is in the hundreds. There would therefore appear to be sufficient interest and available resource to ensure an in-depth evaluation of these bioactive materials that by enhancement or inhibition of inflammation, fibroplasia, epithelization, angiogenesis, connective tissue repair, and contraction may act as the normalizer in nonhealing wounds or the accelerator in normal wounds.

Future Development

Inevitably, new products will continue to become available for wound care in hospitals and the community. There will be extensions to the range of collagen products as well as that of membranes and skin substitutes as research techniques become more sophisticated. Conversely, some products, such as antiseptics and antibacterial materials in their present form, will disappear from the wound-care armamentarium. There is, and will continue to be, an increased interest in the use of biosurgical agents, such as leeches and maggots.

For the foreseeable future, *interactive* materials

will continue to be the first choice for wound management, as they are undoubtedly effective, and their price is competitive when compared to some of the previously described materials and whose use is recommended for wounds requiring specialized treatment. However, there is a real need for more evidence-based information about the comparative efficacies of these interactive materials for wound care to aid the selection of the most appropriate wound-management product to be used on any wound.

Evidence-based practice in wound care has not kept pace with the number of products marketed, and there is a great paucity of reliable information about the effectiveness of individual products or of their comparative effectiveness with products of a similar formulation. At present, it is impossible to select the best hydrocolloid, alginate, or hydrogel or to know that one dressing in a group is superior to another for application to a particular wound type. This has serious implications for both prescribers and patients.

Many of our preconceived ideas of tissue repair will have to be reexamined in the light of the new information these products will reveal. In addition, clinicians need to re-educate themselves with regard to not only the use of bioactive products but also the application of the innovative interactive materials in the management of their patients' wounds. It is a disturbing fact that despite the availability of these technologically and clinically advanced products, many wounds are still dressed with a gauze fabric—an original passive out-of-sight, out-of-mind dressing. The famous remark of the French surgeon, Ambroise Paré (1510–1590) "...que je pensay et Dieu la guarist," meaning, "I dressed (the wound) and God healed it" could well be the current fatalistic philosophy of many healthcare providers and produce a delay in the adoption of new products and procedures.

Ongoing developments, particularly at the cellular level, will hopefully result in successful and speedy healing of most, if not all, wounds with the resultant alleviation of pain and distress in both man and animals, as the management of soft-tissue injuries in animal species is becoming increasingly important, and many research activities are currently being progressed in this area.

Take-Home Messages for Practice

- The reader should understand the differences in formulation and function of passive, interactive, and bioactive materials.
- The reader should be able to compile a practice-based care plan, diagnose the healing stage at each dressing change, and select appropriate materials to ensure that healing progresses satisfactorily to effectively manage the wounds for each patient.

Self-Assessment Questions

1. Which of the following dressings would be suitable to treat a full-thickness burn with moderate exudate?
   - A. Absorbent lint
   - B. Hydrocolloid
   - C. Water vapor permeable film (or polymeric film)
   - D. Foam

2. Glycosaminoglycans belong to which class of wound management products?
   - A. Passive
   - B. Interactive
   - C. Bioactive

3. Which of these growth factors stimulate epidermal cell mitosis?
   - A. TGF-ß
   - B. PDGF
   - C. PDAF
   - D. PDEGF

Answers: 1-C, 2-C, 3-D

References

1. Majno G. *The Healing Hand*. Harvard, Mass: University Press; 1975:115–120.
2. *British Pharmacopoeia*. TSO; London.
3. Bishop WJ. *A History of Surgical Dressings*. London, England: Strangeway Press; 1959:54–57.
4. Elliot JR. Surgical materials. *St Bart Hosp J*. 1954;58:11–14.
5. The Lancet. Elsevier. ISSN: 0140-6736; 1870.
6. Gamgee S. Gauze and cotton tissue. *Lancet*. 1876;10:885.
7. *British Pharmaceutical Codex*. London, England: Pharmaceutical Press; 1923.

8. European Pharmacopoeia 5.0. European Directorate for the Quality of Medicines of the Council of Europe (EDQM). ISBN 92-871-5281-0.

9. Turner TD. Hospital usage of absorbent dressings. *Pharm J.* 1979;222:421–426.

10. Mustoe TA, Cooter RD, Gold MH, et al. International clinical recommendations on scar management. *Plast Reconstr Surg.* 2002;110(2):560–571.

11. Turner TD. Current and future trends in wound management, 2. *Pharm Int.* 1985;6(6):131.

12. Lock DM. Proceedings of the Symposium on Wound Healing; 1979; Helsinki. Sundell B, ed; 103–108.

13. Harding KG. Silastic foam. In: Turner TD, Schmidt RJ, Harding KG, eds. *Advances in Wound Management.* New York, NY: John Wiley & Sons; 1986:41–52.

14. Turner TD. Hydrogels and hydrocolloids. In: Turner TD, Schmidt RJ, Harding KG, eds. *Advances in Wound Management.* New York, NY: John Wiley & Sons; 1986:89–95.

15. Turner TD, Spyratou O, Schmidt RJ. Biocompatibility of wound management products: standardization of and determination of cell growth rate in L929 fibroblast cultures. *J Pharm Pharmacol.* 1989;41(11):775–780.

16. Schmidt R. Xerogel dressings. In: Turner TD, Schmidt RJ, Harding KG, eds. *Advances in Wound Management.* New York, NY: John Wiley & Sons; 1986:65–71.

17. Cherry GW, Ryan TJ. The physical properties of a new hydrocolloid dressing. An environment for healing. In: Ryan TJ, ed. *The Role of Occlusion.* London, UK: Royal Society of Medicine; 1985:61–68.

18. Ovington LG. The well-dressed wound: an overview of dressing types. *WOUNDS.* 1998;10(Suppl A):1A–11A.

19. Chung LY, Schmidt RJ, Andrews AM, Turner TD. A study of hydrogen peroxide generation by, and antioxidant activity of, Granuflex (DuoDERM) Hydrocolloid Granules and some other hydrogel/hydrocolloid wound management materials. *Br J Dermatol.* 1993;129(2):145–153.

20. Flohe L, Beakman R, Grertz H, et al. Oxygen-centered free radicals as mediators of inflammation In: Sies H, ed. *Oxidative Stress.* London, UK: Academic Press; 1985:403–428.

21. Harding CR, Scott IR. Histidine rich proteins (fillagrins): structural and functional heterogenicity during epidermal differentiation. *J Mol Biol.* 1983;170:651–673.

22. Bennett NT, Schultz GS. Growth factors and wound healing: part II. Role in normal and chronic wound healing. *Am J Surg.* 1993;166(1):74–81.

23. Schultz GS, Mast BA. Molecular analysis of the environment of healing and chronic wounds: cytokines, proteases and growth factors. *WOUNDS.* 1998;10(Suppl F):1F–9F.

24. Shah M, Revis D, Herrick S, et al. Role of elevated plasma transforming growth factor-beta1 levels in wound healing. *Am J Pathol.* 1999;154(4):1115–1124.

25. Shah M, Foreman DM, Ferguson MWJ. Control of scarring in adult wounds by neutralising antibody to transforming growth factor ß. *Lancet.* 1992;339(8787):213–214.

Suggested Reading

1. Goldsmith LA, ed. *Biochemistry and Physiology of the Skin,* vol I and II. Oxford, UK: Oxford University Press; 1983.

2. Bucknell TE, Ellis H, eds. *Wound Healing for Surgeons.* London, UK: Balliem, Tindall; 1984.

3. Peacock EE. *Wound Repair.* London, UK: WB Saunders & Co; 1984.

4. Royal Society of Medicine Int Cong, Services No. 88. *An Environment for Healing.* London, UK: Royal Society of Medicine; 1984.

5. Westaby S, ed. *Wound Care.* London, UK: William Heinemann Med. Books; 1985.

6. Sedlarik von KM. Wund–Heilung. Studtgart, Germany, Gustav Fischer Verlag Jena; 1993.

7. Leaper DJ, Harding KG, eds. *Wounds: Biology and Management.* Oxford, UK: Oxford University Press; 1998.

8. Thomas S. Surgical Dressings & Wound Management. Kestrel Health Information, 2012. www.woundsource.com/store

Wound Dressing Product Selection: A Holistic, Interprofessional, Patient-Centered Approach©

Diane L. Krasner, PhD, RN, CWCN, CWS, MAPWCA, FAAN;
R. Gary Sibbald, BSc, MD, MEd, FRCPC (Med, Derm), MACP, FAAD, MAPWCA;
Kevin Y. Woo, PhD, RN, FAPWCA

© 2010 Kestrel Health Information, Inc. Used with permission.

Objectives

The reader will be challenged to:

• Apply a wound dressing product selection framework to clinical practice

• Assess dressing performance parameters for holistic, interprofessional patient-centered care

• Identify web-based resources for up-to-date dressing product information.

Introduction

Many wound care clinicians remember the "good old days" when wound dressing product selection simply involved choosing from a handful of products that were essentially variations on the same theme. There was gauze, impregnated gauze, and filled gauze pads. In the earlier 20th century, clinicians added antimicrobial solutions, creams, and ointments (like Dakin's solution developed during World War I and silver sulfadiazine developed in the 1960s), and the wound care formulary was limited and simplistic.

Fast forward to the 21st century and wound care clinicians are confronted with a totally different situation: hundreds of products, scientific rationale for moist interactive dressings, and an emerging evidence-base for product selection.

Current wound care expertise encompasses numerous dressing-related skills, including:

• *Treating the cause of the wound* and addressing *patient-centered concerns* to set the stage for local wound care

• Properly *assessing the wound* and identifying the dressing requirements

• Selecting *dressings based on their form and function* for an individual wound's needs

• Meeting *setting-specific requirements* for dressing change frequency and maintenance

• Addressing *formulary or healthcare system availability* as well as reimbursement requirements.

Reprinted from Krasner DL, Sibbald RG, Woo KY. Wound dressing product selection: a holistic, interprofessional patient-centered approach©. *WoundSource™: The Kestrel Wound Product Sourcebook.* September 2010. Available at: http://www.woundsource.com/wound-dressing-product-selection-white-paper#. © 2010 Kestrel Health Information, Inc. Used with permission.

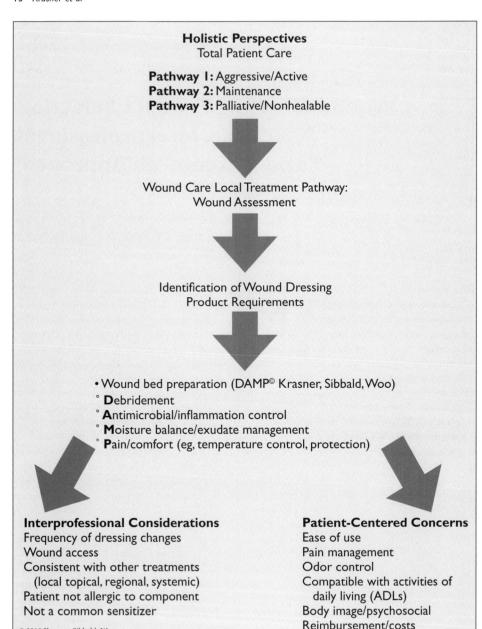

Holistic Perspectives
Total Patient Care

Pathway 1: Aggressive/Active
Pathway 2: Maintenance
Pathway 3: Palliative/Nonhealable

Wound Care Local Treatment Pathway:
Wound Assessment

Identification of Wound Dressing
Product Requirements

• Wound bed preparation (DAMP© Krasner, Sibbald, Woo)
   ° **D**ebridement
   ° **A**ntimicrobial/inflammation control
   ° **M**oisture balance/exudate management
   ° **P**ain/comfort (eg, temperature control, protection)

Interprofessional Considerations
Frequency of dressing changes
Wound access
Consistent with other treatments
   (local topical, regional, systemic)
Patient not allergic to component
Not a common sensitizer

© 2010 Krasner, Sibbald, Woo

Patient-Centered Concerns
Ease of use
Pain management
Odor control
Compatible with activities of
   daily living (ADLs)
Body image/psychosocial
Reimbursement/costs

Figure 1. Conceptual Framework for Wound Dressing Product Selection©.

Wound care product selection today must be as sophisticated and as evidence-based as possible. This chapter presents a conceptual framework for the wound dressing product selection process that is based on 3 principles:

• Holistic perspectives[1]
• Interprofessional considerations[2]
• Patient-centered concerns.[3]

This conceptual framework is illustrated in Figure 1 and is discussed in detail in this chapter.

Wound Dressing Product Selection for the 21st Century

For every complex problem, there is a simple solution, and it is wrong. — H. L. Mencken

Selecting appropriate wound dressing products and supportive care to maximize healing and patient outcomes is a complex process. Dressing and local wound care options based on science and best practices must be filtered by clinical experience and must be consistent with patient preferences, caregiver requirements, and setting/access issues.[4] Additionally, effective dressing selection and local wound care planning involve the perspectives of the entire interprofessional team.[2]

Knowing the performance parameters of dressing categories/individual products and matching these attributes to an individual's wound can optimize the healing process.[5] However, dressings are only one piece of the puzzle. Dressings alone will not promote wound healing, unless the underlying causes for the wound are also addressed (eg, treatment of the wound cause, blood supply, nutrition, patient-centered concerns, local wound care). As the wound changes, the plan of care must change and dressing products may have to be changed. *Appropriate dressing product selection*:

- Optimizes the local wound healing environment
- Reduces local pain and suffering
- Improves activities of daily living and quality of life.

Inappropriate dressing selection can:

- Cause the wound status to deteriorate (eg, wound margin maceration, increased risk of superficial critical colonization or deep infection, skin stripping)
- Increase local pressure or pain, especially at dressing change (dressing removal and cleansing)
- Increase costs with the need for frequent dressing changes or the selection of an inappropriate advanced or active dressing.

National and international wound care guidelines and best practice documents mean that there is no longer a local standard of care. No matter where you practice, you will be held to national/international standards of wound care practice.[6] Some experts have argued that the selection of the wrong dressing is just as problematic as the administration of the wrong drug and the clinician would be just as liable in a court of law. If dressings can be shown to delay the healing process (eg, wet-to-dry gauze dressings in a wound that requires moist wound healing, pain from inappropriate adhesives, failure to treat critical colonization that can lead to deep infection), their use might be deemed negligent by a jury in a court case.

Holistic Perspectives

Wound dressing product selection must be consistent and congruent with the total plan of care for the person with a wound. Four questions that the clinician should consider are:

1. What type of wound is it? What is the underlying etiology/cause and can you treat or correct the cause (eg, pressure, venous, neuropathic, neuroischemic, ischemic)?
2. Is it healable, maintenance, or nonhealable/palliative?[7]
3. Is the wound colonized, critically colonized, or infected in the deep tissue or wound margin?[8,9]
4. Is the plan of care aggressive/active, maintenance, or palliative/nonhealable?

If the overall plan of care for the person is aggressive/active, the dressing plan should be aggressive/active. For example, if a person has an exudating, infected diabetic foot ulcer with osteomyelitis that is being treated with hyperbaric oxygen therapy and serial debridements, a dressing, such as a silver alginate or a silver foam dressing, would be the dressing of choice.[10] On the other hand, if a person is dying and on hospice and the goal of care is to palliate an exudating, infected diabetic foot wound with osteomyelitis, then a topical antimicrobial, such as cadexomer iodine, povidone-iodine, or chlorhexidine or its derivatives (polyhexamethylene biguanide or PHMB), might be a congruent choice.

In clinical practice, occasions occur frequently when patients are too sick to choose an aggressive pathway for their wound care. A common scenario is when a patient is in critical condition in an intensive care unit, on a respirator, immobilized, and anticoagulated and his life hangs in the balance. The patient develops a sacral pressure ulcer that quickly goes from a partial-thickness lesion to a full-thickness wound with eschar. A holistic approach to wound care would lead to the maintenance pathway. Aggressive/active care in a critically ill patient would be unreasonable. Debridement of eschar in an anticoagulated patient with little healing potential is not a reasonable or prudent practice. A more reasonable option is to maintain the wound using a dressing that would protect the area and keep the eschar stable (such as an adhesive foam) until the patient improves (at which point the aggressive/active pathway kicks in) or the patient deteriorates (at which point the palliative/nonhealable pathway is chosen).

Wound Assessment and Identification of Wound Dressing Requirements

Wound care requires a holistic approach, looking at the **whole patient** and not just the **hole in the patient.** The very first step of the assessment should aim to determine the accurate wound diagnosis and the cause of the wound. Despite the importance of dressings, wound healing can only be optimized when the underlying wound cause is corrected. For example, strategies to reduce tissue deformation (pressure, friction, and shear) are crucial to promote healing of pressure ulcers. Patients with venous leg ulcers benefit from venous congestion-improving compression therapies (bandages for healing or support stockings to prevent recurrence). Footwear or devices should be considered to redistribute pressure away from diabetic or other neurotrophic foot ulcers. It is important to remember that wounds are not likely to heal if arterial supply is deficient unless patients undergo bypass or dilation of the affected arteries. Other related factors that may influence wound healing and warrant regular evaluation include nutrition, coexisting medical diseases, and certain medications. When healing is not the realistic objective, moisture is contraindicated; instead, conservative debridement without cutting into living tissue, bacterial reduction, and moisture reduction should be considered.

The first step in wound care is to carefully document the wound characteristics:
- Location
- Size: longest length and the widest width (at a right angle to the longest length or oriented by a head-to-foot perspective)
- Depth as usually measured by a cotton swab or sterile probe
- Undermining and tunneling: location on the clock and extent as measured by a probe
- Wound margin: normal, macerated, erythema, edema, warmth, or increased temperature
- Wound base: by percentage
  - Black-brown firm eschar
  - Brown-yellow soft slough (harmful)
  - Yellow firm tissue that may serve as a foundation for granulation (healthy)
  - Pink, firm, healthy granulation tissue or unhealthy red, friable tissue
  - Exudate:
    - Serous, sanguinous, or pustular or combinations
    - Large, moderate, scant, absent
  - Epithelial edge
  - Sloped purple of advancing, healing epithelial margin
  - Steep slope of stalled chronic wound
- Exposed tissues (tendon, bone) that may not allow granulation on top
- Foreign bodies (eg, gauze fragments, sutures, hardware).

To prepare a wound bed for healing, devitalized and damaged tissue, such as firm eschar, or sloughy materials that promote bacterial growth should be removed or debrided. Topical dressings are used to promote autolytic debridement through the activities of phagocytic cells and endogenous enzymes. Another key function of wound dressings is to manage localized wound infection. All chronic wounds are colonized by bacteria. If bacteria were allowed to proliferate, crossing a critical threshold, local tissue damage can lead to delayed healing. *Many modern dressings contain active antimicrobial ingredients* that are released into the wound surface compartment in an exchange with wound fluid. Dressings with silver are one of the most popular choices of topical agents. Alternatively, bacteria can be entrapped and sequestered in the micro-architecture of a dressing where they may be inactivated. For nonhealable wounds, topical antiseptics dry the wound surface and provide bacterial reduction.

For wounds that have the potential to heal, moisture balance (not too much or too little) is essential for all phases of wound repair. An ideal dressing should be able to keep the wound bed moist for cellular proliferation and migration but at the same time sequester excess drainage to avoid periwound damage.

The major categories of wound dressings are foams, alginates, hydrofibers, hydrogels, and hydrocolloids. These are discussed briefly below.

Foam dressings are designed to wick up a large volume of exudate. The fluid-handling capacity of various foams can be affected by the polyurethane film backing and its ability to transfer moisture vapor out of the dressing but form a barrier to bacterial contamination. Depending on the level of wound exudate, foams have a wear time of 1 to 7 days.

Foams absorb moisture but also give moisture back to a wound if the gradient on the surface becomes dehydrated. This function can lead to periwound maceration, but advanced foam dressings have variable pore sizes that will facilitate partial moisture retention and partial moisture exchange with the wound surface. These second generation foams are less likely to macerate the wound margin. Foams also have been combined with antiseptics (silver, PHMB) and other agents to serve as a delivery vehicle for active therapies at the wound surface (third generation of foam development). Foams that are associated with excessive periwound maceration can be cut to the wound size, fenestrated on the top to wick to a secondary dressing, or changed more frequently.

Alginate dressings are also capable of handling copious exudate, while the gelling effect of these materials will keep the wound base moist. Unlike foams, calcium alginates are bioresorbable (may disappear) and bind fluid to the outside of the fibers rather than the inner pores. Alginates are derived from brown seaweed or kelp. Depending on the species and origin of the calcium alginate (leaf, stem), they may have more gelling (high manuronic acid concentration) or a higher fiber strength (high galuronic acid concentration). These dressings are manufactured in sheets (lateral fluid wicking) or in ropes (vertical fluid wicking). When the alginate is extracted from kelp, it is a sodium hydrogel that can be combined with calcium to form a fibrous structure. When they are applied to the wound, the calcium as part of the alginate is released into the wound and may also trigger the coagulation cascade to facilitate hemostasis. The sodium is exchanged for calcium at the level of the alginate, recreating a sodium alginate hydrogel. In comparison to foams, calcium alginates are less absorptive, but they have

the ability to act as excellent autolytic debriders. Dressings with alginates are often changed daily or as infrequently as 3 times a week.

Hydrofiber dressings consist of carboxymethylcellulose and have a water-hating (hydrophobic) component (methylcellulose) that gives the dressing its tensile strength and a water-loving (hydrophilic) component (carboxy) that acts as a fluid lock. As the dressing absorbs fluid, the hydrofiber is converted into a gel consistency. Hydrofiber dressings are thin and have moderate absorbency, forming a fluid lock. When the hydrofiber is saturated, wound fluid strike-through will occur. These dressings require a secondary dressing to keep them in place because the addition of an adhesive will interfere with the fluid absorption properties of the dressing.

Hydrogel dressings are usually indicated for dry wounds. The major ingredient of hydrogels is water (70% to 90%), which donates moisture into the wound base. The backbone for a hydrogel may be a hydrocolloid, propylene glycol, saline, or other substance. This backbone gives them their viscosity or tack to stay on the wound bed. They are excellent autolytic debriders and preserve moisture balance, largely through donating moisture to the wound surface. They are often changed daily to 3 times a week.

Hydrocolloid dressings consist of a backing (often a film or polyurethane) with carboxymethylcellulose, water-absorptive components (such as gelatin and pectin), and an adhesive. Hydrocolloids are designed for wear times of 1 to 7 days, and for this reason, their absorbency is lower than foams or calcium alginates but similar to hydrogels. When these dressings are used for autolytic debridement, they may need to be changed more frequently and may require the removal of nonviable slough from the surface of the wound to prevent odor or secondary bacterial proliferation under the dressing. These dressings often lower the wound surface pH that may contribute to their antimicrobial effect. Some hydrocolloids leave more residue on the wound surface than others, and this residue may contribute to wound odor under the hydrocolloid dressing.

Film dressings are often used for local protection. The choice of a nonadherent (no adhesive) versus a film with adhesive backing should be determined by the fragility of the surrounding skin.

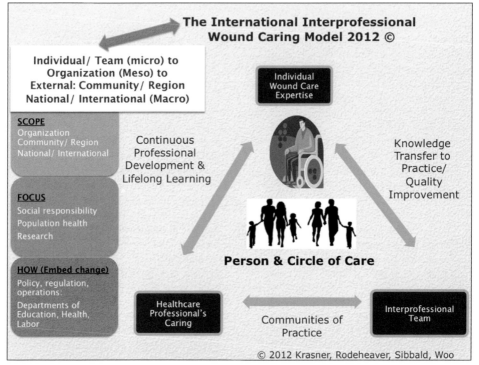

Figure 2. The International Interprofessional Wound Caring Model 2012.
© 2012 Krasner, Rodeheaver, Sibbald, and Woo.

Film materials are semi-occlusive with various degrees of permeability (referred to as the moisture vapor transmission rate or MVTR) that allow a water molecule to pass through the dressing and evaporate into the ambient environment at a variable rate, depending on the MVTR. They are not designed for fluid accumulation below the film. When fluid develops under the dressing, it needs to be evacuated or the dressing changed because the relatively alkaline pH under these dressings with fluid accumulation will promote bacterial proliferation. As an alternative to traditional adhesives (acrylates, hydrocolloids), silicone coatings have been used to reduce local trauma and prevent pain on dressing removal.

Interprofessional Considerations

When different professional groups are involved in a wound patient's care, there may be interprofessional considerations that will have bearing on the dressing selected. Finding a way to accommodate each discipline's unique per-

spectives and needs enhances interprofessional wound care (Figure 2).[2] Here are several common examples:

- In an acute care facility, the surgical team wants to examine a dehisced surgical wound on daily rounds, so a dressing that is changed daily and can be lifted off and replaced without compromising the dressing adherence is the best choice (eg, silicone foam versus adhesive foam or gauze dressing).

- In any setting, the physicians need to measure the output from a draining tube site (eg, nephrostomy tube site). Discontinue absorbent gauze pads (eg, abdominal dressings or ABDs) and use cut-to-fit urostomy pouches to allow accurate measurement of the drainage and protect the periwound skin from maceration and erosion.

- In an outpatient wound center, the hyperbaricist needs to assess the wound daily following hyperbaric treatment. A nonadhesive, daily or between-treatment dressing change is needed (eg, hydrogel, hydrocolloid, or other modern moist interactive dressing).

- In a nursing home, the physical therapy department will begin rehabilitation therapy on a resident with a diabetic foot ulcer. A dressing that minimizes pressure on the wound bed when the resident ambulates is optimal (eg, a piece of alginate rope versus a gauze 2 x 2) with a thin but secure secondary dressing to avoid interfering with the plantar pressure redistribution.

Interprofessional collaboration on dressing selection can prevent complications (such as skin stripping or skin tears) from changing dressings too frequently, having inappropriate adhesive backing or inadequate moisture balance, or lacking required antimicrobial properties. Careful coordination reduces costs and dressing-associated labor.

Another occasion when careful dressing coordination is needed is during wound patient/client transfers from one healthcare setting or service to another, including a discharge home. For example, the optimal dressing for acute care may not be available or reimbursed in long-term care or home care. In the United States, if the person has been a resident in long-term care and is moved to hospice care, the hospice will provide the dressings for the resident while he or she is in the nursing home as part of the per diem hospice benefit. This may necessitate a change of dressing, depending on the hospice dressing formulary.

Finally, is your interprofessional team up to standards? Are you able to provide holistic, patient-centered care? Ask yourself the following 3 questions:

- Does your wound team have the resources (human and otherwise) and knowledge to provide advanced patient-centered wound care?
- Do you have the referral sources in place to meet the needs of selected wound patients (especially their psychosocial and social needs) along with rehabilitation support?
- Does your wound team and dressing formulary enable you to address the needs of special populations (such as bariatric, diabetic, frail elderly, and palliative) in a timely and appropriate manner?

Patient-Centered Concerns

Individualized wound care plans that address specific patient-centered concerns are most likely

| European Pressure Ulcer Advisory Panel: www.epuap.org |
| European Wound Management Association: www.ewma.org |
| World Union of Wound Healing Societies: www.wuwhs.org |
| World Wide Wounds: www.worldwidewounds.org |
| WoundPedia: www.woundpedia.com |
| WoundSource: www.woundsource.com |

Figure 3. Websites with dressing-related information.

to succeed and promote the best outcomes for the patient with a wound. Standardized, "canned" wound care plans often fail because they do not promote patient adherence/coherence. The patient may be labeled "noncompliant" when the real problem is that the care plan has not been properly individualized to the person's specific needs/problems and he or she cannot possibly comply with the routine way. *The road to wound care planning success is paved with careful attention to patient-centered concerns, including pain management, odor control, body image and psychosocial concerns, and reimbursement/cost issues.*

Common examples of patient-centered concerns that impact dressing product selection include:

- Premedicating patients who experience dressing change pain prior to dressing changes and allowing adequate time for the premedication to take effect
- Selecting, when appropriate, nonadherent dressings to reduce pain and trauma at dressing change
- Addressing odor control issues by utilizing absorbent and/or charcoal dressings and adjusting dressing change frequency
- When possible, selecting secondary dressings that enable patients to shower, bathe, and perform other usual activities of daily living
- Choosing dressings that are easy to apply and that address the needs of the person with a wound and his or her circle of care.

Whenever possible, order dressings that are reimbursed by the person's insurance and that are easily purchased/accessed.

Conclusion

When developing wound dressing product formularies and clinical practice guidelines, be sure to follow a formal process that includes a review of relevant existing clinical practice guidelines and regulatory requirements, such as those in the United States from the Centers for Medicare & Medicaid Services. For guidance on this process, readers are referred to *SELECT: Evaluation and Implementation of Clinical Practice Guidelines: A Guidance Document from the American Professional Wound Care Association.*[11]

Two excellent online wound dressing product resources are available to help build a dressing formulary by generic category: WoundSource (Kestrel Health Information, Inc.), www.woundsource.com/product-category/dressings, and World Wide Wounds (United Kingdom), www.worldwidewounds.com. Websites with dressing-related information are listed in Figure 3.

Take-Home Messages for Practice

• Incorporating a wound dressing product selection conceptual model into your practice will assure that your product selection is holistic, interprofessional, and patient-centered.

• Individualized wound care plans that address specific patient-centered concerns are more likely to succeed and promote the best outcomes for the patient with a wound.

• Web-based resources for dressing information help you keep updated and evidence-based.

Self-Assessment Questions

1. Which of the following issues is NOT a patient-centered concern?
   A. Pain at dressing change
   B. Odor
   C. Difficult dressing for the staff and caregivers to apply
   D. Color of dressing calls attention to the fact that the person has a wound

2. Common wound dressing performance parameters that can have a significant impact on a dressing's applicability for a particular wound and a specific patient include all of the following EXCEPT:
   A. Ability to handle exudate
   B. Adhesive with low tack
   C. Packaged in boxes of 10
   D. Daily dressing changes are not required

Answers: 1–C, 2–C

References

1. Sibbald RG, Krasner DL, Lutz JB, et al. The SCALE Expert Panel: Skin Changes at Life's End. Final Consensus Document. October 1, 2009. Downloadable at www.gaymar.com.
2. Krasner DL, Rodeheaver GT, Sibbald RG. Interprofessional wound caring. In: Krasner DL, Rodeheaver GT, Sibbald RG, eds. *Chronic Wound Care: A Clinical Source Book for Healthcare Professionals.* 4th ed. Malvern, PA: HMP Communications; 2007:3–9. www.chronicwoundcarebook.com
3. Osterberg L, Blaschke T. Adherence to medication. *N Engl J Med.* 2005;353:487–497.
4. Sackett DL, Straus SE, Richardson WS, Rosenberg W, Haynes RB. *Evidence-based Medicine: How to Practice and Teach EBM.* 2nd ed. Edinburgh, Scotland: Churchhill Livingston; 2000.
5. Cockbill SME, Turner TD. The development of wound management products. In: Krasner DL, Rodeheaver GT, Sibbald RG, eds. *Chronic Wound Care: A Clinical Source Book for Healthcare Professionals.* 4th ed. Malvern, PA: HMP Communications; 2007:233–248. www.chronicwoundcarebook.com
6. Ayello EA, Capitulo KL, Fife CE, et al. Legal issues in the care of pressure ulcer patients: Key concepts for healthcare providers. A consensus paper from the International Expert Wound Care Advisory Panel. June 22, 2009. Downloadable at www.medline.com.
7. Ferris FD, Al Khateib AA, Fromantin I, et al. Palliative wound care: managing chronic wounds across life's continuum: a consensus statement from the International Palliative Wound Care Initiative. *J Palliat Med.* 2007;10:37–39.
8. Sibbald RG, Woo K, Ayello EA. Increased bacterial burden and infection: the story of NERDS and STONES. *Adv Skin Wound Care.* 2006;19:447–461.
9. Woo KY, Sibbald RG. A cross-sectional validation study using NERDS and STONEES to assess bacterial burden. *Ostomy Wound Manage.* 2009;55:40–48.
10. Krasner DL, Sibbald RG. Dressings and local wound care for people with diabetic foot wounds. In: Armstrong DG, Lavery LA, eds. *Clinical Care of the Diabetic Foot.* 2nd ed. Alexandria, VA: American Diabetes Association; 2010:69–78.
11. SELECT: Evaluation and Implementation of Clinical Practice Guidelines. A Guidance Document from the American Professional Wound Care Association (APWCA). 2009. Downloadable at www.apwca.org.

CHAPTER 14

Interprofessional Perspectives on Individualized Wound Device Product Selection©

Diane L. Krasner, PhD, RN, CWCN, CWS, MAPWCA, FAAN;
R. Gary Sibbald, BSc, MD, MEd, FRCPC (Med, Derm), MACP, FAAD, MAPWCA;
Kevin Y. Woo, PhD, RN, FAPWCA; **Linda Norton,** BScOT, OT Reg (ONT), MScCH

Objectives

The reader will be challenged to:
- Articulate the benefits of interprofessional collaboration to optimize device product selection
- Identify important clinical considerations for compression therapy devices, off-weighting devices, electrical stimulation, ultrasound, hyperbaric oxygen therapy, negative pressure wound therapy, and pressure redistribution surfaces
- Appreciate the complexities of implementing interprofessional individualized selection in clinical practice.

Introduction

Like many aspects of wound care, wound device product selection has become an increasingly complex and sophisticated process over the past several decades. Not only are more products available, but the challenge of matching the appropriate device for a specific patient's profile has become a rising expectation. From pressure redistribution surfaces to negative pressure wound therapy, the process of device selection requires careful interprofessional consideration of the individual's wound as well as his or her holistic, biopsychosocial needs and the setting/environment/access (Figure 1).[1] By utilizing interprofessional collaboration, healthcare teams can "propose" solution(s) that would have been unattainable through single disciplinary means.[2]

The following general categories of wound care-related devices will be reflected in this chapter. Specific category and/or product information can be found at www.woundsource.com.

- Compression therapy devices
- Off-weighting devices (also known as off-loading devices)
- Adjunctive therapies, such as electrical stimulation, ultrasound, and hyperbaric oxygen therapy (HBOT)
- Negative pressure wound therapy (NPWT)
- Pressure redistribution surfaces (also known as specialty beds and support surfaces).

These devices cover a wide range of products: some are prescription; some are over-the-counter (OTC). Many are regulated or classified by the Food & Drug Administration

Reprinted from Krasner DL, Sibbald RG, Woo KY, Norton L. Interprofessional perspectives on individualized wound device product selection©. *WoundSource™: The Kestrel Wound Product Sourcebook.* November 2011. Available at: http://www.woundsource.com/wound-device-white-paper#. © 2011 Kestrel Health Information, Inc. Used with permission.

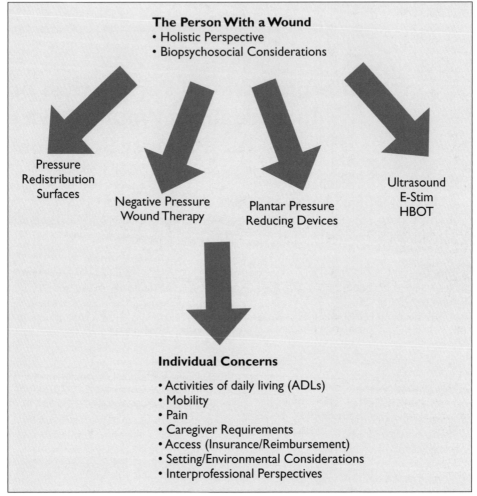

The Person With a Wound
- Holistic Perspective
- Biopsychosocial Considerations

Pressure Redistribution Surfaces

Negative Pressure Wound Therapy

Plantar Pressure Reducing Devices

Ultrasound
E-Stim
HBOT

Individual Concerns

- Activities of daily living (ADLs)
- Mobility
- Pain
- Caregiver Requirements
- Access (Insurance/Reimbursement)
- Setting/Environmental Considerations
- Interprofessional Perspectives

Figure 1. Wound device considerations for the person with a wound. © 2011 Krasner, Sibbald, Woo, and Norton.

(FDA) in the United States or a comparable agency in other countries. In the United States, the Centers for Medicare & Medicaid Services (CMS) may or may not reimburse for devices based on specific policies and criteria (eg, Group 1, 2, and 3 support surface criteria; hyperbaric oxygen therapy coverage policies). Individual medical necessity, if it can be demonstrated by the prescriber, may enable an individual to obtain a reimbursed device under circumstances that usually would not be covered.

Wound care devices may or may not have indications, contraindications, or precautions — just like medications. These are particularly important for such wound devices as NPWT and HBOT. The prescriber (physician or his or her designee, eg, physician's assistant, nurse practitioner) is responsible for knowing the indications, contraindications, and precautions and ascertaining whether a specific device is appropriate for an individual patient. Failure to do so can result in serious adverse outcomes with legal consequences.

Wound Device Product Usage Issues

In addition to labeled product usage guidelines from the manufacturer, facilities often have their own *policies and procedures* or *protocols* for using

National Pressure Ulcer Advisory Panel (NPUAP)
Support Surface Standards Initiative: Terms and Definitions
Version 01/29/2007
http://www.npuap.org/NPUAP_S3I_TD.pdf

Cochrane Review on Support Surfaces
McInnes E, Bell-Syer SE, Dumville JC, Legood R, Cullum NA
Support Surfaces for Pressure Ulcer Prevention.
Cochrane Database Sept Rev. 2008; 4:CD001735

Websites with Device-Related Information

European Pressure Ulcer Advisory Panel	www.epuap.org
European Wound Management Association	www.ewma.org
World Union of Wound Healing Societies	www.wuwhs.org
World Wide Wounds	www.worldwidewounds.org
WoundPedia	www.woundpedia.org
WoundSource	www.woundsource.com

Figure 2. National and international device-related guidelines, resources, and websites.

devices. It is important that such documents be updated on a regular basis; be updated whenever the manufacturer updates its *guidelines* for product use; and reflect national and international best practices and guidelines (Figure 2).[3] All prescribers must be aware of such documents. Legal advisors suggest the facilities should call such documents guidelines instead of policies and procedures or protocols to reflect the need to individualize them for each patient and to reduce legal exposure.[4] All prescribing healthcare professionals should be trained in the use of the device they are prescribing, and if certification courses are available from the manufacturer, having prescribers certified is highly recommended by legal counsel and risk managers. Other process issues with legal ramifications related to device usage include:

- Appropriate orders by appropriate prescribers
- Timely device initiation and discontinuation
- Documentation of device efficacy
- Patient/caregiver education regarding device use, troubleshooting, and who to contact in case of emergency
- Seamless transitioning across the continuum of care.

Devices are frequently rented through a vendor or other external source. These relationships should be acknowledged by written contracts or agreements that specify vendor and facility responsibilities. Issues to consider include:

- Timely delivery and pickup
- Support for problems/device malfunction
- For devices that are purchased and owned by the facility, the process for annual inspection by the manufacturer or in-house bioengineering.

The "lens" through which wound device product selection is viewed, is — in part — a function of our professional training, considerations, and vantage points. Three international thought leaders in wound care will now present their perspectives from the physician, nurse, and therapist perspectives.

The Physician's Perspective on Individualized Wound Device Product Selection

Compression and venous insufficiency ulcers. In the *wound bed preparation paradigm*,[5] members of the interprofessional wound care team need to treat the cause and address patient-centered con-

Type of System Pattern of Pressure	Elastic	Non-elastic
	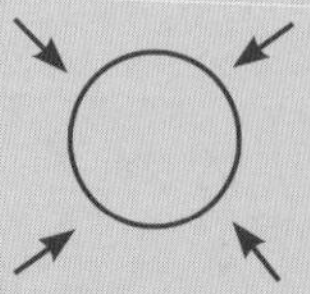	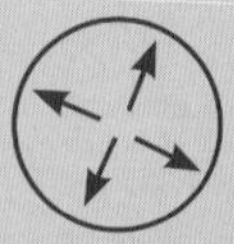
Rest	High Pressure	Low Pressure
Muscle Contraction	High Pressure but less	High Pressure
Low	Single Layer Elastic bandages	Unna Boot
High	Long stretch 4 layer	Short stretch Modified Unna Boot (Duke Boot)

Figure 3. Non-elastic systems have low pressure at rest. © 2007 Sibbald.

cerns before considering the components of local wound care. In the case of venous ulcers, clinicians must rule out arterial disease with an ABPI (ankle brachial pressure index). If the ABPI (ankle systolic pressure over brachial systolic pressure expressed as a ratio) is between 0.8 and 1.2, persons with venous leg ulcers should receive compression bandages for healing and stockings to prevent recurrences post-healing. The Cochrane Review on compression therapy[6] evidence base has concluded:

• Compression increases ulcer healing rates compared with no compression
• Multicomponent systems are more effective than single-component systems
• Multicomponent systems containing an elastic bandage appear more effective than those composed mainly of inelastic constituents.

There are several multilayered elastic and inelastic systems available that deliver high compression.[7] Two elastic systems are the 4-layer bandage systems and long-stretch bandages. For high-compression systems that are inelastic, there is the zinc oxide paste boot (Unna boot) that can be made more rigid with an outer layer of a flexible cohesive bandage (Coban™ over zinc oxide paste bandage = Duke boot) or the Coban™ 2-layer bandage. After healing, it is recommended that patients with venous disease are transitioned into the appropriate compression stockings to help prevent recurrence.

That pain is much more common with venous disease has been discussed by Krasner et al,[8] Woo et al,[9] and the World Union of Wound Healing Societies consensus statements on pain.[10] A patient with pain due to venous edema prior to the application of compression therapy may tolerate an inelastic support system and move up to an elastic system as the pain and edema are controlled. As illustrated in Figure 3,[7] non-elastic systems have low pressure at rest (less squeezing) and may increase patient adherence until edema and pain control have been optimized. If appropriate, an elastic system can then be introduced. Individuals with mixed venous and arterial disease but who have an ABPI between 0.65 and 0.80 should modify their compression therapy with modified product kits delivering lower compression (eg, Profore lite™, Coban 2 lite™).

Plantar pressure redistribution for diabetic and other neuropathic and neuroischemic foot ulcers. Persons with loss of protective sensation are unaware of trauma or injury to the foot. These individuals often develop plantar calluses (increased pressure) and blisters (friction or shear) with the foot sliding or moving in relation to their footwear. These individuals have 3 important components[11,12] to address before considering sharp surgical debridement of the callus. Using the mnemonic **VIP**, they are:

V — Vascular supply. Must be adequate to heal: Palpable pulse or, when the pulse is not palpable, a biphasic or triphasic Doppler signal, toe pressure over 55, or transcutaneous oxygen saturation over 30 mmHg.

I — Infection. There should be no signs of increased surface bacterial burden (any 3 signs from the **NERDS** mnemonic: Non-healing, ↑Exudate, Red friable granulation, Debris on the wound surface or Smell = use a topical antimicrobial) or deep and surrounding tissue infection (any 3 of the **STONEES** mnemonic: ↑Size, ↑Temperature, Os [Latin for bone exposed or probes], New areas of breakdown, Erythema or Edema = cellulitis, or ↑Exudate, Smell = use a systemic antimicrobial). If increased exudate and smell are present, an additional NERDS criteria is needed for a topical antimicrobial or an additional STONEES criteria for systemic antimicrobials or both.[13,14]

P — Plantar pressure redistribution. The gold standard is the contact cast that the patient cannot remove and will download the forefoot where 80% of neuropathic ulcers are usually located. Removable cast walkers (eg, air cast or CROW walker) can be made non-removable by securing them with a fiberglass, flexible cohesive or zinc oxide bandage to increase adherence to treatment. Less expensive alternatives include the half shoe (absent forefoot for forefoot ulcers and absent heel for heel area ulcers) that comprises 10%–15% of neuropathic ulcers. Many of these devices will have a rocker bottom surface. Other custom orthotics and footwear may be ordered in selected cases.[15]

It is also important after the healing of a foot ulcer to order the correct orthopedic deep-toed shoes and orthotics.

The last two treatments in this section are reserved for individuals with chronic wounds that have the cause corrected or compensated and there is adequate blood supply to heal. In addition, local wound care should be optimized: adequate debridement, infection and persistent abnormal inflammation controlled, and moisture balance optimized and still a healable wound is stalled. There are certain indications where acute wounds may have evidence for hyperbaric oxygen therapy and NPWT at an earlier stage.

Hyperbaric oxygen. HBOT is the administration of 100% oxygen at airtight pressures greater than 1 atmosphere absolute (ATA). Adequate tissue oxygen tension is essential to wound healing. Diminished circulation and hypoxia increase lactate production that is deleterious to wound healing. HBOT sessions usually entail approximately 45 to 120 minutes in the chamber once or twice daily for 20–30 sessions. *In-vivo* studies have shown that elevated arterial oxygen tensions can increase regulation of growth factors, decrease regulation of inflammatory cytokines, promote angiogenesis, and exert antibacterial effects in wounds.

Hyperbaric oxygen is often beneficial with overwhelming infection as long as there is enough blood supply to heal and maintain the healing response. Pooled data from 6 randomized controlled trials on diabetic foot ulcers suggested a significant reduction in the risk of major amputation with HBOT,[16] but there was no significant change in wound size reduction and number of healed wounds.

High doses of oxygen are toxic, particularly to the brain and lungs. Other potential drawbacks of HBOT include damage to the ears and sinuses, time and direct cost associated with daily travel to and from the treatment center, and the psychological effect of confinement.

Negative pressure wound therapy. NPWT is the delivery of intermittent or continuous subatmospheric pressure to the wound bed.[17] There have been many interface surfaces between the wound and the NPWT suction device, including gauze or open-celled foam composed of either polyurethane or polyvinyl alcohol that is cut and placed onto the surface of the wound. The foam is then sealed over with a transparent drape to create a closed airtight system. Contraction of the foam dressing exerts a centripetal effect at the wound edges and a mechanical force at the interface of the foam and wound. The suction effect and mechanical stress are transmitted to cellular and cytoskeletal levels, causing deformation of extracellular matrix (ECM) and cells that is postulated to promote cellular proliferation. Other potential advantages of NPWT are:
- Removal of excess interstitial fluid to reduce the intercellular diffusion distance
- Improvement of local wound blood flow

- Potential reduction of bacterial colonization
- Sequestration of excess matrix metallopro- teinases (MMPs) and pro-inflammatory/ab- normal wound exudate.[18]

Armstrong conducted a multicenter, random- ized, controlled trial (N = 162) to examine the effect of NPWT in complex wounds after partial foot amputation to the trans-metatarsal level in patients with diabetes.[19] Fifty-six percent of the patients healed in the NPWT group compared to 39% of the control group (P = .04). Investigations pertaining to the management of acute post- surgical wounds using NPWT also demonstrated positive results.[20,21] Many wound care experts uti- lize NPWT after acute surgical procedures, es- pecially when secondary infection is present (eg, dehiscence of post-sternotomy wounds).

The Ontario Health Technology Advisory Committee performed a systematic review on NPWT[22] in 2010 and concluded:

- NPWT is an effective option in the manage- ment of diabetic foot ulcers
- NPWT is an appropriate option for use following skin grafting of medium-sized (around 30 cm^2) vascular ulcers and burns
- To optimize patient outcomes and safety, ap- propriate guidelines should be adhered to in the application of this technology.

In conclusion, devices are important to facili- tate the treatment of the cause of chronic wounds (compression for venous stasis and plantar pres- sure redistribution for neurotrophic foot ulcers). Other devices (HBOT, NPWT) optimize local wound care for stalled chronic but also healable wounds as well as selected indications in acute wounds.

The Nurse's Perspective on Individualized Wound Device Product Selection

Pressure ulcers are a significant problem across the continuum of healthcare settings. The overall prevalence was 12.3% (N = 92,408) in 2009 ac- cording to a national survey in the United States.[23] The burden of pressure ulcers is significant with the average cost associated with the treatment of deep pressure ulcers and related complica- tions being US $129,248 in acute care. People with pressure ulcers are beset by limited mobil- ity, social isolation, depression, and persistent pain.

In reviews of 53 studies, support surfaces (eg, medical grade sheepskin, high-specification foam mattresses) have been recognized to reduce the incidence of pressure ulcers. Appropriate surfaces or mattresses facilitate pressure redistribution, re- move pressure from injury-prone areas (especially bony prominences), and spread weight evenly to avoid pressure buildup. Foam, gel/water-filled, and low-air-loss mattresses are commonly used. They are considered *reactive* because the effect of pressure redistribution is based on the surface area that the body is in contact with the mattress; the larger the area of the body that is supported by the mattress, the lower the pressure at any given point of contact.

The majority of specialty surfaces are expen- sive, but taking into account the number of ul- cers that can be prevented, the calculated cost of using therapeutic surfaces and other preventative measures is approximately 40 times less than the standard care approach.[24] Amid the wide variety of options, clinicians should understand how to make the selection of the right mattress/surface for the right person (who), the right clinical indication/ circumstances (when), the right length of time (how long), and the right health outcomes (what to expect). Remember, there are 5 rights for the use of therapeutic surfaces. The mnemonic *MAT- TRESSES* (Table 1) highlights 10 key factors that should be considered prior to using a support sur- face to ensure cost-effective use of resources to prevent pressure ulcers.

M — Microclimate and moisture. Increasing attention is drawn to the role of microclimate in pressure ulcer care. Microclimate refers to the en- vironment at or near the skin surface that is influ- enced by the combined effect of skin temperature, humidity/moisture, and air movement. An increase of 1°C in skin temperature results in an approxi- mately 13% increase in tissue oxygen demand, making the skin more vulnerable to mechanical damage. Excess moisture from incontinence, sweat- ing, and wound exudation can cause skin macera- tion, weakening the connections between epider- mal cells and collagen fibers. The interruption of normal barrier function increases skin permeability to irritants and pressure damages. Certainly, heat and moisture accumulation is directly related to air movement at the interface between the skin and the supporting surface. Some of the foam mattresses

Table 1. MATTRESSES

	Indication	Rationale
M	Microclimate and moisture	Low air loss for moisture problems (eg, sweating) and heat accumulation
A	Activity levels	Certain surfaces may hinder mobility in bed and patient's ability to get out of bed
T	Tissue tolerance	Tolerance to pressure and other mechanical forces is determined by local perfusion and oxygen delivery
T	Total body weight	People with extreme body mass indices (BMIs, high or low) are more susceptible to pressure damage
R	Repositioning needs	Lack repositioning surface or difficulty with repositioning
E	Edema	Alternating pressure or pulsating surfaces may reduce edema and promote circulation
S	Shear and friction	Surfaces that conform to the body may prevent sliding and associated shear damage to the tissue
S	Symptom management	Pain, shortness of breath, fatigue, and other associated symptoms
E	Existing pressure ulcer(s)	Existing pressure ulcers indicate that the person is at risk for further skin breakdown
S	Sites	Heels are more prone to pressure ulcers; heels should be managed independently of the support surface

have poor heat properties and tend to "hug" the body, limiting airflow. In contrast, low-air-loss or air-fluidized beds (with vapor-permeable covers) promote air circulation that cools the skin through convection and evaporation of moisture from the skin. This type of mattress may be beneficial for patients with severe burns. Other simple measures to control the microclimate include reducing the layers of pads underneath the patient as well as using incontinent briefs, covering, and clothing that is breathable (avoid plastic). It is important to monitor the skin hydration status to avoid excessive dryness that can also cause skin breakdown.

A — Activity level. Accumulating evidence suggests that people with restricted physical activities and mobility are at risk for pressure ulcers. Norton and colleagues have recently proposed[25] that activity levels should be considered when selecting a

supporting surface. To optimize activities, clinicians must be aware of the potential of certain therapeutic support surfaces (ie, foam, gel-filled, and air-fluidized mattresses) that tend to mold around body contours (envelopment) and allow the body to sink into the surface (immersion), compromising the patient's ability to get in and out of bed and his or her independence.

T — Tissue tolerance. Skin breakdown is inevitable when metabolic demand outstrips the supply of oxygen and vital nutrients. The extent and severity of tissue injury is, however, dependent on a number of intrinsic factors that predispose individuals to the development of pressure ulcers. Some of these key factors are poor nutritional intake, low BMI (BMI < 18.5), hypoproteinemia, low systolic blood pressure, anemia, contractures and prominent bony prominences, vascular disease, neuropathy, and uncontrolled diabetes. Because many of these factors are not addressed by pressure ulcer risk instruments, selection of support surfaces should be individualized, taking assessment of tissue tolerance to injury into consideration.

T — Total body weight. Pressure and other mechanical forces compress, stretch, and distort the normal alignment of the soft tissue, leading to potential injury. The impact of mechanical distortion of the tissue is more pronounced in patients who are emaciated. In one study, the maximum shear force at the coccyx was higher ($P < .01$) in slender than obese individuals when the head of the bed was raised from the supine position.[26] On the other extreme of the body weight spectrum, bariatric patients are also at high risk for pressure ulcer development due to a substantial stress that is put on the skin. Patients with either high or low BMI should be carefully evaluated for a support surface to prevent skin breakdown.

R — Repositioning challenges. While frequent repositioning is deemed essential to manage pressure, it is not always feasible in critically ill patients, as positioning may precipitate vascular collapse or exacerbate shortness of breath (eg, advanced heart failure). A therapeutic surface is recommended for patients who cannot tolerate frequent repositioning or the head of the bed less than 30 degrees (due to dyspnea or to prevent aspiration during enteral feeding). The turning frequency can be reduced by the use of redistributing support surfaces; however, prolonged exposure to low pressure can be equally damaging to tissue. Clinicians must not forget the need for repositioning despite the type of mattresses or specialty surfaces being utilized.

E — Edema. Edema, which stretches the skin and impairs the delivery of oxygen, is considered a risk factor for skin breakdown. By alternating air pressures in compartments of the mattress under the torso and leg that emulates the body's natural intermittent movements, it is hypothesized that the massage movements may reduce edema by improving capillary blood flow and oxygenation to the wound and skin. Further research evidence is needed to substantiate the physiological impact of alternating mattresses. Despite the potential benefits, alternating air mattresses may not be suitable for individuals with spinal instability, motion sickness, protracted pain, and nausea. Individualized assessment is warranted.

S — Shear and friction. Development of pressure ulcers is a dynamic and complex process that involves the combined effect of mechanical forces including shear and friction in addition to pressure. Pressure is defined as the perpendicular force that is applied to the skin, distorting and compressing underlying soft tissues, especially over bony prominences.[27] Shear or shear stress is produced by displacement or deformation of tissue (usually in a diagonal direction), altering the original alignment of tissue as one layer of tissue slides over the deeper structure in opposite directions (bony skeleton moving in an opposite direction to the surface skin). Deformation disrupts the cell structure, obstructs lymphatic drainage, reduces blood flow, and potentiates ischemia.

In contrast, friction describes the resistance to movement created between 2 surfaces, such as the superficial layers of skin and the adjoining support surface. By simply instituting measures to reduce friction, up to 16% of pressure ulcers can be prevented.[28]

S — Symptom management. A support surface is often considered for palliative patients to promote comfort. The primary purpose may not be focused on pressure ulcer prevention but to ensure comfort at the end of life.

E — Existing pressure ulcer(s). Patients with existing pressure ulcers are usually at risk for developing further skin breakdown. For patients who have multiple ulcers, a support surface should be considered due to the lack of appropriate turning surfaces.

S — Sites. One of the areas that is most vulnerable to pressure-related skin damage is the heel. The heel has a pointed shape with a limited surface area of contact to redistribute pressure, and when this is combined with the low subcutaneous tissue volume, this area is prone to pressure damage. Heel tissue is enveloped within the fibrous septa that allow pressure to build up easily and occlude vascular supply. Boots with the heel area cut out to allow the heel to be completely lifted off the surface are useful to prevent and treat pressure ulcers. Many different heel boots and positioning devices are available;

however, no one device works best in all circumstances. Special attention must be paid to potential damage to the lower leg areas where the pressure is redistributed.

The Therapist's Perspective on Individualized Wound Device Product Selection

Reflecting back to the wound bed preparation paradigm,[5] allied health professionals can be especially helpful to manage the cause of wounds while addressing patient-centered concerns. Regardless of the type of wound, until the cause has been addressed, the wound will not progress to closure. The challenge, though, is to address the cause in a way that can be incorporated into the individual's lifestyle. *Evidence-based practice is the integration of the best research evidence with clinical expertise and patient values.*[29] This approach is helpful when considering the prescription of devices to prevent or manage wounds, as the best device is not helpful if the patient does not use it or the care providers do not know how to use or maintain the device.

When interpreting the evidence, clinical expertise is required, as many of the studies have small sample sizes, are completed by the manufacturer, and, in the case of support surfaces, compare therapeutic support surfaces to standard hospital mattresses (ie, foam and coil).[30] These studies also usually only consider an indirect measure (such as interface pressure) rather than an outcome measure (eg, wound prevention or wound closure).[30] In addition, they do not address the impact on the individual's lifestyle or his or her safety. For example, when considering support surfaces in bed, healthcare providers must consider the risk of entrapment. Health Canada[31,32] and the FDA have released documents defining the 7 zones of entrapment and guidance measurements:

1. Within the bed rail
2. Under the rail
3. Between the rail and the mattress
4. Under the rail at rail ends
5. Between split bed rails
6. Between the end of the rail and the side edge of the head or footboard
7. Between the head or footboard and the mattress end.

Prescription of a therapeutic support surface,

whether an overlay or mattress replacement, may impact several of these zones (eg, zone 2, 3, and 7). A standard measuring device is available to check to see if the new support surface increases the risk of entrapment by allowing spaces greater than those outlined in the guideline. The risk of entrapment also may be greater with support surfaces with large air bladders (these are usually found on low-air-loss, alternating, or rotating surfaces). These surfaces tend to collapse the further the individual moves to the edge[33] of the surface, even when a perimeter border is present within the mattress.

When an entrapment risk has been identified, bed rails should only be used with extreme caution and be based on the needs of the individual patient. Some patients find the half bed rail at the head section helpful for repositioning. Another approach for people at high risk is to use an adjustable bed with a very low deck height and a floor mat. This approach allows the bed to be raised to a comfortable height for care providers during care but allows the bed to be low enough to help prevent injury if the person falls out of bed. Foam wedges and other devices are also available to help reduce the risk of entrapment.

In terms of pressure ulcer prevention and management, there is evidence that the use of a pressure management cushion reduces the risk of pressure ulcers and extends the number of pressure ulcer-free days for those who do eventually develop pressure ulcers.[34] It has been demonstrated that higher peak pressures under the ischial tuberosities have been associated with increased pressure ulcer development.[35] One way to evaluate pressure is through use of a pressure-mapping device. This device helps the clinician visualize the interface pressure between the individual and the surface upon which he or she sits. Pressure maps must be interpreted with caution, however, as this technology does not measure shear or consider other factors relevant to the prescription of a seat cushion. Other factors to consider include comfort, postural stability, balance, cost, weight capacity, and maintenance.

When considering an evidence-based approach, the individual's perspectives and values play a pivotal role. The literature suggests that anywhere *between 30% and 70% of devices pre-*

scribed are abandoned by the user.[36] The main reasons for abandonment include:[36]

- Device did not provide the type or extent of assistance required
- Draws unwanted attention to the user
- Individual does not perceive he or she needs the device
- Fit between the individual's environment and the device
- User does not feel his or her opinions were considered
- Training not provided.

In addition, the impact of the device on the person's independence also influences its use. For example, compression stockings are usually prescribed for people with venous insufficiency. Once a venous leg ulcer has closed, however, these stockings can be difficult for people to don and duff independently. Many devices have been designed to assist with this process, however, for people with arthritis or issues with mobility, even when these devices do not foster independence. Many individuals do not want to be dependent on others, as this may increase caregiver burden.

To summarize, an evidence-based approach should be taken in the selection and prescription of equipment to prevent and manage wounds. As the specific devices are often changing, the studies are often conducted by the manufacturers, and the sample sizes are small, studies need to be interpreted with caution. Reviews, such as the **Cochrane Review** on Support Surfaces,[37] and clinical practice guidelines, such as the **Registered Nurses' Association of Ontario** Best Practice Guideline for the Prevention of Pressure Ulcers[38] or the **European Pressure Ulcer Advisory Panel** and **National Pressure Ulcer Advisory Panel** guidelines,[39] may be more helpful for clinicians. Clinical judgment enables the healthcare provider to evaluate new products in relationship to the known evidence and the needs of their individual patients. Patients need education regarding the impact of the device and its use. *The patient's perspective needs to be identified and integrated into the plan of care, as the best device is the one the individual will use.*

Conclusion

This chapter illustrates how by blending the vantage points from different disciplines, a stronger plan of care can be developed for the person with a wound or at risk for developing one. An interprofessional team approach to wound care enhances patient outcomes. When wound device product selection is viewed through multiple professional lenses, patient-centered care is optimized.

Take-Home Messages for Practice

- The challenge of matching the appropriate device for a specific patient's profile has become a rising expectation.
- Wound care devices may or may not have indications, contraindications, or precautions — just like medications.
- Evidence-based practice is the integration of the best research evidence with clinical expertise and patient values.[29] This approach is helpful when considering the prescription of devices to prevent or manage wounds, as the best device is not helpful if the patient does not use it or the care providers do not know how to use or maintain it.

Self-Assessment Questions

1. Effective use of devices involves all of the following EXCEPT:
   A. Appropriate orders by appropriate prescribers
   B. Discontinuing all devices prior to transitioning a person from one care setting to another
   C. Documentation of device efficacy
   D. Patient/caregiver education regarding device use, troubleshooting, and who to contact in case of emergency

2. Factors that negatively influence adherence to wound device use include:
   A. The device draws unwanted attention to the user
   B. Training was not provided
   C. The individual does not perceive that he or she needs the device
   D. All of the above

Answers: 1–B, 2–D

References

1. Krasner DL, Rodeheaver GT, Sibbald RG. Interprofessional wound caring. In: Krasner DL, Rodeheaver GT, Sibbald RG, eds. *Chronic Wound Care: A Clinical Source Book for Healthcare Professionals.* 4th ed. Malvern, PA: HMP Communications; 2007:3–9. www.chronicwoundcarebook.com

2. Miller M, Boix-Mansilla V. Thinking across perspectives and disciplines. Harvard Graduate School of Education, Interdisciplinary Studies Project; Project Zero, 2004.

3. Norton L, Coutts P, Sibbald RG. Beds: practical pressure management for surfaces/mattresses. *Adv Skin Wound Care.* 2011;24(7):324–332.

4. Fife CE, Yankowsky KW, Ayello EA, et al. Legal issues in the care of pressure ulcer patients: key concepts for healthcare providers — a consensus paper from the International Expert Wound Care Advisory Panel. *Adv Skin Wound Care.* 2010;23(11):493–507.

5. Sibbald RG, Goodman L, Woo KY, et al. Special considerations in wound bed preparation 2011: an update©. *Adv Skin Wound Care.* 2011;24(9):415–436.

6. O'Meara S, Cullum NA, Nelson EA. Compression for venous leg ulcers. *Cochrane Database Syst Rev.* 2009;(1):CD000265.

7. Sibbald RG, Alavi A, Norton L, Browne AC, Coutts P. Compression therapies. In: Krasner DL, Rodeheaver GT, Sibbald RG, eds. *Chronic Wound Care: A Clinical Source Book for Healthcare Professionals.* 4th ed. Malvern, PA: HMP Communications; 2007:481–488. www.chronicwoundcarebook.com

8. Krasner DL, Papen J, Sibbald RG. Helping patients out of the SWAMP: Skin and Wound Assessment and Management of Pain. In: Krasner DL, Rodeheaver GT, Sibbald RG, eds. *Chronic Wound Care: A Clinical Source Book for Healthcare Professionals.* 4th ed. Malvern, PA: HMP Communications; 2007:85–97. www.chronicwoundcarebook.com

9. Woo KY, Sibbald RG, Fogh K, et al. Assessment and management of persistent (chronic) and total wound pain. *Int Wound J.* 2008;5(2):205–215.

10. Principles of best practice: Minimising pain at wound dressing-related procedures. A consensus document. Toronto, Ontario, Canada: © WoundPedia Inc 2007.

11. Orsted HL, Searles G, Trowell H, Shapera L, Miller P, Rahman J. Best practice recommendations for the prevention, diagnosis and treatment of diabetic foot ulcers: update 2006. *Wound Care Canada* Reprinted. 2006;4(1):R39–R51.

12. Botros M, Goettl K, Parsons P, et al. Best practice recommendations for the prevention, diagnosis and treatment of diabetic foot ulcers: update 2010. *Wound Care Canada.* 4(1):R39–R51.

13. Sibbald RG, Woo K, Ayello EA. Increased bacterial burden and infection: the story of the NERDS and STONE. *Adv Skin Wound Care.* 2006;19:447–461.

14. Woo K, Sibbald RG. A cross-sectional validation study of using NERDS and STONEES to assess bacterial burden. *Ostomy Wound Manage.* 2009;55(8):40–61.

15. Woo KY, Ayello EA, Sibbald RG. The edge effect: current therapeutic options to advance the wound edge. *Adv Skin Wound Care.* 2007;20(2):99–117.

16. Kranke P, Bennett MH, Debus SE, Roeckl-Wiedmann I, Schnabel A. Hyperbaric oxygen therapy for chronic wounds. *Cochrane Database Syst Rev.* 2004;(2):CD004123.

17. World Union of Wound Healing Societies (WUWHS). *Principles of Best Practice: Vacuum Assisted Closure: Recommendations for Use.* A consensus document. London: MEP Ltd, 2008.

18. Buttenschoen K, Fleischmann W, Haupt U, Kinzl L, Buttenschoen DC. The influence of vacuum assisted closure on inflammatory tissue reactions in the postoperative curse of ankle fractures. *Foot Ankle Surg.* 2001;7:165–173.

19. Armstrong DG, Lavery LA, pour le Diabetic Foot Consortium. Negative pressure wound therapy after partial diabetic foot amputation: a multicentre, a randomised controlled trial. *Lancet.* 2005;366(9498):1704–1710.

20. Luckraz H, Murphy F, Bryant S, Charman SC, Ritchie AJ. Vacuum-assisted closure as a treatment modality for infections after cardiac surgery. *J Thorac Cardiovasc Surg.* 2003;125(2):301–305.

21. Song DH, Wu LC, Lohman RF, Gottlieb LJ, Franczyk M. Vacuum assisted closure for the treatment of sternal wounds: the bridge between debridement and definitive closure. *Plast Reconstr Surg.* 2003;111(1):92–97.

22. Ontario Health Technology Advisory Committee (OHTAC) Recommendations: Negative Pressure Wound Therapy, Dec 2010.

23. VanGilder C, Amlung S, Harrison P, Meyer S. Results of the 2008–2009 International Pressure Ulcer Prevalence Survey and a 3-year, acute care, unit-specific analysis. *Ostomy Wound Manage.* 2009;55(11):39–45.

24. Padula WV, Mishra MK, Makic MB, Sullivan PW. Improving the quality of pressure ulcer care with prevention: a cost-effectiveness analysis. *Med Care.* 2011;49(4):385–392.

25. Norton L, Coutts P, Sibbald RG. Beds: practical pressure management for surfaces/mattresses. *Adv Skin Wound Care.* 2011;24(7):324–332.

26. Mimura M, Ohura T, Takahashi M, Kajiwara R, Ohura N Jr. Mechanism leading to the development of pressure ulcers based on shear force and pressures during a bed operation: influence of body types, body positions, and knee positions. *Wound Repair Regen.* 2009;17(6):789–796.

27. Black JM, Edsberg LE, Baharestani MM, et al; National Pressure Ulcer Advisory Panel. Pressure ulcers: avoidable or unavoidable? Results of the National Pressure Ulcer Advisory Panel Consensus Conference. *Ostomy Wound Manage.* 2011;57(2):24–37.

28. Smith G, Ingram A. Clinical and cost effectiveness evaluation of low friction and shear garments. *J Wound Care.* 2010;19(12):535–542.

29. Kitson A, Harvery G, McCormack B. Enabling the implementation of evidence based practice: a conceptual framework. *Qual Health Care.* 1998;7(3):149–158.

30. McInnes E, Bell-Syer SEM, Dumville JC, Legood R, Cullum NA. Support surfaces for pressure ulcer prevention. *Cochrane Database Syst Rev.* 2008;(4):CD001735.

31. Adult Hospital Beds: Patient Entrapment Hazards, Side Rail Latching Reliability, and Other Hazards, © Minister of Public Works and Government Services Canada 2006, Revised Date: 2008/02/29; Effective Date: 2008/03/17.

32. US FDA Guidance entitled *Hospital Bed System Dimensional and Assessment Guidance to Reduce Entrapment,*

published March 10, 2006. http://www.fda.gov/medi-caldevices/deviceregulationandguidance/guidancedocu-ments/ucm072662.htm.

33. Adult Hospital Beds: Patient Entrapment Hazards, Side Rail Latching Reliability, and Other Hazards, © Minister of Public Works and Government Services Canada 2006, Revised Date: 2008/02/29; Effective Date: 2008/03/17.

34. Brienza D, Kelsey S, Karg P, et al. Randomized clinical trial on preventing pressure ulcers with wheelchair seat cushions. *J Am Geriatr Soc*. 2010;58:2308–2314.

35. Brienza D, Karg PE, Geyer MJ, Kelsey S, Trefler E. The relationship between pressure ulcer incidence and buttock-seat cushion interface pressure in at-risk elderly wheelchair users. *Arch Phys Med Rehabil*. 2001;82:529–533.

36. CAOT Position Statement Assistive Technology and Occupational Therapy (2006), http://www.caot.ca/default.asp?pageid=598.

37. McInnes E, Bell-Syer SEM, Dumville JC, Legood R, Cullum NA. Support surfaces for pressure ulcer prevention. *Cochrane Database Syst Rev*. 2008;(4):CD001735.

38. Registered Nurses Association of Ontario Risk Assessment & Prevention of Pressure Ulcers Guideline Supplement. Registered Nurses Association, Toronto 2011.

39. European Pressure Ulcer Advisory Panel and National Pressure Ulcer Advisory Panel. Prevention and treatment of pressure ulcers: quick reference guide. Washington DC: National Pressure Ulcer Advisory Panel; 2009.

CHAPTER 15

Wound Product Selection Challenges: Developing Strategies for Your Practice Setting

Sue Currence, BSN, RN, CWON;
Diane L. Krasner, PhD, RN, CWCN, CWS, MAPWCA, FAAN

Objectives

The reader will be challenged to:

- Analyze strategies for facilitating the wound product selection process
- Implement new strategies for wound product selection for your practice setting.

Introduction

Developing a comprehensive wound product formulary has never been more challenging. Given the myriad of products, tools, devices, and primers available for today's management of wounds, the selection process can be daunting. The statement "so many wounds, so little time" often comes to mind. In this instance, it could be rephrased to "so many products, so little space." It is the practitioner's challenge to identify and select those products that will best fit the setting in which one practices. Variables that drive the selection process include the organization's contract, purchasing group, and/or reimbursor. This chapter presents strategies to facilitate the wound product selection process.

Discussion

Since Winter's work on moist wound healing almost 6 decades ago, wound management has experienced a revolution in the types and numbers of products available in today's market.[1] Once limited to simple passive fabrics with cotton and viscose inserts, dressings have evolved into more sophisticated, interactive coverings, offering an extensive variety of promises and results.

Additionally, biologically active wound adjuncts, such as topical growth factors and skin substitutes, have emerged as state-of-the-art technology for the advancement and speed of wound resolution.

There are hundreds of products (dressings and devices) currently available to assist with wound healing[2] (see Chap-

Currence S, Krasner DL. Wound Product Selection Challenges: Developing Strategies for Your Practice Setting. In: Krasner DL, ed. *Chronic Wound Care: The Essentials.* Malvern, Pa: HMP Communications, 2014:185–194.

Table 1. Wound Care Product Generic Categories and Examples*

This listing of wound care product examples highlights the importance of generic product categories. Under each generic product category, selected product examples are given (a mix of old and new products) to help familiarize the reader with each category. No endorsement of any product or manufacturer is intended. Within each category, products must be individually evaluated. All products within a category do not necessarily perform equally. Combination products may be listed in more than one category. Refer to manufacturers' instructions for specifics regarding product usage.

* All product names should be considered copyrighted or trademarked regardless of the absence of ® or ™.

1. Alginate Dressings

Examples	Manufacturer
Kaltostat®	ConvaTec
Restore CalciCare	Hollister
SeaSorb®	Coloplast
Sorbsan™	UDL Laboratories

2. Antimicrobial Dressings (see also 22. Silver Dressings)

Examples	Manufacturer
Hydrofera blue®	Hollister
Iodosorb /Iodoflex™ Gel Pad	Smith & Nephew
Kerlix® AMD	Covidien

3. Antimicrobial Solutions

Examples	Manufacturer
Acetic Acid	Multiple
Antibiotic Solutions	Multiple
Antifungal Solutions	Multiple
Chlorpactin WCS-90	United-Guardian
Dakin's Solution	Multiple
SilverStream™	EnzySurge

4. Cleansers

Examples	Manufacturer
a. Saline	Multiple
OTC Spray	
Prescription	
b. Incontinence Cleansers	
PeriFresh™	DermaRite
Peri-Wash®	Coloplast
Soothe & Cool®	Medline
c. Skin Cleansers	
Aloe Vesta®	ConvaTec
Gentle Rain®	Coloplast
Remedy®	Medline
d. Wound Cleansers	
Curasol™	Smith & Nephew
Dermagran® Spray	Derma Sciences
SilverStream™	EnzySurge
Skintegrity™	Medline

Table 1. Wound Care Product Generic Categories and Examples* (continued)

5. Collagen Dressings

Examples	Manufacturer
ChroniCure™	Derma Sciences
Endoform	Hollister
Fibracol® (Collagen/Alginate)	Systagenix
Medifil™/SkinTemp®	BioCore
Puracol™/Puracol™ Plus	Medline

6. Composite Dressings

Examples	Manufacturer
Alldress®	Mölnlycke
CombiDERM™ ACD™	ConvaTec
CovaDerm™/CovaDerm™Plus	DeRoyal
Stratasorb	Medline

7. Compression Bandages/Wraps

Examples	Manufacturer
Unna Boot	Multiple
Dome Paste®	Miles
Elastoplast®	Beiersdorf-Jobst
Setopress®	ConvaTec
SurPress®	ConvaTec

MULTI-LAYERED SYSTEMS	Manufacturer
Circulon™ System	ConvaTec
Dyna-Flex™	Systagenix
FourFlex	Medline
Profore®	Smith & Nephew

8. Conforming/Wrapping Bandages

Examples	Manufacturer
Coban®	3M Healthcare
Kerlix®/ Kerlix® Lite	Covidien
Kling Fluff/Sof-Kling™	Systagenix

9. Contact Layers

Examples	Manufacturer
Mepitel®	Mölnlycke
Profore®	Smith & Nephew
Tegapore	3M Healthcare
Ventex™ Vented Dressing	Covidien

10. Creams/Lotions/Oils (Therapeutic Moisturizers)

Examples	Manufacturer
Aquaphor	Beiersdorf
Biafine®	Ortho McNeil
Remedy™	Medline
Sween Cream®/Sween 24	Coloplast

Table 1. Wound Care Product Generic Categories and Examples* (continued)

11. Devices

Examples	Manufacturer
Electrical Stimulation	Multiple
Hyperbaric Oxygen	Multiple
Negative Pressure Wound Therapy	Multiple
Ultrasound	Multiple

12. Enzymes/Debriding Agents

Examples	Manufacturer
Collagenase Santyl™	Smith & Nephew
Granulex®	UDL Laboratories
Tenderwet	Medline
XENADERM®	Smith & Nephew

13. Foam Dressings (see also Composite Dressings)

Examples	Manufacturer
Allevyn®	Smith & Nephew
Biatain	Coloplast
Lyofoam®/Lyofoam® C/Lyofoam® T	ConvaTec
Mepilex™	Mölnlycke
Optifoam®	Medline
Polymem®	Ferris

14. Gauze Dressings

Examples	Manufacturer
a. Woven	Multiple
b. Nonwoven	Multiple
c. Packing/Packing Strips (Nonimpregnated)	Multiple
d. Debriding	Multiple
e. Impregnated—Sodium Chloride	Multiple
f. Impregnated—Other (eg, hydrogel, honey)	Multiple
g. Nonadherent gauze	Multiple
h. Specialty Absorptive Gauze	Multiple
i. Antimicrobial Gauze	Multiple

15. Growth Factors

Examples	Manufacturer
AutoloGel System™	Cytomedix
Regranex® Gel (becaplermin 0.01%)	Systagenix

16. Honey (Active Leptospermum)

Examples	Manufacturer
Activon	Advancis Medical
MANUKAhd®	ManukaMed
MediHoney®	Derma Sciences
TheraHoney®	Medline

17. Hydrocolloid Dressings

Examples	Manufacturer
Comfeel	Coloplast
DuoDERM®/CGF/Extra Thin	ConvaTec
Exuderm	Medline
Restore™/CX/Extra Thin	Hollister
Tegasorb™/Extra Thin	3M Healthcare

Table 1. Wound Care Product Generic Categories and Examples* (continued)

18. Hydrofiber

Examples	Manufacturer
Aquacel®	ConvaTec
Aquacel® AG	ConvaTec

19. Hydrogel Dressings (see also Impregnated Gauze Dressings)

Examples	Manufacturer
SHEET	
Dermagel®	Medline
Elasto-Gel™	Southwest Technologies
Gentell™	MKM
Vigilon®	Bard
AMORPHOUS	**Manufacturer**
Comfeel® Purilon™ Gel	Coloplast
DuoDERM® Hydroactive Gel (Hydrogel/Hydrocolloid)	ConvaTec
IntraSite® Gel	Smith & Nephew
Saf-Gel®	ConvaTec
Solo-Site®	Smith & Nephew
STRANDS	**Manufacturer**
FlexiGel™ Strands™	Smith & Nephew

20. Impregnated Dressings – see also substrate material eg, gauze, foam, honey and silver

Examples	Manufacturer
Iodoform Packing Strips	Multiple
Antimicrobial Gauze	Multiple
Charcoal	Multiple
Detergent	Multiple

21. Silicone Gel Sheets (scar treatment)

Examples	Manufacturer
Silon	BioMed Sciences
Mepiform	Mölnlycke
Cicacare	Smith & Nephew

22. Silver Dressings

Examples	Manufacturer
Acticoat™	Smith & Nephew
Aquacel™ AG	ConvaTec
Arglaes® Film/Island/Powder	Medline
Contreet	Coloplast
SilvaSorb™	Medline
Melgisorb Ag	Mölnlycke
Silvercel	Systagenix
Silverlon Wound Packing Strips	Argentum Medical

23. Silver Solutions

Examples	Manufacturer
SilverStream™	EnzySurge

Table 1. Wound Care Product Generic Categories and Examples* (continued)

24. Skin Sealants

Examples	Manufacturer
Preppies™	Kendall Healthcare
Skin Prep™	Smith & Nephew
Sure Prep® No Sting Barrier Film	Medline
Cavilon No Sting	3M

25. Transparent Film Dressings

Examples	Manufacturer
Bioclusive™/MVP	Systagenix
OpSite®/Flexifix/Flexigrid/3000	Smith & Nephew
Suresite	Medline
Tegaderm™/HP	3M

26. Wound Fillers

Examples	Manufacturer
Altrazeal™ Transforming Powder Dressing	Uluru
OsmoCyte™ Pillow Wound Dressing	Procyte
Multidex	DeRoyal

27. Wound Pouches

Examples	Manufacturer
Wound Drainage Collector	Hollister
Wound Manager™	ConvaTec
Adult & Pediatric Sized Ostomy Pouches	Multiple

Not Otherwise Classified (NOC)

Product Categories

28. Adhesives	40. Moisturizers
29. Adhesive Removers	41. Ointments
30. Adhesive Skin Closures	42. Perineal Cleansing Foams
31. Adhesive Tapes	43. Sterile Fields
32. Antibiotics	44. Surgical Scrubs
33. Antimicrobials	45. Surgical Tapes
34. Antiseptics	46. Specialty Absorptive Fabrics
35. Bandages	47. Cellular and/or Tissue Based Products
36. Dressing Covers	48. Synthetic & Biosynthetic Dressings
37. Healthcare Personnel Handrinses	49. Maggot Therapy
38. Lubricating/Stimulating Sprays	50. Miscellaneous
39. Moisture Barrier Ointments/Creams/ Skin Protectant Pastes	

© Susan M. Currence & Diane L. Krasner 2014
Used with permission.

ters 13 and 14). Their functions are numerous and offer not only protection but interactive stimulus as well. **(See Table 1 for a listing of wound care product examples by generic category.)**

It is not the intent of this chapter to discuss the extent and roles of these products but instead to help determine the most effective ways in which to select and utilize them.

Identifying the most useful products to employ in one's practice is largely dependent upon the population being served. This of course points to individual practice setting(s), which in most cases are critical/acute, transitional, skilled, or home care. Aside from these specific types of facility or agency settings, the outpatient clinic and private office must also be considered. For instance, the home health wound care provider is obviously limited by the constraints of space: just how many topical agents, wraps, devices, and teaching tools can be stored in one's trunk? A thorough assessment of the practice environment is required before selecting and storing wound care products.

No matter what the setting, the practitioner needs to adhere to a "clearinghouse" process prior to procuring products for use. Most facilities provide a mechanism for approval before allowing new or reformulated products to be added to inventory. They may include such forums as an institutional review board (IRB), a product review or value analysis committee, a proven clinical trial report, and a simple product evaluation. Additionally, the practice facility may require approval from other departments (or cost centers), such as central stores or finance. *Ultimately, the agency or facility has the responsibility of assuring that products are safe and efficacious and that patient outcomes are positive and effective.*

Imposing nonclinical surveillance of any new or alternative technology may seem inconvenient and time consuming, but more often than not, issues are brought to the table that even the most astute practitioner has not considered. For instance, a polyurethane foam dressing may seem absolutely ideal for use in the venous ulcer population of a particular acute care setting, but further investigation reveals that the vendor or manufacturer of that product is not included in that facility's contract status. As a result, the practitioner may have to choose a different absorptive dressing.

All too often, and unfortunately in today's cost-driven environment, an alternative product must be selected and "settled for." If institutional constraints demand the use of wound care options that are inappropriate or inadequate for select populations, the practitioner has the professional responsibility of assuring patient safety by serving as an advocate for the necessary therapy or product.

A case in point: a few years ago, a manufacturer decided it would be extremely user-friendly to prepackage pressure ulcer kits that were designed for Stage 1 through Stage 4 wounds. The kit for any Stage 1 pressure ulcer would include a transparent film dressing, a nonstick gauze dressing for any Stage 2 ulcer, etc. Although the concept appealed to purchasing directors nationwide for the simplicity of ordering/stocking, the clinical outcomes would not be evidence-based. Practitioners realized that no 2 wounds could be treated the same way and debunked the entire promotion as being regressive and injurious to the philosophy/practice of wound care. This example further underscores the philosophy that optimal wound management is individualized and holistic.

Practice Settings

A thorough evaluation of the environment in which wound care is being practiced must be undertaken. A large, urban university facility may be afforded opportunities for product use that smaller, rural settings could not support. Manufacturers usually target larger, well known, or teaching institutions in order to obtain statistically significant numbers to support research-driven or randomized clinical trials. Additionally, their lead investigators are generally recognized by the community as thought leaders and lend further credibility to the product being studied. As a result, cutting-edge wound care products are then utilized in those facilities long before they reach the rest of the community. Growth factors and bioengineered tissue adjuncts, for example, often got their start in such settings.

The smaller acute care setting is often the locale for simple product evaluations. Although these efforts are largely supportive of previous clinical trials, they usually remain testimonial and generally adequate for the grassroots practitioner. In addition, they provide a mechanism for the inclusion of newer technology into a facility's wound care inventory.

Population Analysis

No matter what the setting, an accurate assessment of the population being served must be performed before embarking on either trial or usage. A patient-needs assessment would be the logical starting point prior to examining the products being offered.

Would a negative pressure wound therapy device be sought in a transitional care environment where the extent of tissue damage did not exceed a Stage 2 pressure ulcer? Probably not. Would a simple barrier cream be considered the first line of defense in a critical trauma setting where fistula management was an everyday occurrence? Probably not. How about daily pulsed lavage in the home care setting? Probably not. The importance of matching the dressing to the wound becomes paramount when selecting appropriate products for select populations.[2]

Organizational Contracts and Purchasing Groups

Many product decisions are influenced by organizational contracts or purchasing groups. The leverage that group purchasing offers is often viewed as more valuable than individual choice. This means that while an individual wound care practitioner in an organization may have a preference for 1 particular product or manufacturer, it is often the purchasing agent who is positioned to make the decisions about which manufacturer or distributor will be used for obtaining wound care products. The challenge to wound care practitioners, especially those who practiced in the past and had much more selection freedom, is to optimize the product formulary within the constraints of organizational contracts and purchasing groups. This takes patience, creativity, and somewhat of a paradigm shift in thinking.

Formularies, Procedures and Competencies

Many agencies decide to develop in-house product formularies in order to standardize usage, avoid duplication of products, decrease overutilization, and decrease costs.

There are many excellent references and models of formularies in the literature,[4-8] so no one has to reinvent the wheel. There are also some formularies circulating that you would not want to copy, so readers are advised to use their discretion. For comprehensive dressing and device information in the United States, the reader is referred to WoundSource™ (Kestrel Health Information), www.woundsource.com

Some agencies choose to develop procedures and/or competencies related to their formularies. Again, there are some excellent examples in the wound care literature.[4-8] Having an integrated package of products and performance measures helps to assure optimal patient outcomes.

Conclusion

Identifying the right "tools for the trade" requires forethought and selective integration to attain successful practice outcomes. The development of a system for the consistent, ongoing review and selection of wound care products can be a challenge to any practitioner but is not insurmountable. Thorough assessment of one's patient population is critical; evaluation of agency climate and approval processes is equally important. Blending this mix with product knowledge and planning ultimately results in best wound care practices.

Take-Home Messages for Practice

- Conduct patient-needs assessments to determine the necessary and adequate product inventory for your practice setting.
- Familiarize yourself with the approval processes for trialing, introduction, and procurement of new products in your setting.
- Work in synergy with your purchasing agents, contractors, and vendors to optimize wound product selection.

Self-Assessment Questions

1. All of the following are the MOST appropriate strategies for optimizing wound product selection EXCEPT:

  A. Review manufacturers' product literature

  B. Obtain articles from a review of the literature

  C. Have dinner with the company representative

  D. Network with colleagues to hear their experiences

2. Which of the following constraints has the LEAST impact on product selection?

  A. Cost of product

  B. Organizational contracts

  C. Purchasing groups

  D. Practitioner preference

Answers: 1-C, 2-D

References

1. Thomas A. *Surgical Dressings and Wound Management*. 2nd ed. Hinesburg, Vt: Kestrel Health Information; 2010.

2. *WoundSource™ 2013*. 16th ed. Hinesburg, Vt:Kestrel Health Information. www.woundsource.com

3. Krasner D. Resolving the dressing dilemma: selecting wound dressing by category. *Ostomy Wound Manage*. 1991;35:62–70.

4. Brown P. *Quick Reference Guide to Wound Care: Palliative, Home and Clinical Practices*. 4th ed. Burlington, Mass: Jones & Bartlett; 2013.

5. Bryant RA, Nix DP. *Acute & Chronic Wounds: Current Management Concepts*. 4th ed. St. Louis, MO: Elsevier Mosby; 2012.

6. Collier KS, Protus BM, Bohn CL, Kimbrel JM. *Wound Care At End of Life: A Guide for Hospice Professionals*. Montgomery, AL: HospiScript Services, A Catamaran Company; 2013.

7. Gogia PP. *Clinical Wound Management*. Thorofare, NJ: SLACK; 2011.

8. Kifer ZA. *Fast Facts for Wound Care Nursing: Practical Wound Management in a Nutshell*. New York, NY: Springer Publishing Company; 2012.

CHAPTER 16

Negative Pressure Wound Therapy

Adrianne P. S. Smith, MD;
Kathy Whittington, RN, MS, CWCN;
Robert G. Frykberg, DPM, MPH;
Jean M. de Leon, MD

Objectives

The reader will be challenged to:

- Describe the use of negative pressure wound therapy (NPWT) as a standard in advanced wound care
- Review the appropriate most up-to-date information on the use of NPWT in chronic wound care
- Summarize the current understanding of proposed mechanisms of action for NPWT
- Recognize potential complications related to NPWT usage and determine interventions to reduce risks.

Introduction

"Creativity…consists largely of rearranging what we know in order to find out what we do not know. Hence, to think creatively, we must be able to look afresh at what we normally take for granted."
— George Kneller

egative pressure wound therapy (NPWT) is the process by which negative pressure is distributed across a wound base via a dressing with the specific intent to promote wound healing. Over the centuries, popularity for using negative (subatmospheric) pressure to treat wounds has waxed and waned. In medical literature, negative pressure-based therapies used for wound healing have been referred to as *cupping, pneumatic occlusive therapy, passive hyperemia therapy, active drainage, suction drainage therapy, active aspiration, vacuum drainage, vacuum sealing technique (VST), topical negative pressure (TNP), subatmospheric pressure dressings (SPD), NPWT, vacuum sealing dressing (VSD), irrigation drainage*, and a patent filed in China in 2010 brought it full circle with *reduced pressure wound cupping treatment*. With each advancing generation, healthcare practitioners have observed the wound healing potential of negative pressure interpreted through the limitations of their existing knowledge of medical sciences. Spurred by innovative equipment, advances in healthcare technology, and the artistic ingenuity and technical competency of the practitioner caring for the wounded patient, NPWT has been constrained by the risk of complications, technical difficulties, inappropriate patient selection, and the need to develop a clear, defensible evidence base to support the safe and effica-

Smith APS, Whittington K, Frykberg RG, DeLeon J. Negative pressure wound therapy. In: Krasner DL, ed. *Chronic Wound Care: The Essentials*. Malvern, PA: HMP Communications; 2014:195–224.

cious use of the proposed technique. The advent of new, portable, computer-programmable negative pressure generators, novel treatment materials, newer understandings of *"cellular" healing responses*, and modern cause-effect validation coupled with the healthcare community's burgeoning interest in tissue regeneration created the perfect storm for resurgence of a modern-day platform for NPWT. The utility of NPWT for managing complex wounds, ulcers, burns, postoperative wounds, and non-surgical tissue defects has emerged as a readily available, frequently employed, and internationally adopted therapeutic practice with applicability for acute and chronic wounds in a variety of care settings.[1,2]

The current NPWT platform was built with the full anticipation of eventually using modulations in the negative pressure profile to direct specific cellular responses to improve the healing rate, quantity, and quality of tissue generated. As with all wound care practices, the "evidential clarity and defensibility" for NPWT will be bounded by the capability of the scientific wound care community to understand and judge the merits of the process within the existing conceptual and technological constraints of the era in which they live.

Modern Perspectives of NPWT

"No single achievement in science is possible without the painstaking work of the many hundreds who have built the foundation on which all new work is based." — Nobel Laureate Polykarp Kusch

The current NPWT platform witnessed a surge in popularity when Dr. Louis Argenta and Dr. Michael Morykwas at Wake Forest University developed Vacuum Assisted Closure® (V.A.C.®) Therapy (KCI USA, Inc., San Antonio, Texas) to optimize the benefits of subatmospheric (negative) pressure for wound healing[1,2] with special focus on perfusion and granulation tissue development.[3] This integrated system uses a computerized therapy unit to intermittently or continuously deliver negative pressure through a resilient, open-cell foam surface dressing that is sealed with an adhesive drape. The original tubing design had a terminal pad, sealed in contact with the foam, which delivered wound space pressures and redirected wound exudate into a specially designed, disposable canister.

While the basic components of the NPWT systems remain the same, ongoing research has led to the development of added features and associated benefits for many devices. For example, the Therapeutic Regulated Accurate Care (T.R.A.C.™) Pad used with the V.A.C. Therapy system added pressure sensing ports along the collection tubing to improve monitoring and maintenance of the set target pressure at the wound site as an initial design improvement over the process of inserting the cut end of the collection tube directly into the foam. The SensaT.R.A.C.™ Technology design improvement facilitated increased exudate collection. Improved ability to accurately maintain pressure in a variety of environmental conditions and to alert caregivers through various alarms has contributed to acceptance of NPWT for certification as safe-to-fly on some military air transport vehicles.

Additional refinements have included *Smart Alarms*™ that alert caregivers when corrective action is needed and, in some conditions, interrupt therapy if critical programmed parameters are met. The therapy unit alarms in any of the following conditions:

- The canister is full, missing, or improperly placed
- The tubing is blocked
- The tubing or dressing has air leaks
- Therapy is inactive
- The battery is low.

V.A.C. Therapy is intended to create an environment that *promotes wound healing* by secondary or tertiary (delayed primary) intention by preparing the wound bed for closure, removing exudate and infectious material, reducing edema, promoting granulation tissue formation, and promoting perfusion.[2] V.A.C. Therapy is indicated for patients with chronic, acute, traumatic, subacute, and dehisced wounds; partial-thickness burns; ulcers (such as diabetic or pressure); flaps; and grafts.[4]

NPWT Systems

"Without continual growth and progress, such words as improvement, achievement, and success have no meaning." — Benjamin Franklin

V.A.C. Therapy System, marketed in the United States since 1995, serves as a predicate device for a series of products approved for NPWT. Characteristically described, the current NPWT platform has evolved to include several key components: 1) an electric-powered or non-powered *negative pressure generating "pump"* with continuous and/or intermittent negative pressure modality, 2) *connective tubing* to convey pressure changes to the wound space, provide a conduit to remove exudate, and, in some cases, monitor the pressure delivered to the wound space, 3) a water-impermeable, adhesive-sealed occlusive, *oxygen- and water vapor-semipermeable drape* to protect against pressure loss and wound contamination, 4) an *interface dressing* (with or without a nonadherent intervening contact layer) that interacts with the tissue at the wound base, helps wick exudate from the recesses of the wound, and through which the negative pressure is delivered to the wound space, and 5) an *exudate collection process* to contain exudate removed from the wound.

NPWT System Designs and Innovations

At present, 13 manufacturers of NPWT devices are recognized by the US Centers for Medicare & Medicaid Services (CMS) for reimbursement after undergoing 510K, substantial equivalency determination with the V.A.C. Therapy System as the predicate device. US Food and Drug Administration (FDA)-approved negative pressure pumps span from simple vacuum generators to fully computerized feedback systems, non-powered or electrically powered with and without battery backup, variably capable of generating and monitoring continuous and intermittent negative pressure. *Device alarms* strive to improve the therapeutic safety profile, especially related to identifying situations that may be related to serious and potentially fatal blood loss. NPWT has undergone a tremendous expansion attesting to the extensive applicability of subatmospheric (negative) therapy to multiple clinical situations and care settings. The following generalized, non-comprehensive review of key component modifications is designed to provide insight to the product variation available. Comparative impact of specific therapy and device variances on clinical wound healing outcomes has yet to be fully determined.

Pumps. Prior to the development of computer-regulated pumps, wall suction was used for evacuation of exudate from wounds. While effective for wound exudate management, wall suction techniques create an abrupt drawdown and do not allow for pulsed regulated pressure delivery. Initial modifications on the predicate device were focused on proof of concept and assuring delivery of programmed negative pressure through wound site feedback, monitoring for continuous and intermittent pressure, expanding ranges for negative pressure (-40 mmHg to 230 mmHg) to increase number of approved manufacturers, validating antimicrobial gauze dressing as an appropriate alternative "filler material," decreasing noise, and improving portability. Presumably, modulating pressure cycle times, peak pressure, pressure wave patterns, and treatment regimes influences tissue cellular content, collagen and extracellular matrix deposition, and quantity and rate of generation. "Optimal" tissue healing would be achieved through response-adjusted negative pressure treatment profiles. Previously, lower pressure ranges and gauze were the focus of newer devices to distinguish themselves from the predicate device. Current device improvements seek further portability, ease of use, and universal applicability. Some newer devices are designed for use with both gauze and foam, without preferential styling, thereby securing their utilization independent of the physician's choice of therapy. For instance, XLR8® (Genadyne Biotechnologies, Great Neck, New York) was designed for maximal suitability with low weight (600 g), full-range peak pressure profile capacity (50 mmHg–230 mmHg), continuous and intermittent modality, a built-in Li-Ion battery with minimal 8-hour life, and 3-hour charge time with minimal noise levels.[5]

Power source. Previously, newer models remained electrically powered with a focus on extended battery life. Now attention has turned toward achieving non-powered, alternative energy-sourced devices and devices that are solely battery powered with imminent disposability for short-term, out-of-hospital therapy. Powered and non-powered device clinical safety considerations remain similar to those of the predicate device, even though in the United States non-powered NPWT devices are managed under a separate FDA classification guidance document.[6] The SNaP® Wound Care System (Spiracur Inc., Sunnyvale, California) is an exceptionally light-weight, "ultraportable," non-powered, mechanically generated negative pressure unit that showed special utility for ambulatory, out-of-hospital disaster-injured patients in Haiti where community electricity suffered prolonged disruption.[7]

Portability. Device evolution progressed from remarkably heavy, stationary units to exceptionally lightweight, ultraportable devices, applicable in all care settings from inpatient bedridden to outpatient fully ambulatory. The SNaP device spearheaded this body of devices by switching to a mechanically powered device that maintains a preset constant or intermittent pressure (-75, -100, or -150 mmHg) without electricity or batteries.[8] A novel engineering approach to exceptional portability was achieved through innovative design exemplified by the pocket-sized NPD 1000™ Negative Pressure Wound Therapy device (Kalypto Medical, Mendota Heights, Minnesota) that runs on 3 AA batteries coupled with an antimicrobial combination collection system dressing pad.[9] Other devices followed suit to join the roles of improved portability through "miniaturization," improved economy of size for off-the-shelf availability, and improved "disposability" to optimize application for the post-operative, surgically closed, 7-day treatment, acute wound market (V.A.C.Via™ Negative Pressure Wound Therapy System, KCI USA, Inc.; XLR8 and A4-NWPT pump®, Genadyne Biotechnologies; PICO™ Single Use Negative Pressure Wound Therapy System, Smith & Nephew, Inc., St-Laurent, Quebec, Canada). Accessories also aid portability; for example, car chargers (Vario 18, Medela Inc., McHenry, Illinois) and various out-of-hospital bed connectors, hospital trolley carts, and personal carrying cases provide convenient mobility.[5,10-13]

Device-related clinical safety. Safety considerations for potential complications, such as bleeding, foreign body retention, pain, tissue ingrowth, infection, and exsanguination, exist for all NPWT systems, regardless of care setting, portability, and recommended pressure profiles. Caution should be taken to mitigate potential complications with appropriate patient selection and therapy adjustments, as needed. Alarm types are variable, but most devices have some ability to notify in the event of an air leak and non-delivery of the intended pressure.[4]

Tubing and collection systems (drains). Tube collection systems remove exudate from the wound and deliver negative pressure to the wound space. Across various systems, tubing differs in lumen length and diameter, which affects the rate of exudate removal and the potential for obstruction development. If blockage occurs without clearance, maceration, infection, and wound deterioration may ensue. Some systems use the collection tubing as a simple conduit; others add the benefit of wound space pressure monitoring through the terminal pad (Prevena™ Incision Management System, T.R.A.C. Pad and SensaT.R.A.C., KCI USA, Inc.).[14,15] Another level of advanced negative pressure therapy delivery is achieved through software programming automatic response feedback loops. The Mobility Solutions Miller drains (Miller Digivac Toe and Finger Chambers, Miller Extremity Garments, Miller DermiVex Drain, and Miller Encompass Drain) are body location-specific silicone drains modified for use with gauze interfaces.[16,17] Dressing techniques that assist with digits and unusual contours, even in pediatric populations, have been described.

Canisters. Exudate collection canisters may be open or sealed with gel packs (isolyzers) for solidification of wound exudate. Out-of-hospital disposal of liquid blood-contaminated waste may be limited, depending upon local restrictions imposed by environmental protection regulations. Rules for collection, storage, and disposal of biohazardous materials, both liquid and solid, may apply. The isolyzer assists in converting restricted liquid waste to disposable solid waste to facilitate disposal. One-way valves between canisters and tubing systems prevent backflow of biohazardous materials onto the wound when negative pressure is discontinued. Similarly, some systems may utilize backflow prevention between the pump and the canister connection system to prevent contamination of the pump system and internal filters. Canister sizes vary depending upon the size of the associated pump, desired portability, and wound type being targeted. Canister capacities range from 25 cc to 1500 cc with and without the ability to be emptied and reused. Procedures and policies must be established for reusable products to reduce the likelihood of cross-contamination. Caution must be used with canisters greater than 500 cc as their use may increase the risk of severe fluid loss, dehydration, and exsanguination. Larger canister sizes are not recommended for neonates, infants, children, or adults with low-volume states or problems with coagulation[18] where the removal of a large percent total body fluid volume or coagulation factors may pose a significant risk. Although evidence supports the safe use of NPWT in children, the therapy should be applied to children with caution to ensure safety.[19-21]

Adhesive drape. Most adhesive drapes used with NPWT consist of water vapor-semipermeable polyurethane film coated with a hypoallergenic, pressure-sensitive acrylate adhesive. Drapes seal the environment, maintaining the negative pressure over the wound, create a barrier to outside contaminants, and provide a moist wound healing environment. This allows the underlying wound exudate to condense into a gelatinous coagulum, which supports re-epithelization at the wound margins. There are no distinctions between the drapes used in foam-based systems versus those used in gauze-based systems, and both systems typically require oxygen and water vapor semipermeability to allow for moisture balance and oxygenation of the periwound skin. Many NPWT providers will contract dressing manufacturers to produce a drape with their specific requirements for size, shape, peel tabs, adhesive content, and branding. Since these products are usually essentially equivalent to 3M™ Tegaderm™ Dressings (3M Health Care, St Paul, Minnesota),[22] transparent films are frequently used to repair leaks when the brand-specific drape is not available. Some dressing systems distinguish themselves through attempts to innovate the dressing application process. The NPD 1000 Negative Pressure Wound Therapy device does not require a secondary occlusive drape because the interface dressing and exudate process are integrated within the pad. Additionally, hydrocolloid wafers and stoma paste are often helpful to achieve a seal in difficult-to-dress locations.[23]

Irrigation systems. NPWT *"instillation systems"* also have undergone design changes for programmed wound irrigation treatments with prolonged, intermittent, or continuous profiles.

Although these systems have been used predominantly to treat osteomyelitis and soft tissue infections, they can be used to deliver agents other than antibiotics, such as antimicrobial agents, chemical debriders, anti-inflammatory agents, growth factors, oxygen and energy molecules, chemotherapeutics, "liquefied" cellular and tissue components, and tissue nutritional factors. Appropriate testing to prove the safety and clinical efficacy of expanded indications would be required. This is no small feat, since the medical scientific evidential bar has been set high for demonstrating both mechanisms of action and clinical outcomes. Even with a current, fairly robust clinical retrospective evidence base,[20] achieving full reimbursement approval for NPWT for pediatric indications has been difficult to attain in all countries. The V.A.C. Instill® Therapy Unit (KCI USA, Inc.) and the irrigation systems, Svedman® and SVED® (Innovative Therapies Inc., Gaithersburg, Maryland), are the most commonly used devices.[24]

NPWT pressure treatment modalities. Most manufacturers offer devices with both continuous and intermittent pressure modalities for inpatient and outpatient care settings. Two schools of thought surround the "optimal" negative pressure treatment target: low pressure at -80 mmHg or high pressure at -125 mmHg. Some devices are designed to provide only the lower negative pressure treatment range, while others are designed to treat both the lower and higher ranges. As care setting focus shifts toward alternative care settings/ambulatory out-of-hospital, the trend has shifted to develop NPWT devices specifically designed to target wound types amenable to the continuous pressure modality, simplified operation, and lowered out-of-hospital treatment costs.

NPWT Wound Interface Materials

An interface dressing, with or without a nonadherent intervening contact layer, directly influences 1) microstrain delivery to the tissue surface, 2) exudate removal by helping to wick fluid from the recesses of the wound, and 3) negative pressure modulation as it passes into the wound space and then out to the periwound tissues. The most commonly prescribed NPWT interface dressings are foams composed of either open-cell reticulated polyethylene (PU) foam or polyvinyl alcohol (PVA) foam and an absorbent cotton-blend antimicrobial gauze containing 0.2% polyhexamethylene biguanide hydrochloride (PHMB). Some devices have developed device-specific foams: KCI USA, Inc. with GranuFoam™ and GranuFoam Silver®, Medela Inc. with Avance™ (green foam), Smith & Nephew with RENASYS®-F, and Innovative Therapies Inc. with SVED Svamp® Foam. Most gauze-based dressing kits offer antimicrobial gauze, eg, Kendall™ AMD Antimicrobial Dressings containing 0.2% PHMB (Covidien, Mansfield, Massachusetts).[25] Silverlon® (Argentum Medical, LLC, Chicago, Illinois), a silver-impregnated woven nylon, has received special recognition for utility with NPWT.[26-28] Dressings specifically designed for NPWT systems include the Bio-Dome™ dressing and Bio-Dome EasyRelease (ConvaTec, Inc., Skillman, New Jersey)[29] and the Kalypto collection pad. Adapted for use with any NPWT system, Hydrofera Blue® Bacteriostatic Dressing (Hydrofera, LLC, Willimantic, Connecticut) is a PVA sponge with two broad-spectrum bacteriostatic agents, methylene blue and gentian violet.[30] An intervening nonadherent contact dressing layer (eg, Mepitel® or Mepitel One, Mölnlycke Health Care, Norcross, Georgia) may be applied to any of the dressing systems in an effort to reduce potential complications related to dressing adherence and tissue in-growth.

NPWT foam dressings. PU and PVA are the two most common materials used to create open-cell, hydrophilic or hydrophobic, NPWT foams. Pore size and strut measurements determine the density, tensile strength, and porosity of the foam. Pore diameter, strut (cell or walls of the foam) thickness, and applied negative pressure define the microstrain delivered to the tissue surface.

V.A.C. GranuFoam. The black V.A.C. Granu-Foam PU dressing has reticulated or open pores ranging in size from 400 μm to 600 μm and is considered effective at promoting granulation tissue formation while aiding in wound contraction.[31] It is hydrophobic (or moisture repelling), which enhances exudate removal. Several specialized V.A.C. GranuFoam dressings have also been designed to accommodate the needs of specific wound sites (ie, abdominal cavity, heel, and hand).[32] These facilitate the application of negative pressure to anatomical locations with contours that make it difficult to achieve an airtight seal (Plates 28–31, page 348).

V.A.C. GranuFoam Silver. The V.A.C. GranuFoam Silver Dressing combines the properties of V.A.C. GranuFoam with those of silver. The reticulated or open pores of this dressing have microbonded metallic silver uniformly distributed throughout the dressing, providing continuous delivery of silver.[33] The V.A.C. GranuFoam Silver Dressing is an effective barrier to bacterial penetration and may help reduce infection (Plates 32–35, page 348). Topical silver has broad-spectrum antimicrobial activity. The only silver dressing specifically designed for use with V.A.C. Therapy is the V.A.C. GranuFoam Silver Dressing. This dressing provides continuous release of ionic silver for up to 72 hours and has been shown to be effective against 150 microbial species.[33] A subset of 6 organisms considered clinically relevant was selected for quantitative antimicrobial testing. A sample of the V.A.C. GranuFoam Silver Dressing was added to 50 mL of the challenge organism at approximately 10^5 colony-forming units per milliliter (CFU/mL) and incubated over time. The dressing showed significant antimicrobial activity in as little as 30 minutes after exposure to the organisms. The open-celled, reticulated structure of this dressing allowed for microdeformational changes at the foam-tissue interface in the same manner as the V.A.C. GranuFoam Dressing. A study was conducted on porcine full-thickness wounds treated with either the V.A.C. GranuFoam Dressing or the V.A.C. GranuFoam Silver Dressing to determine if granulation rates would be comparable.[33] There were no significant differences ($P > .05$) in wound granulation rates (as measured using wound volume measurements) between these 2 V.A.C. Therapy dressings. Together, these studies indicate that the properties of the V.A.C. GranuFoam dressing are retained by the V.A.C. GranuFoam Silver dressing, which assists with granulation tissue formation and serves as an effective barrier against microorganism invasion.[34]

V.A.C.® WhiteFoam® Dressing. V.A.C. WhiteFoam PVA dressing is a dense foam with a higher tensile strength that requires higher negative pressures (125 mmHg–175 mmHg) in order to provide adequate distribution of negative pressure throughout the wound. V.A.C. White-Foam is hydrophilic (or moisture maintaining), is premoistened with sterile water, and possesses relatively nonadherent properties.[31] It is generally recommended for use in tunnels and tracts and other situations where special attention is necessary to avoid the possibility of tissue in-growth into the foam.

Hydrofera Blue Bacteriostatic Dressing. Hydrofera Blue Bacteriostatic Dressing ("Blue Foam") is a PVA sponge with two broad-spectrum bacteriostatic agents, methylene blue and gentian violet. These agents are effective against the drug-resistant organisms, methicillin/oxacillin-resistant *Staphylococcus aureus* (MRSA) and vancomycin-resistant *enterococci* (VRE). The foam's open cell structure naturally provides capillary vacuum action to draw excess fluid and exudate from the wound bed. Hydrofera Blue must be moistened with sterile saline or sterile water and squeezed out before application to the wound bed. Color change from blue to white indicates complete release of antimicrobial agents. Case studies support the use of this foam at negative pressure ranges, both low (-80 mmHg) and high (-125 mmHg), to improve chronic wounds without any significant complications.[35,36]

Avance ("Green Foam") Dressings. Avance Foam is open-cell, hydrophobic polyurethane specifically designed for use with the Avance NPWT device at negative pressure (-120 mmHg) to provide the desired 5%–20% microstrain for enhanced cellular proliferation. Preclinical studies conducted by Malmsjö et al compared Avance Foam's biological effects to the predicate V.A.C. GranuFoam (-125 mmHg) and to AMD gauze (-80 mmHg), with and without intervening contact layers, Mepitel and Mepitel One. Specific investigations related to wound bed granulation tissue quantity, tissue in-growth into the filler material, delivery of negative pressure to the wound bed, and blood flow in the wound bed. Malmsjö and colleagues noted a more pronounced granulation tissue formation with foam (green and black) than with gauze. When a wound contact layer was applied, granulation tissue formation was slightly greater under foam than under gauze, with the degree of granulation tissue development being similar for both Avance Foam and V.A.C. GranuFoam. Both foams showed a slightly greater amount of wound contraction as compared with AMD gauze. The two intervening contact layers supported equal degrees of contraction. The wound bed tissue grew into

foam but not into gauze, and the degree of tissue in-growth was similar for both Avance Foam and V.A.C. GranuFoam. The investigators' results confirmed observations that gauze was easier to remove and antimicrobial AMD gauze does not disrupt the wound bed. Moreover, the presence of an intervening contact layer, such as Mepitel and Mepitel One, hinders in-growth and lessens the force needed for removal of foam in NPWT.[37,38]

RENASYS-F foam. The RENASYS-F foam is open-cell, hydrophobic, black, polyurethane foam developed for specific use with the Smith & Nephew RENASYS EZ and RENASYS GO NPWT systems. Smith & Nephew's EZCARE and VISTA systems (formerly BlueSky Medical devices) utilize AMD gauze dressings at negative pressure ranges from 40 mmHg to 80 mmHg, while the RENASYS system platform uses gauze or foam at negative pressure ranges from 40 mmHg to 200 mmHg. Bondojki et al used the RENASYS-F system to treat 18 patients in a prospective, multicenter study with a variety of wound types, including pressure ulcers, diabetic foot ulcers, and traumatic and surgical wounds. Results showed that at the end of the 14.6 day mean treatment duration, 83% of wounds (15/18) had progressed sufficiently to discontinue NPWT. Reductions in wound dimension, exudate level, odor, and nonviable tissue during the therapy with a significant increase in "beefy red" granulation tissue suggested the viability of utilizing the new RENASYS-F foam.[39]

Svamp Foam. Innovative Therapies Inc. (ITI) combines continuous irrigation with negative pressure therapy in its AC electric-powered NPWT systems: the original larger, 5.5 lb, 18-hour battery Svedman device intended for hospital use and the smaller, more portable, 1.9 lb, 14-hour battery SVED device. The proprietary open-celled, hydrophobic black and hydrophilic white PU Svamp Foams may be used with both devices that provide negative pressure therapy prior to, during, or after irrigation. The dry white foam is denser with a higher tensile strength. Irrigation and negative pressure application are achieved by two different pathways within the tubing system, which allows flexibility in the timing of irrigation in relation to the institution of negative pressure. As with other NPWT devices, the ITI systems are intended for use on patients with chronic, acute, traumatic, subacute, and dehisced wounds; diabetic ulcers; pressure ulcers; flaps; and grafts. Antimicrobial and amino acid preparation may be used with the system and all preparations should be used in accordance with the manufacturer's product instructions for use (IFU). Dressings are changed every 48–72 hours and if the irrigation has been discontinued for more than 2 hours, and nonadherent intervening contact layers may be used to reduce patient discomfort with dressing changes. Both continuous (-70 mmHg, -120 mmHg, and -150 mmHg) and intermittent modalities are available with a negative pressure (-25 mmHg) maintained during the off phase of the on-off cycle (5 min/2 min). Visual and audible alarms alert to notify instances of low pressure, air leaks, and full canister as the volume approaches maximum capacity (SVED 300 cc; Svedman 1,200 cc). Teder, Sandén, and Svedman conducted swine model, infected full-thickness wound healing studies to validate their proof of concept to demonstrate that the passage of fluid cleanses both the NPWT pad and the wound. The irrigation systems assisted with avoiding the collection of blood, exudate, or infectious materials, and the negative pressure treatment facilitated granulation tissue development.[40]

Antimicrobial gauze dressings (cotton blends). NPWT systems using moistened gauze typically recommend the Chariker-Jeter Technique where a nonadherent intervening contact layer covers the wound bed; moistened gauze is lightly layered to fill the wound space surrounding a flat, fenestrated drain and enclosed by a transparent polyethylene adhesive drape. The most frequently recommended gauze has a cotton-nylon blend containing 0.2% PHMB, antimicrobial dressing AMD. PHMB is a polymeric, broad-spectrum, cationic antimicrobial agent that impairs the outer membrane of gram-positive and gram-negative bacteria, showing sustained killing activity against MRSA, VRE, *Escherichia coli*, *Pseudomonas aeruginosa*, *Bacteroides fragilis*, *Clostridium perfringens*, and yeasts, such as *Candida albicans*.[25] Studies show antimicrobial gauze dressings with PHMB may expand options for extended occlusive dressing duration without significantly increasing wound bacterial load or human cellular cytotoxicity profiles. If the negative pressure therapy becomes inactive, dressings do not need

to be removed immediately but may be left intact for 24 hours or more depending upon the manufacturer's IFU. Other attributes of PHMB include the reduction of wound pain, odor, and fibrin slough and the prevention of necrotic tissue build-up in chronic wounds.[41,42] Antimicrobial dressings are more commonly used for infection prevention. Dressings may be used clinically to augment treatment of active infections but are not considered stand-alone therapies.

NPWT devices recommending preferential use of AMD Gauze with pressure ranges 60 mmHg–80 mmHg include Prospera® PRO-I™, PRO-II™, and PRO-III™ (Prospera, Fort Worth, Texas), Versatile1™ (BlueSky Medical, Carlsbad, California), EZCARE and V1STA (Smith & Nephew), Exsudex™ (RecoverCare, Louisville, Kentucky), Invia® Liberty™ and Vario (Medela Inc.), Moblvac® (Ohio Medical Corporation, Gurnee, Illinois), A4-NWPT pump (Genadyne Biotechnologies), VENTURI™ AVANTI and VENTURI COMPACT (Tally Medical USA, Lansing, Michigan), and SNaP (Spiracur Inc.).[5,8,13,43–47]

Silverlon Negative Pressure Dressing (nylon). Silverlon NPD (Argentum Medical, LLC), awarded the Frost & Sullivan 2006 Product Innovation Award for the US antimicrobial dressings market, is an absorbent, nonadherent silver nylon product that releases silver for 7 days. The autocatalytic silver-plating process uniformly and permanently coats the entire polymeric substrate surface circumferentially with silver that is readily released in ionic form when contacted by wound exudate. In the presence of moisture, this unique product continuously emits a very high level of ionic silver into the wound bed. The tight nylon weave resists in-growth and adherence while its porous quality permits negative pressure delivery to the tissue without obstructing exudate evacuation. This product serves as the wound contact layer for the Kalypto collection pad. The use of silver as an antimicrobial agent extends back many centuries. Silver has broad antimicrobial activity against both gram-negative and gram-positive bacteria and has demonstrated minimal development of bacterial resistance.

Bio-Dome and Bio-Dome EasyRelease (ConvaTec). This innovative wound dressing, designed for use with the Engenex® NPWT System (licensed from Boehringer Technologies), is comprised of non-woven polyester layers joined by a silicone elastomer, which effectively fills the wound while permitting exudate fluid transport. The Bio-Dome dressing has specifically engineered open pore spaces that resist collapse under negative pressures 30 mmHg–75 mmHg, presenting an unobstructed area for tissue growth influenced by a 5%–20% cellular microstrain tissue-interface pressure. The product's pore structure was designed to lower risks for in-growth and adherence-related pain, bleeding, and foreign body retention with a higher material tensile strength and a lower bioadhesion profile. The silicone elastomer reduces adherence but the Bio-Dome EasyRelease was specifically designed with a flat profile to further reduce tissue adherence and potential in-growth. Studies conducted by Girolami et al demonstrated the ability of the system to reduce aggressive adherence in the wound bed, eliminate risk of foreign body deposits, and reduce pain during removal and re-application while optimizing granulation tissue proliferation.[48] This is the only non-foam-based dressing system purposely designed to further the application of the new NPWT platform focusing on microstrain to specifically direct cellular proliferative responses. The Engenex has unique software programming to provide patient compliance tracking.[49,50]

Kalypto Negative Pressure Device Collection Pad. The Kalypto NPD pad is an innovative combination "all-in-one" styled negative pressure dressing designed for specific use with the Kalypto Medical NPD 1000 lightweight (8 oz) pump. The design allows for maximum portability. The dressing pad has a Silverlon contact nonadherent layer for minimal adherence and antimicrobial activity. The intermediate layer is composed of a two-fiber, non-woven, exudate collection system where absorbent hydrophilic fibers wick fluids into a super absorbent, bonding inner pad. The inner pad is surrounded by a non-woven, semi-occlusive polyurethane film. The indicated negative pressure is delivered to the tissue even though the pad swells as exudate accumulates in the inner core. The periwound margin is protected by a hydrophobic Gore® membrane, which protects against maceration as long as the system fluid limits are not exceeded (25 cc, 50 cc, 75 cc, 140 cc). The hydrogel adhesive

gasket allows for easy application. The pump runs on 3 AA alkaline batteries, provides negative pressures of 40 mmHg–125 mmHg, and offers both continuous and intermittent pressure modes. The Silverlon-generated antimicrobial activity is present with and without active therapy as established by Davis et al[51,52] measuring bacterial clearance in full-thickness wounds inoculated with *Pseudomonas aeruginosa* ATCC 37312 using a porcine model.

The largest reduction in bacterial concentration was seen at 48 hours after inoculation. Case studies in diabetic foot wounds, venous insufficiency, and chronic leg wounds demonstrated the product's ability to support chronic wound healing with minimal complications as long as the fluid handling capacity of the dressing is observed.[52]

Intervening nonadherent contact layers. Early nonadherent contact layers (primary contact dressings) were designed to address the issues of adherence, tissue trauma, and pain. Subsequent evolution added the qualities of avoiding the deposition of fibers, cytotoxic agents, or irritating extractable additives. Both gauze and foam applied directly to the wound surface have been associated with bio-adherence and tissue in-growth. Additives to the materials, such as soft paraffin, oils, or silicone, may alter the adherence of the product. *The application of intervening contact layers reduces negative pressure transduction to the tissue.* The degree of reduction depends upon the product and number of layers applied. Over the years, the development of potential complications and required corrective surgical intervention has prompted a variety of suggested remedies that still influence clinical practice today: careful patient selection, more frequent dressing changes, institution of intervening nonadherent contact dressings, selection of alternative interface materials, lowered treatment pressures, and, in some situations, postponing the use of negative pressure therapy. These remedies should be considered to reduce complications regardless of the interface being applied (gauze, foam, fabricated construct).

Paraffin-coated dressings. Some of the earliest modern-day nonadherent dressings are cotton blends coated with soft paraffin (eg, Vaseline Petrolatum Gauze, Covidien, and Adaptic™ with knotted viscose, Systagenix Wound Management,

Gargrave, United Kingdom). These are manufactured with and without antimicrobials, such as povidone-iodine (eg, Betadine™ gauze, Purdue Frederick, Norwalk, Connecticut) or 3% bismuth tribromophenate (eg, Xeroform™ gauze, Covidien). Available since the 1900s, tulle gras is absorbent cotton coated with balsam of Peru, paraffin, and oils. Plain cotton has been substituted with nylon-blended cotton to improve strength, and balsam of Peru has been replaced with newer, less sensitizing antimicrobials, such as chlorhexidine acetate 0.5% (eg, Bactigras®, Smith & Nephew) and 0.2% PHMB hydrochloride (eg, AMD). The combination of nonadherence and antimicrobial properties increases application duration for some gauze dressings.

Hydrocolloid pectins. Dressings made with hydrocolloid pectins have been used with NPWT (eg, GranuFlux®, ConvaTec) for their increased absorption and ability to "dissolve" into spaces when contacted by exudate yet still be easily removed with rinsing. Generally recommended for open wounds, hydrocolloid wafers used with NPWT-treated wounds help obliterate air spaces between the tissue and the sealing dressing to facilitate the retention of a seal. This is very important for anatomically difficult-to-dress locations. Some products have the added advantage of paraffin and hydrocolloid pectins for increased nonadherence (eg, Urgotul®, Urgo Medical, Chenove, France).

Silicone preparations and other nonadherent materials. Silicone-coated dressings demonstrate improved nonadherent qualities while minimizing irritation or potential allergic reactions. Paraffin has long been an additive to coat materials to decrease adherence. Meshed and woven characteristics of properties of materials may still allow "in-growth," which also affects adherence, ease of removal, and discomfort with extraction. Nonadherent products, such as Mepitel (Mölnlycke Health Care), Jelonet®, Biobrane® (Smith & Nephew), 3M™ Tegapore™, and Adaptic Touch® (Systagenix Wound Management), have become a product staple used under gauze or foam to reduce in-growth and pain during NPWT treatments. While soft silicone is not intrinsically absorbent, it is usually applied to cotton and cotton-blend gauzes to improve the absorptive capacity of the resultant product

while still maintaining the nonadherent quality.

Inappropriate interface materials. Some products are deemed to be inappropriate for use with NPWT systems. Those materials that impede delivery of negative pressure to the wound surface or obstruct full evacuation of wound exudate should be avoided.

Natural sponges. Initially, sponge-based dressings were considered as potential alternative wound dressings because of their ability to conform to a space, fluid capacitance, tensile strength, and availability. However, natural sponges have limited application as NPWT dressings due to their "semi-open cell" communication pattern where some pores do not communicate with others. In a sponge and some "closed cell foams," the fluid channeling may flow into a space that does not allow for complete fluid extraction. Variable pore size and communication make pressure transmission and fluid extraction unpredictable. Consequently, exudate fluids and small particulate infectious materials could become trapped within the body of the sponge and the distribution of negative pressures across portions of a sponge could be compromised.

Perforated plastic film and bordered products. Perforated plastic film composed of polyethylene terephthalate (PET), a thermoplastic polymer resin that does not contain polyethelene, can be used as an NPWT dressing cover; however, the ability of the dressing to function properly will depend upon size and number of perforations.[53] The dressing must allow full exudate extraction while delivering negative pressure. Fenestrated film dressings with absorption layers (eg, TELFA™, Covidien) are available but may not be well suited for NPWT because of impermeable linings. Similarly, composite dressings made from absorbable cotton and polyester blends and water impermeable outer borders were created for "low-adherent" treatments (eg, Melolin® with borders, Smith & Nephew), but the impermeable borders make these dressings unsuitable for NPWT.

NPWT Application: Indications and Complications

"Healthcare providers will compete to offer the best record of patient safety at the lowest prices. Hospitals and patients will benefit from having accurate informa-

Table 1. Indications and contraindications for NPWT Therapy[54]

Indications

• NPWT is intended to create an environment that promotes wound healing by secondary or tertiary (delayed primary) intention by preparing the wound bed for closure, reducing edema, promoting granulation tissue formation and perfusion, and removing exudate and infectious material.
• It is indicated for patients with chronic, acute, traumatic, subacute, and dehisced wounds; partial-thickness burns; ulcers (such as diabetic or pressure); flaps; and grafts.
• NPWT combined with antimicrobial dressings (silver, PHMB, etc) is an effective barrier to bacterial penetration and may help reduce infection in the above wound types.

Contraindications

• Exposed blood vessels, organs, or nerves
• Malignancy in the wound
• Untreated osteomyelitis
• Non-enteric and unexplored fistulas
• Necrotic tissue with eschar present
• Sensitivity to additive materials (eg, silver or antimicrobial agents)

Table 2. Safety precautions for NPWT (as stated in the V.AC. Therapy IFU Safety Information Sheet[54])

Category	Suggested NPWT Treatment
• Exposed vessels and organs	• Cover with muscle flaps or other natural tissue or fine-meshed, nonadherent porous material prior to NPWT • Administer NPWT only in inpatient setting with skilled nursing and close monitoring, when vessels or organs are not completely covered and protected with a thick layer of natural tissue or fine-meshed, nonadherent porous material • Stop NPWT and seek immediate medical intervention if sudden, increased, or hemorrhagic bleeding is observed for any reason or if frank blood is seen in the tubing or in the canister
Inadequate hemostasis • Anticoagulants • Platelet aggregation inhibitors	• If wound hemostasis is tenuous, administer NPWT in inpatient setting with skilled nursing and close monitoring
Non-sutured hemostatic agents • Bone wax • Absorbable gelatin sponge • Spray wound sealant	• Protect against dislodging of agents • Start with lowest negative pressure setting then monitor closely while progressing to target treatment pressure, as tolerated • Administer therapy only in inpatient setting with skilled nursing and close monitoring
Sharp edges or bone fragments	• Eliminate sharp edges or bone fragments from wound • Smooth or cover residual edges to decrease the risk of serious or fatal injury, should shifting of structures occur • Use caution when removing dressing components from wound
Blood vessel erosion due to infection (Note: the depth of infection and degree of weakening are not always readily apparent through direct visual inspection of the exposed vessel)	• Protect with thick layer of natural tissue, such as muscle flap, or nonadherent porous material • Administer therapy in inpatient setting with skilled nursing and close monitoring because there is increased risk of vascular rupture when blood vessel is infected

Table 2. Safety precautions for NPWT (as stated in the V.A.C. Therapy IFU Safety Information Sheet[54])

Category	Suggested NPWT Treatment
Infected wounds	• Change NPWT dressings at least every 12–24 hours if wound is infected • Monitor patient closely if there are any signs of possible infection or related complications • Contact physician for immediate treatment if there are any signs of the onset of systemic infection or advancing infection at the wound site; discontinue NPWT until the infection or complication has been diagnosed and proper treatment has been initiated
Tendons, ligaments, and nerves	• Protect with natural tissues or moist, fine-meshed, nonadherent material
Osteomyelitis (Note: V.A.C. Therapy should not be initiated on a wound with untreated osteomyelitis)	• Debride necrotic, nonviable tissue and infected bone (if necessary) • Initiate antibiotic therapy • Apply when osteomyelitis has been addressed
Foam placement	• Always use NPWT dressings from sterile packages that have not been opened or damaged • Do not place any foam dressing into blind/unexplored tunnels; the V.A.C. WhiteFoam dressing may be more appropriate for use with explored tunnels • Do not force foam dressings into any area of the wound, as this may damage tissue, alter the delivery of negative pressure, or hinder exudate removal • Always count the total number of pieces of foam used in the dressing and document that number on the drape and in the patient's chart; also document the dressing change date on the drape
Foam removal	• Ensure that all foam pieces have been removed from the wound with each dressing change, because NPWT foam dressings are not bio-absorbable • Follow manufacturer's recommended time schedule for dressing changes; foam left in the wound for greater than the recommended time period may foster in-growth of tissue into the foam, create difficulty in removing foam from the wound, or lead to infection or other adverse events
Reaction to acrylic adhesive	• Be aware that patients who are allergic or hypersensitive to acrylic adhesives may have an adverse reaction to the acrylic adhesive coating on the V.A.C. Drape • If a patient has a known allergy or hypersensitivity to such adhesives, or if any signs of allergic reaction or hypersensitivity develop, such as redness, swelling, rash, urticaria, significant pruritus, or bronchospasm, discontinue use and consult a physician immediately
Defibrillation	• Remove the NPWT dressing if defibrillation is required in the area of dressing placement

CHRONIC WOUND CARE: The Essentials

Table 2. Safety precautions for NPWT (as stated in the V.AC. Therapy IFU Safety Information Sheet[54])

Category	Suggested NPWT Treatment
Magnetic resonance imaging (MRI)	• Do not take the V.A.C. Therapy unit into the MR environment because the unit is MR unsafe • Leave V.A.C. GranuFoam dressing in place if therapy will not be interrupted for more than 2 hours • Leave V.A.C. GranuFoam Silver Dressing in place only under certain conditions and if therapy will not be interrupted for more than 2 hours (Note: MR image quality may be compromised if the area of interest is in the same area or relatively close to the position of the V.A.C. GranuFoam Silver dressing)
Hyperbaric oxygen therapy (HBO)	• Remove V.A.C. Therapy unit prior to HBO; the unit is not designed for this environment and should be considered a fire hazard in this environment • Replace dressing with compatible HBO dressing or cover V.A.C. Therapy dressing and tubing with moist cotton, gauze, or towel prior to HBO treatment
Maceration of periwound skin	• Do not allow foam to overlap intact skin • Protect fragile/friable periwound skin with a skin preparation product, additional V.A.C. Drape, hydrocolloid, or other transparent film • Realize that multiple layers of the V.A.C. Drape will decrease the moisture vapor transmission rate, which may increase the risk of maceration

tion about areas of excellence and areas that must be improved." — *Timothy F. Murphy, US Congressman*

All medical devices approved as substantially equivalent to provide NPWT share similar indications and complications as those reported in Table 1 for the V.A.C. Therapy predicate device. As with any medical therapy, potential risks have been reported. The volume of use may skew the number of reports toward the most frequently used device. Understanding the etiology of potential complications assists with mitigating the root cause regardless of the specific product being used. Table 1 lists indications and contraindications for NPWT,[54] and Table 2 presents safety precautions.[54] Although it rarely occurs, bleeding may result from exposed vessels and organs, inadequate hemostasis, inadequate protection of vital structures from sharp edges, or erosion of infected blood vessels. Other reported risks that may or may not be related to NPWT include wound infection, dressing material retention, irritation, and maceration of periwound skin.[54] Pain also has been noted secondary to mechanical stress applied to the wound, chemical contact irrita-

tion, and in-growth of tissue into the dressing material. The use of an intervening nonadherent contact layer or natural tissue should lessen the likelihood of adherence or in-growth to the interface dressing. Decreasing treatment pressure, increasing frequency of dressing changes, and careful patient selection may also lessen the risk of complications.

NPWT Guidelines

General guidelines for NPWT. Several articles describe in detail the general wound care steps associated with the application of NPWT.[55-57] The general process involves the following steps:
- Complete general wound assessment and care
- Debride wound if necessary
- Assess and treat infection
- Assess and protect periwound tissue
- Maintain moist wound environment
- Apply NPWT in accordance with the guidelines and IFU specific for that product and indication (eg, V.A.C. Therapy Clinical Guidelines[31] and V.A.C. Therapy IFU[54])
- Continue therapy until a base of granulation

tissue is robust enough to be maintained after discontinuation of the therapy or epithelization of the wound base.

Guidelines for foam-based NPWT. Articles provide consensus guidelines and/or algorithms that demonstrate how best to incorporate NPWT into the treatment of specific wound types. For example, Andros and members of a multidisciplinary expert panel[58] updated guidelines for the application of V.A.C. Therapy to diabetic foot wounds. This report summarizes clinical evidence, provides practical guidance through a treatment algorithm, offers best practices to clinicians treating diabetic foot wounds, and addresses the appropriate use of V.A.C. Therapy in treating these complex wounds. In 2004, Gupta et al[59] provided guidelines for the treatment of pressure ulcers, including the appropriate use of V.A.C. Therapy. Niezgoda and Mendez-Eastman[60] published an update of these guidelines, including an algorithm to assist in clinical management decisions related to patients with Stage III and Stage IV pressure ulcers and guidelines for incorporating V.A.C. Therapy into a complete clinical program that should include targeted patient education, pressure ulcer prevention, nutrition, aggressive incontinence management, offloading, periwound care, and routine skin surveillance. Other guidelines and algorithms for the use of V.A.C. Therapy also have been published for traumatic wounds, such as the open abdomen,[61] chest wounds,[62] and lower leg trauma.[63] In an international global expert panel, Runkel et al developed recommendations for traumatic wounds and reconstructive procedures and completed a formal consultative consensus involving 422 independent healthcare workers in 2011.[64]

Guidelines for gauze-based NPWT. In 2011, Birke-Sorensen et al reported the determinations of an international consensus panel convened to initiate the steps necessary to determine best practices for treatment variables including treatment pressures, contact layers, and interface dressing selection.[65] Additional information is being published by these and other authors to show the relative risks and benefits of gauze and foam-based dressings for NPWT. In most instances, AMD gauze appears to be similarly beneficial as an NPWT dressing.

Treating Chronic Wounds with V.A.C. Therapy

Diabetic foot wounds. V.A.C. Therapy has been used to treat diabetic foot wounds in randomized and nonrandomized studies (Table 3). Results from small RCTs by McCallon et al[66] and Eginton et al[67] demonstrated the ability of V.A.C. Therapy to reduce wound surface area and volume. Armstrong and Lavery[68] validated these findings in a large RCT in patients with diabetes and partial foot amputation wounds. Of the 77 patients who were randomized to V.A.C. Therapy, 43 (56%) achieved complete wound closure in a median time of 56 days. In a retrospective study, Page et al[69] reviewed the charts of 47 patients with open foot wounds with significant soft tissue defects. Of these patients, 22 (47%) were treated with V.A.C. Therapy. The authors found that V.A.C. Therapy was associated with a reduction in risk of one or more surgical procedures, complications, and admissions related to the treatment of the index wound during the first year after treatment. In another study using administrative claims data from both Medicare and commercial payors in patients with diabetic foot ulcers, the incidence of subsequent amputation was lower in V.A.C.-treated wounds than those treated without NPWT. Of note, while traditionally treated wounds of greater severity/depth had increasing rates of amputation, this trend was not evident for those treated with V.A.C. Therapy.[70] Blume et al conducted a multicenter, randomized, controlled trial, enrolling 342 patients assigned to either NPWT or advanced moist wound therapy (AMWT) that consisted predominantly of hydrogels and alginates, with both treatment groups receiving standard offloading interventions and followed either 112 days or until 100% wound closure by any means. In this study, a greater proportion of diabetic foot ulcers achieved complete closure in the NPWT treatment group (73 of 169, 43.2%) than with the AMWT control (48 of 166, 28.9%) ($P = .007$), without any significant difference in safety profile, including those subjects followed at 6 and 9 months for all wounds achieving 100% closure.[71]

Pressure ulcers. V.A.C. Therapy also has been used to treat Stage III and Stage IV pressure ulcers (Table 4). The findings of 3 RCTs[72-74] demonstrate that V.A.C. Therapy successfully reduced

Table 3. V.A.C. Therapy findings from selected diabetic foot wound articles

First Author (Year)	Study Type	# of V.A.C. Therapy Patients/Wounds Analyzed	V.A.C. Therapy Findings
McCallon[66] (2000)	Randomized, controlled trial	5 patients	• Four patients achieved delayed primary healing in an average of 22.8 days • Wound surface area decreased by an average of 28.4%
Eginton[67] (2003)	Randomized, controlled trial	6 patients with 7 wounds	• Treatment lasted 2 weeks in this crossover design trial • Decreased wound volume 59% and depth 49%
Armstrong[68] (2005)	Randomized, controlled trial	77 patients	• 43 (56%) patients achieved complete wound closure • Median time to wound closure was 56 days • Median time to achieve 76%–100% granulation tissue formation was 42 days
Page[69] (2004)	Comparative, retrospective study	22 patients	• Median time for wound filling was 38 days • Associated with a reduction in risk of one or more surgical procedures, complications, and readmissions related to the treatment of the index wound during the first year after treatment

Table 4. V.A.C. Therapy findings from selected pressure ulcer articles

First Author (Year)	Study Type	# of V.A.C. Therapy Patients/Wounds Analyzed	V.A.C. Therapy Findings
Ford[72] (2002)	Randomized, controlled trial	20 wounds	• Two ulcers healed completely during controlled trial the 6-week treatment phase • Six ulcers underwent flap surgery • 51.8% mean reduction in ulcer volume
Joseph[73] (2000)	Randomized, controlled trial	18 wounds	• 66% reduction in wound depth • 78% final percent reduction in wound volume over time
Wanner[74] (2003)	Randomized, controlled trial	11 patients	• 50% reduction in initial wound volume in a mean (SD) of 27 (10) days • Reduced costs and improved comfort cited by authors as advantages of V.A.C. Therapy
Philbeck[75] (1999)	Retrospective study	43 wounds	• Ulcers averaged 22.2 cm² in area • Average rate of wound closure was 0.23 cm² per day

pressure ulcer size and may have positively affected wound histology. Philbeck et al[75] conducted a retrospective study of Medicare Part B home care patients who had chronic, nonhealing wounds treated with V.A.C. Therapy. The analyzed subset of pressure ulcer patients had an average wound area of 22.2 cm². Their finding that V.A.C. Therapy healed these ulcers at a rate of 0.23 cm² per day supports the findings of the 3 RCTs, which show V.A.C. Therapy to be a successful treatment

Table 5. V.A.C. Therapy findings from other chronic wound or mixed chronic and acute wound RCTs

First Author (Year)	Study Type	# of V.A.C. Therapy Patients/Wounds Analyzed	V.A.C. Therapy Findings
Vuerstaek[76] (2006)	Randomized, controlled trial	30 patients with chronic leg ulcers	• Median total healing time was 29 days • Median wound bed preparation time was 7 days • 90% of ulcers healed within 43 days • Demonstrated cost effectiveness
Braakenburg[77] (2006)	Randomized, controlled trial	32 patients with any type of acute or chronic wound	• V.A.C. Therapy group: 23 (74%) chronic (1 missing value), 2 (7%) acute, and 6 (19%) subacute wounds • An endpoint was a completely granulated wound or a wound ready for skin grafting or healing by secondary intention • Overall median time to healing was 16 days • In subset of 18 diabetic or cardiovascular patients, median wound healing time was 14 days
Moues[78] (2004)	Randomized, controlled trial	29 patients with full-thickness wounds that could not be closed immediately because of infection, contamination, or chronic character	• Wounds stratified by duration: early treated wounds (existing < 4 weeks before hospitalization) and late treated wounds (> 4 weeks) • Overall median time needed to reach "ready for surgical therapy" was 6.00 ± 0.52 days (median ± SEM) • Median time was 5.00 ± 0.85 days for wounds existing < 4 weeks and 6.00 ± 0.99 days for wounds > 4 weeks • The mean rate of wound surface area reduction was 3.8 ± 0.5%/day

for these chronic wounds. Wounds healed faster than standard of care with a higher incidence of closure.

Other V.A.C. Therapy chronic wound studies. In addition to the previously discussed diabetic foot wound and pressure ulcer studies, several RCTs evaluated V.A.C. Therapy in chronic leg ulcers or in study populations that combined chronic and acute wounds (Table 5). Vuerstaek et al[76] conducted an RCT in 60 hospitalized patients with chronic leg ulcers. For the 30 V.A.C. Therapy patients, the median total healing time was 29 days and the median wound bed preparation time was 7 days. Two other V.A.C. Therapy RCTs included chronic and acute wounds in each of the randomized groups. In the Braakenburg et al study,[77] 32 of the 65 patients were treated with V.A.C. Therapy. Twenty-three patients in the V.A.C. Therapy group had chronic

wounds, while the remaining 9 patients had acute or subacute wounds. The median time to healing for the overall V.A.C. Therapy group was 16 days. The median time to healing was 14 days for the subset of 18 V.A.C. Therapy patients with cardiovascular disease or diabetes. The Moues et al RCT[78] evaluated 54 patients with full-thickness wounds that "could not be closed immediately because of infection, contamination, or chronic character." For the 29 patients randomized to V.A.C. Therapy, the median time needed to reach "ready for surgical therapy" was 6.00 ± 0.52 days. The mean rate of wound surface area reduction in V.A.C. Therapy wounds was 3.8 ± 0.5%/day. All of these studies demonstrate that V.A.C. Therapy has been successfully used in the treatment of chronic wounds. NPWT improved the ability to facilitate wound closure in segments of these selected difficult-to-heal populations.

Table 6. V.A.C. Therapy findings from selected skin graft articles			
First Author (Year)	Study Type	# of V.A.C. Therapy Patients/Wounds Analyzed	V.A.C. Therapy Findings
Moisidis[79] (2004)	Randomized, controlled trial	20 wound halves	• Positive results in both qualitative and controlled trial quantitative measures • All wound halves healed without need for further debridement or regrafting • Dressings were well tolerated by the patients
Jeschke[80] (2004)	Randomized, controlled trial	5 patients	• 5 were treated with fibrin glue-anchored Integra and postoperative V.A.C. Therapy • Integra take rate was 98 ± 2% • Mean period from Integra coverage to skin transplantation was 10 ± 1 days
Genecov[81] (1998)	Prospective, controlled trial	10 patients	• 7 of 10 donor sites re-epithelized by Day 7
Carson[82] (2004)	Retrospective study	70 patients	• 86% overall healing rate (60 out of 70 patients) • All 50 skin grafts healed in 11–24 days and remained stable at 6 months

Skin grafts. When skin grafts are used to close wounds, V.A.C. Therapy can assist in preparing the wound bed and bolstering the graft (Table 6). The Moisidis et al RCT[79] studied quantitative graft take and qualitative graft appearance (as determined by an independent evaluator who was blinded to treatment assignment). V.A.C. Therapy grafts achieved positive results quantitatively and qualitatively. In another RCT, Jeschke et al[80] evaluated 12 patients with large defects who underwent Integra™ Bilayer Matrix Wound Dressing (Integra LifeSciences, Plainsboro, New Jersey) grafting for reconstruction. For the 5 patients treated with fibrin glue and V.A.C. Therapy, the Integra take rate was 98 ± 2% and the mean period from Integra coverage to skin transplantation was 10 ± 1 days. The Genecov et al prospective, controlled study[81] reported positive V.A.C. Therapy results in pigs and in humans. For the human subjects, all donor sites demonstrated re-epithelization at 1 week. Finally, in the Carson et al retrospective study,[82] 50 out of 70 patients received skin grafts bolstered by V.A.C. Therapy. All 50 grafts healed and remained stable for at least 6 months. NPWT appears to support improved graft take in selected large defect wounds.

Incision management of acute post-op-erative wounds. The use of NPWT over closed incisional wounds in patients who have a high likelihood of developing infection or mechanical stress-related dehiscence is increasingly being evaluated. Stannard et al studied this application in the prophylactic use of NPWT in high-risk lower extremity fractures.[83] Kilpadi and Cunningham described their experiences with using NPWT to assist with managing closed incisions, noting reduction of hematoma and seroma formation in a porcine model.[84] Clearly, there may be a role for assisting patients in a prophylactic fashion.

Cost effectiveness of V.A.C. Therapy. Various studies have shown that V.A.C. Therapy is cost effective in a variety of care settings. Philbeck et al[75] considered cost in their retrospective study of Medicare home healthcare patients. In a subset analysis of pressure ulcers, the authors used wound closure rates reported by Ferrell et al[85] in 1993 for patients with trochanteric and trunk pressure ulcers averaging 4.3 cm² who were treated with a low-air-loss surface and saline-soaked gauze. Ferrell et al[85] reported that the wounds closed at an average of 0.090 cm² per day. Philbeck et al[75] analyzed patients who were treated with a low-air-loss surface and V.A.C. Therapy and who had

Table 7. V.A.C. Therapy findings from selected acute wound articles

First Author (Year)	Study Type	# of V.A.C. Therapy Patients/Wounds Analyzed	V.A.C. Therapy Findings
Burns			
Kamolz[93] (2004)	Case series	7 patients with bilateral hand burns	• Enhanced perfusion reported in the V.A.C. Therapy-treated hand • Reduction in edema was observed • 5 hands healed without skin grafts • V.A.C. Therapy hand dressing did not need additional splinting
Surgical wounds — dehisced/open abdominal			
Garner[94] (2001)	Case series	14 trauma patients with open abdomens	• Early definitive fascial closure achieved in 13 patients (92%) in a mean of 9.9 ± 1.9 days • A mean of 2.8 ± 0.6 dressing changes were performed
Surgical wounds — sternal wound infections/mediastinitis			
Agarwal[95] (2005)	Retrospective study	103 patients treated after median sternotomy	• 64% had a diagnosis of mediastinitis, while 36% had either superficial infections or a sterile wound • Patients were treated for an average of 11 days • 70 patients (68%) achieved definitive chest closure with open reduction internal fixation and/or flap closure
Subacute wounds			
Argenta[1] (1997)	Case series	94 subacute wounds (overall study evaluated 300 wounds)	• 94 subacute wounds included dehisced wounds, open wounds with exposed orthopedic hardware and/or bone, and other miscellaneous wounds open < 7 days • 26 healed completely • 68 reduced in size and were closed with split-thickness skin grafts, secondary closure, or minor flaps • 37 patients with exposed orthopedic hardware or bone were treated successfully with closure of adjacent muscle and granulation tissue over the bone and hardware

Stage III and Stage IV trochanteric and trunk wounds that averaged 22.2 cm² in area. These wounds closed at an average of 0.23 cm² per day. The average 22.2 cm² wound in this study, treated as described by Ferrell et al, would take 247 days to heal, whereas the same wound would heal in 97 days with V.A.C. Therapy. While acknowledging the fact that larger pressure ulcers typically heal faster than smaller pressure ulcers, the V.A.C. Therapy healing rate described by Philbeck et al

could potentially provide financial benefit associated with a reduced treatment course and patient benefit related to improved quality of life. In another large retrospective study of patients with chronic Stage III and Stage IV pressure ulcers in the home health environment, Schwien et al[86] found that V.A.C. Therapy reduced the number of visits to hospitals and emergent care facilities secondary to wound complications. These studies demonstrate that V.A.C. Therapy is an economical, useful treatment modality for a variety of chronic wounds, rendered in a variety of care settings.[87] Additional negative pressure therapy options have been offered for developed and underdeveloped countries.[88–92]

Treating Acute Wounds with V.A.C. Therapy

More than 125 articles report clinical and scientific results related to V.A.C. Therapy treatment of acute wounds, including burns, dehisced wounds, and subacute wounds. Table 7 briefly summarizes the findings of selected V.A.C. Therapy RCTs, case series, and retrospective studies in each of the aforementioned acute wound categories. Kamolz et al[93] evaluated 7 patients with bilateral hand burns. One hand of each patient was treated with V.A.C. Therapy. The authors reported that V.A.C. Therapy helped to promote perfusion and reduced edema. Garner et al[94] concluded that V.A.C. Therapy can "safely achieve early fascial closure," based on their experiences using V.A.C. Therapy to treat 14 patients with open abdominal wounds. V.A.C. Therapy also has been used to treat sternal wound infections/mediastinitis. In a retrospective review of 103 patients who were treated with V.A.C. Therapy after median sternotomy, Agarwal et al[95] reported that V.A.C. Therapy was administered for an average period of 11 days per patient. The authors also stated that definitive chest closure with open reduction and internal fixation and/or flap closure was achieved for 70 of 103 patients (68%).

In a large case series of 300 wounds, Argenta and Morykwas[1] reported that 26 of 94 subacute wounds healed completely after treatment with V.A.C. Therapy. The remaining 68 subacute wounds reduced in size and were closed using split-thickness skin grafts, secondary closure, or minor flaps. The authors noted that in 37 patients with exposed orthopedic hardware or bone, V.A.C. Therapy successfully achieved closure of adjacent muscle and the formation of granulation tissue over the bone and hardware. Thus, the mechanisms of action that make V.A.C. Therapy a successful treatment for chronic wounds also enable this integrated wound care system to achieve positive results in the treatment of a variety of acute wounds. Additional trials are necessary to determine the economic benefit of adding NPWT to a surgical treatment regime. Certainly, high-risk patients or procedures with increased likelihood of failing would be optimal candidates.

Treating Wounds with Gauze-Based NPWT

Campbell et al[96] performed a retrospective review of 30 patients treated with NPWT using the gauze-based Chariker-Jeter technique[97] at negative pressure (-80 mmHg) to demonstrate the safety and efficacy of NPWT in a long-term care setting with V1STA, Versatile1, and EZCARE devices (Smith & Nephew). Chronic wounds (n = 11), surgical dehiscence (n = 11), and surgical incisions (n = 8) showed significant reduction in wound volume and area to be able to support discontinuation of NPWT after a median 41 days, with an overall median 88% reduction in wound volume, 68% reduction in area, and a 15.1% weekly overall rate of volume reduction, comparing comparably with foam-based systems. Hurd et al reported 80% pain-free dressing changes and 96% lack of tissue damage with dressing changes in a long-term care facility.[98] Dunn et al validated factors associated with positive and negative outcomes in patients treated with gauze-based NPWT; these outcomes were similar to those noted with foam dressings.[99] Gauze- and foam-based NPWT products appear to produce similar proportions of closed split-thickness skin graft (STSG) wounds according to Fraccalvieri et al; however, the wounds closed with a foam-based (-125 mmHg) system applied on average at 25.9 days as compared to a gauze-based (-80 mmHg) system applied on average at 24.7 days were less pliable with a thicker scar beneath the graft.[100] Dunn et al noted a 96% overall STSG take, increase in granulation tissue to 90% median wound area, and a decrease in non-viable tissue (20%–0%) for wounds treated with gauze-based NPWT (-80 mmHg) for 12 days pre-treatment and 5 days post-treatment.[101] Landsman et al demonstrated the effectiveness of a mechanically powered gauze-based dressing system used to treat diabetic lower extremity wounds.[102] Non-inferiority clinical studies performed by Dorfshar et al demonstrated that gauze-based dressings show similar changes in wound volume and surface area as those observed with foam-based therapies in a clinical inpatient setting.[103] Availability of dressing materials, familiarity with product use, required dressing change intervals, and cost may influence a given practitioner's selection.

Mechanisms of Action for NPWT

A clear understanding of how a therapy works is crucial for making the best use of that treatment. Ongoing research into the mechanisms of action for NPWT continues to clarify the effects that produce the overall wound healing outcome. The combined effects of direct mechanical stress on the cell and alterations in the cell's environment unite to promote a positive wound healing response.

Granulation tissue formation. For healing to occur, the wound defect must fill with granulation tissue. Granulation tissue is composed of new blood vessels, fibroblasts, inflammatory cells, myofibroblasts, endothelial cells, and extracellular matrix. In experiments where V.A.C. Therapy was used to treat porcine surgical wounds, it appeared that V.A.C. Therapy assisted in the formation of granulation tissue.[2] Armstrong and Lavery[68] conducted a large RCT of 162 patients with complex diabetic foot amputation wounds. Their study assessed the time to achieve 76%–100% granulation in patients initially presenting with 0%–10% granulation at baseline. Results from the study indicated that V.A.C. Therapy patients achieved this level of granulation in a mean of 42 days. It is believed that mechanical forces resulting from V.A.C. Therapy and their effect on biochemical processes promote granulation tissue formation.

Mechanical forces. Virtually all aspects of cell physiology may be affected by mechanical stimulation. The cellular response to strain has long been known to result in increased tissue formation. Classic examples are the use of the Ilizarov or distraction osteogenesis technique in hard tissue and tissue expanders in soft tissue.[104,105] With V.A.C. Therapy, externally applied forces may be subdivided into 1) macrostrain and 2) microstrain and microdeformations.[106,107]

Macrostrain. When V.A.C. Therapy is applied, air is evacuated from the dressing via the vacuum, and the tissue is drawn up against the foam. The foam's mechanical properties initially resist the force of the tissue against it, but as the air continues to be evacuated and the tissue force pulling inward exceeds that of the foam pushing outward, the foam compresses, and the wound becomes smaller.

By applying this bulk tissue deformation, or macrostrain, NPWT draws the wound edges together and supports wound healing by decreasing the size of the defect to be filled with granulation tissue.

Microstrain and microdeformations. Microdeformations are caused by negative pressure-induced microstrain of the tissue. The negative pressure draws the tissue surface into the foam pores, promoting cellular stretch and proliferation, which may lead to a decrease in wound size. When the foam-tissue interface is more closely examined, microdeformations can be clearly seen once the vacuum is applied. These microdeformations occur due to microstrains that result in 1) tissue being compressed below the struts and 2) tissue being stretched into the foam pores between the foam struts.

Micromechanical forces have long been known to be responsible for the *induction of cell proliferation and division*.[106,108–110] Other cellular responses to micromechanical forces include gene expression,[111] extracellular matrix (ECM) deposition,[111,112] migration,[113] and differentiation.[108] In general, it is theorized that the cells sense these changes in their local environment through transmembrane signaling proteins known as integrins. The integrins transmit signals to the intracellular molecules, which then transmit the signals to the nucleus, leading to changes in gene transcription.[114,115] The resulting cellular proliferation and ECM production result in decreased wound size.

Saxena et al[106] reported that V.A.C. Therapy and open-celled polyurethane foam produced tissue strains in the average range of 5%–20%. These values are consistent with those shown to result in increased cellular proliferation in bench studies.[109,116] Furthermore, the theoretical models developed by Saxena et al[106] correlated well to actual deformations seen in clinical wounds that had been treated for 4–7 days with V.A.C. Therapy. Greene et al[107] investigated the effect of V.A.C. Therapy-induced microdeformations on capillary formation in chronic wounds. The authors performed an intra-wound comparison of tissue samples with and without exposure to the V.A.C. Therapy. The level of cellular microstrain is believed to be directly related to pore diameter of the interface of the dressing structure, strut thickness, and applied pressure. Wound tissue samples in contact with the GranuFoam Dressing (causing microdeformations) showed increased microvessel density, suggesting improved cellular proliferation and angiogenesis.[107] These changes were attributed to the properties of foam in these early trials specifically designed to investigate foam as an interface material.

Collagen deposition. Provisional matrix models have been generated to evaluate the impact of NPWT on cellular division and migration, extracellular matrix deposition, apoptosis, and angiogenesis.[117] Parameters, such as pressure profile and interface material, show a marked influence on the development of key tissue components, such as collagen deposition, cellular composition, and vascularity *in vitro*.[100,118] The full clinical impact of these findings has yet to be validated *in vivo*, where many other factors influence clinical outcomes and high pressures, or the influence of interface materials may potentially adversely influence tissue quality.[119,120]

Extracellular matrix deposition (hyaluronic acid). Hyaluronic acid makes up approximately 80% of the extracellular matrix (ECM). Increased levels of hyaluronic acid may be a factor in the increased levels of granulation tissue formation shown in studies using V.A.C. Therapy.[68,73] Hyaluronic acid is an important non-sulfonated glycosaminoglycan in the ECM. It is an extremely hygroscopic molecule that provides the tissue with resilience to compressive forces. Hyaluronic acid also may have a protective effect on tissues due to its ability to scavenge free radicals.[121] In tissues biopsied from human mucosal wounds, Oksala et al[122] demonstrated that hyaluronic acid levels rose early before decreasing at Day 7 post wounding. In a porcine full-thickness wound model, granulation tissue was biopsied at Day 9 post wounding and analyzed for hyaluronic acid.[123] High levels of hyaluronic acid were measured in the tissue biopsied after 9 days of V.A.C. Therapy.

Infection management. Bacteria colonize all wounds. Infection occurs when the presence of replicating organisms increases to a high titer level, which then leads to the production and accumulation of bacterial toxins and proteases that impair wound healing. Chronic wound infection is associated with reduced fibroblast presence and improper collagen deposition.[124] It is therefore important to control wound infection to ensure optimal wound healing.

Exudate management. A goal in proper wound bed preparation is to provide exudate management.[125] Extensive evidence exists in the wound healing literature to indicate that the presence of edema in the wound bed can negatively impact wound healing. Removal of excess interstitial fluid by NPWT results in decreased tissue turgor, decreased intercapillary distance, increased lymphatic flow, and improved inflow of nutrients to and removal of waste by-products and proteases from the tissue. The ability of V.A.C. Therapy to favorably impact edema removal has been reported experimentally and clinically in diverse wound types, such as chronic wounds, burns, and acute traumatic wounds.[1,93,126] Caution should be taken to avoid dehydration, coagulopathies, and protein nutritional deficits with excessive exudate removal.

Enhanced perfusion. Adequate perfusion is extremely important to the healing process. Nutrients (including oxygen) that are essential for wound healing are transported to the wound via the blood. Improved perfusion also allows for the removal of cellular waste products, such as carbon dioxide. Initial preclinical studies by Morykwas et al[2] showed that compared to baseline levels, intermittent application of V.A.C. Therapy with the GranuFoam Dressing resulted in more than a 4-fold increase in perfusion. Subsequent studies have confirmed the increase in perfusion associated with V.A.C. Therapy.[127-129]

While the aforementioned studies show the immediate effect of V.A.C. Therapy on perfusion, Kamolz et al[93] showed that increased perfusion also may continue later into the wound healing continuum. It is commonly known that certain burn injuries can progress from partial-thickness to full-thickness burns within a few days of injury and that compromised microcirculation is a contributing factor.[130] In a study of 7 patients with bilateral hand burns, Kamolz et al[93] used video angiography to measure perfusion in the burns. They found that use of V.A.C. Therapy was associated with hyperperfusion and that this may have been a contributing factor to the prevention of burn progression. Five of the 7 V.A.C. Therapy-treated hand wounds healed without skin grafts.

NPWT "filler material" debate. Wound dressing materials are the topic of considerable debate. Yet, one of the most important scientific questions needs to be better addressed: the relevant physics of negative pressure on filler substance and its affect to either augment or diminish pressure distribution throughout the entire tissue plane. In an interdependent fashion, the negative pressure profile and the interface material alter exudate evacuation and tissue microstrain and thereby influence the rate, quantity, and quality of tissue generated. Interface material is not simply "filler material;" it impacts distribution of negative pressure within the wound space, modulates pressure waveforms, and dampens peak pressures delivered to tissue surfaces and extending into surrounding periwound tissue planes. The amount and viscosity of the fluid being evacuated also affects negative pressure delivery, and for some materials, this "fluid effect" is further amplified by variability introduced by the dressing material. Gauze, as compared to open-cell foam, is thought to be more likely to alter the programmed pressure based upon the amount of material used, packing density, method of packing, and interaction between the applied layers. The unique open-cell PU and PVA foams created for the modern NPWT platform were designed to transduce negative pressure to the wound surface with minimal pressure alteration regardless of the exudate quantity or quality, amount of filler material used, layers applied, or orientation of insertion. Foam facilitates delivery of negative pressure profiles in a very "exacting" fashion. The specially designed foams can be easily sized for most wounds and are readily available at a relatively low cost.

On the other hand, gauze is an abundant, inexpensive, and familiar wound dressing material. It can be easily molded around irregular contours and packed into wounds and tunnels and is now readily available in economical, antimicrobial, low-bioadherent, noninflammatory product lines utilized for some NPWT wound types, especially where lower peak pressure and the use of a nonadherent contact layer is required to reduce adherence, in-growth, bleeding, and pain. Many believe gauze has a tendency to "mat and wad" during application and under negative pressure, which may affect fluid evacuation and pressure transduction, especially in larger wounds. In confirmation, Anesäter et al performed a series of studies to examine the effect of material type (foam or gauze) and size (small or large)

on wound contraction and tissue pressure in a porcine full-thickness peripheral wound model under exposure to negative pressure ranges (-20 mmHg to -160 mmHg).[119] NPWT application caused a decrease in tissue pressure at 0.1 cm from the wound margin and an increase at 0.5 cm from the wound margin. Tissue pressure at 0.5 cm was higher with smaller amounts of foam, and smaller amounts of foam also caused significantly more wound contraction. In contrast, gauze created intermediate contraction unrelated to the amount of "filler" material used.

In summary, foam is more likely to deliver programmed pressure profiles, but not all clinical situations require that level of "exactness." Gauze or large amounts of foam generate less contraction, which could be less painful and less likely to cause strain-related bleeding, while small amounts of foam would be most beneficial when maximal wound contraction and granulation tissue development are needed. Researchers are still trying to ferret out the interplay between mechanical pressure modulations and tissue responses.

High versus low NPWT peak pressure debate. Recent studies highlight the existence of *3 zones of perfusion established by NPWT*: 1) the wound bed, 2) the wound margin, and 3) the periwound tissue.[119,128] The current NPWT platform dictates a specific range of microstrain at the wound base and derived its justification based upon measurements of increased blood flow in the periwound tissue and the resulting amount of granulation tissue developed.[1,2] Higher peak negative pressure (-125 mmHg) optimized flow in the periwound tissue and supported a significant increase in granulation tissue development. Lower peak negative pressures (-80 mmHg) generated lower levels of periwound tissue perfusion. Studies showed marginal tissue perfusion increased with increasing negative pressure to a plateau then decreased as additional negative pressure was instituted. Hypoxia (low oxygen content) and ischemia (low perfusion pressure) develop at different levels of pressure for different types of tissue. High levels of negative pressures can lead to hypoxia at the wound margin, and excessive pressures cause ischemic tissue breakdown, apoptosis, and necrosis. Certainly, prolonged hypoxia and ischemia have been associated with tissue necrosis; however, intermittent hypoxia and "mild ischemia" are both recognized stimuli for hypoxia-inducing factor (HIF) and other biomolecules that signal wound healing cascades. It is interesting to note that the "hypoxia and potential ischemia" may be associated with at lower overall pressure at that 0.1 cm tissue plane because the applied energy source is a negative (suction) pressure. At present, there is insufficient information to fully interpret the relative importance of wound base, marginal, and distal blood flow in tissue under the influence of negative pressure forces.

Negative pressure profiles and tissue quality. Studies show that higher levels of peak pressure (-125 mmHg) and intermittent modality have been associated with more granulation tissue developed at a faster rate in full-thickness wounds with adequate vasculature for perfusion and a source for fibroblast cells needed for fibroplasias.[1-3] Multiple factors influence the choice of negative pressure therapy parameters. These may relate to the health of the patient, quality of the tissue being treated, amount of exudate, tissue oxygen and perfusion, and other treatment modalities being used. A practitioner may prefer to use higher negative pressure in a large, well vascularized, highly exudative, post-operative, dehisced hip wound but choose a lower pressure level (-80 mmHg) for a dehisced, infected, abdominal wound with substantial amounts of poorly perfused fat tissue in an elderly patient with diabetes. Hypoxic, ischemic fat tissue may develop necrosis at higher pressure settings. Optimal negative pressure should be high enough to draw the wound margins toward each other without creating adverse tension, deliver sufficient tissue microstrain (5%–20%) to activate cellular division to create the desired amount and quality of collagen-ECM mix deposited, and effectively evacuate inflammatory exudate from the wound space to "perfect" the wound environment.

In an effort to adopt evidence-influenced practice models, some practitioners have utilized bedside diagnostics for perfusion (hand-held Doppler) and oxygenation (transcutaneous oxygen, TCPO2) along with patient comfort levels to guide treatment pressure profiles. While Doppler and TCPO2 assessments are not practical for commonplace application today, newer technology may assist with bedside perfusion and oxygenation verification to inform treatment choices

in the future. Additional diagnostics are being developed and marketed to test wound environment matrix metalloproteinases and other inflammatory mediators. Nonetheless, up to this point, there has been a well established **medical practice of reducing the peak negative pressure and slowing the rate of draw down to reduce pain, bleeding, and other potential complications**. Those choices are made at the presumed potential loss of comparative granulation tissue generated. More information is needed to establish how those choices impact the actual rate and quality of tissue generated.

More scientific-focused research is required. Clearly, wound surface microstrain directly influences cellular proliferation, apoptosis, extracellular matrix deposition, and inflammatory mediator profiles; however, the relative importance of that influence to impact final clinical outcomes has yet to be fully delineated. Negative pressure profile may be manipulated to deliver different levels of strain by modulating peak pressure, pressure waveforms, pressure modality (continuous or intermittent), duration and frequency of application, and selection of different interfaces for transduction. Additionally, a host of non-pressure-related factors influences final clinical wound healing outcomes[125] (Table 8). Several key areas need further investigation and definition: 1) interplay between mechanical stress and inflammatory mediator reduction alters the cell's biomolecular profile either directly (microstrain) or indirectly through environmental changes (exudate evacuation) and their effects are interdependent; 2) pressure profile alterations related to dressing materials in the wound space; 3) tissue growth response (fibroplasias, angiogenesis, and collagen-ECM deposition) resulting from varied pressure profiles applied at different times throughout the human wound healing cycle; 4) tissue growth response in relation to varied pressure profiles depending upon initial tissue type (fat, muscle, tendon/ligament, bone); and 5) tissue growth response where various soluble additives are provided (ie, antimicrobials, nutrients, oxygen, nitric oxide, growth factors, cytokines, collagen, ECM, and cells). A great amount of additional research is warranted. In lieu of the current insufficient level of "evidential clarity" and minimal number of comparative clinical trials, it would be premature to designate a "best" dressing or "best"

Table 8. Factors impacting wound healing

NPWT Device-Related Factors

- Interface materials to distribute pressure and interact with the underlying tissues
- Presence or absence of an intervening nonadherent layer
- Pressure profile
  - Peak negative pressure (maximum)
  - Pressure modality — continuous versus intermittent
  - Pressure wave forms — rapidity of pressure onset ("draw down")
  - Treatment regimes — application frequency and overall duration

Wound-Specific Factors

- Etiology of tissue injury (eg, incision, contusion, blast, thermal, pressure, moisture)
- Location, size, shape, depth
- Exposed vital structures (eg, bone, blood vessels, tendons)
- Tissue nutritional state
- Local vascular status and perfusion
- Local tissue inflammatory status
- Infectious status (local, systemic, biofilm, abscess, suppuration)
- Existing cells, extracellular matrix (ECM), and structural support tissues
- Local oxygenation and tissue energy
- Tissue fluid — edema, drainage, exudate
- Temperature, moisture, and pH

General Health-Related Factors

- Overall physical health and emotional status
  - Medical diseases and disorders
  - Medications, prescribed, over-the-counter, herbals, homeopathic
  - Psychiatric and emotional health
- Socio-economic status and ability to access appropriate care

Recommended Treatments and Interventions

- Debridement — selective and non-selective
- Antibiotic, antimicrobial, anti-inflammatory agents
- Offloading therapy and the ability to mitigate future recurrent trauma
- Compression and manual massage therapy — continuous and intermittent pneumatic
- Oxygenation and perfusion support
- Nutritional supplementation
- Temperature and moisture management
- Case management
- Physical therapeutics
- Tissue-based therapy components (eg, growth factors, cytokines, collagen, hyaluronic acid, cells)
- Exogenous energy provision — electric, electromagnetic, infrared, ultrasound, or vibratory

pressure. In all likelihood, it will not be one "best" for all clinical situations.

Conclusion

NPWT has widespread clinical acceptance. A substantial body of evidence reports its clinical utility in the treatment of chronic and acute wounds. NPWT is intended to create an environment that promotes wound healing by secondary or tertiary (delayed primary) intention by preparing the wound bed for closure, reducing edema, promoting granulation tissue formation and perfusion, and removing exudate and infectious material. It is indicated for patients with chronic, acute, traumatic, subacute, and dehisced wounds; partial-thickness burns; ulcers (such as diabetic or pressure); flaps; and grafts. NPWT design innovations have accelerated provider adoption and improved patient compliance, care setting appropriateness, and realized healthcare system cost reductions. Ease of use coupled with positive clinical healing outcomes fueled a rapid, widespread adoption and penetration of NPWT across the spectrum of surgical and non-surgical medical specialties. Modification toward improved lightweight portable to ultra-portability compact modeling, visible and audible alarms, wound site pressure monitoring feedback, and flight certification approval facilitated NPWT expansion across inpatient, out-of-hospital, ambulatory care, disaster preparedness, and military transport care settings. Improved healing times, pain reduction, and fewer restrictions to mobility with potentially fewer interruptions in patient work schedules encourage positive patient adherence and adoption. Focused awareness of potential risks and complications with structured mitigation strategies should support continued positive safety standing. Further research into clinical efficacy, health outcomes, cost effectiveness, and mechanisms of action will assist in defining future NPWT utilization.

Take-Home Messages for Practice

- NPWT is a proven, clinically effective, and safe process that promotes healing for acute and chronic wounds.
- NPWT provides a mechanical strain that alters cellular proliferation, extracellular matrix deposition, and local perfusion; additionally, the removal of exudate facilitates the reduction of inhibitory mediators.
- Mechanical strain and inflammatory exudate removal act interdependently to positively impact wound tissue healing response.
- The type of material at the interface is not as important as the modification of NPWT pressure profiles and tissue growth responses.
- Adding nonadherent intervening contact dressings at the tissue-material interface helps mitigate complications.

Self-Assessment Questions

1. Which of the following is not an indication for use of NPWT?
   A. Chronic wounds and ulcers (such as diabetic or pressure)
   B. Acute, traumatic, subacute, and dehisced wounds
   C. Full-thickness burns
   D. Flaps and grafts

2. Peak pressure may alter which of the following?
   A. Cellular proliferation
   B. Collagen deposition
   C. Local arterial blood flow
   D. All of the above

3. Which of the following mechanisms of action relate to NPWT?
   A. Promoting edema
   B. Inhibiting granulation tissue formation and perfusion
   C. Wound space expansion
   D. Decreasing exudate and infectious material

4. What dressing has the best likelihood of reducing NPWT-related pain?
   A. Gauze
   B. Foam
   C. Bio-Dome
   D. Intervening nonadherent contact layer

Answers: 1-C, 2-D, 3-D, 4-D

References

1. Argenta LC, Morykwas MJ. Vacuum-assisted closure: a new method for wound control and treatment: clinical experience. *Ann Plast Surg*. 1997;38(6):563–576.

2. Morykwas MJ, Argenta LC, Shelton-Brown EI, McGuirt W. Vacuum-assisted closure: a new method for wound control and treatment: animal studies and basic foundation. *Ann Plast Surg*. 1997;38(6):553–562.

3. Morykwas MJ, Simpson J, Punger K, Argenta A, Kremers L, Argenta J. Vacuum-assisted closure: state of basic research and physiologic foundation. *Plast Reconstr Surg*. 2006;117(7 Suppl):121S–126S.

4. Sullivan N, Snyder DL, Tipton K, Uhl S, Schoelles KM. Negative Pressure Wound Therapy Devices. Technology Assessment Report. Available at: http://www.ahrq.gov/clinic/ta/negpresswtd/negpresswtd.pdf. Accessed February 1, 2012.

5. Genadyne Biotechnologies. XLR8® Negative Pressure Wound Therapy. Available at: http://www.genadyne.com/productoverview.php?category=wound_therapy. Accessed January 29, 2012.

6. US Department of Health and Human Services, Food and Drug Administration, Center for Devices and Radiological Health. Guidance for Industry and FDA Staff: Class II Special Controls Guidance Document: Non-powered Suction Apparatus Device Intended for

Negative Pressure Wound Therapy (NPWT). Available at: http://www.fda.gov/downloads/MedicalDevices/DeviceRegulationandGuidance/GuidanceDocuments/UCM233279.pdf. Accessed February 1, 2012.

7. Fong KD, Hu D, Eichstadt S, et al. The SNaP system: biomechanical and animal model testing of a novel ultra-portable negative-pressure wound therapy system. *Plast Reconstr Surg*. 2010;125(5):1362–1371.

8. Spiracur Inc. SNaP® Brochure. Available at: http://spiracur.com/for-clinicians/trainingifu/. Accessed January 29, 2012.

9. Kalypto Medical. Guidelines for Use of the NPD 1000™ Negative Pressure Wound Therapy System from Kalypto Medical®. Available at: http://www.kalyptomedical.com/clinical.php. Accessed January 29, 2012.

10. V.A.C. Via™ Negative Pressure Wound Therapy System [instructions for use]. San Antonio, TX: KCI USA, Inc; 2010.

11. Genadyne Biotechnologies. A4-NPWT. Available at: http://www.genadyne.com/productoverview.php?category=wound_therapy. Accessed January 29, 2012.

12. PICO™ Single Use Negative Pressure Wound Therapy System [instructions for use]. St-Laurent, Quebec, Canada: Smith & Nephew, Inc; 2011.

13. Vario [instructions for use]. McHenry, IL: Medela Inc; 2011.

14. Prevena™ Incision Management System [instructions for use]. San Antonio, TX: KCI USA, Inc; 2010.

15. SensaT.R.A.C.™ Technology [information sheet]. San Antonio, TX: KCI USA, Inc; 2009.

16. Miller MS, Ortegon M, McDaniel C. Negative pressure wound therapy: treating a venomous insect bite. *Int Wound J*. 2007;4(1):88–92.

17. Kasukurthi R, Borschel GH. Simplified negative pressure wound therapy in pediatric hand wounds. *Hand (N Y)*. 2009 Jun 27. [Epub ahead of print]

18. US Food and Drug Administration. FDA Safety Communication: UPDATE on Serious Complications Associated with Negative Pressure Wound Therapy Systems. Available at: http://www.fda.gov/MedicalDevices/Safety/AlertsandNotices/ucm244211.htm. Accessed August 26, 2011.

19. Schiestl C, Neuhaus K, Biedermann T, Böttcher-Haberzeth S, Reichmann E, Meuli M. Novel treatment for massive lower extremity avulsion injuries in children: slow, but effective with good cosmesis. *Eur J Pediatr Surg*. 2011;21(2):106–110.

20. Baharestani M, Amjad I, Bookout K, et al. V.A.C. Therapy in the management of paediatric wounds: clinical review and experience. *Int Wound J*. 2009;6 Suppl 1:1–26.

21. Halvorson J, Jinnah R, Kulp B, Frino J. Use of vacuum-assisted closure in pediatric open fractures with a focus on the rate of infection. *Orthopedics*. 2011;34(7):e256–e260.

22. 3M Health Care. The expanding family of Tegaderm™ Brand Dressings [brochure]. St Paul, MN: 3M Health Care; 2005.

23. Rock R. Get positive results with negative-pressure wound therapy. *American Nurse Today*. 2011;6(1):49–51.

24. Giovinco NA, Bui TD, Fisher T, Mills JL, Armstrong DG.

Wound chemotherapy by the use of negative pressure wound therapy and infusion. *Eplasty*. 2010 Jan 8;10:e9.

25. Shah CB, Swogger E, James G. Efficacy of AMD™ dressings against MRSA and VRE [white paper]. Montana State University, Bozeman, MT. Mansfield, MA: Covidien (formerly Tyco Healthcare Group LP). September 2008.

26. Rodriguez A, To D, Hansen A, Ajifu C, Carson S, Travis E. Silver dressings used with wound vacuum assisted closure: is there an advantage? Available at: http://www.silverlon.com/studies/dressing_vac_closure.pdf. Accessed August 28, 2011.

27. Krieger BR, Davis DM, Sanchez JE, et al. The use of silver nylon in preventing surgical site infections following colon and rectal surgery. *Dis Colon Rectum*. 2011;54(8):1014–1019.

28. Deitch EA, Marino AA, Gillespie TE, Albright JA. Silver-nylon: a new antimicrobial agent. *Antimicrob Agents Chemother*. 1983;23(3):356–359.

29. Penny HL, Dyson M, Spinazzola J, Green A, Faretta M, Meloy G. The use of negative-pressure wound therapy with bio-dome dressing technology in the treatment of complex diabetic wounds. *Adv Skin Wound Care*. 2010;23(7):305–312.

30. Hydrofera Blue® [instructions for use]. Willimantic, CT: Hydrofera, LLC.

31. Kinetic Concepts Inc. V.A.C.® Therapy™ Clinical Guidelines: A Reference Source for Clinicians. San Antonio, TX: Kinetic Concepts Inc; 2005.

32. Kinetic Concepts Inc. KCI 2006 Product Source Guide. San Antonio, TX: Kinetic Concepts Inc; 2006.

33. Ambrosio A, Barton K, Ginther D. V.A.C. GranuFoam Silver Dressing. A new antimicrobial silver foam dressing specifically engineered for use with V.A.C. Therapy [white paper]. San Antonio, TX: KCI Licensing, Inc; 2006.

34. Payne JL, Ambrosio AM. Evaluation of an antimicrobial silver foam dressing for use with V.A.C. therapy: morphological, mechanical, and antimicrobial properties. *J Biomed Mater Res B Appl Biomater*. 2009;89(1):217–222.

35. Peterson DJ, Hermann K, Niezgoda JA. Effectively managing infected wounds with Hydrofera Blue™ and negative pressure wound therapy. Available at: http://www.hydrofera.com/documents/product_literature/hydrofera_blue/hydrofera_blue_NPWT.pdf. Accessed February 2, 2012.

36. Niezgoda JA. Combining negative pressure wound therapy with other wound management modalities. *Ostomy Wound Manage*. 2005;51(2A Suppl):36S–38S.

37. Malmsjö M, Ingemansson R. Effects of green foam, black foam and gauze on contraction, blood flow and pressure delivery to the wound bed in negative pressure wound therapy. *J Plast Reconstr Aesthet Surg*. 2011;64(12):e289–e296.

38. Malmsjö M, Ingemansson R. Green foam, black foam or gauze for NWPT: effects on granulation tissue formation. *J Wound Care*. 2011;20(6):294–299.

39. Bondjoki S, Reuter C, Rangaswamy M, et al. Clinical efficacy of an alternative foam-based negative pressure wound therapy system. Presented at the Symposium on Advanced Wound Care in Anaheim, CA, September

23–25, 2010.

40. Teder H, Sandén G, Svedman P. Continuous wound irrigation in the pig. *J Invest Surg.* 1990;3(4):399–407.

41. Gray D, Barrett S, Battacharyya M, et al. PHMB and its potential contribution to wound management. *Wounds UK.* 2010;6(2):40–46.

42. Gilliver S. PHMB: a well-tolerated antiseptic with no reported toxic effects. *J Wound Care*/Activa Healthcare Supplement. 2009:S9–S14.

43. Prospera® Negative Pressure Wound Therapy [brochure]. Fort Worth, TX: Prospera; 2008.

44. V1STA Negative Pressure Wound Therapy [quick reference guide]. Largo, FL: Smith & Nephew; 2007.

45. EZCARE Negative Pressure Wound Therapy [quick reference guide]. Largo, FL: Smith & Nephew; 2007.

46. Talley Medical. VENTURI™ Negative Pressure Wound Therapy Clinical Guidelines Manual. Romsey, Hampshire, England: Talley Group Limited; 2009.

47. Hirsch T, Limoochi-Deli S, Lahmer A, et al. Antimicrobial activity of clinically used antiseptics and wound irrigating agents in combination with wound dressings. *Plast Reconstr Surg.* 2011;127(4):1539–1545.

48. Girolami S, Sadowski-Liest D. Bio-Dome™ technology: the newest approach to negative pressure wound therapy. Presented at the Symposium on Advanced Wound Care & Wound Healing Society Meeting in Tampa, FL, April 28–May 1, 2007.

49. Hill L, McCormick J, Tamburino J, et al. The effectiveness of engenex™: a new NPWT device. Presented at the Symposium on Advanced Wound Care & Wound Healing Society Meeting in Tampa, FL, April 28–May 1, 2007.

50. Mitra A, Weyrauch B, Bentley L. Engenex™ and Foundation Based Healing™ [white paper]. Available at: http://www.boehringerwound.com/Engenex%20and%20Foundation%20based%20Healing.pdf. Accessed February 2, 2012.

51. Davis SC, Perez R, Gil J, Valdes J. A pilot study to determine the effects of a negative pressure device on full thickness wounds inoculated with *Pseudomonas aeruginosa* [white paper]. Available at: http://www.kalyptomedical.com/clinical.php. Accessed February 2, 2012.

52. Page J, Woodruff D. The performance of a negative pressure device on chronic wounds of the lower leg and foot. A pilot study [white paper]. Available at: http://kalyptomedical.com/clinical.php. Accessed June 6, 2011.

53. Timoney MF, Zenilman ME. How we manage abdominal compartment syndrome. Available at: http://www.contemporarysurgery.com/pdf/6410/6410CS_REVIEW.pdf. Accessed March 5, 2012.

54. Kinetic Concepts Inc. Instructions for Use: V.A.C.® Therapy Safety Information (for V.A.C.® GranuFoam®, V.A.C.® GranuFoam® Silver™ and V.A.C.® WhiteFoam™ Dressings). San Antonio, TX: Kinetic Concepts Inc; 2006.

55. Venturi ML, Attinger CE, Mesbahi AN, Hess CL, Graw KS. Mechanisms and clinical applications of the vacuum-assisted closure (VAC) device: a review. *Am J Clin Dermatol.* 2005;6(3):185–194.

56. Kaufman MW, Pahl DW. Vacuum-assisted closure therapy: wound care and nursing implications. *Dermatol Nurs.* 2003;15(4):317–326.

57. Short B, Claxton M, Armstrong DG. How to use VAC therapy on chronic wounds. *Podiatry Today.* 2002;15(7):48–54.

58. Andros G, Armstrong DG, Attinger CE, et al. Consensus statement on negative pressure wound therapy (V.A.C. Therapy) for the management of diabetic foot wounds. *Ostomy Wound Manage.* 2006;52(6 Suppl):1–32.

59. Gupta S, Baharestani M, Baranoski S, et al. Guidelines for managing pressure ulcers with negative pressure wound therapy. *Adv Skin Wound Care.* 2004;17(Suppl 2):1–16.

60. Niezgoda JA, Mendez-Eastman S. The effective management of pressure ulcers. *Adv Skin Wound Care.* 2006;19(Suppl 1):3–15.

61. Kaplan M, Banwell P, Orgill DP, et al. Guidelines for the management of the open abdomen. *WOUNDS.* 2005;17(Suppl 1):S1–S24.

62. Orgill DP, Austen WG, Butler CE, et al. Guidelines for treatment of complex chest wounds with negative pressure wound therapy. *WOUNDS.* 2004;16(Suppl B):1–23.

63. Hardwicke J, Paterson P. A role for vacuum-assisted closure in lower limb trauma: a proposed algorithm. *Int J Low Extrem Wounds.* 2006;5(2):101–104.

64. Runkel N, Krug E, Berg L, et al; International Expert Panel on Negative Pressure Wound Therapy (NPWT-EP). Evidence-based recommendations for the use of Negative Pressure Wound Therapy in traumatic wounds and reconstructive surgery: steps towards an international consensus. *Injury.* 2011;42 Suppl 1:S1–S12.

65. Birke-Sorensen H, Malmsjo M, Rome P, et al; International Expert Panel on Negative Pressure Wound Therapy (NPWT-EP). Evidence-based recommendations for negative pressure wound therapy: treatment variables (pressure levels, wound filler and contact layer) -- steps towards an international consensus. *J Plast Reconstr Aesthet Surg.* 2011;64 Suppl:S1–S16.

66. McCallon SK, Knight CA, Valiulus JP, Cunningham MW, McCulloch JM, Farinas LP. Vacuum-assisted closure versus saline-moistened gauze in the healing of postoperative diabetic foot wounds. *Ostomy Wound Manage.* 2000;46(8):28–34.

67. Eginton MT, Brown KR, Seabrook GR, Towne JB, Cambria RA. A prospective randomized evaluation of negative-pressure wound dressings for diabetic foot wounds. *Ann Vasc Surg.* 2003;17(6):645–649.

68. Armstrong DG, Lavery LA; Diabetic Foot Study Consortium. Negative pressure wound therapy after partial diabetic foot amputation: a multicentre, randomised controlled trial. *Lancet.* 2005;366(9498):1704–1710.

69. Page JC, Newswander B, Schwenke DC, Hansen M, Ferguson J. Retrospective analysis of negative pressure wound therapy in open foot wounds with significant soft tissue defects. *Adv Skin Wound Care.* 2004;17(7):354–364.

70. Frykberg RG, Williams DV. Negative-pressure wound therapy and diabetic foot amputations: a retrospective study of payer claims data. *J Am Podiatr Med Assoc.* 2007;97(5):351–359.

71. Blume PA, Walters J, Payne W, Ayala J, Lantis J. Comparison of negative pressure wound therapy using vacuum-assisted closure with advanced moist wound therapy in the treatment of diabetic foot ulcers: a multicenter randomized controlled trial. *Diabetes Care.* 2008;31(4):631–636.

72. Ford CN, Reinhard ER, Yeh D, et al. Interim analysis of a prospective, randomized trial of vacuum-assisted closure versus the Healthpoint system in the management of pressure ulcers. *Ann Plast Surg.* 2002;49(1):55–61.

73. Joseph E, Hamori CA, Bergman S, Roaf E, Swann NF, Anastasi GW. A prospective, randomized trial of vacuum-assisted closure versus standard therapy of chronic non-healing wounds. *WOUNDS.* 2000;12(3):60–67.

74. Wanner MB, Schwarzl F, Strub B, Zaech GA, Pierer G. Vacuum-assisted wound closure for cheaper and more comfortable healing of pressure sores: a prospective study. *Scand J Plast Reconstr Surg Hand Surg.* 2003;37(1):28–33.

75. Philbeck TE Jr, Whittington KT, Millsap MH, Briones RB, Wight DG, Schroeder WJ. The clinical and cost effectiveness of externally applied negative pressure wound therapy in the treatment of wounds in home healthcare Medicare patients. *Ostomy Wound Manage.* 1999;45(11):41–50.

76. Vuerstaek JD, Vainas T, Wuite J, Nelemans P, Neumann MH, Veraart JC. State-of-the-art treatment of chronic leg ulcers: a randomized controlled trial comparing vacuum-assisted closure (V.A.C.) with modern wound dressings. *J Vasc Surg.* 2006;44(5):1029–1038.

77. Braakenburg A, Obdeijn MC, Feitz R, van Rooij IA, van Griethuysen AJ, Klinkenbijl JH. The clinical efficacy and cost effectiveness of the vacuum-assisted closure technique in the management of acute and chronic wounds: a randomized controlled trial. *Plast Reconstr Surg.* 2006;118(2):390–397.

78. Moues CM, Vos MC, van den Bemd GJ, Stijnen T, Hovius SE. Bacterial load in relation to vacuum-assisted closure wound therapy: a prospective randomized trial. *Wound Repair Regen.* 2004;12(1):11–17.

79. Moisidis E, Heath T, Boorer C, Ho K, Deva AK. A prospective, blinded, randomized, controlled clinical trial of topical negative pressure use in skin grafting. *Plast Reconstr Surg.* 2004;114(4):917–922.

80. Jeschke MG, Rose C, Angele P, Füchtmeier B, Nerlich MN, Bolder U. Development of new reconstructive techniques: use of Integra in combination with fibrin glue and negative-pressure therapy for reconstruction of acute and chronic wounds. *Plast Reconstr Surg.* 2004;113(2):525–530.

81. Genecov DG, Schneider AM, Morykwas MJ, Parker D, White WL, Argenta LC. A controlled subatmospheric pressure dressing increases the rate of skin graft donor site reepithelialization. *Ann Plast Surg.* 1998;40(3):219–225.

82. Carson SN, Overall K, Lee-Jahshan S, Travis E. Vacuum-assisted closure used for healing chronic wounds and skin grafts in the lower extremities. *Ostomy Wound Manage.* 2004;50(3):52–58.

83. Stannard JP, Volgas DA, McGwin G 3rd, et al. Incisional negative pressure wound therapy after high-risk lower extremity fractures. *J Orthop Trauma.* 2012;26(1):37–42.

84. Kilpadi DV, Cunningham MR. Evaluation of closed incision management with negative pressure wound therapy (CIM): hematoma/seroma and involvement of the lymphatic system. *Wound Repair Regen.* 2011;19(5):588–596.

85. Ferrell BA, Osterweil D, Christenson P. A randomized trial of low-air-loss beds for treatment of pressure ulcers. *JAMA.* 1993;269(4):494–497.

86. Schwien T, Gilbert J, Lang C. Pressure ulcer prevalence and the role of negative pressure wound therapy in home health quality outcomes. *Ostomy Wound Manage.* 2005;51(9):47–60.

87. de Leon JM, Barnes S, Nagel M, Fudge M, Lucius A, Garcia B. Cost-effectiveness of negative pressure wound therapy for postsurgical patients in long-term acute care. *Adv Skin Wound Care.* 2009;22(3):122–127.

88. Perez D, Bramkamp M, Exe C, von Ruden C, Ziegler A. Modern wound care for the poor: a randomized clinical trial comparing the vacuum system with conventional saline-soaked gauze dressings. *Am J Surg.* 2010;199(1):14–20.

89. Lerman B, Oldenbrook L, Eichstadt SL, Ryu J, Fong KD, Schubart PJ. Evaluation of chronic wound treatment with the SNaP wound care system versus modern dressing protocols. *Plast Reconstr Surg.* 2010;126(4):1253–1261.

90. Armstrong DG, Marston WA, Reyzelman AM, Kirsner RS. Comparison of negative pressure wound therapy with an ultraportable mechanically powered device vs. traditional electrically powered device for the treatment of chronic lower extremity ulcers: a multicenter randomized-controlled trial. *Wound Repair Regen.* 2011;19(2):173–180.

91. Hutton DW, Sheehan P. Comparative effectiveness of the SNaP™ Wound Care System. *Int Wound J.* 2011;8(2):196–205.

92. Campbell AM, Kuhn WP, Barker P. Vacuum-assisted closure of the open abdomen in a resource-limited setting. *S Afr J Surg.* 2010;48(4):114–115.

93. Kamolz LP, Andel H, Haslik W, Winter W, Meissl G, Frey M. Use of subatmospheric pressure therapy to prevent burn wound progression in human: first experiences. *Burns.* 2004;30(3):253–258.

94. Garner GB, Ware DN, Cocanour CS, et al. Vacuum-assisted wound closure provides early fascial reapproximation in trauma patients with open abdomens. *Am J Surg.* 2001;182(6):630–638.

95. Agarwal JP, Ogilvie M, Wu LC, et al. Vacuum-assisted closure for sternal wounds: a first-line therapeutic management approach. *Plast Reconstr Surg.* 2005;116(4):1035–1043.

96. Campbell PE, Smith GS, Smith JM. Retrospective clinical evaluation of gauze-based negative pressure wound therapy. *Int Wound J.* 2008;5(2):280–286.

97. Chariker ME, Jeter KF, Tintle TE, Bottsford JE. Effective management of incisional and cutaneous fistulae with closed suction wound drainage. *Contemporary Surgery.* 1989;34:59–63.

98. Hurd T, Chadwick P, Cote J, Cockwill J, Mole TR, Smith JM. Impact of gauze-based NPWT on the patient and nursing experience in the treatment of challenging wounds. *Int Wound J.* 2010;7(6):448–455.

99. Dunn R, Hurd T, Chadwick P, et al. Factors associated with positive outcomes in 131 patients treated with gauze-based negative pressure wound therapy. *Int J Surg.* 2011;9(3):258–262.

100. Fraccalvieri M, Zingarelli E, Ruka E, et al. Negative pressure wound therapy using gauze and foam: histological, immunohistochemical and ultrasonography morpho-

logical analysis of the granulation tissue and scar tissue. Preliminary report of a clinical study. *Int Wound J.* 2011;8(4):355–364.

101. Dunn RM, Ignotz R, Mole T, Cockwill J, Smith JM. Assessment of gauze-based negative pressure wound therapy in the split-thickness skin graft clinical pathway-an observational study. *Eplasty.* 2011;11:e14.

102. Landsman A. Analysis of the SNaP Wound Care System, a negative pressure wound device for treatment of diabetic lower extremity wounds. *J Diabetes Sci Technol.* 2010;4(4):831–832.

103. Dorafshar AH, Franczyk M, Gottlieb LJ, Wroblewski KE, Lohman RF. A prospective randomized trial comparing subatmospheric wound therapy with a sealed gauze dressing and the standard vacuum-assisted closure device. *Ann Plast Surg.* 2011 Jun 27. [Epub ahead of print]

104. Ilizarov GA. The tension-stress effect on the genesis and growth of tissues. Part I. The influence of stability of fixation and soft-tissue preservation. *Clin Orthop Relat Res.* 1989;(238):249–281.

105. Ilizarov GA. The tension-stress effect on the genesis and growth of tissues: Part II. The influence of the rate and frequency of distraction. *Clin Orthop Relat Res.* 1989;(239):263–285.

106. Saxena V, Hwang CW, Huang S, Eichbaum Q, Ingber D, Orgill DP. Vacuum-assisted closure: microdeformations of wounds and cell proliferation. *Plast Reconstr Surg.* 2004;114(5):1086–1098.

107. Greene AK, Puder M, Roy R, et al. Microdeformational wound therapy: effects on angiogenesis and matrix metalloproteinases in chronic wounds of 3 debilitated patients. *Ann Plast Surg.* 2006;56(4):418–422.

108. Danciu TE, Gagari E, Adam RM, Damoulis PD, Freeman MR. Mechanical strain delivers anti-apoptotic and proliferative signals to gingival fibroblasts. *J Dent Res.* 2004;83(8):596–601.

109. Huang S, Ingber DE. Shape-dependent control of cell growth, differentiation, and apoptosis: switching between attractors in cell regulatory networks. *Exp Cell Res.* 2000;261(1):91–103.

110. Ikeda M, Takei T, Mills I, Kito H, Sumpio BE. Extracellular signal-regulated kinases 1 and 2 activation in endothelial cells exposed to cyclic strain. *Am J Physiol.* 1999;276(2 Pt 2):H614–H622.

111. Chiquet M, Renedo AS, Huber F, Flück M. How do fibroblasts translate mechanical signals into changes in extracellular matrix production? *Matrix Biol.* 2000;22(1):73–80.

112. MacKenna D, Summerour SR, Villarreal FJ. Role of mechanical factors in modulating cardiac fibroblast function and extracellular matrix synthesis. *Cardiovasc Res.* 2000;46(2):257–263.

113. Katsumi A, Naoe T, Matsushita T, Kaibuchi K, Schwartz MA. Integrin activation and matrix binding mediate cellular responses to mechanical stretch. *J Biol Chem.* 2005;280(17):16546–16549.

114. Shyy JY, Chien S. Role of integrins in cellular responses to mechanical stress and adhesion. *Curr Opin Cell Biol.* 1997;9(5):707–713.

115. Wang N, Naruse K, Stamenovic D, et al. Mechanical behavior in living cells consistent with the tensegrity model. *Proc Natl Acad Sci U S A.* 2001;98(14):7765–7770.

116. Chen CS, Mrksich M, Huang S, Whitesides GM, Ingber DE. Geometric control of cell life and death. *Science.* 1997;276(5317):1425–1428.

117. McNulty AK, Schmidt M, Feeley T, Kieswetter K. Effects of negative pressure wound therapy on fibroblast viability, chemotactic signaling, and proliferation in a provisional wound (fibrin) matrix. *Wound Repair Regen.* 2007;15(6):838–846.

118. Wilkes R, Zhao Y, Kieswetter K, Haridas B. Effects of dressing type on 3D tissue microdeformations during negative pressure wound therapy: a computational study. *J Biomech Eng.* 2009;131(3):031012.

119. Anesäter E, Borgquist O, Hedström E, Waga J, Ingemansson R, Malmsjö M. The influence of different sizes and types of wound fillers on wound contraction and tissue pressure during negative pressure wound therapy. *Int Wound J.* 2011;8(4):336–342.

120. Goutos I, Ghosh SJ. Gauze-based negative pressure wound therapy as an adjunct to collagen-elastin [corrected] dermal template resurfacing. *J Wound Care.* 2011;20(2):55–56,58,60.

121. Chen WY, Abatangelo G. Functions of hyaluronan in wound repair. *Wound Repair Regen.* 1999;7(2):79–89.

122. Oksala O, Salo T, Tammi R, et al. Expression of proteoglycans and hyaluronan during wound healing. *J Histochem Cytochem.* 1995;43(2):125–135.

123. McNulty AK, Feeley T, Schmidt M, Norbury K, Kieswetter K. Glycosaminoglycan composition of granulation tissue from wounds treated with negative pressure wound therapy or moist wound therapy. Presented at the Symposium on Advanced Wound Care in San Antonio, TX, April 30–May 3, 2006.

124. Bucknall TE. The effect of local infection upon wound healing: an experimental study. *Br J Surg.* 1980;67(12):851–855.

125. Schultz GS, Sibbald RG, Falanga V, et al. Wound bed preparation: a systematic approach to wound management. *Wound Repair Regen.* 2003;11(Suppl 1):S1–S28.

126. DeFranzo AJ, Argenta LC, Marks MW, et al. The use of vacuum-assisted closure therapy for the treatment of lower-extremity wounds with exposed bone. *Plast Reconstr Surg.* 2001;108(5):1184–1191.

127. Timmers MS, Le Cessie S, Banwell P, Jukema GN. The effects of varying degrees of pressure delivered by negative-pressure wound therapy on skin perfusion. *Ann Plast Surg.* 2005;55(6):665–671.

128. Wackenfors A, Sjögren J, Gustafsson R, Algotsson L, Ingemansson R, Malmsjö M. Effects of vacuum-assisted closure therapy on inguinal wound edge microvascular blood flow. *Wound Repair Regen.* 2004;12(6):600–606.

129. Wackenfors A, Gustafsson R, Sjögren J, Algotsson L, Ingemansson R, Malmsjö M. Blood flow responses in the peristernal thoracic wall during vacuum-assisted closure therapy. *Ann Thorac Surg.* 2005;79(5):1724–1731.

130. Zawacki BE. The natural history of reversible burn injury. *Surg Gynecol Obstet.* 1974;139(6):867–872.

CHAPTER 17

Risk Assessment in
Pressure Ulcer Prevention

Barbara J. Braden, PhD, FAAN;
Shirley Blanchard, PhD, ABDA, OTR/L, FAOTA

Objectives

The reader will be challenged to:

- Envision the appropriate use of risk assessment tools in a program of prevention of pressure ulcers
- Analyze interventions to reduce the intensity and duration of pressure in both bedfast and chairfast patients
- Propose a plan for evaluating a program of prevention of pressure ulcers
- Conceptualize occupational therapys contribution to the prevention of pressure ulcers.

Introduction

In recent years, a consensus has developed that the incidence of pressure ulcers in a facility or agency is an important indicator of quality of care. Unfortunately, as nurses and other healthcare professionals adjust to the increasing acuity of patients being cared for in every setting, they are suffering a sort of sensory overload. As more problems compete for their attention and less time is available to analyze the implications of all the data they collect, certain basic assessments and interventions are sometimes overlooked.

Pressure ulcer risk assessment and prevention seems to have been among these overlooked problems.[1,2] There is also evidence that a program of prevention guided by risk assessment can simultaneously reduce the institutional incidence of pressure ulcers by as much as 60% while reducing the costs of prevention.[3] *One way to assure optimal risk assessment and effective prevention is through collaboration with multiple disciplines.* The 2 disciplines most often involved in risk assessment and prevention are nursing and occupational therapy, but this collaboration has been minimally addressed in the literature. While nurses are primarily responsible for risk assessment, occupational therapists offer unique skills in the identification of special risks related to seating surfaces, instruction in pressure relief, and prescription of positioning devices and wheelchair seating. This chapter will pay significant attention to the contributions of both nursing and occupational therapy to effective prevention.

Braden BJ, Blanchard S. Risk assessment in pressure ulcer prevention. In: Krasner DL, ed. *Chronic Wound Care: The Essentials*. Malvern, Pa: HMP Communications, 2014:225–242.

Table 1. A clinician's guide to research terminology	
Validity	Synonymous with accuracy; does the tool accurately identify those who are risk for pressure ulcers and those who are not?
Predictive validity	To what extent does the tool accurately identify those who will or will not develop pressure ulcers?
Reliability	Synonymous with consistency; to what extent does the tool consistently produce the same score in identical situations?
Interrater reliability	To what extent do different raters consistently assign the same score to the same patient?
Sensitivity	The percentage of people who develop a pressure ulcer that were previously identified by the tool as being at risk
Specificity	The percentage of people who do not develop a pressure ulcer and were previously identified as not being at risk

Table information adapted. Courtesy of Luther Kloth, PT, MS, FAPTA, CWS, FACCWS.

Norton Scale

Physical Condition		Mental Status		Activity		Mobility		Incontinence	
4	Good	4	Alert	4	Ambulant	4	Full	4	Not controlled
3	Fair	3	Apathetic	3	Walks with help	3	Slightly limited	3	Occas. controlled
2	Poor	2	Confused	2	Chairbound	2	Very limited	2	Usually urinary
1	Very Bad	1	Stuporous	1	Bedfast	1	Immobile	1	Double

Figure 1. The Norton Scale.

Choosing a Risk Assessment Tool

Risk assessment is not confined to the problem of pressure ulcers. Risk assessment is part of the prevention of many diseases. Risk assessment tools are analogous to screening tests, which are used to detect incipient disease in persons who are asymptomatic. An assortment of screening tools has been used or proposed to determine whether patients are at risk for pressure ulcer development. These tools vary from simple (rating scales, serum albumin, serum transferrin) to complex (thermography, laser Doppler flowmetry, ultrasound).

The US Preventive Services Task Force recommends certain criteria in qualitatively evaluating the appropriateness of screening tests.[4] The first criterion is related to the effectiveness of the treatment for the condition predicted: Does the treatment do more good than harm? Is it more effective in asymptomatic patients than it is in symptomatic patients? Is there good evidence of that effectiveness? The second criterion relates

to the burden of suffering, should the disease be contracted, in terms of mortality, morbidity, discomfort, dissatisfaction, or destitution. The third criterion relates to quality of the test in terms of reliability, validity, acceptability, safety, simplicity, and cost (Table 1). It is clear that risk assessment for pressure ulcer prevention is appropriate, given the first 2 criteria. The third criterion as it relates to risk for pressure ulcer development will require further exploration.

In looking at the various screening tools available, the paper and pencil rating scales possess the best balance of characteristics (eg, reliability, validity, acceptability, safety, simplicity, and cost). Indices such as serum albumin or serum transferrin, while somewhat lower in patients who develop pressure ulcers, are not valid predictors of pressure ulcer development.[5] The more complex tools, such as laser Doppler flowmetry and ultrasound, have higher costs, lack simplicity and practicality of use, and are less accurate as pre-

The Braden Scale for Predicting Pressure Sore Risk.

Patient's Name _____	Evaluator's Name _____			Date of Assessment				

SENSORY PERCEPTION ability to respond meaningfully to pressure-related discomfort	**1. Completely Limited** Unresponsive (does not moan, flinch, or grasp) to painful stimuli, due to diminished level of consciousness or sedation. OR limited ability to feel pain over most of body	**2. Very Limited** Responds only to painful stimuli. Cannot communicate discomfort except by moaning or restlessness OR has a sensory impairment which limits the ability to feel pain or discomfort over ½ of body.	**3. Slightly Limited** Responds to verbal commands, but cannot always communicate discomfort or the need to be turned. OR has some sensory impairment which limits ability to feel pain or discomfort in 1 or 2 extremities.	**4. No Impairment** Responds to verbal commands. Has no sensory deficit which would limit ability to feel or voice pain or discomfort..				
MOISTURE degree to which skin is exposed to moisture	**1. Constantly Moist** Skin is kept moist almost constantly by perspiration, urine, etc. Dampness is detected every time patient is moved or turned.	**2. Very Moist** Skin is often, but not always moist. Linen must be changed at least once a shift.	**3. Occasionally Moist:** Skin is occasionally moist, requiring an extra linen change approximately once a day.	**4. Rarely Moist** Skin is usually dry, linen only requires changing at routine intervals.				
ACTIVITY degree of physical activity	**1. Bedfast** Confined to bed.	**2. Chairfast** Ability to walk severely limited or non-existent. Cannot bear own weight and/or must be assisted into chair or wheelchair.	**3. Walks Occasionally** Walks occasionally during day, but for very short distances, with or without assistance. Spends majority of each shift in bed or chair	**4. Walks Frequently** Walks outside room at least twice a day and inside room at least once every two hours during waking hours				
MOBILITY ability to change and control body position	**1. Completely Immobile** Does not make even slight changes in body or extremity position without assistance	**2. Very Limited** Makes occasional slight changes in body or extremity position but unable to make frequent or significant changes independently.	**3. Slightly Limited** Makes frequent though slight changes in body or extremity position independently	**4. No Limitation** Makes major and frequent changes in position without assistance.				
NUTRITION usual food intake pattern	**1. Very Poor** Never eats a complete meal. Rarely eats more than ⅓ of any food offered. Eats 2 servings or less of protein (meat or dairy products) per day. Takes fluids poorly. Does not take a liquid dietary supplement OR is NPO and/or maintained on clear liquids or IV's for more than 5 days.	**2. Probably Inadequate** Rarely eats a complete meal and generally eats only about ½ of any food offered. Protein intake includes only 3 servings of meat or dairy products per day. Occasionally will take a dietary supplement. OR receives less than optimum amount of liquid diet or tube feeding	**3. Adequate** Eats over half of most meals. Eats a total of 4 servings of protein (meat, dairy products per day. Occasionally will refuse a meal, but will usually take a supplement when offered OR is on a tube feeding or TPN regimen which probably meets most of nutritional needs	**4. Excellent** Eats most of every meal. Never refuses a meal. Usually eats a total of 4 or more servings of meat and dairy products. Occasionally eats between meals. Does not require supplementation.				
FRICTION & SHEAR	**1. Problem** Requires moderate to maximum assistance in moving. Complete lifting without sliding against sheets is impossible. Frequently slides down in bed or chair, requiring frequent repositioning with maximum assistance. Spasticity, contractures or agitation leads to almost constant friction	**2. Potential Problem** Moves feebly or requires minimum assistance. During a move skin probably slides to some extent against sheets, chair, restraints or other devices. Maintains relatively good position in chair or bed most of the time but occasionally slides down.	**3. No Apparent Problem** Moves in bed and in chair independently and has sufficient muscle strength to lift up completely during move. Maintains good position in bed or chair.					

© Copyright Barbara Braden and Nancy Bergstrom, 1988			Total Score				

Figure 2. The Braden Scale for Predicting Pressure Sore Risk.
© 1998 Barbara Braden and Nancy Bergstrom
Used with permission.

dictors than the paper and pencil rating scales. Two rating scales have been recommended by the Agency for Healthcare Research and Quality (AHRQ) panel in its *Pressure Ulcer Prevention Guidelines*.[6] The Norton Scale[7] (Figure 1) and the Braden Scale[8] (Figure 2) were judged to have undergone sufficient testing to justify their use in making clinical judgments.

The parameters examined to establish the validity of this type of screening tool are sensitivity (ability to identify true positives while minimizing false negatives) and specificity (ability to identify true negatives while minimizing false positives). The Norton Scale has been reported to have good sensitivity but low to moderate specificity at a score of 14.[9,10] The Braden Scale [8,11–13] has demonstrated good sensitivity and specificity in a variety of settings at cutoff scores that range from 16 to 18. The Braden Scale has also been

demonstrated to have excellent interrater reliability when used by registered nurses, but a much lower level of reliability when used by licensed practical nurses or nursing assistants.[11,12]

These risk assessment tools measure broad categories of factors that most commonly put patients at risk and that can be committed to interval ratings (eg, 1–4). Other factors enter into pressure ulcer risk, however. Some of the risk factors that have been found to predict who develops pressure ulcers and who does not are advanced age, low diastolic blood pressure, elevated body temperature, and inadequate current intake of protein.[5] Other factors are also thought to contribute to risk but have not been adequately studied include smoking, vasoactive drugs, and elevated cortisol levels due to exogenous or endogenous corticosteroids.[14]

In addition, specific patient populations may

Table 2. AOTA practice framework	
Occupational Therapy Practice Framework	**Braden Scale Score**
Sensory perception (ability to perceive sensation, pain, pressure via mechanoreceptors) Motor and sensory function of dermatomes and myotomes.	Sensory perception: ability to respond to meaningful pressure related
Bowel and bladder (continence and hygiene following toileting)	Moisture: degree to which skin is exposed to moisture
Basic Activities of Daily Living (grooming, self-feeding, dressing from a upright or seated position) Functional Independence Measure Modified Falls Efficacy Scale Canadian Occupational Performance Measure	Activity: degree of physical activity
Bed mobility Wheelchair mobility Functional mobility Mobility-related ADLs (access to essential areas, transfers to bed, bath tub, commode, or car)	Mobility: ability to change and control body position
Eating: mastication and bolus formation Swallowing: 4 stages of swallowing Self-Feeding: plate to mouth pattern	Nutrition: usual food intake pattern
Pressure Relief (push-ups, lateral weight shifts, or forward raises) Range of motion, strength to perform pressure relief and transitional movements	Friction and shear: level of assistance required to move

have unique characteristics that are not measured by existing risk assessment tools. For example, spinal cord rehabilitation units have a population that is fairly homogeneous with respect to sensory perception, mobility and activity, thus limiting the predictive capacity of those subscale scores. Other predictors may have to be considered, and specialized tools may prove more useful.[15,16]

Pressure Mapping as a Specialized Tool

Occupational therapists may utilize the Braden or Norton Scale to predict pressures ulcer risk and pressure mapping to determine and prioritize the site of the risk. According to Harrison and Loukras, "Pressure is defined as Pressure = Force/Area. Therefore, an effective method of reducing pressure is to increase the area of contact, resulting in pressure reduction. Load distribution can be achieved by providing support distally on the anterior thigh and laterally across the buttocks and by accommodating the bony prominences of the anatomical seating surface."[17] Pressure mapping is a pressure sensor system that utilizes computer aided design/computer aided manufacturing (CAD/CAM) to identify a patient's pressure distribution when seated. An advantage of pressure mapping is that a graph or chart provides a representation of pressure areas. A disadvantage is that movement causes the pressure distribution to change.[18,19] Stinson et al[20] recorded 2 sets of pressure maps of 15 occupational therapists with experience in pressure mapping and 50 occupational therapy students with no practical experience in pressure mapping. Subjects ranked both sets of maps in terms of best to poorest distribution of pressure. Pressure maps, average interface pressure (mmHg) and maximum interface pressure (mmHg) were rank-ordered. Results suggest that pressure map interface pressure was a reliable method in identifying pressure risks. There was significant agreement ($P < 0.001$) between groups of operators and reliability extended over the range of seating surfaces. Thus, pressure mapping is a reliable assessment for interpreting interface pressure in seating and may be used to guide treatment intervention.

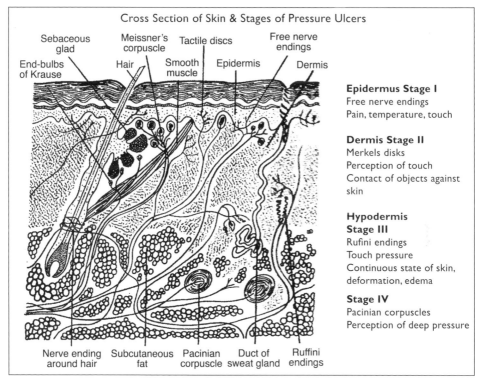

Figure 3. Layers of the skin and sensory perceptual structures associated associated with each pressure ulcer stage.

Using Risk Assessment in Prevention Programs

At-risk patients should be identified on admission to healthcare facilities and home care services. The activity subscales of either the Norton Scale or the Braden Scale can be used to determine whether patients require a full assessment for pressure ulcer risk. Following the admission assessment, reassessment should take place 48 hours later and at periodic intervals depending on the rapidity with which the condition changes as well as whenever a major change occurs in the condition.

Special vigilance is required during acute illness and during the first 2 weeks following admission to long-term care, as these are times of high risk for pressure ulcer development. In one prospective study of nursing home residents, investigators followed new admissions for 3 months and found that 80% of those who developed a pressure ulcer did so within 2 weeks

of admission and 96% did so within 3 weeks of admission.[5] *Thus, an appropriate schedule for reassessment of pressure ulcer risk in nursing homes might be every week for 4 weeks followed by routine quarterly assessments.*

In hospital settings, reassessments are often performed daily in intensive care units (ICUs) and every other day in general medical-surgical units. If this schedule is burdensome, it may be sufficient to assess on admission and 48 hours later. In home care, screening should probably be done with every registered nurse visit as the frequency of these visits is generally predicated on the severity of illness or the lability of the condition of the patient.

Clinicians should keep in mind that the risk assessment tools are intended to supplement their judgment but not replace it. Additional factors should be considered when patients are assessed for risk of pressure ulcer development. Nurses and other practitioners should also keep in mind that patients who are rapidly improving (eg, young

Table 3. Protocols by level of risk

Mild Risk (15–18)*

- Turning schedule
- Maximal remobilization
- Protect heels
- Manage moisture, nutrition, friction, and shear
- Pressure reduction support surface if bed- or chair-bound

*If other major risk factors are present, advance to next level of risk

Moderate Risk (13–14)*

Turning schedule with 30° rule
+
All interventions for mild risk

High Risk (10–12)*

- Frequency of turning and facilitate 30-degree lateral turns with foam wedges
- Supplement turning with small shifts
+
All interventions for mild risk

Very High Risk (>_ 9)

- Consider static air overlay if adequate monitoring possible
- Consider use of low-air-loss bed if patient has additional risk factors ameliorated by low-air-loss beds OR uncontrolled pain OR severe pain exacerbated by turning
+
All interventions for mild risk

*low-air-loss beds do not substitute for turning schedules

---

persons recovering from surgery) are probably at low risk, although their scores at the time may indicate otherwise. Likewise, persons whose level of function and health is declining may be at higher risk than their scores would indicate.

Occupational Therapists and Risk Assessment

Occupational therapy practitioners providing services in the ICU, acute care, rehabilitation, long-term care, and home health may utilize the Braden Scale score or the Norton Scale score provided by the nursing staff as a first step when determining the cause of pressure ulcer risks. In recent times, more occupational therapy practitioners are using the Braden Scale as a primary assessment tool to aid in predicting pressure ulcer risks. There are several reasons why the Braden

Scale score is utilized in occupational therapy practice. First, occupational therapy practice is guided by the American Occupational Therapy Association's Practice Framework (PFW).[21] The PFW guides practice intervention and identifies specific areas that need to be addressed prior to treatment intervention. The Braden Scale score mirrors the PFW and is comprised of specific occupational therapy performance areas, skills, and patient factors. Performance areas include activities of daily living (ADLs) and performance skills address strength and range of motion (ROM) necessary to achieve mobility and perform self-pressure relief (Table 2). Patient factors include cognitive and neuromusculoskeletal structures that may affect attention span and sensory receptors, which are responsible for the perception of pain and pressure that directly impact skin integrity during seating and positioning. Figure 3 represents a cross section of skin and mechanoreceptors that may be compromised depending on the stage of pressure ulcer (Stages I–IV). Second, occupational therapists need to follow guidelines for reimbursement laid out by the Centers for Medicare and Medicaid Services (CMS) in the Advanced Determination of Medicare Coverage for Durable Medical Equipment (mobility, seating, positioning). Claims reviewers recommend the use of evidence-based assessment tools, such as the Braden Scale and pressure mapping,[22] to aid in making a determination regarding occupational therapists' recommended pressure relieving devices (eg, as wheelchair bases, seat backs, and cushions). Third, reviewers also require an International Classification of Diseases, Ninth Revision, Clinical Modifications (ICD-9-CM) code that represents the medical necessity for providing intervention; occupational therapy practitioners may utilize the PFW and the Braden Scale score to select appropriate primary and secondary ICD-9-CM codes. For example, a patient diagnosed with chronic obstructive pulmonary disorder (COPD) or congestive heart failure (CHF) would have a primary diagnosis code of 496, an occupational therapy treatment diagnosis of lower extremity edema of 457.1, a compromised sensation code of 780, and a Braden Scale score of "high risk" (10–12).[23] Because patients with COPD or CHF are often immobilized

Table 4. Turning schedules

These turning schedules may be used to organize care on nursing units with large numbers of patients who are at risk for pressure ulcers. Patients on a team or unit can be assigned to 1 of 3 schedules in a balanced manner, eg, if 6 patients are at risk, 2 would be assigned to each of the 3 schedules. These schedules may have to be adjusted to each day, depending on other components of the patient's schedule.

Direction of Turn	Schedule 1	Schedule 2	Schedule 3
1. Back (breakfast and bath)	7:00–9:00	7:30–9:30	8:00–10:00
2. Right side	9:00–11:00	9:30–11:30	10:00–12:00
3. Back (lunch)	11:00–1:00	11:30–1:30	12:00–2:00
4. Right side	1:00–3:00	1:30–3:30	2:00–4:00
5. Left side	3:00–5:00	3:30–5:30	4:00–6:00
6. Back (dinner)	5:00–7:00	5:30–7:30	6:00–8:00
7. Left side	7:00–9:00	7:30–9:30	8:00–10:00
8. Right side	9:00–11:00	9:30–11:30	10:00–12:00
9. Left side	11:00–1:00	11:00–1:30	12:00–2:00
10. Back	1:00–3:00	1:30–3:30	2:00–4:00
11. Right side	3:00–5:00	3:30–5:30	4:00–6:00
12. Left side	5:00–7:00	5:30–7:30	6:00–8:00

secondary to compromised physical conditioning, they may develop edema in the same areas where pressure ulcers develop.[24] Pitting edema develops in dorsal, sacral, and peripheral extremities that are in a dependent position. Edema increases capillary pressure and inhibits transport of nutrients to the cells. "The presence of interstitial fluid increases the distance from the capillary to the cell. The rate of diffusion of nutrients is reduced by the reciprocal of the square root of that distance; this is calculated as field theory. Thus local edema doubles the capillary-to-cell distance and decreases the supply of nutrients."[24] Finally, when occupational therapists couple the Braden Scale score with a comprehensive seating assessment, pressure mapping, or the use of a pressure sensor, the practitioner is able to prescribe appropriate wheelchair bases, cushions, and back supports.

Preventive Protocols Based on Level of Risk

Preventive interventions should become more frequent and/or intense as risk increases. Braden and Bergstrom[8] have made specific recommendations based on level of risk (Table 3). There is evidence that this approach leads to more effective and less expensive care.[3,25,26] This likely occurs

because appropriate assessment of risk allows the clinician to limit interventions to those persons who are at risk, to reserve intensive and costly interventions to those who are most in need, and to identify and address specific problems or factors that contribute to that level of risk.

Reducing the Exposure to Pressure

Turning schedules. Close attention should be paid to an individualized turning schedule. Sample turning schedules that account for periods when the patient must be on his or her back, such as during meals and morning care, can be seen in Table 4. These schedules can be further altered to meet individual patient needs. Repositioning should be done with assistance and with attention to good body mechanics, such as using pillows and pads to protect bony prominences.

To protect the heels when the patient is supine, pillows should be used to support the entire length of the legs, ending at the ankles and suspending the heels above the mattress. The heels must be checked frequently to ensure that, as the pillows compress, they remain free of pressure. If use of the pillows is not effective in protecting the heels, consult physical therapy or occupational therapy to construct devices that adequately protect the heels from excessive pressure. Pressure-

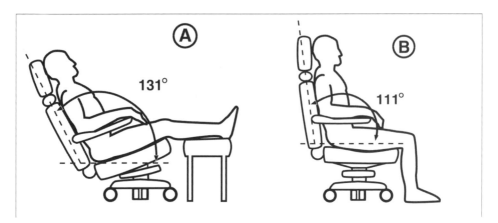

Figures 4a and 4b. Chair positioning. Adated from Defloor T, Grypdonck MH. Sitting posture and prevention of pressure ulcers. *Appl Nurs Res. 1999;12(3):136–142.*

relieving ankle-foot orthoses are often used to prevent pressure on the heels.

At higher levels of risk or for emaciated patients, turning schedules should include either increased frequency of turns or assisted frequent, small shifts in body weight. Lateral turns should not exceed 30 degrees[27] and, if at all possible, the head of the bed should not be elevated beyond 30 degrees. Foam wedges are helpful in lateral positioning and can be used to increase the frequency of repositioning by pulling it out slightly every 30 minutes to 1 hour. If narcotics or sedatives are being used, extra attention should be paid to turning during those times of heavy sedation. A turning schedule linked to meal time may be posted at the head of the patient's bed to facilitate interdisciplinary and inter-shift communication.

When patients can tolerate the prone position (ie, lying horizontally with the face down) it should be added to the turning schedule, as it allows the most common sites of pressure ulcer formation (eg, sacrum, trochanters, heels) to be totally relieved of pressure while also preventing flexion contractures of the hips. Careful padding and positioning are required if the prone position is employed. Prone positioning is contraindicated in patients who have a gastrointestinal tube or nasogastric tube due to the high probability of regurgitation and aspiration. In addition, partial or full paralysis of the diaphragm or trunk may impede adequate respiration in the prone position.

Attention must also be paid to effective chair positioning, as very high interface pressure and shearing forces can develop with poor posture or seating surfaces. Defloor and Grypdonck[28] found that a chair position with the back tilted slightly backward, with the leg supported on a rest and the heel extending over the end of the rest, resulted in the lowest interface pressures at the sacrum and ischial tuberosities (Figure 4a). If this position cannot be achieved with the available seating, an upright posture with feet resting on the floor in a chair equipped with arm rests should be used (Figure 4b).

Wheelchair Positioning

There are many different types of and brands of wheelchairs that may be used to aide in pressure relief, positioning and mobility. Common areas of pressure loading secondary to wheelchair seating include the scapula and spine, elbow and forearm, knee and calf (politeal fossa), buttocks, and heel and foot. Pressure, friction and shearing must be considered when selecting a wheelchair. The frame, back, and seat comprise the seating system. Seating systems are attached to a wheeled base for mobility. Goals of seating and positioning include evenly distributing pressure over a large surface, preventing friction and shear, and providing a stable support surface.

Pressure ulcers tend to develop when the amount of pressure that can be tolerated reduces blood flow to capillary beds to between 30 and 100 mmHg. The amount of pressure exerted on the patient's buttocks, sacrum or other anatomical structures by the seating system must be determined prior to prescribing the final wheelchair seat and back. Braden Scale scores, pressure mapping, and pressure monitoring aid in determining the best wheelchair seat and cushion for pressure relief.

A majority of wheelchairs prescribed for consumers will be manual, tilt in space, or recline. The type of wheelchair prescribed depends on the physical (strength, ROM, sensation) and cognitive ability (cause and effect, memory, problem solving, and level of self-care participation) of the patient.

Manual (mobility-based) wheelchairs may be self-propelled with the upper and lower extremities or by an assistant. Various wheelchair seats and backs may be added to manual bases for pressure relief to bony prominences. A standard or manual wheelchair does not have a tilt or recline feature, so there is increased loading on the ischial tuberosities. When the vinyl or nylon seat and back upholstery become stretched out secondary to wear, the back and seat may become slung, adding to the hammock effect of seating. Hammocking of the wheelchair seat and back increases musculoskeletal deformities, including posterior pelvic tilt (sacral sitting), anterior pelvic tilt, scoliosis, obliquity, and a combination of deformities referred to as windswept. A key factor in reducing pressure ulcers associated with manual wheelchair sitting is to have the patient move off the area. Patients who have adequate upper extremity strength and ROM are encouraged to perform self-pressure relief. Pressure relief to the ischial tuberosities, greater trochanters, sacrum, buttocks, popliteal area, and upper extremities may be achieved through performing push-ups, lateral weight shifts from sided to side, and forward raises.

Remobilization of the immobile. When a patient is found to have deficits in activity or mobility, the nurse should always be alert to the patient's potential to become remobilized. During an episode of illness, it is easy for an elderly person to be less active than is optimal and to enter into a spiral of deconditioning and decline. This leads to a myriad of complications beyond increased pressure ulcer risk. A physical therapy consultation may be helpful in determining the degree to which remobilization is possible and beginning the process of remobilization. The physical therapist, the occupational therapist, the nurse, and, if possible, the patient should collabo-

rate in developing a plan that is clear about the responsibilities that each one holds in the process of remobilization.

In cases for which the return to full mobility is not possible, the patient can be taught to make small shifts in body position. This includes things such as moving the legs and shifting weight from one buttock to another. If the person is wheelchair-bound, he or she needs to be taught to perform a variation of the push-ups. To perform this push-up, lock the wheelchair or brakes, make sure the armrests are locked to the wheelchair, grasp the armrest with respective right and left hands, and push down of the armrest. This will result in the buttocks being lifted or pushed up from the wheelchair seat. Wheelchair push-ups should be performed every 15 minutes throughout the time spent in the wheelchair.[24,29]

Performing lateral weight shifts requires good balance and strength. The patient places his or her elbows on the left or right side of the wheelchair armrests and turns to the left or right side and shifts the weight off the buttocks of the respective side. The hips and buttocks should be lifted at least 1 inch off the chair (seat) surface; the patient should lean far enough to the side to allow a hand to guide under the buttock or thigh. Lateral weight shifts should be performed every 15 minutes throughout the time spent in the wheelchair.[24,29]

Forward weight shifts or raises may also be performed from a manual wheelchair. The patient with good balance removes his or her feet from the wheelchair footrests and places them onto the floor. The trunk is positioned in forward flexion and the elbows rest on the distal thighs or knees until the buttocks are lifted off the wheelchair seat. A duration of every 15 minutes throughout the time spent in the wheelchair is congruent with pressure relief time recommended for push ups and lateral weight shifts. Forward raises should be performed by patients who have adequate balance, strength, ROM, and knowledge of cause and effect.

The elbow or wrist may also be hooked around the wheelchair push-handle allowing, the patient to lean to the opposite side or forward. Patients who cannot perform wheelchair push-ups or forward raises because of balance or other safety reasons should perform lateral weight shifts in bed using a bed rail.

Table 5. Pros and cons of manual recline and tilt wheelchair positioning systems		
Type of Seating system	**Pros**	**Cons**
Manual or Standard Wheelchair	• Self-propelled • Use upper- and lower-extremity for propulsion • Self-pressure relief • User positioned in upright-position	• Force of gravity increases falling forward or to the side • Hammocking of wheelchair seat and back • Increased associated musculoskeletal deformities
Recline System	• Distributes pressure • Easier intermittent catheterization • Transfers easier with back of wheelchair reclined	• Increased pressure over sacral area • Molded system increases shear forces • Disrupted postural alignment increases shear forces • Limited knee or hip ROM pulled out of position
Tilt System	• Comfort • Increased sitting tolerance • Minimal shear forces	• Constant hip flexion limits bladder emptying • Prolonged hip and knee flexion increases potential for contracture • Interferes with use of lap tray

Adapted from Lange[30] and Perr.[62]

Because patients using manual wheelchairs are expected to participate in pressure relief using one or more of the aforementioned types of pressure relief either manually or aided by an assistant, clinicians may want to increase the possibility of adherence by designing a weight shift schedule. Providing a reminder such as an auditory cue (eg, an alarmed wrist watch) or a vibratory cue (eg, a vibrating PDA) placed in an area of normal sensation may also be an effective reminder to perform pressure relief.

Weight shifts may also be achieved by using a tilt-in-space or recline feature of a wheelchair. A 45-degree tilt allows adequate pressure relief. Tilt and recline wheelchairs or seating systems may also aid in pressure relief, seating stability, comfort, and rest (Table 5). Some seating systems combine tilt and recline features.[30]

Recline systems open the seat to back angle, which allows the patient to lie down and back and return to an upright position. Shearing and friction are often associated with wheelchair repositioning. When a reclining back of a wheelchair is raised or lowered, the patient's skin tends to adhere to the surface of the wheelchair seat or back. Friction may occur when the skin slides over skin during repositioning of the wheelchair or when performing transfers. Recent gains in seating technology include low- or no-shear backs for reclining wheelchairs.

"Tilt-in-space systems allow the patient to drop back without changing anatomical angles (bending at the hips and knees)."[30] Tilt systems are used for patients who have increased tone, orthopedic limitations (contractures), or forward head postures, which compromise speech, swallowing, or eye gaze.

Use of special support surfaces. Support surfaces include overlays (mattress or wheelchair seating), mattress replacements, or specialty beds. Mattress overlays and mattress replacements may be classified as either static (eg, foam, gels) or dynamic (eg, alternating pressure surfaces). Specialty beds are classified as either low-air-loss or air-fluidized. The comparative effectiveness of these surfaces is difficult to evaluate, but findings converge on these areas: a) almost any surface tested reduced interface pressure below those seen with a standard hospital mattress;[31-33] b) foam overlays that were 2–3 inches thick did not compare favorably to other pressure-reduction surfaces,[34] including thicker foam surfaces;[35] c) foam mattresses with flat surfaces are more effective than those with convoluted foam surfaces;[36] d) static air overlays, if properly maintained, are some of the most effective overlays at reducing interface pressure, performing nearly as well or equally well as specialty beds;[37-39] e) air-fluidized beds and low-air-loss beds result in substantial pressure reduction and appear to be beneficial in healing pressure ulcers, though results are not always dramatic,[40-43] and f) rotating beds show no apparent benefit over standard hospital or ICU beds.[44,45] Two excellent integrated reviews of existing research related to efficacy of various pressure reduction surfaces by Whittemore[46] and Reddy et al[47] are suggested for those requiring more detailed information.

If the patient is bed-bound, an overlay or replacement support surface to decrease interface pressure over bony prominences is recommended.[6] If the Braden Scale score is below 9 or the patient has intractable or severe pain exacerbated by turning, use of a low-air-loss bed may be indicated. *It is important to remember that turning will still be necessary to prevent pressure ulcers and other complications of immobility. However, the nurse must be clear about the goal of care for these patients. When the patient is terminal and the goal of care is provision of comfort, a rigorous schedule of turning is not appropriate.*

Patients who are chair-bound also require special support surfaces, as the interface pressures that develop at the sacrum and ischial tuberosities when seated on a hard surface are much higher than those experienced in a supine position. Few studies have been published on chair seating surfaces, but a recent study comparing 4 surfaces (2 static air, 1 foam, and 1 water-cushion) found that the static air cushions provided the best pressure reduction.[28]

Wheelchair Support Surfaces

The type of wheelchair back and cushion will depend on the needs of the patient, prior history of pressure ulcers, awareness of sensation, and ability to perform pressure relief. Occupational therapists prescribe wheelchair cushions to prevent the risk of sitting acquired pressure ulcers

(SAPUs). Periodic reassessments of the effectiveness of the base of support is performed for long-term tertiary prevention. An ideal cushion distributes pressure evenly over a large surface area, is lightweight, requires minimal maintenance, and provides even pressure distribution which facilitates circulation. Research consistently suggests that no one cushion is universally effective for all patients.[18,48-50]

Various strategies are used to select wheelchair cushions including an individual needs assessment, Braden or Norton scale scores, medical history and comprehensive review of systems (eg, neuromuscular skeletal, sensory, cognitive, vision), results of pressure mapping, physical conditioning (ability to perform self-pressure relief, activity tolerance, and energy expenditure) and how the wheelchair and seating surface will be used to accommodate lifestyle and occupational (functional) performance.

For able-bodied persons sitting is not static but dynamic, and posture is generally modified approximately every 15–20 minutes. For persons immobilized by disabling conditions, wheelchair cushions are prescribed to compensate for inadequate pressure relief, increase sitting tolerance, and allow maximum participation and performance of ADLs. Wheelchair cushions provide a firm base of support, minimize the hammocking effect or slung wheelchair seat, and promote postural alignment. Thus, associated deformities (eg, posterior pelvic tilt, obliquity, and scoliosis) are reduced.

All wheelchair users benefit from pressure relieving cushions. Medicare classifies wheelchair cushions into 4 basic types: a) a 1-inch cushion; b) a 2-inch cushion; c) a pressure-equalization cushion; and d) a custom-molded seat. To qualify for a 1- to 2-inch cushion, the wheelchair user must sit in the wheelchair at least 4 hours per day. Pressure equalization cushions are prescribed for patients meeting the following criteria: 1) the patient is unable to perform self-pressure relief; 2) skin is insensate under the ischial tuberosities; 3) abnormal tone increases buttock migration or sliding; 4) muscle atrophy impedes ability to shift weight; 5) age-related changes diminish strength of the skin and reduce circulation with increase risk of skin breakdown; 6) orthopedic deformities increase pressure over bony prominences; and 7) diabetes compromises circulation in the lower

Table 6. Comparison of wheelchair cushions				
1 - Excellent	2 - Good		3 - Fair	4 - Poor
Characteristics	**Foam**	**Fluid/Gel**	**Air**	**Custom**
Availability	1	1–2	1–2	4
Can be customized	2	2	2	1
Numerous choices	1	2	2	3
Comfort	2	2–3	1	1
Stable base of support	3	1	2–3	1
Low maintenance	1	3	3	1
Easy to clean	4	1	1	1
User friendly	1	3	3	1
Durable	4	2	2	1
Skin breakdown protection	3–4	1	1	1
Shear protection	3–4	1	1	3–4
Prevents heat buildup	3	4	1	3
Allows good air circulation	4	4	1	4
Lightweight	1	3–4	1	4
Cost	1	3	3	4
Adapted from Schmidt[63]				

extremities while seated.[51]

The composition of wheelchair cushions has changed based on technology, evaluation of pressure between the cushion and the seating surface, type of wheelchair base, and the lifestyle of the consumer. Practitioners are more knowledgeable about wheelchair cushions and are using evidence-based practice to match the patient's risk factors for pressure ulcers to positioning needs and the most effective seating system based on occupation and lifestyle.[52] "New technologies are reintroducing the concept of offloading–translating pressure to muscular areas, such as gluteal and posterior thigh and eliminating pressure from the ischial tuberosities and coccyx."[48,30] When offloading is combined with computerized pressure mapping, the clinician gains a sound understanding of the magnitude of pressure resulting from the buttock and seat interface.

Cushions are selected based on their ability to provide pressure relief and prevent pressure ulcers. Other considerations include weight, height, contour, shape, size, stability versus emersion, composition of materials, cover material, maintenance, and cost.[48] Cushions also provide comfort through shock absorption and vibration reduc-tion. Repetitive shock and vibration may result in pain in the back and pelvis, increased fatigue, and reduced sitting tolerance. Cushions may reduce friction and shear between the wheelchair and the buttocks and aid in minimizing the development of heat and moisture at the seat interface.[53]

Practitioners must also consider cushion density, stiffness, resilience, dampening, and envelopment. Interface pressure depends on the properties of stiffness, dampening, and enveloping. Stiffness is defined as the depth at which the patient sinks into the cushion. Dampening refers to the cushion's ability to soften and reduce the impact of tissue loading during activity. Enveloping is the cushion's ability to surround or contain the buttocks. Interface pressure mapping assists in the evaluation of envelopment.[50]

Cushions may be classified as linear and nonlinear. Linear systems (eg, foam) conform to the weight of the individual, and nonlinear cushions are custom-contoured or modular.[53] Cushions may be static (pressure-reducing) or dynamic (pressure-relieving). Static cushions are used when the risk of developing pressure ulcers is low to high, and dynamic cushions are used with high risk or existing pressure ulcers.[54]

Custom-contoured cushions maximize contact with the support surface, provide pressure relief, and accommodate fixed-orthopedic deformities, such as pelvic obliquity. Contoured cushions are constructed by pushing foam up underneath a planar surface, resulting in a pressure distribution that is shaped like the person. Vacuum molding creates a negative impression that is recorded digitally and utilizes pressure mapping to guide cushion fabrication. Contoured cushions provide a stable base of support and are durable. Patients may experience shear and heat build-up depending on the surface coating.

The most commonly prescribed cushions are gel, air, flotation, or a combination of different shapes and materials. For example, "floam" is a newer technology that is lighter than gel; viscosity is stable with temperature changes, and the cushion is durable up to 3–5 years with proper care. Some cushions are constructed of thermoplastic material in which the cells resemble a honeycomb; the perforated walls of the cushion add ventilation and provide pressure relief and are easily laundered.[55]

Foam cushions are lightweight, have varying degrees of density (firm or soft), and may be open- or closed-cell. Foam used for pressure relief may be layered with varying levels of density (pound weight), which helps to maintain shape. Foam is temperature-sensitive, so it is important to use foam that is resistant to temperature changes. Foam cushions less than 6–7 cm deep tend to bottom out more quickly than those that are 10–11 cm deep. Advantages in selecting foam include its numerous choices, its low cost, its light weight, its degree of comfort, and its low maintenance. Foam is not easy to clean, and it provides fair pressure relief.[48,54]

Cushions that utilize air are lightweight. They require regular maintenance and consistent monitoring, and they are easily punctured. Air cushions are based on flotation technology and provide excellent pressure relief. Pressure reduction and positioning occur when the body is immersed into the surrounding air sacs depending on the profile of the cushion (eg, high or low or wedged), stability or base of support may be compromised. Air minimizes heat build-up and moisture. Lower interface pressures are achieved with nonstretch cushion cover materials; cushion cover materials may limit immersion based on the degree of stretch.[48,54]

Gel cushions are heavier than air and foam and are temperature sensitive. Polymer gels reduce shear as the material moves with the skin; therefore, immersion is limited and aids in cooling the skin. Polymer gels may be used in combination with foam-based cushions. Fluid gels promote immersion and reduce shear because bony prominences move within the fluid. Bottoming out may occur as a result of repetitive immersion.[48,54] Table 6 illustrates the comparison of properties between foam, gel, air, and custom cushions.

Wheelchair seat backs may also cause pressure ulcers over the vertebral spine (eg, the apex of kyphosis) and spine of the scapula. Assessments used to determine pressure ulcer risk associated with seat cushions may also be used for seat backs. Seat backs may be constructed of gel or foam, and they may be modular or contoured. For patients experiencing lateral flexion of the trunk, padded lateral supports may be used to reduce pressure to the ribs. Correcting scoliosis may require three points of interface contact between the lower ribs, shoulder, and hip and may result in pressure ulcers. Practitioners attempting to correct fixed deformities of the spine may need to consider using a tilt-in-space wheelchair base.

Managing moisture. Exposure of the skin to excessive moisture from any source can weaken the outer layers and increase the opportunity for skin injury. Incontinence is a common cause of skin maceration and breakdown. A variety of interventions aimed at reducing or eliminating incontinent episodes is available to clinicians, including use of bladder training, prompted voiding, or other behavioral methods.[56,57] After each incontinent episode, the nurse should use a very mild soap to cleanse the skin, rinse thoroughly, and pat the skin dry before applying a commercial moisture barrier. Absorbent underpads or briefs should be used, checked frequently, and changed as needed. The use of thin, plastic-backed underpads should be avoided, as these keep the mattress dry while the patient sits in a pool of urine or liquid stool.

Diarrhea is very caustic to the skin and can lead quickly to skin breakdown. An attempt should be made to determine the cause of the diarrhea and eliminate that cause. Such diarrhea may be related to hyperosmolar tube feedings or

Table 7. Formulas for program evaluation		
Prevalence	=	# with pressure ulcers # surveyed during study
Nosocomial rate	=	# with ulcers during study - # with ulcers on admission # of patients surveyed during study
Severity Index	=	([length + width]/2) x stage
Severity Index for Hospital	=	total severity index for all pressure ulcers total # with pressure ulcers

impaction. If intervention to stop the diarrhea does not bring quick results, a fecal incontinence pouch should be used while further attempts at control are made.

Perspiration can be problematic when it is constant, trapped between skin folds, or held close to the skin through contact with nonbreathable support surfaces. Absorbent materials should be used beneath the patient and next to the patient's skin. Use of absorbent powders is generally not advisable, as the powder may collect in skin folds and become a source of injury. If perspiration is the result of a nonbreathing support surface, an alternative surface should be sought.

Friction and shear. Friction and shear are very harmful to the skin and make it particularly susceptible to the effects of pressure. Dinsdale[58] used swine to investigate the effects of friction. He found that, in the absence of friction, a pressure of 290 mmHg was required to produce ulceration while a pressure of only 45 mmHg would produce ulceration in skin pretreated with friction.

Several interventions may be used to prevent or ameliorate exposure of the skin to friction and shear. The use of a trapeze or turning sheet may be used to assist movement in bed. Ankle and heel protectors, while doing nothing to relieve pressure, may be very helpful in protecting these areas from friction. In some instances, hydrocolloid dressings may be used over a particular prominence that is being exposed to friction.

Shearing can occur in the sacral area when the head of the bed is elevated or the patient slumps in a chair. *For those who are bedfast, maintaining the elevation of the head of the bed at or below 30 degrees will prevent shearing as well as excess pressure at the sacrum. This may not be possible at all times, but the duration of higher elevations should be minimized in persons*

at higher levels of risk. When slumping in a chair is problematic, a recliner or special chair that allows for slight backward recline with elevated legs should be considered.

Nutritional repletion. Both long-term and short-term problems with nutrition make patients more prone to pressure ulcer development. It appears that an even slightly lower than optimal dietary intake of protein is an especially strong risk factor.[5] It is possible that immediate nutritional repletion, particularly for protein intake, may provide some protection. If the patient has good liver and renal function, it may be helpful to increase protein intake beyond 100% of the Food and Drug Administration (FDA)'s recommended daily allowances (RDA) and increase general caloric intake so as to spare the protein from being used for energy. Although there is no direct evidence that vitamin deficiencies increase the risk for developing pressure ulcers, it is known that vitamins A and C and zinc are important in building new tissue and healing injured tissue. Nutritional supplementation with these vitamins and minerals may be helpful.

When there are problems with nutrition, a consultation with a registered dietitian should be considered. This is particularly important when the patient is being fed enterally to ensure adequacy of the feeding for the individual patient's needs. If the patient develops diarrhea, a change to a feeding with a lower osmolality, higher fiber content, and/or lower volume may be sufficient to treat the diarrhea. Bacterial contamination from the feeding equipment should be considered as a potential contributing factor. Occasionally, antidiarrheal medication may be necessary.

Evaluating a Program of Prevention

Developing an evaluation plan for a program of prevention is important for a variety of reasons.

Table 8. Stratification of data by pressure ulcer stage and level of risk								
		Total Pts.	PU-	PU+	Stage 1	Stage 2	Stage 3	Stage 4
Not at risk	#	700	700	0				
Low Risk	#	170	110	60	45	15	0	0
	%		65%	35%	26%	9%		
Mod. Risk	#	75	35	40	20	20	0	0
	%		47%	53%	27%	27%		
High Risk	#	35	5	30	5	21	4	0
	%		14%	86%	14%	60%	12%	
Very High Risk	#	20	0	20	5	7	4	4
	%			100%	25%	35%	20%	20%

Note: All percentages represent percents of the total number of patients at that level of risk.

One important but seldom recognized reason is that the act of periodically evaluating progress and giving feedback to nursing staff has been shown to enhance the effectiveness of the overall program. For example, one Midwestern tertiary care hospital, using a continuous quality improvement strategy that allowed for this periodic feedback, cut the nosocomial rate of pressure ulcers from 18.7% to 6.4% over 3 years.[3]

Baseline data are important to the accurate measurement of the impact of the program of prevention. While many clinical facilities/agencies have sophisticated management information systems that enable them to determine how many pressure ulcers had been documented by the nursing staff in a previous time period, a point-prevalence study is a better method for obtaining an accurate baseline. This is because prior to implementation of a formal program of prevention, the nursing staff may not be attentive to certain pressure ulcers, particularly partial-thickness lesions. This inattentiveness leads to under-documentation and, therefore, underestimation of the problem. A point-prevalence study will provide more accurate information.

The purpose of a point-prevalence study is to determine the percentage of patients with pressure ulcers in the facility or agency at 1 point in time (usually 1 day). Conducting such a study requires a team of nurses who have been trained to stage and measure pressure ulcers. All nursing units participating in the program of prevention should be part of the point-prevalence study. If possible, each patient currently in the facility should be examined for the presence or absence of pressure ulcers on that day. If the facility is too large to inspect the skin of all patients, a large random sample should be selected for study.

If a patient is found to have one or more pressure ulcers, an estimate of wound severity should be recorded. Scores on formal wound assessment tools, such as the PUSH (Pressure Ulcer Scale for Healing) or the PSST (Pressure Sore Status Tool), may be used.[59,60] If these are not available or are too time-consuming for purposes of a point-prevalence study, the stage, size (length and width), and location of each should be recorded on the data collection sheet. From these data, a severity index may be calculated for each ulcer and for the facility (Table 7). The nurse should also note whether any of the admissions assessments indicated the presence of any ulcers, as this information will allow one to estimate the percent of nosocomial ulcers found.

A chart review should be conducted at the same time as the point-prevalence study. The chart review usually consists of calculating the percentage of times the risk assessment score is charted on admission notes and noting evidence of implementation of preventive interventions on the care plan and in the charting. The results of both should be reported to nursing staff on various units. In most facilities, the association between the point-prevalence study and the chart review will be obvious; nursing units having the lowest prevalence, nosocomial rate, and severity index are usually the units on which the staff is most diligent in performing risk assessment and implementing preventive measures. Units that have high nosocomial rates and low compliance with protocols are usually targeted for additional education or assistance in strengthening their care procedures.

The baseline point-prevalence study should be conducted as close to the time of start-up as possible. This means the study should be conducted a few weeks before the facility-wide educational programs are initiated. After the staff has been educated, the point-prevalence study should be conducted at specific intervals, such as every 6 months.

Because the case mix in a facility or hospital may change based on season and other factors, it is advisable to stratify nosocomial data by level of risk and severity. The most straightforward method for doing this involves using the levels of risk by Braden Scale score (Table 8) and the stages of pressure ulcers. This type of table should be pre-

pared at the conclusion of each point-prevalence study and used to examine trends. The desirable outcomes are that both nosocomial rates and severity would decrease at each level of risk.

Self-Assessment Questions

1. Patients should be assessed for pressure ulcer risk at which of the following intervals?
   A. An admission assessment is sufficient
   B. An admission assessment and a repeat assessment in 24 hours
   C. An admission assessment and a repeat assessment in 48 hours and every other day thereafter
   D. An admission assessment and a repeat assessment in 48 hours and at intervals based on severity and lability of the patient's illness

2. Which of the following methods for collecting baseline prevalence and nosocomial data

---

Take-Home Messages for Practice

- While not all pressure ulcers are preventable, many are. The cost and human suffering associated with treatment of pressure ulcers is tremendous and, for the most part, unnecessary. Prevention of pressure ulcers requires a systematic approach that begins with risk assessment and ends with appropriate preventive measures being delivered in a timely manner to those who are in need. Primary, secondary, and tertiary prevention of pressure ulcers may be achieved through the interprofessional collaboration of nursing, occupational therapy, and physical therapy. Prevention regimes should focus on a plan that includes increasing physical activity, which increases oxygen and nutrients to the tissues. Increased strength may contribute to better weight shifts and reduced comorbidities. Skin that is too dry is fragile, moisture leads to maceration, and heat increases metabolic rate, resulting in increased oxygen demand and will potentiate the possibility of ischemia. Skin over the ischia, sacrum/coccyx, trochanters, heels, ankles, knees, spine, scapula, and elbows should be inspected twice a day.

- A long-handled skin assessment mirror may be used by persons with spinal cord injuries (eg, paraplegia and C6-C8 tetraplegics); higher-level spinal cord injured persons require caregiver assistance for skin inspection. Malnourished persons are typically underweight and may develop ischemia over bony prominences. In contrast, obesity may limit participation in weight shifts and increase friction and shear during transfers[61]. Remember that appropriate wheelchair seat bases, cushions, and backs aid in reducing pressure, providing alignment and a stable base of support, and increased activity tolerance and participation in occupational performance (ie, functional activity). Push-ups and lateral and forward weight-shift routines are also effective ways to prevent pressure ulcers. A careful reading of this chapter should supply the clinician with the necessary information to initiate a formal, research-based program of prevention in his or her facility.

---

was recommended in this chapter as a way to evaluate outcomes of a pressure ulcer prevention program?

    A. A 1-year retrospective review of hospital research prior to implementation

    B. Continuous prospective data collection during the first 6-month period following training of nursing staff and/or the implementation of a program of prevention

    C. Point-prevalence by direct observation and estimates of nosocomial rates obtained prior to training or implementation of a program of prevention

    D. Point-prevalence by direct observation and estimates of nosocomial rates obtained by the American Occupational Therapy Association during the first 6-month period following implementation of a program of prevention

3. Tilt-in-space wheelchair bases are effective in preventing pressure sores. The tilt-in-space system may be used for all of the following conditions EXCEPT:

    A. Orthopedic limitations (contractures)

    B. Hypertonicity

    C. Dysphagia

    D. Bladder emptying

4. Wheelchair seat cushions offer a stable base of support, prevent spinal deformities, and support pressure relief. Which of the following spinal deformities may be associated with wheelchair seat hammocking?

    A. Posterior pelvic tilt

    B. Scoliosis

    C. Obliquity

    D. Kyphosis

    E. All of the above

Answers: 1-D, 2-C, 3-D, 4-E

References

1. Xakellis GC, Frantz RA, Arteaga M, Nguyen M, Lewis A. A comparison of patient risk for pressure ulcer development with nursing use of preventive interventions. *J Am Geriatr Soc*. 1992;40(12):1250–1254.

2. Bergstrom N, Braden B, Kemp M, Champagne M, Ruby E. Multi-site study of incidence of pressure ulcers and the relationship between risk level, demographic character-

istics, diagnoses, and prescription of preventive interventions. J Am Geriatr Soc. 1996;44(1):22–30.

3. Bergstrom N, Braden B, Boynton P, Bruch S. Using a research-based assessment scale in clinical practice. *Nurs Clin North Am*. 1995;30(3):539–551.

4. O'Malley MS, Fletcher SW. US Preventive Services Task Force. Screening for breast cancer with breast self-examination. A critical review. *JAMA*. 1987;257(16):2196–2203.

5. Bergstrom N, Braden B. A prospective study of pressure sore risk among institutionalized elderly. *J Am Geriatr Soc*. 1992;40(8):747–758.

6. Panel for the Prediction and Prevention of Pressure Ulcers, ed. Pressure Ulcers in Adults: Prediction and Prevention. Clinical Practice Guideline Number Three. Rockville, Md: US Department of Health and Human Services. Agency for Health Care Policy and Research;1992. AHCPR Publication No. 92-0047.

7. Norton D, McLaren R, Exton-Smith AN, eds. An Investigation of Geriatric Nursing Problems in Hospitals. London, UK: National Corporation for the Care of Old People; 1962.

8. Braden BJ, Bergstrom N. Pressure reduction. In: Bulechek GM, McCloskey J, eds. Nursing Interventions: Essential Nursing Treatments. 2nd ed. Orlando, Fla: WB Saunders Co.; 1992.

9. Goldstone LA, Roberts BV. A preliminary discriminant function analysis of elderly orthopaedic patients who will or will not contract a pressure sore. Int J Nurs Stud. 1980;17(1):17–23.

10. Goldstone LA, Goldstone J. The Norton Score: An early warning of pressure sores? J Adv Nurs. 1982;7(5):419–426.

11. Bergstrom N, Braden BJ, Laguzza A, Holman V. The Braden Scale for predicting pressure sore risk. *Nurs Res*. 1987;36(4):205–210.

12. Braden BJ, Bergstrom N. Predictive validity of the Braden Scale for pressure sore risk in a nursing home population. *Res Nurs Health*. 1994;17(6):459–470.

13. Braden BJ, Bergstrom N. Clinical utility of the Braden Scale for Predicting Pressure Sore Risk. *Decubitus*. 1989;2(3):44–46,50–51.

14. Braden B, Bergstrom N. A conceptual schema for the study of the etiology of pressure sores. *Rehabil Nurs*. 1987;12(1):8–12,16.

15. Salzberg CA, Byrne DW, Cayten CG, van Niewerburgh P, Murphy JG, Viehbeck M. A new pressure ulcer risk assessment scale for individuals with spinal cord injury. *Am J Phys Med Rehabil*. 1996;75(2):96–104.

16. Garber SL, Rintala DH, Hart KA, Fuhrer MJ. Pressure ulcer risk in spinal cord injury: Predictors of ulcer status over 3 years. *Arch Phys Med Rehabil*. 2000;81(4):465–471.

17. Harrison P, Loukras J. FOAM: a support medium for wheelchair cushions. Dow Chemical Product Development.

18. Garber SL. Wheelchair cushions for spinal cord-injured individuals. *Am J Occup Ther*. 1985;39(11):722–725.

19. Pfaff K. Seating science: pressure sensor systems and CAD/CAM technology are providing added precision in customized seating and positioning. Team Rehab Report. July-August 1993:31–33.

20. Stinson MD, Porter-Armstrong AP, Eakin PA. Pressure mapping systems: Reliability of pressure map interpreta-

tion. *Clin Rehabil*. 2003;17(5):504–511.

21. Youngstrom MJ, Brayman SJ, Anthony P, et al. Occupational therapy practice framework: domain and process. *Am J Occup Ther*. 2002;56(6):609–639.

22. Center for Medicare and Medicaid Services. Medicare coverage of power mobility devices (PMDs): power wheelchairs and power operated vehicles. US Department for Health and Human Services (HHS). Centers for Medicare and Medicaid Services. April, 2006; Publication No. 100-04:1–9.

23. Bowie MJ, Schaffer RM. Understanding ICD-9-CM: A Worksheet. Clifton Park, NY:Thomson-Delmar Learning; 2006.

24. Sine R, Liss SE, Roush RE, Holcomb JD, Wilson O. Basic Rehabilitation Techniques: A Self-Instructional Guide. Gaithersburg, Md: Aspen; 2000.

25. Richardson GM, Gardner S, Frantz RA. Nursing assessment: impact on type and cost of interventions to prevent pressure ulcers. *J Wound Ostomy Continence Nurs*. 1998;25(6):273–280.

26. Xakellis GC, Frantz R, Lewis A. Cost of pressure ulcer prevention in long-term care. *J Am Geriatr Soc*. 1995;43(5):496–501.

27. Seiler WO, Stahelin HB. Decubitus ulcers: Preventive techniques for the elderly patient. *Geriatrics*. 1985;40(7):53–60.

28. Defloor T, Grypdonck MH. Sitting posture and prevention of pressure ulcers. *Appl Nurs Res*. 1999;12(3):136–142.

29. Easton K. Gerontological Rehabilitation Nurses. Philadelphia, Pa: WB Saunders Co.; 1999.

30. Lange ML. Focus on tilt and recline systems. OT Pract. 2000;5:21–22.

31. Bliss MR, McLaren R, Exton-Smith AN. Preventing pressure sores in hospital: Controlled trial of a large-celled ripple mattress. Br Med J. 1967;1(5537):394–397.

32. Goldstone LA, Norris M, O'Reilly M, White J. A clinical trial of a bead bed system for the prevention of pressure sores in elderly orthopaedic patients. *J Adv Nurs*. 1982;7(6):545–548.

33. Jacobs MA. Comparison of capillary blood flow using a regular hospital bed mattress, ROHO mattress, and Mediscus bed. *Rehabil Nurs*. 1989;14(15):270–272.

34. Stapleton M. Preventing pressure sores: An evaluation of three products. *Geriatr Nurs (Lond)*. 1986;6(2):23–25.

35. Krouskop TA, ed. The Effect of Surface Geometry on Interface Pressures Generated by Polyurethane Foma Mattress Overlays. Houston, Tex: Institute for Rehabilitation and Research, The Rehabilitation Engineering Center; 1986.

36. Krouskop TA, Noble PS, Brown J, Marburger R. Factors affecting the pressure-distributing properties of foam mattress overlays. J Rehabil Res Dev. 1986;23(3):33–39.

37. Hedrick-Thompson J, Halloran T, Strader MK, McSweeney M. Pressure-reduction products: Making appropriate choices. *J ET Nurs*. 1993;20(6):239–244.

38. Maklebust J, Siggreen MY, Mondoux L. Pressure relief capabilities of the Sof.Care bed and the Clinitron bed. *Ostomy Wound Manage*. 1988;21:32,36–41,44.

39. Sideranko S, Quinn A, Burns K, Froman RD. Effects of position and mattress overlay on sacral and heel pressures in a clinical population. *Res Nurs Health*. 1992;15(4):245–251.

40. Allman RM, Walker JM, Hart MK, Laprade CA, Noel LB, Smith CR. Air-fluidized beds or conventional therapy for pressure sores. A randomized trial. *Ann Intern Med*. 1987;107(5):641–648.

41. Bennett RG, Bellantoni MF, Ouslander JG. Air-fluidized bed treatment of nursing home patients with pressure sores. *J Am Geriatr Soc*. 1989;37(3):235–242.

42. Jackson BS, Chagares R, Nee N, Freeman K. The effects of a therapeutic bed on pressure ulcers: an experimental study. *J Enterostomal Ther*. 1988;15(6):220–226.

43. Ferrell BA, Osterweil D, Christenson P. A randomized trial of low-air-loss beds for treatment of pressure ulcers. *JAMA*. 1993;269(4):494–497.

44. Keogh A, Dealey C. Profiling beds versus standard hospital beds: effects on pressure ulcer incidence outcomes. *J Wound Care*. 2001;10(2):15–19.

45. Gentilello L, Thompson DA, Tonnesen AS, et al. Effect of a rotating bed on the incidence of pulmonary complications in critically ill patients. *Crit Care Med*. 1988;16(8):783–786.

46. Whittemore R. Pressure-reduction support surfaces: a review of the literature. *J Wound Ostomy Continence Nurs*. 1998;25(1):6–25.

47. Reddy M, Gill SS, Rochon PA. Preventing pressure ulcers: a systematic review. JAMA. 2006;296(8):974–984.

48. Fisher K. Well-seated. *Rehab Manage*. 2006;19(3):28–30.

49. Garber SL, Dyerly LR. Wheelchair cushions for persons with spinal cord injury: an update. Am J Occup Ther. 1991;45(6):550–554.

50. Swaine JM. Seeing the difference: Interface pressure mapping displays a new view for wheelchair cushion selection. Rehab Manage. 2003;16:26,28,30–31.

51. Walls G. Choosing the right cushion: when selecting the most effective wheelchair cushion, different materials should be considered with the guidance of an experienced seating team. Rehab Manage. 2002;15:32–36.

52. Morress C. Bottom up or top down?: An occupation-based approached to seating. OT Practice. 2006;11(16):13–17.

53. Fitzgerald SG, Thorman T, Cooper R, Cooper RA. Evaluating wheelchair cushions: the variety of types and the absence of standards make choosing the right cushion no easy feat. *Rehab Manage*. 2001;14:42, 44–5.

54. Collins F. Seating: assessment and selection. J Wound Care. 2004;9–12.

55. Bibow M. Under your skin. New Mobility. 1996:32–33.

56. Foster P. Behavioral treatment of urinary incontinence: a complementary approach. Ostomy Wound Manage. 1998;44(6):62–70.

57. Eustice S, Roe B, Paterson J. Prompted voiding for the management of urinary incontinence in adults. *Cochrane Database Syst Rev*. 2000(2):CD002113.

58. Dinsdale SM. Decubitus ulcers: role of pressure and friction in causation. *Arch Phys Med Rehabil*. 1974;55(4):147–152.

59. Bates-Jensen BM, Vredevoe DL, Brecht ML. Validity and reliability of the Pressure Sore Status Tool. *Decubitus*. 1992;5(6):20–28.

60. Cuddigan J, Frantz RA. Pressure ulcer research: Pressure ulcer treatment. A monograph from the National Pressure Ulcer Advisory Panel. *Adv Wound Care*. 1998;11(6):294–300.

Support Surfaces: Tissue Integrity, Terms, Principles, and Choice

Cynthia Ann Fleck, RN, BSN, MBA, APN/CNS, ET/WOCN, CWS, CFCN, DNC;
Stephen Sprigle, PhD, PT

Objectives

The reader will be challenged to:

- Analyze the classes of support surfaces and their characteristics
- Appraise the 5 extrinsic risk factors that can be affected by a support surface
- Select support surfaces specific to patient needs.

Introduction

In the pursuit of prevention and management of skin and tissue breakdown, support surface selection remains an important decision for the clinician. Pressure ulcers are caused by a myriad of intrinsic and extrinsic factors. *Support surfaces can have significant influence over extrinsic factors, such as pressure, shear, friction, moisture, and temperature.* These factors directly impact deformation of the soft tissue, blood flow, tissue ischemia and necrosis, and pressure ulcer development, especially in the immobile patient. The manner by which support surfaces manage these extrinsic factors can be used by clinicians as they select support surfaces for their patients.

By definition, pressure ulcers are caused by localized pressure, which deforms soft tissue and occludes capillaries causing ischemia, which can lead to cell and tissue death.[1,2] Clinicians typically use the term "pressure" to reflect normal pressure or interface pressure—the force-per-unit area that acts perpendicular to the tissue. The forces that result in normal pressure on the tissues are typically due to gravity: body weight is resting on the supporting surface. With respect to support surfaces, this normal loading may be the most significant but not the only force that impacts tissue integrity.

While commonly used together, shear and frictional forces are not the same thing, but both can contribute to pressure ulcer development. Friction is a force that opposes the movement of 2 bodies in contact, such as the sliding of the buttocks on a bed surface. The term "shear"

Fleck CA, Sprigle S. Support surfaces: tissue integrity, terms, principles, and choice. In: Krasner DL, ed. *Chronic Wound Care: The Essentials*. Malvern, Pa: HMP Communications, 2014:243–258.

can refer to either shear stress—the force acting tangentially on an area of an object—or shear strain—the deformation of an object in response to shear stresses. With respect to support surfaces, shear strain results from all the forces that cause the deformation of the body's tissues, including normal, shear, and frictional forces. Shear stress on tissue has been documented as adversely affecting tissue integrity.[3–6]

Moisture and temperature can also increase the risk of skin breakdown. The ability of a support surface to dissipate heat affects the temperature and moisture of the buttock tissues. Moisture and temperature are often linked because an increase in temperature typically results in moist skin through sweating. Obviously, many other sources of moisture and wetness can put skin at risk. Increasing evidence suggests that an increase in tissue temperature increases tissue's susceptibility to pressure ulcers.[7,8] Furthermore, any increase of moisture, whether from sweating or another source, will increase the coefficient of friction of the skin.[9,10] Excessive moisture can also macerate tissue, resulting in a reduced ability to withstand external forces.

Various clinical strategies exist to manage these extrinsic factors, especially for patients exhibiting the 2 greatest risk factors for pressure ulcers: lack of mobility and lack of sensation. Turning and repositioning are the most effective ways to counteract impaired mobility. However, the accepted protocol of turning and repositioning a patient every 2 hours may not be enough.[11] An individualized care plan must be developed that includes support surfaces as integral components to prevention and management of pressure ulcers.

The purposes and indications for use of a support surface are to prevent skin breakdown in the immobile and high-risk patient, to prevent further breakdown, to promote healing and granulation in the patient with an existing wound, and to address pain management and comfort issues in patients experiencing chronic pain (eg, end-stage cancer). Fortunately, a wide variety of surfaces are available. While clinicians cannot be expected to know everything about every product, an understanding of how to judge support surface performance and of the different options will result in a more informed selection.

Considerations When Selecting Support Surfaces

In 1995, Krouskop and van Rijswijk[12] gathered pressure ulcer experts to determine and identify important features that reflect support surface performance and usability. The list included:
- Redistribution of pressure
- Moisture control
- Temperature control
- Patient and product friction control
- Infection control
- Flammability
- Life expectancy
- Fail safety
- Product service requirements.

One can readily see the extrinsic risk factors along with other important and practical criteria. This chapter will discuss many of these criteria in hopes of defining the various tradeoffs in performance that are inherent to the selection of support surfaces.

Redistribution of Pressure

The damaging effects of pressure on the body depend on both the magnitude and duration of that pressure.[13] The body can withstand higher pressures for shorter amounts of time. This relationship drives the design of active support surfaces as well as clinical turning schedules.

Many researchers have attempted to determine the pressures at which tissue ischemia occurs with widely varying results. Some studies related measures of blood pressure to blood flow occlusion[14–17] and others documented differences in occlusion pressures in the presence and absence of shear forces.[4,5] Taking these results together, one can deduce that the pressures needed to cause ischemia differ from person to person and from body site to body site. If one accepts this conclusion, pressure ulcer prevention strategies must become more individualistic and reflect the current understanding of clinical and physiological situations that influence the load-bearing integrity of tissues.

Envelopment is the ability of a support surface to conform around the contours of the body to redistribute pressure. The ability of a support surface to envelop the body can be adversely impacted by the surface tension of the material or cover. A low surface tension environment will allow the surface to deform and the engaging body to sink in, accommodating bony prominences and displacing body weight. The surface should deform, not the body and soft tissues. Surface tension can be increased by tight bed linens or support surface cover.

Determining if a support surface offers adequate pressure distribution is difficult. Regular monitoring of localized, post-ischemic erythema is always required. The measurement of interface pressures is one approach that is gaining in popularity. This is a simple, noninvasive method of comparing and determining the force-per-unit area that acts between the body and the support surface. The approach typically uses an array of pressure sensors between the subject and the support surface. While a detailed description of interface pressure measurement is beyond the scope of this chapter, a few important issues should be remembered.

Clinicians should concentrate on the interface pressures under bony prominences that are more at-risk for pressure ulcer development. One must remember, however, that pressures are dependent on the position in bed, so the measurements should ideally be repeated in supine and side lying as well as in other positions commonly adopted by the patient. Finally, since these devices measure interface pressure, the interface between the person and surface must reflect clinical use. If a person typically lies upon a towel, incontinence pad or "chux," or multiple fabrics, these should be in place during measurement as they, most likely, will affect the pressures on the body.

Patient and product friction control. As previously mentioned, the presence of shear impacts the tissue's ability to withstand pressures. However, because friction cannot be avoided, clinicians must assess the impact on the specific patient. Some support surfaces and covers are manufactured with material that is inherently low in friction, which may prove beneficial to the person. However, some patients may be adversely impacted by very low friction surfaces if they hinder sitting up in bed, transferring, or bed mobility.

Temperature and moisture control. Excessive skin moisture and temperature are contributors to tissue damage. Temperature and moisture are often linked because an increase in body surface temperature leads to sweating, which elevates mois-

ture. Maintaining normal skin temperature and moisture may be important in certain patients to preserve skin integrity.

Support surfaces dissipate heat and moisture with varying abilities. Surfaces made from foam tend to elevate temperatures more than those topped with gel or a viscous fluid. Air cushions are hard to judge since their impermeable cover has a huge impact on temperature. Some support surfaces are designed to exchange air, which permit more temperature and moisture control. A person's activity on a cushion also impacts temperature. Regular movement helps dissipate heat from the body-support surface interface. A judicious clinical guideline follows: if a person regularly sweats on a particular surface, others should be investigated.

As stated, moisture can result from sweating and many other sources. Support surface covers have a huge impact on how this moisture is managed. Cushions that permit airflow via a breathable cover and cushioning material are better able to dissipate moisture than cushions that do not. Some "incontinence" covers are breathable: they are made from fabric that prevents water passage but allows airflow. These have advantages over covers that block both air and water flow but at a higher cost.

Support Surface Categories

The many designs of support surfaces complicate simple groupings or categorization. By definition, all support surfaces must meet a medical need, as do all types of durable medical equipment. One simple manner to divide support surfaces is active and reactive surfaces.

Reactive support surfaces redistribute pressures by deflecting or deforming in response to the load from the body. The goal of these surfaces is to allow the body to immerse, thereby accommodating the bony prominences by increasing the contact area between the body and support surface. By definition, increasing contact area will reduce overall pressure given a constant body weight. The different materials used in support surfaces redistribute pressures a little differently as will be discussed later in the chapter. Reactive surfaces can be powered or non-powered.

Active support surfaces purposely offload or re-direct forces away from the areas of the body.

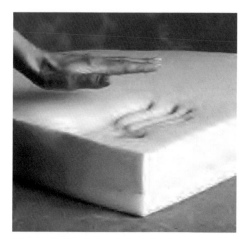

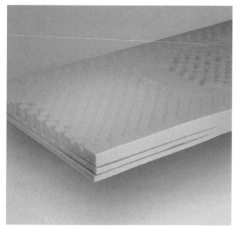

Figure 1. Example of viscoelastic or "memory" foam.

Figure 2. Example of a foam overlay.

Typically, these surfaces are comprised of compartments, which alternatively reduce loading on one or more areas thereby supporting the body on the remaining compartments. These are powered systems that have pumps, blowers, or some other electro-mechanical system.

Support surfaces may or may not be combined with a bed frame and associated hardware. Overlays are designed to be placed directly on top of an existing mattress. Mattress replacements are designed to be placed on the bed frame. Different features can be incorporated into overlays, replacements, and full bed systems that define their use and performance. Some of the more common features include low air loss, alternating pressure, air fluidized, and lateral rotation. The National Pressure Ulcer Advisory Panel offers the following definitions of each feature.[18]

Low air-loss systems provide airflow to assist in managing the microclimate (moisture and heat) of the skin. Support surfaces with alternating pressure provide pressure redistribution via cyclic changes in loading and unloading as characterized by frequency, duration, amplitude, and rate of change parameter. Air fluidized systems provide pressure redistribution by means of a fluid-like medium created by forcing air through beads as characterized by immersion and envelopment. Lateral rotation systems provide rotation about a longitudinal axis as characterized by degree of patient turn, duration, and frequency.

The use of support surfaces can be organized into 2 distinct purposes with respect to pressure ulcers: prevention and treatment. *Overall, surfaces designed for prevention tend to be of a simpler design. Prevention surfaces can be reactive or active. Some are single material surfaces, but a few incorporate combinations of materials. Surfaces designed for patients with pressure ulcers, most often, severe ulcers, can also be active or reactive but exhibit more complex designs to provide advanced performance.*

Overlays. Overlays are placed directly on top of existing hospital or home care mattresses and are available in foam, air, gel, viscous fluid, water, or some combination of these materials. They range in height, usually up to 4 inches.

Foam overlays. Several characteristics of foam are important for effective pressure redistribution, such as base height, density, and indentation force deflection.[19] Base height refers to the height of the foam from the base to where the convolutions begin. Density is the weight per cubic foot (the amount of foam in a product) and reflects the foam's ability to support a subject's weight. Indentation force deflection (IFD) is a measurement of stiffness and is determined by the number of pounds required to indent a sample of foam with a circular plate to a depth of 25% of the thickness of the foam. Indentation force deflection reflects foam's ability to deflect and conform to distribute the subject's body weight.

CHRONIC WOUND CARE: The Essentials

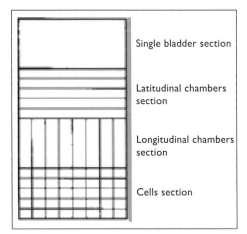
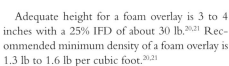

Single bladder section

Latitudinal chambers section

Longitudinal chambers section

Cells section

Figure 3. Air cell/chamber configurations.

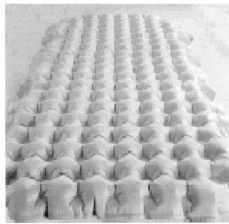

Figure 4. Example of an air-filled non-powered overlay.

Adequate height for a foam overlay is 3 to 4 inches with a 25% IFD of about 30 lb.[20,21] Recommended minimum density of a foam overlay is 1.3 lb to 1.6 lb per cubic foot.[20,21]

Foam products, including overlays and mattress replacements, can be comprised of various types of foam. In a general sense, foam can be divided into elastic or viscoelastic.[18] Elastic foam acts like a spring. It deflects in proportion to the load applied to it. As previously mentioned, the amount of deflection per unit force defines the stiffness of foam. Like a spring, elastic foam has resilience, so it will recover once the load is removed. Viscoelastic foam has time-dependent qualities, so it deflects in relation to both the load applied and the rate of that loading (Figure 1). Viscoelastic foam exhibits creep and stress relaxation and thus has much less resilience than elastic foam. In other words, it relaxes after being compressed, so it does not push back against the skin. However, this advantageous feature has a tradeoff. The creep characteristics of viscoelastic foam also make it susceptible to bottoming out. Many foam products use a combination of elastic and viscoelastic foam to take advantage of the respective benefits of each.

The manufacture's guidelines should state the body weight limit and the estimated length of use for a foam overlay. It may be advantageous to pressure map new foam products. This process of pressure mapping should continue at regular intervals to determine their ability to offer effective pressure reduction. This offers a practical means to determine whether the product meets performance claims throughout the warranty period.

Advantages of foam overlays include cost effectiveness (one time patient charge), no set-up cost, low maintenance, portability, light weight, availability in many sizes, and ability to be customized (Figure 2).

Disadvantages of foam overlays include limited life span; absorption of fluids from incontinence, perspiration, and exudate; infection control issues (if not covered by plastic protective covers); weight limit; disposal problems, which create environmental concerns (is there the ability to recycle?); single patient use; and lack of effectiveness.[22]

Air overlays. Air overlays can be described as non-powered and powered. Non-powered overlays are designed so that air is enclosed in interconnected air cells, a single bladder, or latitudinal or longitudinal tubes (Figure 3 and 4).[23] These systems can be comprised of multitude zones to address different bony prominences (ie, occiput, scapulae, sacrum, and heels) or as a single bladder system that is more likely to cause peak pressures. The more resolution a product has, the more likely it will reduce and evenly distribute pressures. In addition, pressure and pain reduction is contingent upon adequate immersion of the body into such a product.

Powered alternating pressure (AP) overlays

consist of columns or chambers of air that are alternately inflated and deflated by an air pump. The air pressure fluctuates as one column or chamber inflates and another deflates, creating areas of low and high pressure. These systems work on the theory that while one area of the body might be experiencing a high peak pressure, another area has a very low pressure. As these areas inflate and deflate at specific intervals, this creates an environment for reactive hyperemia. Published studies on the efficacy of AP overlays report conflicting results; some show effectiveness, while others do not.[24-26]

Advantages of air overlays include ease of cleaning, durability, ease of repair, portability and light weight, cost effectiveness, low maintenance, ability to adjust to individual patient, ability to synthesize fluid without the weight, provision of custom environment for each bony prominence by zoned products, and provision of distribution of pressures by products with greater resolution.

Disadvantage of air overlays include requirement of electricity for powered products; limited use of dynamic/battery-powered products during power failures; high risk of damage by sharp objects; necessity of set up and monitoring to determine proper inflation and adjustment; environmental concerns caused by disposal problems (is there the ability to recycle?).

Water overlays. Water-filled overlays are polyvinyl bladders that are filled with water. The theory behind water beds and overlays is that of Pascal's law, which states, "The weight of a body floating on a fluid system is evenly distributed over the entire supporting system."[27] However, by encasing water in a bladder, the patient does not realize total immersion and could suffer from high pressure forces due to hammocking and uneven distribution of pressure. The engaging body should displace the water without bottoming out.

Advantages of water overlays include cost effectiveness, ease of cleaning, and coolness in temperature.

Disadvantages of water overlays include heavy weight; inability to raise the head of the bed unless the mattress has separate compartments; potential to be over- or under-filled; water temperature becoming too cold without a heater; motion of fluid may be undesirable to patients and unstable for procedures, such as CPR; potential to

be punctured, which may also present a safety hazard; and possible hammock effect.

Mattress replacements. These products are designed to take the place of standard hospital mattresses while providing more pressure reduction compared to standard mattresses. They are placed directly on the existing bed frame. Mattress replacements vary in design and medium. Most are constructed of foam, gel, air, water, or some combination of these materials. Those comprised of foam may have layers and combinations of different densities of foam for various areas of the body.

The base height of a foam mattress replacement should be 5 inches or greater.[28] The density of a mattress replacement is between 1.35 lb and 1.8 lb per cubic foot.[28] A 25% IFD between 25 lb and 35 lb is recommended.[28] Mattress replacements are usually covered with durable, waterproof, bacteriostatic covers similar to standard hospital mattresses.

For all mattress replacements, the manufacturer's guidelines should be consulted for maximum weight of the engaging patient as well as the life span of the product. Most mattress replacements hold a warranty that is between 2 and 5 years. Some warranties are as long as 5 to 10 years or lifetime warranties. *It may be advantageous to date each mattress (with an indelible marker) and pressure map new foam products upon delivery. Pressure mapping should continue at regular intervals as the mattress replacement ages to determine the product's ability to offer effective pressure reduction throughout its life.* This procedure will also offer a practical way to determine whether the product meets its stated warranty/guarantee and, in the long run, save the facility money.

Some mattress replacements need to be turned and flipped over periodically while others should not be turned or flipped due to their compositions. To keep the warranty intact, it is important to know and understand the manufacturer's requirements.

Purchasing of mattress replacements typically requires a large capital expenditure by the institution. Some people hypothesize that renting support surfaces reduces costs and utilization, but some studies refute that belief. One randomized, controlled clinical trial with economic evaluation by Inman and colleagues concluded that purchas-

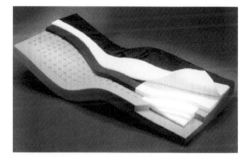

Figure 5. Example of a multidensity foam mattress replacement.

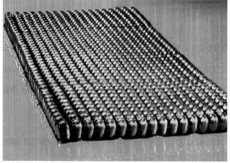

Figure 6. Example of a reactive non-powered overlay.

ing options were more cost effective for their facility.[29] Clark also advocated the purchase of foam mattress replacement systems in lieu of standard hospital mattresses in his 650-bed hospital study.[30]

Advantages of mattress replacements include low maintenance requirements, theoretical reduction in the use of pressure reduction overlays, multiple patient use, and provision of automatic pressure reduction.

Disadvantages of mattress replacements include high initial expense to purchase, potential for delay in obtaining more appropriate level of support surface, possibility of not performing as desired throughout the life expectancy of the product, and potential disposal issues.

Figure 5 shows an example of a multidensity foam mattress replacement.

Reactive, non-powered advanced systems. These support surfaces typically rely on a combination of materials to better redistribute pressures. Both overlays and mattress replacements may fall under this category. These advanced systems do not require electricity to operate, and some designs exhibit a low surface tension, allowing the surface to conform to any shape; thereby, the product deforms to accommodate bony prominences (Figure 6). This allows for maximum surface contact and equalization of pressure. Additionally, these systems are designed to provide low friction and shear due to the consistency of their medium.

Non-powered, air-filled surfaces offer zoned, adjustable environments that can be customized to the body shape and bony prominences of the subject. Unlike a single bladder support surface, this zoned approach minimizes the chance of

bottoming out and allows pressure to be adjusted for each body segment. These products may be rented or purchased.

Advantages of reactive, non-powered, advanced support surfaces include no need for electricity; convenient rental agreement secures set-up, service, and pickup; less expensive than most other therapeutic systems; easy set-up, use, cleaning, and maintenance; durability and ease of repair; air-filled products are adjustable, zoned, and can be customized to each individual patient and body segment; assimilate well into care environment, with no noise that may agitate patients; no need for storage or disposal of existing mattresses if an overlay is used; multiple patient use is possible; and air-filled products are light weight and portable. With air-filled products, individual sections can be replaced without replacing the entire support surface, and customization is possible by adding an air-flow module for moisture and temperature control or a bariatric kit for obese patients.

Disadvantages of non-powered viscous fluid or gel beds include heaviness and necessity for periodic kneading to address movement of gel and bottom-out potential. With air-filled products, regular monitoring to determine proper adjustment is required and the risk of puncture necessitates caution in use; regular assessment to prevent bottoming out is necessary. Other disadvantages include the necessity to store the existing mattress if a mattress replacement is used and potential daily rental fees, which can increase overall costs in addition to the possibility of the gel becoming hardened and causing pressure in a cold environment or storage situation.

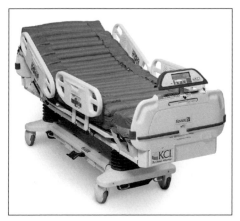

Figure 7. Example of a fully integrated low air-loss system.

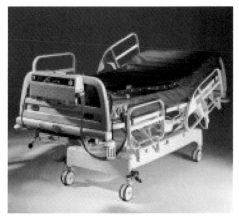

Figure 8. Example of an alternating pressure mattress replacement.

Advanced Features of Powered Support Surfaces

Low air-loss therapy. ***These support surfaces enhance air circulation or flow for improved moisture and temperature control (microclimate) in addition to providing low interface pressures.*** They should provide diffuse airflow through the top and across the entire support surface, which directly or indirectly interfaces with the patient. One study defines "true" low air loss as an air flotation support surface capable of dissipating a minimum of 200 g of moisture per 24 hours from the patient-bed boundary via a continuous flow of fresh air in sufficient proximity and volume so that the body can regulate skin temperature through heat evaporation.[31] The National Pressure Ulcer Advisory Panel's (NPUAP) Support Surface Initiative has criteria for low air-loss and moisture dissipation. The widest variety of support surface products falls into this category, so extra care should be taken in product selection, and attention to design and performance is suggested.

Low air-loss products are comprised of connected air pillows that are supplied with a predetermined amount of continuous airflow that is supplied by a pump. This airflow can be controlled to provide low interface pressure as well as moisture and temperature control. The clinician should consider whether the product is comprised of a single bladder or a zoned environment.

Low air-loss support surfaces are available as overlays, mattress replacements, and full bed sys-

tems (Figure 7). They may be rented or purchased.

Advantages of low-air loss include provision of moisture and temperature control; possible customization for each individual patient depending on number of zones and adjustment features in pump/blower; potential convenience of rental agreement, which secures set-up, service, and pickup; disposal or storage of an existing mattress is not necessary, if mattress overlay is used; and durability and ease of repair.

Disadvantages of low air-loss include use of electricity, which is a hidden expense;[32] limited use of dynamic/battery-powered products during power failures; noisy motors; daily rental fees, which can increase overall costs; inability to accommodate very obese patients in some circumstances; larger-than-standard sizes are not always available; storage of an existing mattress may be necessary; and full-bed (specialty bed) systems are the most costly of low air-loss support surfaces.

Evidence indicates that low air-loss surfaces have been shown to improve prevention and treatment outcomes compared to conventional treatment and non-powered foam alternatives.[25,33]

Powered flotation and alternating pressure. ***These are powered mattress replacement products characterized by air pumps or blowers, which provide either sequential inflation and deflation of the air cells or a low interface pressure throughout the mattress*** (Figure 8).

Powered flotation systems vary in the height of the air chambers and proximity of the air chambers to one another, and air pressure provides adequate patient lift, reduces pressure, and prevents bottoming out.

Alternating pressure mattresses vary widely in design and performance. The number of cells, their inflated and deflated height, and the frequency of air cycling can impact performance. This wide variation may explain the conflicting results of research into AP technology.[25,33]

Fleurence used a modeling approach to assess cost effectiveness of alternating pressure mattresses and overlays and showed that they were more cost effective for the treatment of superficial and severe pressure ulcers and prevention of pressure ulcers, respectively, than standard hospital mattresses.[26]

Advantages of powered flotation and alternating pressure include convenience of rental agreements, which secure set-up, service, and pickup; ability to use with multiple patients; and durability and ease of repair.

Disadvantages of powered flotation and alternating pressure include use of electricity, which is a hidden expense; noisy motors; limited use of dynamic/battery-powered products during power failures; daily rental fees (if leased), which can increase overall costs; inability to accommodate very obese patients in some cases; larger-than-standard sizes are not available; and storage of an existing mattress may be necessary.

Air-fluidized or high air-loss systems. **These products employ the circulation of filtered air through silicone-coated ceramic beads creating the characteristics of fluid** (Figure 9).[18,34] This technology is comprised of small silicone-coated beads in a tank-like environment that is covered by a permeable sheet. The ceramic beads become dynamic when a high rate of airflow is forced through them, allowing the patient to float on the sheet with two-thirds of the body immersed and enveloped in the beads.[35]

Air-fluidized systems are utilized to manage large amounts of excessive skin and wound moisture as well as burns and provide a low friction and shear environment. High airflow against the skin and tissue can dry moist wound dressings and desiccate the wound bed. An occlusive wound dressing or non-permeable under pad may be utilized or another form of therapeutic support surface may need to be investigated if

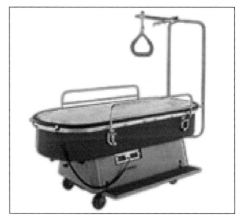

Figure 9. Example of an air-fluidized bed system.

these challenges exist. Air-fluidized beds are the heaviest and most costly of the therapeutic support surfaces.

High air-loss bed systems circulate and warm the room air, which may cause heat accumulation and increased room temperature. Air-fluidized beds are not recommended for patients with pulmonary disease or with unstable spines due to the inability to raise the head of the bed and the relative instability of the surface.

Although some evidence indicates that high air-loss beds enhance pressure ulcer healing rates,[36] occipital and calcaneous skin resting surface interface pressure may remain sufficient to occlude capillary perfusion. Occipital and calcaneous ulcers have been reported to develop in patients while on the high air-loss surfaces.[37] These systems have traditionally been recommended as a last resort, if all else fails, and for patients with burns, tissue grafts and flaps, or multiple Stage III and Stage IV pressure ulcers; however, recent research suggests that less costly pressure-relieving support surfaces (ie, non-powered pressure reducing systems and low air-loss systems) can be used with an equal therapeutic benefit.[38,39]

Advantages of air-fluidized beds include ability to manage high volumes of excessive skin and wound moisture; maintenance of low friction and shear environment; convenience of rental agreement, which secures set-up, service, and pickup; and ability to provide pain reduction in some patients.

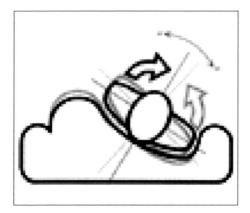

Figure 10. Schematic of lateral rotation.

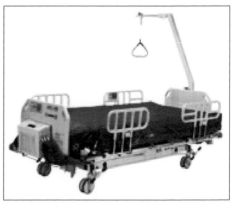

Figure 11. Example of a bariatric low air-loss bed system.

Disadvantages of air-fluidized beds include expensive rental or purchasing fees; potential dehydration of patients by the continuous warm, dry air circulation; difficulty of transfers and bedside care due to tank's edge; inability to raise head of bed, which may require the use of foam wedges, which in turn may interrupt therapy; difficulty moving product due to size and weight (1,600 lb or more), which may not be appropriate for certain environments (ie, home care); potential expense of electricity; and potential adverse side effects, such as corneal abrasions.

Alternative hybrid air-fluidized and low air-loss combination products have been developed to decrease the disadvantages of air-fluidized therapy, making it more acceptable to both the patient and the clinician.

Hybrid support surfaces. **Hybrid support surfaces offer combinations of low air-loss and kinetic or percussion therapies, alternating pressure, or air-fluidized and low air-loss therapies.**

The combination of low air-loss and air-fluidized therapies offers the ability to effectively raise and lower the head of the bed while maintaining air-fluidized therapy, as the upper one-third of the system is comprised of low air-loss therapy and the lower two-thirds of air-fluidized therapy.

Lateral rotation. **Lateral rotation offers rotation from side to side about a longitudinal axis as characterized by degree of patient turn, duration, and frequency** (Figure 10). It is believed to provide passive pulmonary secretion mobilization thus decreasing complications of immobility, such as

atelectasis and pneumonia; preventing deep vein thrombosis and pulmonary emboli due to venous stasis; and reducing urinary tract infections by preventing urinary stasis. Lateral rotation does not take the place of turning and repositioning the patient. It can be intrusive and unpleasant to the patient due to the continual movement.

Bariatric support surfaces. Obese patients, defined as those having a larger than average body mass index (>40 body mass index [BMI]), may need a bariatric support surface to provide safety and protection. These special bed frames and surfaces are generally wider, utilize a reinforced frame, have side rails that tilt outward, feature a built-in scale, and offer a chair feature that allows the head of the bed to be put at a 45-degree angle and the foot of the bed to be positioned directly down.

Special non-powered or low air-loss therapeutic overlays or mattress replacements can be added to address the obese patient's pressure, shear, friction, and moisture issues (Figure 11). An important caveat for all support surfaces is ascertaining the patient weight limit of that particular product. This is particularly true for bariatric systems.

Continuity of Care

Support surface needs should be considered along the continuum of care. Pressure reduction in the seated position, whether in a wheelchair, geriatric chair, easy chair, or automobile, is sometimes even more important since the seated posture dramatically decreases the surface area over which the engaging body is in contact. In the

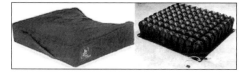

Figure 12. Examples of therapeutic seat cushion support surfaces.

seated position, approximately 70% of the body's weight is distributed over a small area of space. Three bony prominences, the sacrum, coccyx, and bilateral ischial tuberosities (ITs), further increase the likelihood of pressure ulcer development in the seated position. Approximately 47% of pressure ulcers occur on these 3 areas.[40] *If the patient sits upright, the care plan should reflect the need for a pressure reduction seat cushion comprised of air, foam, gel, or a combination of these mediums (Figure 12). Likewise, a plan for weight shifts should be incorporated, allowing blood flow to reach the occluded area.*

Other areas of pressure-reduction concern include stretchers, gurneys, operating room and exam tables, as well as managing tissue loads at the heel. The pressure ulcer incidence of intraoperatively acquired pressure ulcers has been reported to be as low as 12% and as high as 66%.[41] By utilizing an effective pressure-reduction device in the operating room, pressure ulcer incidence can be decreased to 3%–8%.[28] A patient who is at risk for pressure ulcers can develop breakdown as a result of pressure, shear, and friction from these surfaces, depending on the duration of use and procedure being done.

Heels provide a particular dilemma in that they not only present a penetrating bony prominence and a thin layer of subcutaneous fat tissue,[42] they can additionally present with compromised circulation, further complicating their risk for breakdown.

Unacceptable products that should be avoided for pressure redistribution include those comprised of sheepskin (genuine or synthetic), 2-inch foam "egg crate" type overlays or cushions, and invalid rings or "donut-type" cushions. These measures constitute comfort measures only.

Practice Setting, Clinician, Cost, and Patient Considerations

Practice environment criteria. Choosing support surfaces for facilities, agencies, and home care settings should involve an interprofessional team approach. Although team members may vary depending on the setting, team members should generally include all interested and knowledgeable participants in the patient's plan of care. Headed up by a specialist with expertise in wound management and skin care, the committee should include, but not be limited to, staff nurses from various clinical areas, a materials management and/or purchasing member, an infection control professional, a seating and positioning professional (ie, physical and/or occupational therapist), a member of the financial management staff or administrator, and a case manager or discharge planner.

No single support surface has the ability to address all of the institution's requirements. Rather, a range of categories should be available to speak to both preventative and therapeutic needs. The following questions should be considered when selecting support surfaces for an agency:

• What are the collective needs of the patient population?
• Does the institution or department deal with high-acuity, high-risk, critically ill patients?
• Do patients exhibit any unique needs?
• What size are the patients?
• What extrinsic risk factors are causing the breakdown?
• What is the pressure ulcer prevalence rate?
• What is the nosocomial pressure ulcer incidence rate?

Prevalence and incidence rates will help isolate areas of high risk and provide a big-picture view of patient and institutional need. An institution with a wide variety of patients will require several support surfaces.

Other concerns within the institution and home involve questions regarding who will set up and operate the devices. Are company personnel available 24 hours a day, 7 days a week? Are the products simple to use? How is the product maintained or disposed? Is the support surface durable and repairable? Is it easy to clean? Who will clean it? How about infection control issues? Are special linens necessary?

Cost is another matter to consider. Questions, such as, "How much does the product cost?" and "Are there additional associated costs, such as electrical power consumption?" are of supreme importance. Another item to deal with is how a power failure will be addressed. Some support surfaces are available for rental and others for purchase. Factors, such as clinician's time and ease of repair and service, are of extreme significance. A rental agreement addresses the indirect cost of staff time to set-up, maintain, periodically check, and discontinue support surfaces. The cost of rental and purchase should be factored. Many preventative support surfaces are a one-time purchase item. This can be of particular importance to a large facility that may need to consider capital budget concerns.

Manufacturer and provider information should be collected from the companies supplying the support surfaces. The company's reputation for service, set-up time, delivery, and availability should be further investigated. Ask for a list of independent clinicians who are willing to discuss their experiences with the product considered. Other important questions include: Is service adequate? What is the corresponding warranty/guarantee? What type of clinical education support is provided? Is there independent clinical research available to determine product effectiveness and interface pressure measurement? An evaluation plan should be developed that includes a trial period.

Patient-needs criteria. After the practice environment issues have been addressed, selection of those specific support surfaces for individual patients must be made. Development of an institution or facility protocol for both prevention and treatment of pressure ulcers and use of specific support surfaces should then be developed. Bergstom and her colleagues reported that support surface choice established by classifying patients using a pressure ulcer risk assessment, such as the Braden Scale, created both successful and cost-effective outcomes.[43] Risk-based prescription of support surfaces has also been shown cost effective by others.[29] Algorithms, decision trees, and decision guidelines are often useful. First and foremost, goals need to be established for each patient. The goals for treatment of a pressure ulcer of a young, newly injured, quadriplegic patient may be different from our goals for

treatment of a pressure ulcer of an end-stage lung cancer patient.

Several factors should be investigated when considering support surfaces specific to patient need. The patient's risk assessment, overall condition, and disease process should be taken into account as well as his or her mobility, sensory perception, and pain the patient experience. Does the disease process or current therapy dictate the necessity to place the patient in certain positions? The ability to customize the support surface, no matter what position the patient takes, is important, as is the ability to adjust to each individual body segment. In what types of activities does the patient participate? Are there activities of daily living that could be contributing to the pressure, shear, friction, and moisture factors that encourage pressure ulcers? What about the patient's support surface needs? Are they short term or long term? Is this a product that the patient might need for a chronic condition or for the rest of his life? In the case of a home care patient, is the home environment suited for the space, size, and structural needs of the support surface?

A therapeutic support surface can additionally be used as an adjunct to pain management. Redistributing pressure from the body's frame, as well as managing heat and moisture, offer comfort and relief to patients experiencing chronic pain. Conformation to the body's contours helps to equalize soft tissue pressure, diminish ischemia, promote healthy blood flow, and can decrease the experience of pain. Dallum and her associates showed that pain was significantly lower in patients using support surfaces for pressure reduction.[44]

The patient's reimbursement source is of paramount importance when choosing a support surface. For example, Medicare Part B has distinctive medical policy coverage and payment rules, which dictate coverage criteria for specific support surfaces. Documentation is therefore critical. Does the support surface meet the criteria for the patient's insurance, reimbursement, or private pay? Can the patient afford a co-pay in the case of Medicare B and some private insurance? Will the support surface be available in the next healthcare setting? In other words, is it portable? How about any hidden costs, such as electricity, the patient will incur?

Important matters to consider when using support surfaces include pressure and time, so turning and repositioning the patient continues to be paramount. *Despite support surface use, patients still need to be turned and repositioned according to protocol, or at a minimum of every 1 to 2 hours, no matter how effective the surface.* Kosiak postulated that turning and repositioning take place at 1- to 2-hour intervals based on his study of healthy subjects.[45] Keep in mind, the elderly with less resilient skin may not be able to tolerate a single position for 2 hours without damage. This protocol should therefore be customized to each patient. Range of motion and prevention of contractures and other problems is not accomplished by any surface, so good care must prevail.

A minimum of linen and incontinence pad use is recommended with every support surface. The closer the patient body is to the therapy (the support surface), the better the product will be able to prevent and heal ulcers. Layering of multiple or tight linens and incontinent pads is not suggested. Finally, checking for "bottoming out" or "hitting bottom" on a support surface should be ascertained on a regular basis. The patient's body must be immersed, yet float or be suspended in the surface. If not, a part of his or her body (usually the trunk and/or pelvis) can sink to the bottom of the product with no medium between the body and the surface. A simple hand check can be done by placing one's hand between the patient's bony prominences and the surface, making certain there is "wiggle room," or enough depth to support the patient's body.

Conclusion

Support surface selection will continue to challenge the healthcare provider until we develop a ubiquitous master plan of criteria that consistently demonstrates excellent outcomes. This is currently in the works as the NPUAP Support Surface Initiative; a group of interested parties (clinical personnel, manufacturers, scientists, and researchers) are currently developing consistent language, terminology and definitions, and life span and tissue integrity management criteria. The state of the science for determining support surface product effectiveness is growing with the addition of high-tech interface pressure mapping, laser Doppler blood velocimetry, and transcutaneous oxygen tension measurement. The process of support surface selection continues to be refined and clarified as more is discovered about gauging effectiveness. Further outcome-focused research on the relative effectiveness of specific support surfaces is needed.

It is important to consider that support surfaces are only one component of a comprehensive pressure ulcer treatment plan. If the ulcer(s) does not show progress toward healing, the entire care plan should be reevaluated before the support surface is changed. Accordingly, it is important for the clinician to be aware of support surface categories and decision-making factors in order to make an informed and effective choice.

Take-Home Messages for Practice

- Support surfaces are specialized devices for pressure redistribution designed for management of tissue loads, microclimate, and/or other therapeutic functions.

- External pressure, especially over the bony prominences, has been identified as the major etiology in pressure ulcer development. Additional associated origins consist of the degree of shear and friction forces and the further effects of temperature and moisture. All of these factors can be affected by, and are correlated to, the characteristics of the support surface selected for an individual.

- Support surface selection is one of many important decisions the clinician and team must assess, plan, implement, evaluate, and discuss.

Self-Assessment Questions:

1. A support surface can affect all of the following EXCEPT:
   A. Pressure
   B. Shear
   C. Albumin level
   D. Moisture

2. Support surfaces include:
   A. Beds and mattresses
   B. Seat cushions
   C. Operating room tables
   D. All of the above

3. An immobile patient at high risk for pressure ulcers who requires good microclimate control would be best treated on which type of support surface:
   A. Low air-loss mattress or bed
   B. Water mattress
   C. Non-powered, air-filled support surface
   D. None of the above

Answers: 1-C, 2-D, 3-A

References

1. Kosiak M. Etiology and pathology of ischemic ulcers. *Arch Phys Med Rehabil.* 1959;40(2):62–69.
2. Panel for the Prediction and Prevention of Pressure Ulcers. Clinical Practice Guideline Number 3: Pressure Ulcers in Adults: Prediction and Prevention. Rockville, Md: US Department of Health and Human Services. Agency for Health Care Policy and Research; 1992.
3. Dinsdale SM. Decubitus ulcers: role of pressure and friction in causation. *Arch Phys Med Rehabil.* 1974;55(4):147–152.
4. Bennett L, Kavner D, Lee BK, Trainor FA. Shear vs. pressure as causative factors in skin blood flow occlusion. *Arch Phys Med Rehabil.* 1979;60(7):309–314.
5. Goossens RH, Zegers R, Hoek van Dijke GA, Snijders CJ. Influence of shear on skin oxygen tension. *Clin Physiol.* 1994;14(1):111–118.
6. Bennett L, Lee BY. Pressure versus shear in pressure sore causation. In: Lee BY, ed. *Chronic Ulcers of the Skin.* New York, NY: McGraw Hill; 1985:39–56.
7. Patel S, Knapp CF, Donofrio JC, Salcido R. Temperature effects on surface pressure-induced changes in rat skin perfusion: implications in pressure ulcer development. *J Rehabil Res Dev.* 1999;36(3):189–201.
8. Kokate JY, Leland KJ, Held AM, et al. Temperature-modulated pressure ulcers: a porcine model. *Arch Phys Med Rehabil.* 1995;76(7):666–673.
9. Visscher MO, Chatterjee R, Ebel JP, LaRuffa AA, Hoath SB. Biomedical assessment and instrumental evaluation of healthy infant skin. *Pediatr Dermatol.* 2002;19(6):473–481.
10. Egawa M, Oguri M, Hirao T, Takahashi M, Miyakawa M.

The evaluation of skin friction using a frictional feel analyzer. *Skin Res Technol.* 2002;8(1):41–51.
11. Clark M. Repositioning to prevent pressure sores—what is the evidence? *Nurs Stand.* 1998;13(3):58–64.
12. Krouskop T, van Rijswijk L. Standardizing performance-based criteria for support surfaces. *Ostomy Wound Manage.* 1995;41(1):34–45.
13. Same as 1
14. Ek AC, Gustavsson G, Lewis DH. Skin blood flow in relation to external pressure and temperature in the supine position on a standard hospital mattress. *Scand J Rehabil Med.* 1987;19(3):121–126.
15. Holloway GA, Daly CH, Kennedy D, Chimoskey J. Effects of external pressure loading on human skin blood flow measured by 133Xe clearance. *J Appl Physiol.* 1976;40(4):597–600.
16. Lassen NA, Holstein P. Use of radioisotopes in assessment of distal blood flow and distal blood pressure in arterial insufficiency. *Surg Clin North Am.* 1974;54(1):39–55.
17. Sangeorzan BJ, Harrington RM, Wyss CR, Czerniecki JM, Matsen FA. Circulatory and mechanical response of skin to loading. *J Orthop Res.* 1989;7(3):425–431.
18. NPUAP. Support Surface Terms and Definitions Draft Statement. Available at: http://www.npuap.org. Accessed August 31, 2006.
19. Krouskop TA, Noble PS, Brown J, Marburger R. Factors affecting the pressure-distributing properties of foam mattress overlays. *J Rehabil Res.* 1986;23(3):33.
20. Krouskop T. Scientific aspects of pressure relief. Lecture presented at the 1989 International Association for Enterostomal Therapy Annual Conference, Washington, DC, 1989.
21. Krouskop TA, Garber SL. The role of technology in the prevention of pressure sores. *Ostomy Wound Manage.* 1987;16:45.
22. Pase MN. Pressure relief devices, risk factors, and development of pressure ulcers in elderly patients with limited mobility. *Adv Wound Care.* 1994;7(2):38–42.
23. Fleck CA. Support surfaces: criteria and selection. In: Krasner DL, Sibbald RG, Rodeheaver GT, eds. *Chronic Wound Care: A Clinical Source Book for Healthcare Professionals.* 3rd ed. Wayne, Pa: HMP Communications; 2001:665.
24. Conine TA, Daechsel D, Choi AK, Lau MS. Costs and acceptability of two special overlays for the prevention of pressure sores. *Rehabil Nurs.* 1990;15(3):133–137.
25. Cullum N, McInnes E, Bell-Syer SE, Legood R. Support surfaces for pressure ulcer prevention. *Cochrane Database Syst Rev.* 2004;(3):CD001735.
26. Fleurence RL. Cost-effectiveness of pressure-relieving devices for the prevention and treatment of pressure ulcers. *Int J Technol Assess Health Care.* 2005;21(3):334–341.
27. The Columbia Encyclopedia. 6th ed. King of Prussia, Pa: University Press; 2001.
28. Hoyman K, Gruber N. A case study of interdepartmental cooperation: operating room-acquired pressure ulcers. *J Nurs Care Qual.* 1992;Suppl:12–17.
29. Inman KJ, Dymock K, Fysh N, Robbins B, Rutledge FS, Sibbald WJ. Pressure ulcer prevention: a randomized controlled trial of 2 risk-directed strategies for patient surface assignment. *Adv Wound Care.* 1999;12(2):73–80.

30. Clark M. Changing pressure-redistributing mattress stocks: cost and outcomes. *Br J Nurs.* 2005;14(6):S30–S31.

31. Bodine OH, Flam E. Low air-loss support surfaces: myths and facts. Second Annual NHHCE presentation; 1995.

32. Weaver V, McCausland D. Revised Medicare policies for support surfaces. A review. *J WOCN.* 1998;25(1):26–35.

33. Cullum N, Deeks J, Sheldon TA, Song F, Fletcher AW. Beds, mattresses and cushions for pressure sore prevention and treatment. *Cochrane Database Syst Rev.* 2000;(2):CD001735.

34. Bergstrom N, Bennett MA, Carlson CE, et al. Clinical Practice Guideline Number 15: Treatment of Pressure Ulcers. Rockville, Md: US Department of Health and Human Services. Agency for Health Care Policy and Research; 1994. AHCPR Publication 95-0653.

35. Viner C. Floating on a bed of beads. *Nurs Times.* 1986;82:62.

36. Ochs RF, Horn SD, van Rijswijk L, Pietsch C, Smout RJ. Comparison of air-fluidized therapy with other support surfaces used to treat pressure ulcers in nursing home residents. *Ostomy Wound Manage.* 2005;51(2):38–68.

37. Parish LC, Witkowski JA. Clinitron therapy and the decubitus ulcer: preliminary dermatologic studies. *Int J Dermatol.* 1980;19(9):517–518.

38. Economides NG, Skoutakis VA, Carter CA, Smith VH. Evaluation of the effectiveness of two support surfaces following myocutaneous flap surgery. *Adv Wound Care.* 1996;8(1):49–53.

39. Sharp-Pucci M. Evaluation center study and report on the comparative efficacy of different classes of support surfaces. Blue Cross and Blue Shield, 1998.

40. Agris J, Spira M. Common sites for pressure ulcers and frequency and ulceration per site. *Clin Symp.* 1979;31(5):2.

41. Scott SM, Mayhew PA, Harris EA. Pressure ulcer development in the operating room. *AORN J.* 1992;56(2):242–50.

42. Abu-Own A, Sommerville K, Scurr JH, Coleridge Smith PD. Effects of compression and type of bed surface on the microcirculation of the heel. *Eur J Vasc Endovasc Surg.* 1995;9(3):327–334.

43. Bergstrom N, Braden B, Boynton P, Bruch S. Using a research-based assessment scale in clinical practice. *Nurs Clin North Am.* 1995;30(3):539–550.

44. Dallam L, Smyth C, Jackson BS, et al. Pressure ulcer pain: assessment and quantification. *J Wound Ostomy Continence Nurs.* 1995;22(5):211–218.

45. Kosiak M. Etiology of decubitus ulcers. *Arch Phys Med Rehabil.* 1961;42(1):19–28.

CHAPTER 19

Compression Therapies

R. Gary Sibbald, BSc, MD, MEd, FRCPC (Med, Derm), MACP, FAAD, MAPWCA;
Afsaneh Alavi, MD, FRCPC (Derm); **Linda Norton**, BScOT, OT Reg (ONT), MScCH;
A.C. Browne, MB, MICGP; **Patricia Coutts**, RN

Objectives

The reader will be challenged to:

- Select appropriate compression therapy for edema control and ulcer healing considering arterial circulation, pain, and other patient-related factors
- Differentiate between inelastic (support) and elastic systems of compression
- Analyze the types of stockings/hosiery available to maintain edema control and prevent ulcer recurrences.

Introduction

Venous leg ulcers account for 40%–70% of chronic lower-extremity wounds.[1] As the population ages, the proportion of pure venous ulcers is decreasing with more patients presenting with mixed venous and arterial disease. Compression therapy, in the form of bandaging, is the cornerstone of management in the absence of any significant arterial disease.[2] Compression therapy is contraindicated in decompensated chronic congestive heart failure and peripheral vascular disease where arterial disease predominates over a co-existing venous component.[3]

In a 2006 comprehensive systematic review update of the 2001 systematic review, Cullum et al[4] reassessed the evidence for compression therapy. The authors tabulated the randomized, controlled trials that compared the effectiveness of various compression systems and alternative therapies for the treatment of venous ulcers. Some important findings are summarized in Table 1.

In this systematic review, compression bandaging facilitated faster healing of venous ulcers compared to no compression. The review also concluded that the multilayer elastic systems were superior in the 5 studies that qualified for inclusion. High compression also produced higher venous ulcer healing rates than low compression with single-layer bandaging. There was no difference in trials with the 4-layer bandage compared to other equivalent multilayer bandaging systems. A high compression stocking was also more effective combined with a thromboembolic stocking under-layer than a short-stretch system for venous ulcer healing. This

Sibbald RG, Alavi A, Norton L, Browne AC, Coutts P. Compression therapies. In: Krasner DL, ed. *Chronic Wound Care: The Essentials*. Malvern, Pa: HMP Communications, 2014:259–270.

Table 1. Cochrane systematic review (update 2006)[4]

Comparison of healing rates	# of RCTs with a positive result
Compression > no compression	4 out of 6
Multilayer: elastic > nonelastic	5 out of 5
High multilayer > single layer	4 out of 4
4 layer = other high multilayer	3 out of 3
Equal elastomeric (multilayer)	4 out of 4
HC stocking + TED > short stretch	1 trial

may be predictable, because short-stretch bandage effect depends on the skill of the bandage applier, and as the edema is reduced, the bandage will loosen or fall down. Often, this bandaging system has to be reapplied frequently.

There is a 3-class bandage classification system in the United Kingdom: retention, nonelastic, and elastic. Retention bandages include continuous cotton bandage rolls, such as Kling® (Johnson & Johnson Wound Management, Somerville, NJ) or Kerlix® (Kendall HealthCare, Mansfield, Mass). Retention-type bandages may not provide compression but are designed as secondary dressings to keep the primary wound dressings in place and provide protective padding. The second type of bandages, *nonelastic (support) bandages,* includes the short-stretch bandages, such as Comprilan® (BSN-JOBST, Inc, Charlotte, NC), and bandages impregnated with zinc oxide or gelatin, such as Viscopaste® (Smith & Nephew, Largo, Fla). The third type of bandages, *elastic bandages,* can be divided into low, medium, or high compression subclasses. The low elastic subgroup includes Tubigrip® (ConvaTec, Princeton, NJ). This product is a tubular rolled bandage in different sizes that can be cut and applied with 1 or more layers. A single layer will provide approximately 8 mmHg, and 2 layers will provide approximately 16 mmHg.[5] A simple elastic nonadhesive bandage applied in a spiral would provide approximately 14 mmHg

to 17 mmHg compression at the ankle. A noncohesive elastic bandage (eg, Tensopress™, Smith & Nephew) is in its relaxed state when it is taken out of the package, and when fully stretched, it will reach the stopping distance. For a maximum application of elastic energy, the bandage should be applied at half stretch between the relaxed and stopping distance. The bandage should start at the base of the toes, usually includes a heal lock, and is applied to just below the knee with no gaps visible. Moderate elastic systems combine 1 or 2 under-layers with a cohesive elastic bandage (18 mmHg–24 mmHg). The high compression elastic systems often combine 1 or 2 padding under-layers with an elastic mid-layer and a cohesive layer on top. The elastic layer can be applied in a spiral for slightly lower compression or in a figure-of-8 to apply higher pressures around the ankle. The last cohesive layer is usually applied using a spiral technique at 50% or full stretch with a 50% overlap of each layer.

In summary, the main conclusions from the most recent systematic review of compression therapy have remained unchanged:[4]

- High compression was better than low compression in the treatment of venous edema provided there is no co-existing significant arterial disease
- There was no clear difference in the effectiveness of the different types of multilayer high compression systems
- There may be an advantage of elastic systems over nonelastic systems
- The increased use of any correctly applied high compression treatment should be promoted.[2]

The Cochrane site provides periodic updates on a number of reviews in wound care and can be accessed at the Cochrane site: http://www.cochrane.org/reviews/ en/ab000265.html (you may need an institutional or personal license for access).[4] It is important to remember that this evidence base must be interpreted for clinical practice. Not all patients tolerate all compression systems, and there may be other contraindications to both elastic and inelastic systems. For example, patients with significant lower leg pain may tolerate inelastic systems with a lower pressure at rest and can be transitioned to an elastic system with pain control.

Table 2. Vascular assessment criteria for treatment

ABPI	Toe Pressure	Toe Brachial Index	Ankle Doppler Waveform	TcPO₂	Diagnosis
> 0.8	> 80 mmHg	> 0.6	Normal/Triphasic	> 40 mmHg	No arterial disease
> 0.6	> 50 mmHg	> 0.4	Biphasic/Monophasic	30 mmHg–39 mmHg	Some arterial disease: Modify compression
> 0.4	> 30 mmHg	> 0.2	Biphasic/Monophasic	20 mmHg–29 mmHg	Arterial disease predominates
< 0.4	< 30 mmHg	< 0.2	Monophasic	< 20 mmHg	High risk for limb ischemia

Vascular Assessment: Doppler Ankle to Brachial Pressure Index (ABPI)

A thorough vascular assessment should be performed prior to considering the use of any compression therapy on a patient. The presence or absence of pedal pulses should be determined, but this alone is inadequate as a vascular assessment. In addition to clinical assessment, clinicians should perform a Doppler assessment. The ankle to brachial pressure index (ABPI) helps identify any coexisting arterial disease.[5–7] Moffatt and O'Hare[8] have demonstrated that if clinicians rely on the presence of a palpable pulse alone (approximately 80 mmHg for the foot), they will misclassify 17%–20% of patients who have significant arterial disease. Portable Doppler with 4-MHz to 8-MHz probes can be utilized in the community or ambulatory clinic to measure the arterial ABPI.[5–7]

The following steps are required for obtaining ABPI:

1. Patient should be in supine position 15 minutes before the procedure
2. Obtain the brachial blood pressure in both arms and use the higher systolic pressure
3. Apply the blood pressure cuff around the ankle just above the malleoli
4. Apply ultrasound gel over the dorsum of the foot to obtain a dorsalis pedis pulse and over the notch below the medial malleolus to obtain tibialis posterior pulse (probe should be at a 45-degree angle pointing upward to meet blood flow)

5. When the pulse signal is audible, inflate the sphygmomanometer until the signal disappears
6. Slowly release the cuff until the pulse signal is heard representing the systolic pressure
7. Divide the ankle systolic pressure by brachial systolic pressure (eg, 80 [ankle] ÷ 100 [brachial] = 0.8 ABPI).

The Doppler is more accurate than a stethoscope, but in the presence of calcified arteries (commonly seen in people with diabetes), falsely elevated readings of systolic dorsalis pedis and posterior tibial pressures may occur. In these patients, toe pressure analysis and waveforms will be more reliable.[9–11] Depending on the patient's history, clinical examination, and the ABPI, one can decide the type and level of compression therapy that may be required. In patients with an ABPI > 0.8 (toe pressure usually > 80 mmHg) high compression (30 mmHg–40 mmHg or higher) can be applied. An ABPI between 0.6–0.8 (toe pressure usually > 50 mmHg) is considered borderline or indicative of some arterial insufficiency, and modified low level compression can be applied. For patients with an ABPI < 0.6 and toe pressure < 50 mmHg, no compression should be used.[12] Refer to Table 2 for a guideline for interpreting the ABPI.[10] Patients with an ABPI between 0.6–0.8 may have claudication with prolonged walking; for patients with an ABPI of 0.4–0.6 claudication often occurs with walking short distances; those with an ABPI between 0.2–0.4 have pain with leg elevation; and an ABPI < 0.2 is associated with potential rest pain.

How is the Ideal Compression Bandage Determined for Individual Patients?

Ideal compression is determined by the modified Laplace's law. According to this law, sub-bandage pressure is determined by the number of layers of bandage applied and the tension by which it is applied. This is also influenced by the leg circumference and the width of the bandage:

Laplace's law:
Sub-bandage pressure =

$$\frac{T \text{ (tension)} \times N \text{ (number of layers)} \times C \text{ (constant)}}{C \text{ (circumference of limb)} \times W \text{ (bandage width)}}$$

In Laplace's law, the circumference of the limb is in the denominator of this equation—the larger the circumference, the less the compression. This is why a relatively thin ankle will achieve 25 mmHg–45 mmHg with the same bandage that will give only 15 mmHg–20 mmHg compression to a larger circumference leg just below the knee. In summary, obtained compression is the inverse of the circumference with smaller circumferences receiving higher compression. In addition, narrow bandage widths will also give greater compression (also an inverse relationship).

Laplace's law also tells us that the bandage tension is important. An elastic bandage comes out of the package in the relaxed state. As it is stretched as far as it can go, the bandage reaches the stopping distance (and a loss of elastic energy), making it a support system. As previously stated, proper bandage technique requires any elastic bandage to be applied halfway between the relaxed state and stopping distance, maximizing the elastic energy in both directions. Some bandage systems have indicator systems that will determine 50% or higher levels of stretch (for example, rectangles become squares). It is also known that the more layers present, the greater the compression. If there is extra bandage left by the time the knee is reached, do not apply extra elastic layers at the knee. This increases the compression proximally. If this is done, the venous blood is sent back down to the foot. Instead, some bandages may be cut, or the bandage can be rewrapped

with greater overlap between the layers to utilize the extra bandage length. Inelastic bandage techniques may criss-cross and go up and down the leg. It is important that the clinician be familiar with each of the systems to determine the appropriate adjustments needed to accommodate extra bandage length.

Padding may be used to even out the leg circumference in irregular shaped legs, effectively redistributing the pressure in a uniform fashion. Padding may also be used to protect bony prominences of the pretibial and Achilles areas.[13]

Role of the Calf Muscle Pump

Good calf muscle pump function is important in the healing of venous leg ulcers. High venous pressures are found in patients with venous leg ulcers often due in part to the partial or complete failure of the calf muscle pump.[14] Major injuries, neurological disease, vascular insufficiency, bone and joint pain, as well as an altered gait can all adversely impact the calf muscle pump.[15] Calf muscle pump function can also be affected by ankle range of motion, as ankle dorsiflexion of 90 degrees occurs in the normal walking pattern.[9]

As activation of the calf muscle pump is a critical component of leg ulcer healing,[9] regular exercise, such as walking, as well as exercises to increase ankle mobility should be prescribed.[15] Referral to an occupational or physical therapist for those patients who have difficulty adhering to an exercise program or who have limitation in joint mobility[16] should be considered A physical or occupational therapist can assist the patient to find an alternative form of exercise that will foster adherence as well as employ techniques to improve joint range of motion.

Mechanism of Compression versus Support (Figure 1)

There is a difference between compression and support. Compression is an elastic system with high pressure at rest and high but less pressure with muscle contraction. A support system is relatively rigid (inelastic), giving little pressure at rest and high pressure with muscle contraction against fixed resistance. Despite the differences in these 2 systems, the nomenclature is often used in a less precise and interchangeable fashion.

Three- and 4-layer, as well as long-stretch

	Compression	Support
Type of system pattern of pressure	*Elastic*	*Nonelastic*
	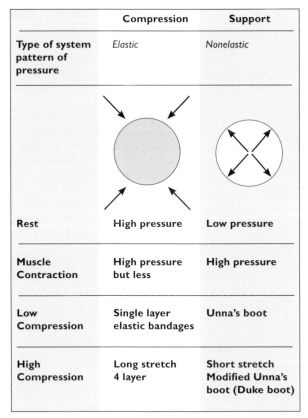	
Rest	**High pressure**	**Low pressure**
Muscle Contraction	**High pressure but less**	**High pressure**
Low Compression	**Single layer elastic bandages**	**Unna's boot**
High Compression	**Long stretch 4 layer**	**Short stretch Modified Unna's boot (Duke boot)**

Figure 1. Compression is an elastic system with high pressure at rest and high but less pressure with muscle contraction. A support system is relatively rigid (inelastic) giving little pressure at rest and high pressure with muscle contraction against a fixed resistance.

elastic compression systems, control edema with elastic energy and high resting pressure. Support systems (short stretch, Duke boot/modified Unna's boot) have low resting pressures, and their mechanism of action is through exerting pressure against a fixed resistance.

Various high compression systems are available. High compression systems have been used with increasing frequency to treat venous ulcers in the absence of any co-existing arterial disease. High compression systems include 4-layer systems[17] and long-stretch systems.

High Compression/4-Layer Systems

The 4-layer system (Profore™, Smith & Neph-

ew) is a high pressure elastic bandage consisting of:

- Layer 1: natural cotton padding roll that is applied in a spiral bandage technique
- Layer 2: light, conformable bandage; a crepe layer is applied in a spiral bandage technique
- Layer 3: light compression bandage; an elastic bandage is applied in a figure-of-8 fashion at 50% stretch
- Layer 4: flexible cohesive bandage; a cohesive elastic bandage applied in a spiral with 50% overlap of each layer and 50% stretch (keeps the bandage in place without slippage).

The first, second, and fourth layers are applied in a spiral fashion, and the third layer is applied in a figure-of-8. A figure-of-8 wrapping style will give 10 mmHg to 15 mmHg more compression than a spiral technique using the same bandage.[9] The third layer is responsible for approximately 17 mmHg of the 42.5 mmHg sustained pressure obtained from the bandage during a 1-week average wear time.

Multilayer bandages are somewhat bulky but are usually comfortable. They should not be used if significant coexisting arterial disease is noted (Doppler ABPI < 0.8). They are designed for single use but, because they reduce the number of follow-up visits, can be cost effective and efficient. Multilayer bandages are not recommended for ankle circumferences of < 18 cm (unless the third layer is omitted), because high ankle pressures in excess of 60 mmHg may be obtained, resulting in the potential for local skin breakdown and pain. With ankles > 26 cm in circumference, an extra third layer should be added; otherwise, a lesser level of compression at the ankle will be achieved. *Four-layer bandages are considered to be the gold standard of compression therapy and represent a major advance over previous methodologies.* They combine the advantages of 4 layers (that help to minimize bandaging error) with the elastic properties of a cohesive layer (that prevents slippage). Patients with fragile skin, loss of muscle tone, and severe pain may not tolerate multilayer bandage systems. High elastic pressure at rest can cause the fragile skin of people with rheumatoid arthritis or neuromuscular conditions with loss of muscle tone to develop new areas of breakdown.

Other High Compression and Support Systems

A long-stretch bandage (SurePress™ and Seto-Press®, ConvaTec; Tensopress™, Smith & Nephew) consists of an orthopedic wool under-layer and a long-stretch elastic system (so named due to the long stopping distance or maximum stretch ability compared to the relaxed state). One system (SurePress) has small rectangles printed in the center of the bandages that become squares when the bandage is applied at a 50% stretch for ankle circumferences between 18 cm and 26 cm. For ankle circumferences above 26 cm, a two-thirds stretch is recommended, allowing the larger rectangles in the middle of the bandage to become squares. The long-stretch system, like a 4-layer bandage, may give too much compression to a smaller ankle (< 18 cm circumference) and not enough compression for ankles > 26 cm. One practical advantage of this system is that the elastic layer can be reused, replacing only the orthopedic wool layer with each reapplication, facilitating regular review of an unstable, possibly infected wound. It is also less bulky than a 4-layer system and is cost effective.[18] This is a good option for patients who want to do their own bandage wrapping. A major disadvantage is the propensity of this bandage to slip, especially in the champagne bottle-shaped legs of chronic venous ulcer patients.

Long-stretch bandages can be washed carefully, perhaps up to 18 to 20 times, but should be replaced if they lose their elasticity. The orthopedic wool must be replaced with each application. Pressures at the ankle average about 35 mmHg. To avoid slippage, nonelastic tubular gauze netting is helpful. Alternatively, a layer of petrolatum on the leg prior to the application of orthopedic wool will also minimize slippage in both elastic systems.

There are 2 other elastic high compression systems that have been recently introduced to some markets: Proguide® (Smith & Nephew), which combines a pad with a single layer elastic cohesive layer, and 3M™ Coban™ (3M Health Care, Saint Paul, Minn). Further studies and expert opinion are going to be required before these are accepted in everyday practice.

The short-stretch bandage, Comprilan® (available in the United States through BSN-JOBST, Inc), has little elastic energy and mostly acts as a support system. *This is the gold standard in many countries of continental Europe.*[19] This inelastic bandaging system technique does not need to start at the tip of the toes but often starts on the ankle, with a complicated overlapping system with 2 separate bandages. In the authors' clinic, an orthopedic wool or continuous bandage is recommended as a primary layer. A 6-cm bandage is applied on the foot with two-thirds overlap in a spiral. An 8-cm bandage is then used in a similar fashion from the ankle to below the knee.[20] This simplified technique allows reproducible bandaging in community and other care settings with minimal slippage. A flexible, cohesive bandage (eg, Coban) can be used to fix the bandage and minimize slippage, but if this is applied at full stretch or becomes bunched, a high local pressure may be obtained. Alternatively, a cotton cohesive bandage without a major elastic component has been developed (Easifix®, Smith & Nephew). Because short-stretch bandaging is so effective at reducing edema, bandages need to be changed more frequently (every 24 to 72 hours) unless they are applied with a cohesive outer layer, such as Easifix. Short-stretch systems are excellent for thin ankles (< 18 cm in circumference) and edematous feet. The balloon foot is often due to too much compression at the ankle, impairing edema drainage from the foot. Short stretch is useful with decreased muscle tone or muscle atrophy. There is low pressure at rest, preventing new areas of breakdown. The bandage can be washed 10 or more times. Short-stretch bandages can also be modified depending on edema level noted after removal of the bandages. Increased therapeutic action can be achieved with narrower bandaging or an increased overlap. Conversely, wider bandages with less overlap will have decreased clinical edema reduction. Their drawback is that they take considerable training and skill to apply cor-

Table 3. Cochrane systematic review: compression for preventing recurrence of venous ulcers 2006	
Comparison of recurrence rates	**# of RCTs**
Compression hosiery > no compression	2 out of 2
High compression = moderate compression hosiery (higher patient adherence rates)	1 trial (300 patients)
Two types of medium compression hosiery are equal	1 trial (166 patients)

rectly. A short-stretch bandage may also be useful for mixed arterial and venous disease where the resting pressure is low. The nonelastic systems are also useful for patients with pain and can be tolerated in some individuals where elastic systems become problematic and painful. When the major leg edema and pain have decreased, these patients may be switched to appropriate elastic systems when necessary.

The gold standard for support therapy in the United States has been the modified Unna's boot (Uniflex®, ConvaTec; Viscopaste®, Smith & Nephew) or Duke boot.[21] Professor Unna, a German dermatologist, introduced zinc oxide paste bandages in 1896. In their modern form, wet zinc oxide bandages are applied in a continuous spiral fashion or using an interrupted strip technique with 50%–80% overlap.[12] The patient should be reminded to keep his or her foot in the dorsiflexed position during the wrapping. The Duke boot adds a hydrocolloid wafer over the wound and a flexible cohesive bandage as an outer layer. The flexible cohesive bandage is often applied at full stretch as an extra layer to reinforce the boot, increase the support, and even out irregular areas of the zinc oxide paste layer. The 4-layer elastic system and the inelastic Duke boot have the same outer layer, but the 4-layer system has the flexible cohesive bandage applied at 50% stretch.

Each of the 4 high compression/support systems has advantages and disadvantages, and each patient will benefit from different systems. Patients should be checked for edema control, comfort, local wound discharge, and new areas of breakdown. Remember to address patient-centered concerns when selecting a compression system.

Pain is common with venous disease[22] and should be addressed (see Chapter 9). Constant pain may be due to infection or superficial or deep phlebitis. The cause of the pain must be treated, but patients also need co-existing edema control. This may be achieved initially with short-stretch systems, which do not cause pressure at rest, minimizing additional pain from the bandage. These patients may then progress to the elastic systems. Local practices may reflect tradition, or therapy may be dictated by drug tariffs, reimbursement plans, or institutional formularies. Knowledge of bandage characteristics can optimize treatment. There is no doubt that 1 bandage system is not optimal for all patients, and clinics providing several options can often optimize patient care outcomes.

Low Compression

Patients with ABPIs ranging from 0.6 to 0.8 have mixed arterial/venous disease and may still benefit from compression for the venous component of their ulcers. Edema control must be balanced against decreasing arterial circulation. Although sub-bandage pressure locally may be well below adjacent arterial pressures, distal arterial digit perfusion may be significantly reduced, leading to critical ischemia. These patients may complain of local pain, and clinical examination may reveal signs of vascular compromise (cold foot/dusky erythema).[23] For these patients, a simple single-layer elastic bandage or short-stretch system may be sufficient. Patients should be told to remove this if any discomfort develops. Bandages can be modified and a layer of padding used underneath when tolerated. This will, however, increase compression. Other ways to increase

Table 4. Level of compression stockings[12]

US standard	UK standard
Class I: 20 mmHg–30mmHg (light)	14 mmHg–17mmHg
Class II: 30 mmHg–40 mmHg (light)	18 mmHg–24 mmHg
Class III: 40 mmHg–50 mmHg (light)	25 mmHg–35 mmHg
Class IV: 50 mmHg–60 mmHg	N/A

compression if edema control is not adequate include changing the bandage from a spiral to a figure-of-8 all the way up the leg. Be cautious with these patients, because edema may represent clinical signs of congestive right heart failure, low albumin, or other medical causes.

Compression Hosiery and Stockings

In general, bandaging is for healing, and compression hosiery or stockings are for maintenance and preventing recurrence. Thromboembolic stockings are designed for bedrest and compression stockings for ambulatory patients.[24]

Once healing has been achieved with compression bandaging, patients should be advised to wear compression hosiery for life (unless co-existing arterial disease exists) in order to maintain healing. Compression stockings have elasticity providing compression at rest and also with muscle contraction. Results of 2 randomized, controlled trials have qualified for a recent Cochrane review on the prevention of venous ulcers with compression hosiery.[24] The results are listed in Table 3.

Various types of compression hosiery on the market meet varying patient needs. The qualified healthcare provider ordering the stockings has several decisions to make. As the prescriber, you must decide several things.[25] The first decision is to determine the appropriate stocking strength based on the ABPI and patient considerations (will they wear them and can they put them on). Dress support stockings may be used for prominent veins without edema (very light, 8 mmHg–15 mmHg; light, 16 mmHg–20 mmHg). Once the venules become leaky or venous edema de-

velops, the patient will often require hosiery of 25 mmHg pressure (Class 1, 20 mmHg–30 mmHg pressure). When lipodermatosclerosis (woody fibrosis or nonpitting edema) develops with chronic disease, the capillaries are leaky to fibrin, and 30 mmHg to 40 mmHg pressure (Class 2) is often required. The development of lymphedema requires even higher pressure stockings of strengths > 40 mmHg (Class 3)[26,27] (Table 4).

The qualified clinician should next decide on the length. Knee-high stockings may be with or without toes and with or without a grip. Mid-thigh, full-thigh, or pantyhose variations are available for men and women. One can choose the type, such as natural latex or synthetic. If the clinician chooses natural latex hosiery, the wear time is longer, but the chance of allergic reaction is much higher.

Support stockings are not a good option as initial treatment because of rapid change in the leg's circumference.[12] It is better to order compression stockings when the limb circumference has been stabilized. Also, stocking should be applied immediately after getting up in the morning before local edema has a chance to accumulate. The other challenge is severe lipodermatosclerosis that can be associated with an inverted champagne bottle-shaped leg. Fitting a stocking on an irregularly shaped leg such as this is a challenge.

Patients often complain of compression hosiery application difficulties. The healthcare team should advise patients on how they can overcome these difficulties. For example, various assistive devices are available for use with the high pressure stockings. These include small devices that go up the leg and larger devices that allow the patient to step into a prestretched stocking (Stocking Don-ner®, BSN-JOBST, Inc). Other patented devices, such as rip-stop nylon (Easy Slide®, Sigvaris, Inc, Peachtree, Ga), can be used with open or closed-toed stockings. Another suggestion for patients having problems applying high-pressure hosiery is a nylon or cotton under sleeve with a compression stocking on top. By using an under sleeve, the compression will increase by approximately 10 mmHg. This illustrates Laplace's law: with the addition of more layers, we have increased the total compression. The patient may also find applying 2 low-strength stockings on top of each other easier than applying 1 high-pressure stocking. This often gives the patient greater flexibility. Another tip is to use a zippered stocking (Jobst Ulcer Care™, BSN-JOBST, Inc). The wearer can pull the zipper down at night and pull it up in the morning. Patients with arthritis may put a key ring on the zipper and use a hook to pull the zipper up. The zippered stockings are often used with a nylon under sleeve to increase pressure and protect the stocking. For those patients who experience the tourniquet effect at the knee or edema just above the stocking, a knee-length stocking with grip or elastic bandage above the stocking may be used. Most patients prefer knee-high stockings. If a large amount of edema occurs above the knee, local hemorrhage may result from this large pressure gradient differential. These patients may not only require the grip as described but also mid-thigh or full-length stockings. Full pantyhose are available as well in maternity designs for women or in a chap style for men. For patients with lymphedematous legs, there is a unique, nonelastic, sustained compression system utilizing Velcro® adjustable straps (CircAid® Thera-Boot, Coloplast Corp, Minneapolis, Minn). The tabs may be tightened as the edema changes. With lymphedema, the 4-layer bandage is modified with an extra third layer. Patients may be referred to a specialist center for intermittent pneumatic compression[28] with a lymphedema pump.

Anti-thrombolic anti-embolism hose (Thromboembolic Stockings TED®, Kendall HealthCare) provides low level compression, but it does not provide calf muscle support during ambulation. Anti-embolism hose is a single-layer stocking designed for patients on bed rest.

It is important to emphasize to patients that they must wear their stockings at all times except while sleeping. The recurrence rate is high for an individual with a venous ulcer who is not adherent to the treatment plan. It is important that the healthcare team and patient work together to design an effective program. When stockings loose their elasticity, they must be replaced. Many patients require more than 1 stocking to facilitate daily use. Clinicians should examine patients with their stockings on as part of their ongoing evaluation and to assess adequate edema control. Elderly patients with arthritis may have difficulty in applying the stockings, so a lower compression may be easier to manage than the ideal compression.

Adherence with Treatment Recommendations

The best compression therapy system is the one the patient will wear. Even after the wound has healed, patients must use "compression for life" to minimize recurrence. However, clinicians must always watch for newly developing arterial disease. Coaching patients with leg ulcers toward adherence with compression therapy and healthy lifestyles can improve health and quality of life in patients and should be undertaken without delay.[5] The latest Cochrane review reminds us that a lower compression stocking is better than non-adherence or leaving the stocking in the drawer.

Conclusion

As the population ages, venous ulcers are more common—22% of the population have their first ulcers by age 40, and 72% have ulcers by the age of 60.[9] Recurrent ulcers were seen in 72% of treated subjects, suggesting the importance of support or compression therapy for life.[9] Healthcare professionals need to differentiate between elastic and inelastic bandaging systems to achieve the best possible compression for patient-centered concerns including pain, quality of life, and ideal edema control. It is essential to use a handheld Doppler or perform a thorough vascular assessment prior to prescribing any compression therapy. The clinical decision is a compromise between the patient's concerns and best evidence. Clinicians must make their patients their partners in the treatment plans and reinforce the importance of adherence with the particular compression

Take-Home Messages for Practice

• Compression is the gold standard for the treatment of venous ulcers

• High compression is ideal for patients with venous ulcers in the absence of significant arterial disease

• Compression therapy needs to be modified for patients with mixed arterial and venous disease, and is contraindicated in arterial predominant disease

• Any form of high compression therapy has been shown to be beneficial. The clinician needs to assess the advantages and disadvantages of the various elastic and inelastic systems (slight advantage to elastic systems in recent studies)

• Bandaging is for healing and compression stockings or hosiery is for maintenance and to lower the incidence of recurrences

• Thromboembolic stockings are for bed rest patients and compression stockings are for the ambulatory patient.

therapy prescribed to prevent recurrence. Ongoing patient education (continuous and repetitive) is most likely to increase the rate of success.

Self-Assessment Questions

1. Compression therapy is indicated in which of the following conditions?
   A. Patient with symptomatic congestive heart failure
   B. Patient with peripheral vascular disease
   C. Patient with ABPI > 0.8 and toe pressure > 80 mmHg
   D. Toe pressure < 40 mmHg

2. Support stockings are used mainly:
   A. To heal ulcers
   B. For patients on bed rest
   C. For patients with arterial predominant disease
   D. For control of venous edema and prevention of ulcer recurrence

3. Which of the following bandages provide non-elastic (support) compression therapy?

A. 4-layer bandage (Profore)

B. Zinc oxide impregnated bandage (Visco-paste)

C. Long-stretch bandage (SurePress)

D. Cohesive bandage (Coban)

Answers: 1-C, 2-D, 3-B

References

1. Margolis DJ, Berlin JA, Strom BL. Risk factors associated with the failure of a venous leg ulcer to heal. *Arch Dermatol.* 1999;135(8):920–926.

2. Fletcher A, Cullum N, Sheldon TA. A systematic review of compression treatment for venous leg ulcers. *BMJ.* 1997;315(7108):576–580.

3. Williams RJ, Wertheim D, Melhuish J, Harding KG. How compression therapy works. *J Wound Care.* 1999;8(6):297–298.

4. Cullum N, Nelson EA, Fletcher AW, Sheldon TA. Compression for venous leg ulcers. *Cochrane Database Syst Rev.* 2000;(3):CD000265.

5. Williams IM, Picton AJ, McCollum CN. The use of Doppler ultrasound 1: arterial disease. *Ostomy Wound Manage.* 1993;4.

6. Stubbing NJ, Bailey P, Poole M. Protocol for accurate assessment of ABPI in patients with leg ulcers. *J Wound Care.* 1997;6(9):417–418.

7. Moffatt C. The principles of assessment prior to compression therapy. *J Wound Care.* 1998;7(7 Suppl):6–9.

8. Moffatt C, O'Hare L. Ankle pulses are not sufficient to detect impaired arterial circulation in patients with leg ulcers. *J Wound Care.* 1995;4(3):134–138

9. Sibbald RG. Venous leg ulcers. *Ostomy Wound Manage.* 1998;44(9):52–64.

10. Sibbald RG, Orsted HL, Coutts PM, Keast D. Preparing the wound bed: update 2006. *Wound Care Canada.* 2006;4(1):15–29.

11. Martson W, Vowden K. Compression therapy: a guide to safe practice 2003. *EWMA Position Document.* 2003:11–17.

12. Doughty D, Holbrook R. Lower extremity ulcers of vascular etiology. In: Bryant R, Nix D, eds. *Acute and Chronic Wounds: Current Management Concepts.* 3rd ed. Saint Louis, Mo: Mosby; 2005:258–306.

13. Weir D. Pearls of compression. In: Falabella A, Kirsner R, eds. Wound Healing. *Informa Healthcare;* 2005:423–437.

14. Oduncu H, Clark M, Williams RJ. Effect of compression on blood flow in lower limb wounds. *Int Wound J.* 2004;1(2):107–113.

15. Virani T, Santos J, McConnell H, et al. *Assessment & Management of Venous Leg Ulcers.* Toronto, Ontario, Canada: Registered Nurses Association of Ontario; 2004.

16. Osterberg L, Blaschke T. Adherence to medication. *N Engl J Med.* 2005;353(5):487–497.

17. Blair SD, Wright DD, Backhouse CM, Riddle E, McCollum CN. Sustained compression and healing of chronic venous ulcers. *BMJ.* 1988;297(6657):1159–1161.

18. Franks PJ, Posnett J. *Cost effectiveness of compression therapy*

2003. EWMA Position Document. 2003:11–17.

19. Duby J, Hoffman D, Cameron J, et al. A randomized trial in the treatment of venous leg ulcers comparing short-stretch bandages, four-layer bandage system, and a long-stretch bandage system. *WOUNDS*. 1993;5:276–279.

20. Hofman D, Poore S, Cherry GW. The use of short-stretch bandaging to control edema. *J Wound Care*. 1998;7(1):10–12.

21. Hendricks WM, Swallow RT. Management of stasis leg ulcers with Unna's boot versus elastic support stockings. *J Am Acad Dermatol*. 1985;12(1 Pt 1):90–98.

22. Krasner D. Painful venous ulcers: themes and stories about their impact on quality of life. *Ostomy Wound Manage*. 1998;44(9):38–49.

23. Moffatt C. Issues in the assessment of leg ulceration. *J Wound Care*. 1998;7(9):469–473.

24. Nelson EA, Bell-Syer SE, Cullum NA. Compression for preventing recurrence of venous ulcers. *Cochrane Database Syst Rev*. 2000;(4):CD002303.

25. Jones JE, Nelson EA. Compression hosiery in the management of venous leg ulcers. *J Wound Care*. 1998;7(6):293–296.

26. Bello YM, Phillips TJ. Management of venous ulcers. *J Cutan Med Surg*. 1998;3(Suppl 1):S6–S12.

27. Gniadecka M, Karlsmark T, Bertram A. Removal of dermal edema with class I and II compression stockings in patients with lipodermatosclerosis. *J Am Acad Dermatol*. 1998;39(6):966–970.

28. Smith PC, Sarin S, Hasty J, Scurr JH. Sequential gradient pneumatic compression enhances venous leg ulcer healing: a randomized trial. *Surgery*. 1990;108(5):871–875.

Offloading Foot Wounds in People with Diabetes

David G. Armstrong, DPM, PhD, MD;
Nicholas J. Bevilacqua, DPM, FACFAS;
Stephanie C. Wu, DPM, MS

Objectives
The reader will be challenged to:
- Analyze the mechanical etiology of neuropathic diabetic foot wounds
- Utilize selection criteria for the use of various offloading modalities
- Distinguish the attributes and negative aspects of the most commonly utilized offloading modalities.

Introduction

In general, foot ulcers in people with diabetes result from repetitive moderate stress applied to the plantar aspect of the foot while walking.[1] This mechanism of injury commonly occurs because neuropathy provides a permissive environment for these wounds to occur. Without the ability to adequately respond to noxious stimuli, patients without protective sensation may sustain a breach of the skin, the way sensate persons wear holes in their stockings. As there are no current means available to completely ameliorate the effects of neuropathy, the present tenet for treating and preventing wounds focuses on the redistribution of pressure.

Although many offloading modalities are currently utilized, only a small number of case series exist describing the frequency and rate of wound healing associated with these modalities. This review describes the most commonly used modalities and the evidence that supports their employment.

Total Contact Casts

Total contact casts (TCCs) are considered by most diabetic foot specialists to be the gold standard offloading modality.[2] Plaster casting to treat neuropathic foot wounds was first described by Milroy Paul and later popularized in the United States by Dr. Paul Brand at the Hansen's Disease Center in Carville, Louisiana.[3] The technique has come to be known as TCC because it employs a well-molded, minimally padded cast that maintains contact with the entire plantar aspect of the foot and the lower leg. TCCs have been shown to reduce pressure at the site of ulceration by 84%–92%,[4] and there

Armstrong DG, Bevilacqua NJ, Wu SC. Offloading foot wounds in people with diabetes. In: Krasner DL, ed. *Chronic Wound Care: The Essentials.* Malvern, Pa: HMP Communications, 2014:271–278.

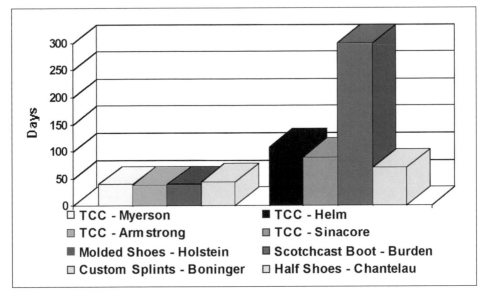

Figure 1. Healing times by offloading modality.

is a large body of work that supports the TCC's clinical efficacy. TCC is quite effective in treating a majority of noninfected, nonischemic plantar diabetic foot wounds, with healing rates ranging from 72%–100% over a course of 5–7 weeks.[5–10] Averaged throughout gait, peak plantar pressures are highest in the forefoot, while they tend to be generally less significant in the rearfoot and medial arch. Shaw[11] and Armstrong[12] have noted that a large proportion of the pressure reduction that occurs in the forefoot of the TCC is transmitted along the cast wall or to the rearfoot. This supports the postulate of several authors who have suggested that the TCC is effective because it permits walking by uniformly distributing pressures over the entire plantar surface of the foot.[3,5–8,13–15] Figure 1 illustrates healing times of different offloading modalities compared to TCCs.

Total contact casts are effective for a number of other reasons besides their ability to offload. They potentially protect the foot from infection and may help reduce or control edema, which can impede healing.[16] However, the most important attribute of this modality may be its ability to ensure appropriate patient adherence. In other words, because the device is not easily removable, the patient has no option other than to comply with the regimen prescribed by the clinician.

The above-described advantages make the TCC an attractive choice to offload the diabetic foot ulcer. However, there are a number of potential negative attributes that may dissuade some clinicians from using this modality. Most centers do not have a skilled healthcare professional or cast technician available with adequate training or experience to safely apply a TCC. Since improper cast application can cause skin irritation and in some cases even frank ulceration, this can be its single biggest negative feature. TCCs do not allow patients, family members, or healthcare providers to assess the foot or wound on a daily basis. Patients have difficulty sleeping comfortably and they cannot bathe easily without getting the cast wet. Certain designs of TCCs may exacerbate postural instability (Figure 2).[17] In addition, TCCs are generally contraindicated for wounds with ischemia, soft-tissue infections, or osteomyelitis.[18] Total contact casts are best for offloading the forefoot and may not be appropriate for heel ulcers because they may apply extra pressure on the posterior foot.[12]

Removable Cast Walkers and the "Instant" Total Contact Cast

The removable cast walker (RCW) offers several potential advantages over the traditional

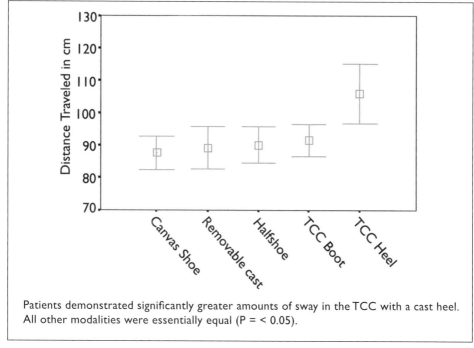

Patients demonstrated significantly greater amounts of sway in the TCC with a cast heel. All other modalities were essentially equal (P = < 0.05).

Figure 2. Postural instability in ulcer treatment modalities.[19] The total contact cast, when applied with a walking heel, may cause significantly more postural instability than one applied without a heel. Casts applied without heels have comparable stability profiles with many other common offloading modalities.

Reprinted with permission from WOUNDS. 2000;12(6 Suppl B):32B.

TCC. Removable walkers are, as their name implies, easily removed for self-inspection of the wound and application of topical therapies that require frequent administration. Patients can bathe and sleep more comfortably when wearing these devices. Because they are removable, they can be used for infected wounds as well as superficial ulcers.

Data from gait laboratory studies suggest that the amount of pressure reduction for certain RCWs is equivalent to TCCs.[4] Figures 3 and 4 illustrate mean peak pressure for ulcers under the metatarsal heads using various offloading techniques. In two randomized controlled trials comparing the proportion of healed ulcers treated with the TCC compared with other readily available and popular devices (RCWs, half shoes, and therapeutic depth inlay shoes), TCC healed a higher proportion of wounds compared to other

modalities.[16,19] This was an interesting finding because certain types of RCWs, including one used in one of the above-mentioned trials, often reduce pressure on the plantar aspect of the foot as well as TCCs.[19] If patients do not heal as well in the RCW, and yet the RCW offloads pressure about as well as the TCC, a logical explanation for the RCW's less effective clinical performance is that patients are simply not wearing these devices.[20] Because patients can remove RCWs easily, the best feature of this device is also, paradoxically, its potential downfall. The patient's ability to remove the RCW eliminates the element of "forced adherence," which is the finest attribute of the TCC. Patients may remove the RCW for dressing changes, sleeping, and showers, but they can also choose to use the walker only when they leave the house or walk excessively.

Armstrong et al postulated that although the

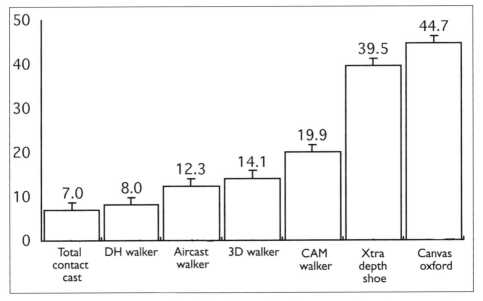

Figure 3. Mean peak pressure (N/cm^2) for ulcers under the metatarsal heads among various removable cast walkers.[20]

DH Walker (Centec Orthopaedics, Camarillo, Calif) is also licensed under the name Easy Step Pressure Relief Walker (Kendall Orthopedics, Mansfield, Mass)

CAM Walker (Darco International, Inc., Huntington, WV)

Aircast Walker (Aircast, Summit, NJ)

3D Walker (DeRoyal Orthopedic, Powell, Tenn)

Reprinted with permission from WOUNDS. 2000;12(6 Suppl B):34B.

RCW and TCC may offload equally well, patients, because of their dense neuropathy, might not be wearing their devices and not strictly adhering to their pressure-offloading regimen. In a recently conducted study, Armstrong et al evaluated the activity of patients with diabetic foot ulcers and their adherence to their offloading regime. This study, using accelerometers worn on the patients' waist and hidden in the RCW, suggested that patients wore their offloading device for less than 30% of their total daily activity.[20] This disappointing result has prompted a search for a simpler solution.

Understanding that TCCs are technically difficult and time consuming to apply, in light of the previous data, Armstrong et al have suggested that a potential alternative might be to make the RCW less easily removable. *This simple concept, termed an "instant total contact cast,"[21] (iTCC) involves simply wrapping the RCW with either a layer of cohesive bandage or plaster/fiberglass (Figure 5); thereby, making it more difficult for patients to remove.* The iTCC may have the benefit of adequate offloading as well as adding an element of "forced compliance" to the prescribed course of pressure reduction.

Two recent randomized controlled trials support the above-mentioned postulate. In the first study, subjects given an iTCC appeared to heal as readily at 12 weeks as patients given a standard TCC (80% iTCC versus 74% TCC).[22] A second study performed in parallel with this project compared the iTCC with a standard RCW. This study suggested substantial differences in healing at 12 weeks between the irremovable and removable devices (83% versus 52%).[23]

Scotchcast Boot

The Scotchcast boot is an alternative plaster of Paris cast and was developed when fiberglass ma-

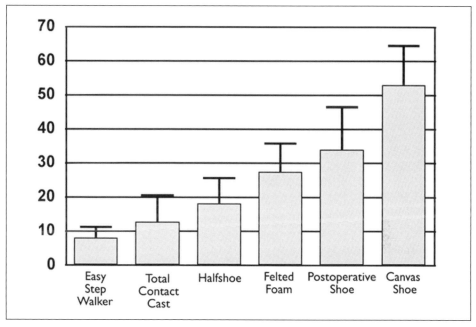

Figure 4. Mean peak pressure for ulcers under the metatarsal heads.[28]

Reprinted with permission from WOUNDS. 2000;12(6 Suppl B):32B.

terials were introduced. As a substitute for plaster of Paris, Scotchcast is much lighter with high-integral strength.[24] The basic functions of the cast are to reduce the pressure on the lesion, maintain patient mobility, and protect the remaining foot.

The Scotchcast boot is a well-padded cast cut away by the ankle and made either removable or nonremovable by cutting away the cast over the dorsum of the foot and making a closure of padding and tape with Velcro straps. Windows are cut over the ulcers as needed. A removable heel cap of fiberglass is added for large heel ulcers. The boot is worn with a cast sandal to increase patient mobility, keeping the patient ambulant while protecting the ulcer from any pressure.

Once the ulcer has healed, the patient can gradually start increasing the wear time of normal protective footwear while decreasing the wear time of the Scotchcast boot. The patient usually keeps the boot and the sandal, as this can be worn if an ulcer recurs.

The main advantages of this type of casting is that it is removable, allowing regular inspection and redressing of the wound. However, this ad-vantage is also one of the disadvantages (ie, potential for non-adherence). An alternative cast for the nonadherent patient would be a nonremovable Scotchcast boot.

Although the Scotchcast boot has been used successfully for more than a decade in several UK clinics, predominantly treating neuropathic and sometimes neuroischemic ulcers, no comparisons of healing rates between this type of cast and the more standard casts, such as the TCC, exist. Preliminary data of healing rates ranging from 61% to 88% with a mean healing time of between 10 and 13 weeks have been reported.[24,25] As with other modalities, a comparison study is warranted to investigate the efficacy of this cast against other currently used methods of offloading.

Halfshoes

Originally designed to decrease pressure on the forefoot postoperatively,[26] the halfshoe has become quite popular for treating foot wounds in people with diabetes. These devices are inexpensive and easy to apply. Chantelau and co-workers retrospectively evaluated 22 patients who

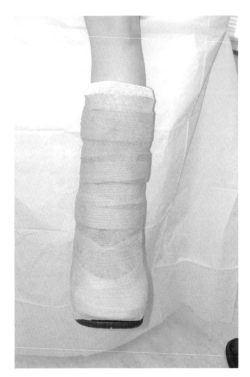

Figure 5. Instant total contact cast (iTCC).

received the halfshoe compared with 26 who received "routine wound care" and crutch-assisted gait. The results from this study suggested that more patients healed faster when using the halfshoe (70 versus 118 days) and that they developed fewer serious infections requiring hospitalization than those receiving standard therapy (4% versus 41%).[26] In a gait laboratory study comparing halfshoes to both TCCs and removable cast walkers, halfshoes were much less effective at reducing pressure than TCCs and certain removable cast walkers.[4] Just as is the case with removable cast walkers and the other modalities described in this review, studies evaluating outcomes, patient satisfaction, costs, and complications are needed to completely study this modality compared to other frequently utilized devices.

Healing Sandals

Applying a rigid rocker to the sole of a specially designed sandal may theoretically limit dorsiflexion of the metatarsophalangeal joints,

thereby limiting plantar progression of the metatarsal heads during propulsion in gait. In addition, the molded nature of a "healing sandal" provides a greater distribution of metatarsal head pressures and may theoretically provide for a shorter pressure-time integral. This device is lightweight, stable, and reusable. It does, however, require a significant amount of time and experience to produce the rigid-sole rocker design and other modifications. Most facilities do not have the time or expertise to modify these devices. Finally, these devices do not work as well as many other modalities that take less effort to produce.[27] Recently, a cross between a healing sandal and a removable cast walker has been introduced. This device, known as the MABAL shoe, is removable, but perhaps maintains more contact with the foot than does a standard healing sandal. In a study by Hissink et al, this device showed a similar time to healing when compared to studies of TCC.[28] However, this potentially promising device also has many of the downfalls of the contact cast and healing sandal, as it requires special expertise for its fabrication and application.

Felted Foam

Felted foam is another frequently used offloading technique,[29] which is fashioned by fixing a bilayered felt-foam pad over the plantar aspect of the foot with an aperture corresponding to the ulcer site. There is always a concern when applying an aperture around a wound that "the edge effect" will increase shear and vertical forces at the wound's periphery.[30] This approach is frequently used at some diabetes centers with anecdotal reports of success,[31,32] but to date, there are no controlled studies at these centers describing outcomes associated with this padding technique.

In 1997, Fleischli et al[33] conducted a study comparing the offloading ability of TCCs, halfshoes, RCWs, rigid postoperative shoes, and felted foam accommodative dressings. The results of this project suggested that TCCs and certain RCW achieved the best reduction of plantar pressures at the site of neuropathic ulcerations. The halfshoe finished a distant third, followed by the felted foam dressing and surgical shoe.

Crutches, Walkers, and Wheelchairs

It would stand to reason that completely

offloading a foot with crutches, walkers, or wheelchairs would be very effective in promoting healing in the diabetic wound. However, the vast majority of patients for whom these devices are prescribed do not have the upper body strength, endurance, or will power to use these devices when they do not perceive any limitation in function in their ulcerated limb. Additionally, it should be noted that some of these devices can, in fact, place the contralateral limb at risk for ulceration by increasing pressure to the unaffected side.[34] In the case of wheelchairs, it is prudent to understand that most patients' domiciles are not designed for wheelchair access; thus, reducing their utility in the place where they may potentially be most active—at home.

Therapeutic Footwear (Depth Inlay Shoes)

Many patients are prescribed therapeutic shoes in an effort to assist in pressure reduction and wound healing. However, these devices have not proven to be effective in this role. Gait laboratory studies suggest that therapeutic shoes allow up to 900% more pressure in areas of the forefoot compared to TCCs and some RCWs.[4] Furthermore, even the most optimistic studies using shoes as a primary offloading mechanism suggest that half of noninfected, nonischemic, superficial wounds (University of Texas Grade 1A[35,36]) will heal at 12 weeks.[37] *Therefore, the true value of therapeutic shoes and insoles might be in the prevention of ulceration and not offloading an active ulceration.*

Conclusion

It is important to understand that while the recent past history of treatment of wounds in general—and wounds in people with diabetes specifically—has been marked by some exciting advances on the high-technology front, it is in fact the low-technology systematic aspects of care that must assume priority. We often are heard saying, "It's not what one puts on a wound that heals it, but what one takes off." Appropriate wound care, debridement, and pressure reduction have and will continue to be the cornerstones of treatment. The key to successful pressure reduction possibly lies more in patient adherence than in the prescribed offloading devices. Persons with diabetes who have lost the "gift of pain" may not always adhere to the offloading regimen. Combining an effective, easy-to-use offloading device that ensures patient compliance with advanced wound healing modalities may form a formidable team in healing ulcers and potentially averting lower-limb amputations.

Take-Home Messages for Practice
- With sufficient vascular supply, appropriate debridement, and infection control, the primary mode of healing a diabetic neuropathic foot ulcer is pressure dispersion.
- The key to successful pressure reduction possibly lies more in patient adherence than in the prescribed offloading devices.

Self-Assessment Questions

1. Which of the following devices provides the greatest amount of pressure reduction at the site of ulceration?
   A. Instant total contact cast
   B. Scotchcast boot
   C. Healing sandal
   D. Halfshoe

2. All of the following are essential for wound healing except:
   A. Appropriate wound care
   B. Pressure reduction
   C. Debridement
   D. Antibiotics

Answers: 1-A, 2-D

References

1. Boulton AJM. The importance of abnormal foot pressure and gait in causation of foot ulcers. In: Connor H, Boulton AJM, Ward JD, eds. *The Foot in Diabetes.* Chichester, UK: John Wiley and Sons; 1987:11–26.
2. American Diabetes Association. Consensus development conference on diabetic foot wound care. *Diabetes Care.* 1999;22(8):1354.
3. Coleman W, Brand PW, Birke JA. The total contact cast: a therapy for plantar ulceration on insensitive feet. *J Am Podiatr Med Assoc.* 1984;74:548–552.
4. Lavery LA, Vela SA, Lavery DC, Quebedeaux TL. Reducing dynamic foot pressures in high-risk diabetic subjects with foot ulcerations. A comparison of treatments. *Diabetes Care.* 1996;19(8):818–821.
5. Armstrong DG, Lavery LA, Bushman TR. Peak foot

pressures influence the healing time of diabetic foot ul-cers treated with total contact casts. *J Rehabil Res Dev.* 1998;35(1):1–5.

6. Walker SC, Helm PA, Pulliam G. Chronic diabetic neu-ropathic foot ulcerations and total contact casting: heal-ing effectiveness and outcome probability (abstract). *Arch Phys Med Rehabil.* 1985;66:574.

7. Walker SC, Helm PA, Pulliam G. Total contact casting and chronic diabetic neuropathic foot ulcerations: heal-ing rates by wound location. *Arch Phys Med Rehabil.* 1987;68:217–221.

8. Sinacore DR, Mueller MJ, Diamond JE. Diabetic plan-tar ulcers treated by total contact casting. *Phys Ther.* 1987;67:1543–1547.

9. Myerson M, Papa J, Eaton K, Wilson K. The total contact cast for management of neuropathic plantar ulceration of the foot. *J Bone Joint Surg.* 1992;74A(2):261–269.

10. Helm PA, Walker SC, Pulliam G. Total contact casting in diabetic patients with neuropathic foot ulcerations. *Arch Phys Med Rehabil.* 1984;65:691–693.

11. Shaw JE, Hsi WL, Ulbrecht JS, Norkitis A, Becker MB, Cavanagh PR. The mechanism of plantar unloading in total contact casts: implications for design and clinical use. *Foot Ankle Int.* 1997;18:809–817.

12. Armstrong DG, Stacpoole-Shea S. Total contact casts and removable cast walkers: mitigation of plantar heel pres-sure. *J Am Podiatr Med Assoc.* 1999;89:50–53.

13. Boulton AJM, Bowker JH, Gadia M, et al. Use of plaster casts in the management of diabetic neuropathic foot ul-cers. *Diabetes Care.* 1986;9(2):149–152.

14. Kominsky SJ. The ambulatory total contact cast. In: RF Frykberg, ed. *The High Risk Foot in Diabetes Mellitus.* 2nd ed. New York, NY: Churchill Livingstone, 1991:449–455.

15. Lavery LA, Armstrong DG, Walker SC. Healing rates of diabetic foot ulcers associated with midfoot fracture due to Charcot's arthropathy. *Diabet Med.* 1997;14:46–49.

16. Mueller MJ, Diamond JE, Sinacore DR, et al. Total con-tact casting in treatment of diabetic plantar ulcers. Con-trolled clinical trial. *Diabetes Care.* 1989;12(6):384–388.

17. Lavery LA, Fleishli JG, Laughlin TJ, et al. Is postural instability exacerbated by off-loading devices in high risk diabetics with foot ulcers? *Ostomy Wound Manage.* 1998;44(1):26–34.

18. Wu SC, Crews RT, Armstrong DG. The pivotal role of offloading in the management of neuropathic foot ulcer-ation. *Curr Diab Rep.* 2005;5(6):423–429. Review.

19. Armstrong DG, Nguyen HC, Lavery LA, van Schie CH, Boulton AJ, Harkless LB. Offloading the diabetic foot wound: a randomized clinical trial. *Diabetes Care.* 2001;24(6):1019–1022.

20. Armstrong DG, Lavery LA, Kimbriel HR, Nixon BP, Boulton AJ. Activity patterns of patients with diabetic foot ulceration: patients with active ulceration may not adhere to a standard pressure off-loading regimen. *Diabe-tes Care.* 2003;26(9):2595–2597.

21. Armstrong DG, Short B, Espensen EH, Abu-Rumman PL, Nixon BP, Boulton AJ. Technique for fabrication of an "instant" total contact cast for treatment of neu-ropathic diabetic foot ulcers. *J Am Podiatr Med Assoc.* 2002;92:405–408.

22. Katz IA, Harlan A, Miranda-Palma B, et al. A random-ized trial of two irremovable off-loading devices in the management of plantar neuropathic diabetic foot ulcers. *Diabetes Care.* 2005;28(3):555–559.

23. Armstrong DG, Lavery LA, Wu S, Boulton AJ. Evaluation of removable and irremovable cast walkers in the healing of diabetic foot wounds: a randomized controlled trial. *Diabetes Care.* 2005;28: 551–554.

24. Burden AC, Jones GR, Jones R, Blandford RL. Use of the "Scotchcast boot" in treating diabetic foot ulcers. *Br Med J (Clin Res Ed).* 1983;286(6377):1555–1557.

25. Knowles A, Boulton AJM. Use of Scotchcast boot to heal diabetic foot ulcers. Presented at: the 5th European Con-ference of Advanced Wound Care; 1996; London, Eng-land.

26. Chantelau E, Breuer U, Leisch AC, Tanudjada T, Reuter M. Outpatient treatment of unilateral diabetic foot ulcers with "half shoes." *Diabet Med.* 1993;10:267–270.

27. Giacalone VF, Armstrong DG, Ashry HR, et al. A quan-titative assessment of healing sandals and postoperative shoes in offloading the neuropathic diabetic foot. *J Foot Ankle Surg.* 1997;36(1):28–30.

28. Hissink RJ, Manning HA, van Baal JG. The MABAL shoe: an alternative method in contact casting for the treatment of neuropathic diabetic foot ulcers. *Foot Ankle Int.* 2000;21(4):320–323.

29. Guzman B, Fisher G, Palladino SJ, Stavosky JW. Pressure-removing strategies in neuropathic ulcer therapy. *Clin Podiatr Med Surg.* 1994;11(2):339–353.

30. Armstrong DG, Athanasiou KA. The edge effect: how and why wounds grow in size and depth. *Clin Podiatr Med Surg.* 1998:105–108.

31. Myerly SM, Stavosky JW. An alternative method for reducing plantar pressures in neuropathic ulcers. *Adv Wound Care.* 1997;10(1):26–29.

32. Ritz G, Kushner D, Friedman S. A successful technique for the treatment of diabetic neurotrophic ulcers. *J Am Podiatr Med Assoc.* 1992;82(9):479–481.

33. Fleischli JG, Lavery LA, Vela SA, Ashry H, Lavery DC. 1997 William J. Stickel Bronze Award. Comparison of strategies for reducing pressure at the site of neuropathic ulcers. *J Am Podiatr Med Assoc.* 1997;87(10):466–472.

34. Armstrong DG, Liswood PL, Todd WF. The contralat-eral limb during total contact casting: a dynamic pres-sure and thermometric analysis. *J Am Podiatr Med Assoc.* 1995;85(12):733–737.

35. Armstrong DG, Lavery LA, Harkless LB. Validation of a diabetic wound classification system: the contribution of depth, infection, and ischemia to risk of amputation [see comments]. *Diabetes Care.* 1998;21(5):855–859.

36. Oyibo SO, Jude EB, Tarawneh I, et al. A comparison of two diabetic foot ulcer classification systems. *Diabetes.* 2000;49 (Suppl 1):A33.

37. Gentzkow GD, Iwasaki SD, Hershon KS. Use of Der-magraft, a cultured human dermis, to treat diabetic foot ulcers. *Diabetes Care.* 1996;19:350–354.

CHAPTER 21

Surgical Repair in Advanced Wound Caring

Dean P. Kane, MD, FACS

Objectives

The reader will be challenged to:
- Justify the role of surgical wound repair in the spectrum of wound management
- Differentiate the reconstructive options in surgical wound healing
- Distinguish the difference between a skin graft and tissue flap.

Introduction

Today's wound healing environment remains compromised by reimbursement disincentives, which are cost shifting more chronically ill patients to lesser skilled facilities, including the home. Less surgery is being offered as patients are found more catabolic and in less than optimal states for reconstructive options. On the other hand, there is greater awareness and knowledge of the factors that can positively impact healing potential.[1] Marked technological strides in stimulatory growth factors and biologic skin substitutes have reduced cost and improved healing when used appropriately.

Surgery, with the ultimate goal of hastened healing, pain reduction, durable repair, and less healthcare costs, is offered in those relatively few patients whose catabolic states have been reversed and whose wounds are of such size and clinical magnitude they otherwise would not heal. Advanced wound caring now includes compassionate patient management for those whose wounds will not heal.

It is prudent for the modern wound care specialist to appreciate more global views of chronic wound healing. The human ecosystem survives within a galaxy of overlying environments.

World Orders: The Big Picture

Anabolic growth, catabolic aging, and disease-oriented decline are best described by the subcellular nanoenvironment. Within the cellular environment, DNA transcribes RNA, and RNA translates cellular messengers and structural proteins. These cellular messengers come in many shapes

Kane DP. Surgical repair in advanced wound caring In: Krasner DL, ed. *Chronic Wound Care: The Essentials*. Malvern, Pa: HMP Communications, 2014:279–292.

and sizes. Growth factors, hormones, cytokines, interleukins, eicosanoids, and other chemical transmitters distribute instructions intra-, extra-, and intercellularly.

The intercellular environment, or "microenvironment," determines cell health. Without a balance of nutrients, oxidants, and antioxidants, each cell will not function optimally. Each cell has a particular form and function and works in concert with other cells orchestrated by intercellular messengers.

Those cells with similar function compose each "minienvironment." These minienvironments may include organs or, for the purposes of this discussion, chronic wounds. *Each chronic wound has a different environment based on location, pathologic entity, and comorbidities of the individual patient.* A diabetic neuropathic ulcer has a different world of environments than a pressure ulcer or nonhealing malignancy, yet they are all part of the human constellation.

The "macroenvironment" includes the constellation of organs in each unique patient. Aging and organ system decline appear to be regulated by intra- and intercellular messengers, as well as the harmony or disharmony of the external environment, including social, financial, familial, and health opportunities.

The pathophysiology of each wound and recognition of those significant comorbidities unique to each patient must be reversed in order to optimize healing. A domino effect of catabolic decline accelerates when wounds are not viewed globally. Only after this big picture of a chronic wound is appreciated will optimal outcomes and surgical management of the chronic wound be achieved.

History

Wound healing dates back to the caveman. The "gestures" inscribed into the Sumerian clay tablet of 2100 BC[2,3] including incantations, charms, and potions had little direct effect on the healing of injuries. The Edwin Smith Papyrus in 1600 provides the first written documentation of wound healing. The ancient physicians of Egypt, Greece, India, and Europe provided debridement and cleansing, removal of foreign bodies, covering and protection, drainage, and wound closure to hasten healing and protect their patients from limb loss and loss of

life.[2] The first written documentation of wound care dates back to the Ebers Papyrus in 1534 BC where bleeding vessels were "burnt with fire."[2]

Wound healing evolved through centuries of caustic and gentle treatments often carried out on the battlefield of history's famous field surgeons where amputation was reasoned to obviate gangrene and death.[4]

Wound healing, however, is mostly dependent on the body's natural ability to heal itself. Boiling oil, hot cautery, and scalding water were aggressive 14th century responses to injuries caused by gunpowder and bullets. Ambroise Paré espoused salves and gentle care in the 1500s. Metals, such as silver, were used in wounds during the 1800s. Not much has changed in 3,600 years; however, a better understanding of the wound healing process, occlusive, moist environments, and surgical reconstruction has hastened the wound healing process to achieve the body's first priority, a healed barrier from the outside environment.

Surgical Versus Nonsurgical Wound Healing

Most wounds, given the opportunity, will heal by secondary intent or round wound healing. If the wound is greater than the size of a quarter (2.5 cm in diameter) and/or is on a pressure-bearing site, the wound may heal secondarily, but without durable cover, it will eventually split, erode, bleed, or become infected endlessly. If the wound and the patient can tolerate it, surgical closure or linear wound healing is recommended.

When a wound is fully excised, a new acute wound has been created with removal of all infected, senescent cells and tissues. Primary closure or approximation of wound edges uses undermining to create random adjacent flaps. Visually, the wound is closed linearly. Linear wound healing is hastened as the tissue components are placed in apposition at the repair site and only collagen needs to hold the wound together. Since it takes 6 weeks in the immunocompetent patient to achieve 60% tensile strength (Figure 1), splinting and protection of the wound against stress are recommended for at least that period of time.

The essence of modern day surgical reconstruction is to carry prefabricated tissues into the prepared wound site for repair. This may include the plumbing (vessels), electrical conduits (nerves

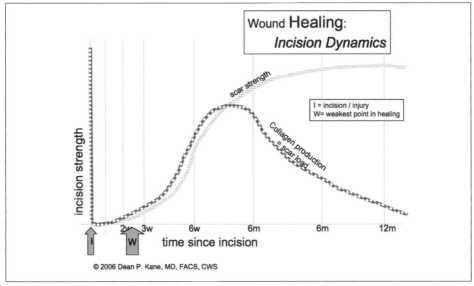

Figure 1. Postoperative linear wound strength.

for sensation and proprioception), fill, and durable cover. This may be as complex as a free tissue transfer (free flap), which may carry all layers of tissue, including tendons, muscle, fascia, and skin. For wounds of lesser clinical magnitude, surgical options range from simple to complex, providing the missing components according to the clinical stage of injury. This may include the foundation of the wound (bone, cartilage, muscle, or subcutaneous tissue), the walls (structure and scaffolding) of the wound, or its roof (skin).

The Most Common Wounds

Each wound is created by a unique physiologic event. Accurate diagnosis of the cause of the wound is essential in order to create the appropriate management plan. The wound specialist should seek the consultation of a plastic surgeon when he or she believes that a wound will not spontaneously heal given an optimized wound environment or the risk of such wound may complicate the patient's life or limb. Surgical closure is called for when a more efficacious outcome is expected by a more intensive surgical approach.

Pressure ulcers. Also called decubitus ulcers, bed sores, and pressure sores, these wounds occur when unrelieved pressure causes soft tissue necro-sis between the underlying chair or bed surface and the overlying bony prominence. More than $1.3 billion in healthcare costs were spent treating an estimated 2.1 million pressure ulcers[5] in 1990. Patients with central neurologic maladies, such as stroke or Parkinson's disease, as well as peripheral nerve injuries, including such polyneuropathies as diabetes or spinal cord lesions (paraplegics and quadriplegics), have a high risk of immobility, and therefore, pressure ulcer formation is common.

In addition to local pressure relief and considerations for reconstruction, the total management scheme includes nutrition, hydration, pain control, pressure-relieving or pressure-reducing surfaces, and a turning schedule that adequately maintains patient mobility and tissue perfusion.

The outward signs of pressure ulcer formation are typically described as the "tip of the iceberg." The redness, blistering, or small necrotic eschar first visualized on the outer skin overlying sacral, ischial, trochanter, scapular, posterior heel, elbow, and occipital ulcers are always smaller than the underlying cone-shaped zone of necrosis, which includes epidermis, dermis, subcutaneous fat, fascia, and muscle. If the zone of necrosis due to unrelieved pressure is deep enough, it will participate with the underlying periosteum, bone, and joint.

Rapid coagulation necrosis with infection of soft tissue planes may occur. If this becomes a source of infection and sepsis, surgical debridement and drainage of infected tissues are required. Topical and systemic antibiotics may be recommended. Local care is indicated and if consistent with the patient's overall plan of care may include staged debridement of necrotic tissue until such time that the wound has progressed through the inflammatory stages of wound healing and has achieved a clean granulation base free of infection, which hastens the realization of wound healing goals.

Both surgical and nonsurgical options should be considered to achieve closure of a wound. Occasionally, given the appropriate environment, wounds go on to complete healing by secondary intent. Surgical alternatives are considered when reconstruction will hasten the healing process, provide greater pain reduction, and/or reduce costs. The risk/benefit ratio must be clearly discussed with the patient and family.

Flap reconstruction provides well vascularized composite tissue resurfacing, lending greater durability to sites with bony prominences. Many patients are not appropriate candidates for such surgical options (eg, patients with multiorgan failure causing malnutrition, immobility, and multiple pressure ulcers). For these individuals, the secondary goals of wound care, which are to promote a stable, chronic, aseptic wound, comfort measures, and reduced pain, are essential. Appropriate candidates for flap reconstruction may require interim periods of rehabilitation, including activities of daily living (ADLs), in order to regain nutrition, strength, range of motion, and mobility. During this time, the wounds are stabilized after debridement and drainage of infection. Once optimized, these patients with better prognostic outcomes would undergo excision of the ulcer, including the underlying bone, to create an acute noninfected, round wound. The patients would then immediately undergo myofasciocutaneous flap reconstruction, filling the defect and closing the donor site in a linear fashion. Six weeks following flap reconstruction when surgical wound strength is reasonable, these patients may continue their rehabilitation to optimize function.

Patients who have the highest pressure ulcer acuity include people with diabetes, incontinence, or sacral pressure ulcers. These patients frequently become septic, necessitating broad-spectrum antibiotic coverage for the multibacterial flora at the time of debridement. Should fecal incontinence continue, a diverting colostomy or newer internal or external collection devices/options should be considered in order to reduce chronic, septic recurrences whether or not flap reconstruction is offered.

Many well vascularized and durable flaps are available based on the axial circulation of the region. Gluteal myocutaneous and gluteal fasciocutaneous flaps are used in the sacral region. Tensor fascia lata fasciocutaneous flaps reconstruct hip ulcers. Biceps femoris myocutaneous flaps fill ischial sores. Latissimus dorsi myocutaneous and lumbar fasciocutaneous flaps cover scapula wounds.

Posterior heel wounds are often the most difficult pressure ulcers to heal due to the end arterial blood supply based on the peroneal vessels laterally and the posterior tibial vessels medially of the foot, especially in the arterially insufficient patient. Once the dermal blood supply has been interrupted by full-thickness necrosis, no collateral circulation is available, and healing by secondary intent frequently fails. Debriding these types of wounds may lead to wet gangrene due to distal peripheral vascular disease. In these cases, it is recommended the clinician lift the heel off all hard surfaces using a splint or pillow under the calf. The wound also should be desiccated with an antiseptic, such as povidone iodine. Many patients with posterior heel dry gangrene will subsequently lose their limbs to wet gangrene if not monitored often. A stable, chronic, dry wound may be the best option for many of these patients. The use of a splint itself also may cause a pressure or traumatic injury; the surfaces in contact with the skin should be watched carefully for any signs of pressure or erosion.

Most pressure ulcers occur on the sacrum while the patient is in a lying or partially upright position. Pressure ulcers of the trochanter occur while the patient is in a side-lying position. Pressure ulcers of the ischium occur while the patient is in a sitting position. Depending on immobility, contractures, and neurologic incompetence (including spasticity), other sites of pressure ulcers and necrosis include the occiput, scapulae, elbows, knees, ankles, iliac crest, and buttocks.

Those patients with some of the poorest outcomes for healing and greatest morbidity are protein and/or calorie malnourished. Patients with albumin levels less than 2.5 mg/dL carry a morbidity 4 times greater than normal and a mortality 6 times greater.[6] Recommendations are made to postpone reconstruction while protein, vitamin, and mineral stores are replenished.

Lower-extremity ulcers. Lower-extremity ulcers include arterial, venous, diabetic, vasculitic, skin-malignant, and other chronic wounds. Many pathophysiologic and comorbid processes occur together, so accurate diagnosis remains the initial step in appropriate wound management.

Arterial ulcers. Arterial ulcers develop from inadequate arterial perfusion to the lower extremity. These ulcers may compound pressure ulcers and diabetic neuropathic ulcers. They may also exacerbate venous ulcers and traumatic wounds. If isolated, arterial ulcers typically present with gangrene or necrosis of the most distal aspects of the leg and foot. The wounds themselves appear to be round and punched out from lack of end arterial perfusion. Many patients experience claudication or ischemic pain during their presentation. Increased rubor or erythema of the extremity is noted as collateral circulation occurs at the subdermal level.

If a lack of circulation is palpated or determined by Doppler, noninvasive testing, such as arterial pulse volume recordings, is indicated to identify the level of arterial occlusion. This testing may lead to arteriogram and subsequent angioplasty or revascularization. A treatment plan must be coordinated between the vascular surgeon and the reconstructive surgeon. If infection is present, debridement to reduce the septic burden is necessary, while improved perfusion is rendered. Once increased blood supply is provided and the wound is free of infection with healthy and clean granulation tissue, reconstructive options can be offered. Split-thickness skin grafts, full-thickness skin grafts, and flap reconstructions may be considered. While revascularization is often short lived, healing the wound during the interval of good perfusion may avert limb loss. If unable to be revascularized, these patients are best off undergoing amputation prior to unrelieved

ischemic pain. This reduces the likelihood of the phantom limb pain syndrome, which could negatively impact their lives on a daily basis.

Venous ulcers. Venous insufficiency is seen in a large proportion of the ambulatory population. Venous drainage of the lower-extremity returns to the heart through deep and superficial veins that are connected by veins perforating the deep fascial layer. These perforating veins have valves that drain blood from the superficial to the deep venous system but not vice versa, unless they become incompetent from phlebitic obstruction in the deep venous system. Pelvic masses and obesity may worsen deep venous obstruction, causing chronic swelling and lymphedema.

The majority of venous insufficiency ulcers maintain epithelial islands within the irregular distal leg wounds, and when properly managed, these islands will re-epithelize without surgical intervention. On occasion, split-thickness skin grafts are necessary. These grafts may be performed as outpatient procedures as long as the patient has adequate home support to maintain leg elevation and minimize ambulation during the 3 to 6 weeks of skin graft healing.

Split-thickness skin grafts are typically harvested from the lateral thigh, although other donor sites are available. Current techniques allow for expansion of these grafts prior to placing them on the noninfected, well granulated wound bed. Five to 7 days of compression are necessary, and most patients are maintained on prophylactic antibiotics while the dressings are in place. Seven days of healing provide minimal, if any, collagen anchoring of the skin grafts to their beds, and immediate ambulation after initial take of the skin grafts will lead to skin graft loss. These patients require compression and elevation for 3 to 6 weeks, depending on their level of activity following venous stasis ulcer skin grafting.

Diabetic neurotropic ulcers. Diabetic wounds are multifactorial in origin. Patients with long-term diabetes develop polyneuropathy creating motor, sensory, and proprioceptive abnormalities. Skin surfaces become insensate, and foot clawing creates abnormal joint positions, placing greater pressure over bones and joints previously unaccustomed to such stresses. Combined with vascular disease and immunosuppression, patients with diabetes have a higher incidence of pressure ulcers, traumatic injury, and infected progressive wounds than the normal population.

Neurotropic infections in people with diabetes commonly take longer to heal due to the delayed introduction of macrophages as well as diminished leukocyte migration, which prolongs the inflammatory phase. This process allows for progressive bacterial invasion and results in longer hospital stays. Once infection and osteomyelitis or pyarthrosis are controlled, reconstruction is dependent on wound location. For weight-bearing surfaces, durable tissue in the form of flaps is recommended. Nonweight-bearing surfaces may be allowed to heal by secondary intent or, depending on their size, grafted with split- or full-thickness skin.

With the majority of diabetic wounds originating within the toe web spaces or plantar metatarsal phalangeal joint prominences, amputations should be limited and used only for extensive soft-tissue injury in the face of systemic sepsis. In these cases, patience is a virtue. Saving a patient's limb will protect the patient's function as well as prevent stress on the remaining leg, plantar surfaces, posterior heels, and pressure areas during ambulation, sitting, and lying. While amputation may be a quicker opportunity for wound healing, it also accelerates the deterioration of functional outcomes for these patients. The incidence of pressure ulcers from greater instability and immobility leads to sepsis and early death. Transmetatarsal, Ray, Syme, below-knee, or above-knee amputations should be the last resort.

Skin cancers. Nonhealing, bleeding wounds, whether heaped with granulation tissue, pigmented, or punched out and exuding, must be suspected as possible skin cancers, particularly those noted on sun-exposed body surfaces. These lesions should be biopsied for definitive diagnosis and, depending on the pathologic result, widely excised and reconstructed.

Basal cell. Basal cell cancers are less aggressive and rarely metastatic. Large basal cell cancers can become quite deforming and can invade the underlying bone. Options include wide excision with skin grafting or random flaps. Full-thickness skin grafts and adjacent-tissue, random-flap reconstruction provide the best color and texture match when considering the exposed areas of the face, neck, and hands. Other options include

Mohs micrographic surgery with similar reconstructive options or radiation therapy.

Squamous cell. Squamous cell cancers tend to be more ulcerating and may be highly metastatic. Chronic pressure ulcers and burn scars of prolonged duration have been known to degenerate into squamous cell carcinomas (Marjolin's ulcer). They necessitate wide excision with wound closure. Again, if on the face, reconstructing the anatomic defect with skin matched for color, texture, and quality will provide the greatest aesthetic appearance. If these wounds appear on pressure-bearing areas, a durable myofasciocutaneous flap is indicated. Regional lymph node dissection may be necessary to assess for metastatic disease.

Melanomas. Melanomas are the most fatal types of skin cancer. If extensive, they may appear as pigmented or nonpigmented, ulcerated, necrotic lesions on any body surface. Incisional or excisional full-thickness (not shave) biopsies are necessary for diagnosis. Depending on tissue depth, prognosis and treatment management options should be discussed with the patient/family. Distal extremity lesions with possible cure often require Ray amputation or partial-limb amputation. Surgical and medical oncology recommendations are requested for this uniquely individual problem.

Surgical wounds. Postoperative surgical wounds will usually heal when placed in traditional midline or well-vascularized sites. Many wounds are complicated by infection, tobacco use, diabetes, and other circulatory-limiting problems. Initially, epidermolysis and erythema may be noted. As wound healing deteriorates, full-thickness necrosis, serous drainage, infected exudate, and ultimately wound dehiscence, occur.

Consideration to optimize healing should be given to reduce tension across the surgical site and to improve perfusion, nutrition, and free radical destruction. Hydration, vitamins, protein and caloric repletion, as well as nonsteroidal anti-inflammatory drugs should all be considered.

Early intervention, such as revision of the wound closure back to bleeding edges of the nonhealing surgical incision, may prevent wound dehiscence. Debridement and local care that allow for healing of the wound by secondary intent or by other approaches ascending the reconstructive ladder should be entertained (Table 1).

Table 1. The reconstructive ladder of surgical wound healing options[4]
Free tissue transfer flap
Myofasciocutaneous flap
Random flap
Skin graft (split and full thickness)
Wound approximation (primary and secondary)
Based on the technical complexity and clinical staging of the wound, surgeons must consider the fastest, most cost-effective, durable, least painful, most functional, and best aesthetic reconstructive option appropriate for the patient's needs.

Surgical Reconstructive Options

Split-thickness skin grafts. When large superficial injuries occur, a split-thickness skin graft is indicated to resurface the wound. Healing is rapid and stable, providing the defect with epithelial and partial dermal components. As with all reconstructive options, a donor site wound remains, as does the defect site. Split-thickness skin grafts leave behind epithelial cells in the dermal adnexal appendages, such as sweat glands and hair follicles, to repopulate the donor surface. If the donor site is void of such adnexal appendages as is seen in elderly patients with no hair-bearing thigh skin, a secondary chronic wound at the donor site can be expected. In such a case, consideration should be made for full-thickness skin grafting or expanded meshed split-thickness skin grafting to both the defect and the donor site.

Skin graft take is a process by which the harvested paper-thin layer of skin now devoid of circulation becomes attached and viable to the defect site. Plasmatic imbibition and a transfer of cell fluids, nutrients, and toxins occur during the first 3 days. Inosculation, a process whereby the cut capillary edges of the skin graft match up with those of the recipient site, begins the process of revascularization. Initially, arterioles attach, causing congestion of the split-thickness skin graft. Greater tissue weight is noted as well as cyanosis and swelling. When the venules have approximated and tissue decongestion occurs, the skin graft turns pale pink and becomes viable.

It takes up to 3 weeks of collagen formation

to develop 30% tensile strength and up to 6 months for 90% tensile strength (Figure 1). Clinically, those skin grafts that have initially taken but subsequently failed may have occurred due to the misconception that a taken skin graft is fully healed. Should the patient be remobilized, remember the graft is not fully durable until scar or collagen anchoring of the skin graft has occurred (3–6 weeks).

Full-thickness skin grafts. A full-thickness skin graft includes the epidermis and full-thickness dermis. On occasion, composite grafts also include underlying fat or fascia. These grafts replace a total skin deficit as might occur with a skin cancer excision on the nose. Full-thickness skin grafts will contract less and blend better due to equal texture and color if donated from surrounding redundant tissues. Due to their extra thickness and perfusion needs, full-thickness skin grafts need longer immobilization in order to take. On occasion, epidermolysis may occur due to delayed perfusion of the epidermal layer. Re-epithelization will occur because of the adnexal appendages left in the full-thickness skin grafts.

Random flaps. Adjacent tissue reconstruction is the next level in wound construction complexity. Flaps based on the random circulation of the subdermal capillary plexus under the skin allow for undermining and advancement or flap creation and rotation of the skin and subcutaneous tissues (Figure 2).

Random flaps are useful in any portion of the body from the scalp to the toes where redundancy of tissue in 1 direction will allow for linear closure of the donor site and advancement or rotation of tissues to fill the defect. Due to the random nature of the circulation, areas of greater vascularity, such as the face and neck, will allow for more disproportionate length and width dimensions of the flap. Generally on the trunk and lower extremities, length of the flap and base width must be equal in order to achieve circulation to the tip of the random flap.[7–9]

Axial flaps. More complex on the reconstructive ladder is the axial flap (Figure 3). When larger or deeper defects, such as Stage IV, V (injury including bone), and VI (open joints) wounds occur, thicker, better vascularized, and more durable flaps will be necessary (Plates 25–27, Page 347). Transferring a tongue of tissue based on its

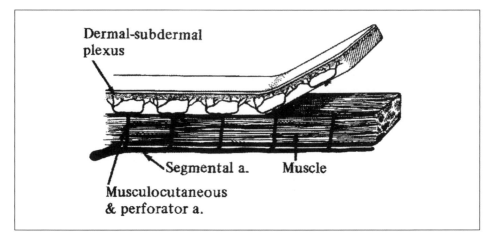

Figure 2. Random pattern skin flap.

Reprinted with permission from Grabb WC, Smith JW. *Plastic Surgery*. 3rd ed. Little, Brown and Company; 1979:39.

own blood supply yet leashed to its origin is the concept of transferring skin, subcutaneous tissue, fascia, muscle, and bone as a flap. These myofasciocutaneous flaps are useful in reconstruction of oral, face, and neck cancers and traumatic extremity injuries. The rectus abdominus myocutaneous flap is a well-recognized breast reconstruction following mastectomy.

Free tissue transfer flaps. State-of-the-art techniques, including microrevascularization, have allowed for composite tissues to be transferred from a body area, such as the face or back, to the defect site. Supple, well vascularized fascia or muscle tissue may be transferred as a free flap to defects in the leg, which would have otherwise progressed to limb loss (Figure 3). These free tissue transfers are more technically challenging but are now the basis for complex oral and maxillofacial reconstructions from cancer. Traumatic reconstructions of the legs and dynamic reconstructions for patients with nerve injuries or hand dysfunctions are other examples of the use of free tissue transfers.

Postoperative Surgical Care

Common sense should be the guide regarding postoperative wound care. Understanding the concepts of the wound healing curve will provide the basis of wound healing dynamics and appropriately timed therapeutic intervention (Figure 4).[9]

While skin graft take is occurring, immobili- zation of the wound site is mandatory to allow for adherence and neovascularization. Disruption of the partial- or full-thickness skin graft due to sliding or direct pressure forces will cause separation of the graft from its vascularized bed with seroma, hematoma, fibrin, or purulent secondary effects. Immobilization with the use of splinting, restricted motion, and at times pinning or external fixation across joints may be necessary. A sterilized wound bed and antibiotics should be maintained to reduce skin graft loss due to infection. Assessment should be made at first dressing removal (5–7 days), and topical dressings should be applied according to wound-dressing matching schemes.

Considering the need for collagen anchoring of the skin graft to its bed, 3–6 weeks of protected care may be necessary until the tensile strength between the skin graft and its bed will prevent further disruption. Lower-extremity surgery will necessitate longer immobility and greater protection using firm compressive dressings and continuous elevation of the site. Other skin-grafted wounds closer to and including the head region will require less immobility and are usually already elevated.

Random adjacent tissue transfers and all flaps require elevation, pressure relief, immobilization, and reduction of shearing forces. These round wounds have been reconstructed in linear fashion. While these flaps are vascularized, they also

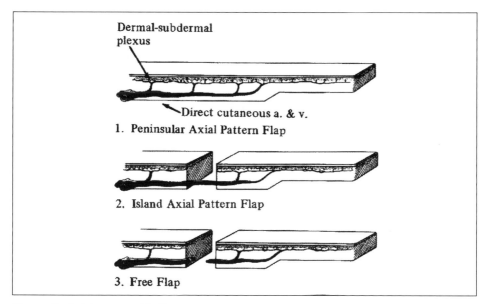

Figure 3. Axial pattern skin flaps.

Reprinted with permission from Grabb WC, Smith JW. *Plastic Surgery.* 3rd ed. Little, Brown and Company; 1979:39.

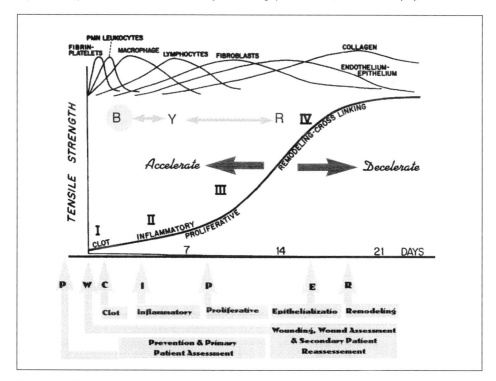

Figure 4. The wound healing curve noting acceleration (left shift) of the wound healing process and deceleration (right shift).

develop neovascularization from their wound bed and wound edges. Any disruption between the overlying flap and underlying wound bed will cause similar wound healing problems including seroma, hematoma, fibrin separation, and purulent consequences, endangering the flaps viability. While linear wound healing is certainly faster than round wound healing, the incision line should be protected from infection, incontinence of urine and stool, and tension. Suture selection is imperative to provide the appropriate time for collagen deposition and remodeling of the scar to reduce wound dehiscence. The weakest point in time of the incision is when the suture strength is weakest (2–3 weeks) and at the beginning of collagen production (2 weeks) (Figure 1). External suture or staple removal timing is dependent on the wound site. Pressure bearing areas and sites of dependency, such as pressure ulcer flap reconstructions or lower-extremity wound flap reconstructions, necessitate at least 6 weeks of wound approximation to approximate 60% tensile strength before attempting to stress the incision line. Three weeks, approximating 30% tensile strength of suture or staple reinforcement, is provided for major trunk and upper extremity flap reconstructions (Figure 1). When consideration is made regarding the aesthetic appearance of the scar in the less stressed regions of the face and neck or in smaller reconstructive sites, sutures may be removed at 5–7 days when layered dermal closure has also been performed. In addition, the current use of skin glue to retain skin approximation without the use of staples and sutures will maintain strength across the incision line for an extra 2–3 weeks.

These grafts or flaps may be rescued by directing medical or surgical attention to the adverse problem if wound disruption, infection, underlying collection of fluids, or vascular compromise occurs during the early wound healing phases.

Postoperative Graft and Flap Assessment

Assessment for reconstructive wound healing failure is timed according to the risk of its occurrence as well as the magnitude of the problem that such a complication might create. If the magnitude of the deformity or the risk of secondary deformity is great, such as loss of a free, latissimus, or rectus abdominus myofasciocutaneous flap, assessment may be necessary in the intensive care unit every hour using visibility as a guide or more refined technology, such as Doppler flow meters, laser Doppler flow meters, transcutaneous pO_2 sensors, temperature probes, and others. Small flaps and skin grafts may need reevaluation at 5 days when sutures are to be removed and then daily or weekly depending on the magnitude of the secondary defect.

Flap and Skin Graft Failure

Even with valiant attempts for wound closure, underlying problems may cause flap or skin graft failure. Flap or skin graft failure proceeds through a series of events that, if caught early enough, may be reversed. The cardinal signs of flap failure include:

- Swelling (hyperpermeability)
- Erythema (hyperemia)
- Cyanosis (venous congestion)
- Epidermolysis (partial-thickness necrosis)
- Demarcation necrosis (full-thickness necrosis)
- Wound separation (loss of vascularity, fibrin/collagen attachments).

With flap failure, the cardinal signs of infection may become superimposed on the cardinal signs of flap failure. These include:

- Rubor (redness)
- Calor (warmth)
- Dolor (pain)
- Tumor (induration).
- Functio laesa (organ dysfunction), ie, Vichow's pentad as seen in flap failure.

These may then become more complicated by progressive infection: contamination, colonization, cellulitis, and sepsis.

Flap rescue. The rescue of failing flaps is dependent on the critical observation and management plan to reverse the physical and physiologic cause of the causative event (Table 2).

The "essential cannons of wound healing" include adequate circulation and a robust anabolic immune system.

Immunocompromise occurs with inadequate calories and protein, minerals, anti-oxidants, and vitamins to maintain hemostasis, debridement, and structural and repair functions of wound healing. Nutrition is absolutely essential to the reversal of catabolic effects, immunosuppression, morbidity, and mortality.[10] The added energy re-

Table 2. Rescue of failing surgical flaps

Physiologic conditions of graft/flap failure	Graft/flap rescue
Reduced or lack of perfusion	
Inadequate hydration	*IV hydration* volume expansion: lactated ringers, whole blood transfusion
Vasospasm	*Vasodilatation* lidocaine 1% topical to blood vessels
arterial	sublingual calcium channel blocker, L-arginine; sympathetic blockage: epidural anesthesia; antihistamines: cimetidine, ranitadine, others
venous	topical/sublingual nitroglycerin
pain (catecholamine release)	pain control: analgesics, steroids
Inflammatory edema	Membrane stability: IV or oral steroids, NSAIDs
Hypercoagulability	
Platelet aggregation and degranulation	*Platelet deaggregation: ASA 84mg/day* (⇑*prostacyclin*, ⇓*thromboxane*)
Venous obstruction	*Leeches (local anticoagulation)*
Hyperperfusion injury, due to free radical formation and xidants	Antioxidants; free radical scavengers: melatonin, super oxide dismutase, glutathione, others
Hypo-oxygenation	Stop all nicotine products, nasal oxygen, hyperbaric oxygen, topical oxygen
Infection	Anti-infectants *antibiotics, antifungals, antivirals*
Physical causes of graft/flap failure	**Graft/flap rescue**
Twist or tension of vascular pedicle	Release or untwist flap pedicle; release extension (ie, flexion across the surgical site)
Swelling of flap or surrounding tissues	Reduce tension: release sutures, elevate body site

quirements and mechanical and physiologic stress will strain the success of a wound reconstruction, including flaps and grafts. Reassessment of all wound healing parameters is necessary when a failing flap or skin graft is found.

Volume expansion and increased cardiac output will assist in arterial perfusion of the flap and wound. When a kinked arterial and venous blood supply is considered, "take-down" of the flap for re-evaluation and untwisting of the pedicle or re-anastamosis of the microvascular approximation are necessary. Lidocaine without epinephrine may reverse arterial vasospasm. Nitroglycerin as an intravenous infusion, sublingual tablet, paste, or transdermal patch may reduce venous congestion. Today, medicinal leaches that secrete hirudin, an antithrombin anticoagulant, as they ingest pooled venous blood are used. Pain control is recommended to reduce the elevated epinephrine levels associated with surgical and ischemic discomfort.

The inflammatory and coagulability cascades have been described in Chapters 8 and 12 and other chapters of this textbook. Aspirin and other nonsteroidal, anti-inflammatory medications are useful in reducing the vasospastic, fibrin-clotting actions associated with the complement, arachidonic, and other inflammatory cascades at the risk of excess bleeding. Cell membrane stability and reduction in edema are also assisted with the use of intravenous or oral steroids. Simply elevating the extremity may reduce edema and venous congestion. Antioxidants, such as vitamins A, C, and E as well as alpha-lipoic acid, are useful in neutralizing the membrane, protein, and nucleic acid injuries attributed to free radical formation.

Oxygenation is necessary as an anti-infective and for cell metabolism. Nasal oxygen, topical oxygen, and hyperbaric oxygen have all found their niche in reversing the failing flap.

Should infection be the source of skin graft or flap failure, irrigation and drainage to reduce bioburden may revive the graft or flap. Secondary bacterial infections may occur following viral or fungal colonization. Antiviral and antifungal medications will need to be considered in addition to topical antiseptics and oral/intravenous antibiotics.

A combined rescue approach must be considered early and aggressively. Once permanent injury has occurred, the flap or graft is dead, and chronic wound healing pathways persist.

Summary

A greater global appreciation of wound healing is necessary, including overlapping environments kept in anabolic repair by chemical transmitters, (eg, hormones, cytokines, growth factors, and others) in order to achieve a durable, healed wound. Current goals for wound care include the reversal of wound progression in order to save limb and life. Thereafter, healing, function, and aesthetics are desired outcomes. Many present-day patients with chronic, debilitating, neurologic maladies, malnutrition, and immobility may never heal a chronic wound nor are they suitable candidates for reconstruction. For these patients, compassionate, local management and dignified, holistic care are reasonable alternatives that should be provided. Surgical reconstructive options should be considered for selected patients whose length of healing would be extraordinarily long (months or years) and whose health status is appropriate for rapid healing.

Take-Home Messages for Practice

- Surgical alternatives from simple to complex are considered when reconstruction will hasten the healing process, provide greater pain reduction, and/or reduce costs.
- Adequate nutrition and vascular competence are essential to wound healing.
- Reversal of catabolism (immobility, anti-inflammatory medications, anti-infectives) is as critical as anabolic stimulation (nutrition, topical wound care, growth factors) in wound healing.
- Compassionate care is acceptable in those patients whose wounds will not heal.

Self-Assessment Questions

1. The cardinal signs of inflammation include all of the following EXCEPT:
   A. Rubor (redness)
   B. Calor (warmth)
   C. Pallor (ischemia)
   D. Tumor (induration)

2. The cardinal signs of flap failure include:
   A. Swelling, erythema, cyanosis, epidermolysis, necrosis, dehiscence
   B. Hemostasis, inflammation, proliferation, remodeling
   C. Imbibition, inoculation, neovascularization
   D. All of the above

3. Reconstructive options for wounds include all of the following EXCEPT:
   A. Amputation
   B. Split- and full-thickness skin grafts
   C. Random and axial flaps
   D. Vascularized flaps of skin, fat, muscle, and bone

4. Which of the following comorbidities would be LEAST likely to delay wound healing?
   A. Diabetes
   B. Peripheral vascular disease
   C. Venous insufficiency
   D. Osteoarthritis

Answers: 1-C, 2-A, 3-A, 4-D

References

1. Krasner DL, Sibbald RG. Nursing management of chronic wounds: best practices across the continuum of care. *Nurs Clin North Am.* 1999;34(4):933–953.

2. Majno G. *The Healing Hand: Man and Wound in the Ancient World.* Cambridge, Mass: Harvard University Press; 1975:570.

3. Lionelli GT, Lawrence WT. Wound dressings. *Surg Clin North Am.* 2003;83(3):617–638.

4. Helling TS, McNabney WK. The role of amputation in the management of battlefield casualties: a history of two millennia. *J Trauma.* 2000;49(5):930–939.

5. Bergstrom N, Bennet MA, Carlson CE, et al. Clinical Practice Guideline Number 15: Treatment of Pressure Ulcers. Rockville, Md: US Department of Health and Human Services. Agency for Health Care Policy and Research; 1994. AHCPR Publication 95-0652.

6. Demling RH, DeSanti L. Use of anticatabolic agents for burns. *Curr Opin Crit Care.* 1996;2:482–491.

7. Mathes SJ, Nahai F. *Clinical Applications for Muscle and Myocutaneous Flaps.* St Louis, Mo: CV Mosby; 1982.

8. Demling RH, DeSanti L. Involuntary weight loss and the nonhealing wound: the role of anabolic agents. *Adv Wound Care.* 1999;12(1 Suppl):1–16.

9. Schilling J. Wound healing. *Surg Round.* 1983:46–62.

10. Kinney J. Energy requirements of the surgical patient. In: Ballinger W, ed. *Manual of Surgical Nutrition.* Philadelphia, Pa: WB Saunders; 1975.

CHAPTER 22

The Role of Oxygen and Hyperbaric Medicine

**Robert A. Warriner, III†, MD, FCCP, FACWS, FAPWCA*;
James R. Wilcox, RN, BSN, ACHRN, CWCN, CFCN, CWS, WCC, DAPWCA, FCCWS;
Richard Barry, BBA, CHT-A**

Objectives

The reader will be challenged to:

- Analyze the impact of local tissue hypoxia on wound healing and response to infection
- Distinguish the physiological benefits to wound healing provided by oxygen delivered by different mechanisms
- Assess the physiological and pharmacological benefits of hyperbaric oxygen treatment to wound healing
- Select appropriate patients for adjunctive hyperbaric oxygen treatment provided in an integrated wound care setting
- Implement essential aspects of safe hyperbaric patient management in the practice setting.

Introduction

Hyperbaric oxygen treatment (HBOT) as adjunctive therapy to aggressive surgical debridement and antibiotic therapy for necrotizing soft tissue infection dates back to the 1960s. Clinicians took advantage of the specific benefits of elevating tissue oxygen levels in the presence of these anaerobic, exotoxin-producing wound infections to improve limb and tissue salvage and overall survival. Subsequent experience and research in other wound healing problems, including radiation bone and soft tissue injury, acute traumatic ischemias, various types of ischemic reperfusion injury states, and a wide range of chronically hypoperfused and hypoxic wounds, has led to the development of the current recommendations for the clinical use of HBOT as outlined in the 12th edition of *Hyperbaric Oxygen Therapy Indications*,[1] which was published by the Undersea and Hyperbaric Medical Society in 2009. Over the past 10 years, a new understanding of the pharmacology of hyperbaric oxygenation of tissues and randomized, controlled, clinical trials of HBOT in radiation tissue injury and refractory diabetic ulcer healing and limb salvage have enhanced the acceptance of adjunctive HBOT for the mainstream management of complex problem wounds.

Adequate molecular oxygen is required for a wide range of biosynthetic processes essential to normal wound healing. Molecular oxygen is required for hydroxylation of proline during collagen synthesis and cross linking as well as provision of substrate for the production of reactive oxygen species during the respiratory burst occurring within leukocytes that have

Warriner RA, Wilcox JR, Barry R. The role of oxygen and hyperbaric medicine. In: Krasner DL, ed. *Chronic Wound Care: The Essentials*. Malvern, PA: HMP Communications; 2014:293–302.

phagocytized bacteria within the wound. While short-term hypoxia is one stimulus for angiogenesis in wound healing, adequate local oxygen levels are required to sustain an effective angiogenic response and for the reconstruction of an adequate dermal matrix. Recent research has shown that oxygen also plays an important role in the cell signaling events necessary for tissue repair, which further explains the fragile dynamic between oxygen availability and the increased demands for oxygen during recovery from tissue injury.[2]

When oxygen availability to a wound is reduced by hypoperfusion from macrovascular arterial disease, microvascular failure, local edema, or infection, wound healing is invariably impaired. *Periwound hypoxia* can be objectively determined by transcutaneous PO2 measurement.[3] When identified, periwound hypoxia should be addressed with further vascular assessment and interventions to improve large vessel perfusion, reduce tissue edema, and improve microvascular homeostasis by maintaining normovolemia and vasomotor tone and with therapeutic oxygen administration. The method of administration determines the potential beneficial effects of additional oxygen administration in support of wound healing.

Supplemental Oxygen Breathing at One Atmosphere

Additional oxygen can be provided therapeutically by increasing the inspired oxygen concentration above 21% by use of a nasal cannula or a simple facemask. The maximum achievable intra-arterial PO2 breathing 100% oxygen at 1 ATA (atmospheres absolute) is approximately 670 mmHg. In well perfused tissues, supplemental oxygen breathing at 1 ATA may transiently reverse mild local tissue hypoxia secondary to edema or mild hypothermic vasoconstriction but has not been shown to reduce postoperative wound infections[4] or improve collagen deposition.

Topical Oxygen

HBOT is not provided by devices that apply oxygen at 1 ATA over the surface of the wound, by devices that provide a small pressure differential (usually around 1.04 ATA) by enclosing an appendage in an inflatable bag or plastic cylinder, or by devices providing a surface oxygen blow-

over using a micro-oxygen concentrator device. None of these devices are considered by the US Food and Drug Administration to provide hyperbaric oxygen, and the misused terminology has led to significant confusion in both the literature and in discussion of the potential merits of oxygen applied by some manner to the wound surface. Two recent reviews[5,6] addressed the potential for topical oxygen to benefit wound healing. While *in-vitro* research has suggested some rationale for topical oxygen,[7] critical questions have yet to be answered. Topical oxygen appears to increase wound surface and subsurface PO2 values but only to a relatively shallow depth. Topical oxygen produces a gradient opposite of what is produced during HBOT, and it is unclear how this reverse gradient might drive the direction of angiogenesis and tissue growth. Clinical trials and case series to date have produced positive and negative effects,[8-12] unlike the consistently positive results seen with HBOT for chronic lower-extremity wounds and diabetic limb salvage cases. The Undersea and Hyperbaric Medical Society published a position statement[13] that discussed these concerns. The proposed recommendations for topical oxygen in lower-extremity wounds[6] require further validation before they are widely accepted in clinical practice.

An alternative to oxygen delivered by low-flow blowover or topical oxygen under pressure is a dressing that might deliver oxygen to the wound surface typically through incorporation of hydrogen peroxide into the dressing core structure. There is little evidence to suggest any benefit on wound healing other than potential suppression of wound surface microorganisms.

Hyperbaric Oxygen

HBOT is defined as *breathing 100% oxygen in an environment of elevated atmospheric pressure typically ranging from 2.0 to a maximum of 3.0 ATA or 2 to 3 times normal atmospheric pressure.* This can occur in a *monoplace (single-patient) chamber* typically compressed with 100% oxygen or, less frequently, in a *multiplace (multiple-patient) chamber* typically compressed with air with the patient breathing 100% oxygen through a specially designed hood or mask. Intravascular PO2 values are in excess of 1700 mmHg.[14]

HBOT provides additional oxygen to the

hypoxic wound and supports wound healing through a variety of mechanisms. The immediate effects of HBOT occurring during treatment improve wound "metabolism" in the setting of acute or chronic local hypoxia. These relatively short-lived effects in support of wound healing include the following:

1) Improved local tissue oxygenation, leading to improved cellular energy metabolism
2) Increased collagen and other extracellular matrix protein deposition and epithelization
3) Decreased local tissue edema due to vasoconstriction of vessels in nonischemic tissues
4) Improved leukocyte-bacterial-killing (adequate leukocyte count critical for benefit)
5) Suppressed exotoxin production
6) Increased effectiveness of antibiotics that require oxygen for active transport across microbial cell membranes.

These effects, while important, would not by themselves account for the degree of improvement in wound healing seen in most diabetic foot ulcers treated with HBOT.

Over the past 15 years, research has led to a somewhat different understanding of the role of HBOT, which has focused on the role HBOT plays in altering the balance of reactive oxygen (ROS) and reactive nitrogen (RNS) species within the wound, fundamentally altering the wound environment and its healing response. In this context, HBOT also must be thought of as providing oxygen as a cell-signaling agent.[15,16] Achieving these effects beneficial to wound healing requires that a minimum PO_2 of around 200 mmHg be achieved in the periwound tissues. The effects include:

1) Enhanced growth factor and growth factor receptor production (especially platelet-derived growth factor [PDGF] and vascular endothelial growth factor [VEGF], helpful in wound matrix reconstruction and angiogenesis)
2) Altered leukocyte β-integrin receptor sensitivity (helpful in mitigating ischemia-reperfusion injury, which occurs in many chronic and some acute wound settings)
3) Reduced inflammation and apoptosis (at least in some acute ischemic wound models)
4) Activated stem cell metabolism and release into the circulation from bone marrow reservoirs.

These physio-pharmacological changes have been observed both *in vitro* and *in vivo*.[17-20] It is interesting to note that the ROS- and RNS-mediated pathways that can be enhanced by HBOT can have both positive and negative effects on wound healing. The biochemical environment of the wound when exposed to HBOT probably determines these effects. Perhaps in the future we will be better able to characterize these conditions within the wound or ulcer bed as a means to better select specific patients who will respond optimally to HBOT for limb salvage.

Clinical Experience with HBOT in Wound Healing

Prior to 2010, the strongest clinical evidence for HBOT in diabetic limb salvage was the randomized, controlled, clinical trial reported by Faglia et al.[21] This study involved 68 patients randomized to HBOT and standard care groups. Revascularization was provided to all patients where indicated by arteriographic findings. A team comprised of members who were blinded to the core intervention made the surgical decisions. The HBOT group required 3 major amputations (3/35 or 8.6%), while the standard care group required 11 major amputations (11.33, 33%) with a $P = .016$.

Following a review of the Faglia et al study and an independent, evidence-based review in 2002, the Centers for Medicare & Medicaid Services approved HBOT for Wagner grade 3 and greater diabetic foot ulcers. A 2004 Cochrane review concluded that HBOT significantly reduced the risk of major amputation in diabetic foot ulcer patients.[22] In cost-effectiveness studies, Guo et al[23] and the Canadian Diabetes Association[24] demonstrated that HBOT reduced anticipated major amputations and was cost-effective on a long-term basis.

In a *meta-analysis of HBOT* in wound healing and limb salvage, Goldman[25] evaluated published randomized, controlled, clinical trials and observational studies of various designs using the **GRADE criteria** for assigning levels of evidence. Thirty-five studies (excluding the 2010 Löndahl et al study[26]) met the inclusion criteria of original human studies with diabetes-related wound healing, tissue salvage, or limb salvage as the clinical endpoint. Thirty-three of the studies reported positive efficacy, 1 was equivocal, and 1 was negative with a low strength of evidence. In all, 4,057 patients with diabetes were included in the studies reviewed. When the endpoint was limb salvage, HBOT provided a 3-fold reduction in the risk of amputation when compared to conventional wound care alone, providing GRADE level 1 evidence.

The most recent clinical trial of hyperbaric oxygen in diabetic ulcers was published by Löndahl et al in Sweden.[26] The randomized, single-center, double-blind, placebo-controlled, clinical trial was completed at the Institution for Clinical Sciences in Lund, Lund University. Ninety-four patients with Wagner grade 2, 3, or 4 ulcers of greater than 3 months' duration with adequate perfusion or with non-reconstructable peripheral arterial disease were randomized into 2 groups. Patients were treated with 2.5 ATA air or 2.5 ATA 100% oxygen for 85 minutes in a multiplace chamber with a coded gas delivery system. Treatments were administered 5 days per week for 8 weeks (40 treatments) with a study duration of 10 weeks and a 1-year follow-up. This was an intention-to-treat analysis with a primary endpoint of ulcer healing. Complete healing was achieved in 37/94 patients at 1 year, 25/48 (52%) in the HBOT group and 12/42 (29%) in the placebo group ($P = .03$). Subgroup analysis of patients completing > 35 HBOT sessions showed healing in 23/38 (61%) in the HBOT group versus 10/37 (27%) in the placebo group ($P = .009$).

Finally, the Wound Healing Society Clinical Practice Guidelines for diabetic foot ulcer care[27] give HBOT a 1A level of evidence recommendation, and the ischemic ulcer guidelines[28] give it a level IIB recommendation.

Indications for HBOT in Wounds

The Undersea and Hyperbaric Medical Society[3] provides recommendations for the use of HBOT based on a selected expert panel's review of relevant published clinical and experimental data. This report and other published reviews define the specific wound etiologies that may be expected to benefit from intermittent HBOT exposure, including:

• Acute thermal burns
• Clostridial myonecrosis
• Other necrotizing soft tissue infections

• Compromised skin grafts and flaps
• Crush injury and compartment syndrome
• Other acute traumatic ischemias
• Osteoradionecrosis
• Soft tissue radionecrosis
• Refractory osteomyelitis
• Other wounds with demonstrated peri-wound hypoxia, particularly in patients with diabetes mellitus and chronic ischemic ulcers.

Selection of Patients for HBOT

HBOT is best justified within a consistently applied patient selection process that takes into consideration those factors suggested to impact response to this therapy.[29,30] The most critical of these factors is sufficient local blood flow to support the local elevation of tissue PO_2 that is possible during the HBOT exposure. The following should be considered in the initial treatment decision:

• Is the clinical presentation of the wound consistent with the published experience of wounds in which HBOT has been demonstrated to be beneficial?
• Is hypoxia as measured by $PtcO_2$ present in tissue adjacent to the wound?
• Does the periwound tissue respond to an increase of inspired oxygen concentration, indicating at least minimally sufficient periwound blood flow to allow a therapeutic increase in local oxygen tension during HBOT?

Based on these considerations, the hyperbaric physician follows a process similar to the following to determine which patients with problem wounds are appropriate candidates for adjunctive HBOT delivered as a component of total wound care:

1. An appropriate wound etiology associated with local hypoxia or persistent infection is identified.
2. Periwound hypoxia is demonstrated by $PtcO_2$ measurement whenever possible. The equipment for this testing is readily available, and an excellent review article described in detail the principles for performance of the test and interpretation of the results obtained. Multiple electrode sites should be selected whenever possible, including sites adjacent to and in the normal anatomical distribution

of blood flow to the wound. PtcO2 measurements have been shown to be of value in predicting wound healing success or failure and in the evaluation of peripheral arterial occlusive disease.[3]

3. All patients considered for adjunctive HBOT undergo a complete medical and nursing evaluation to determine the risks of treatment and the medical and care issues that will have to be addressed by the hyperbaric medicine team. Glycemic control and prevention of hypoglycemia associated with HBOT are of particular importance. Absolute contraindications (untreated pneumothorax, some concomitant chemotherapeutic agents) should be identified and the patient excluded from treatment. Relative contraindications (factors that increase CNS or pulmonary oxygen toxicity risk, such as high fever, some drugs, such as bleomycin, cis-platin, and factors that increase the risk of otic or pulmonary barotrauma, such as reactive airway disease) should be identified and the patient's condition optimized prior to treatment whenever possible. The hyperbaric physician should determine the appropriateness of the treatment for each patient with respect to the best likely achievable outcome. Cost-effectiveness studies based on medical economic modeling have demonstrated the cost and clinical value position of HBOT in diabetic limb salvage.[31,32] While the personal economic impact of daily visits to an outpatient healthcare facility for HBOT and wound care have not been assessed by study, one can consider the impact and the potential value of the outcome as similar to that experienced by cancer patients undergoing protracted radiation therapy treatment. Londahl demonstrated that HBOT improved long-term health-related quality of life.[33]

4. HBOT is initiated. Treatments for wound healing are typically 90 minutes of 100% oxygen breathing at 2.0 ATA in monoplace chambers or 2.4 ATA in multiplace chambers. Air breathing breaks are usually provided, particularly when treatment pressures are greater than 2.0 ATA, to reduce the risk of central nervous system oxygen toxicity.

Treatments for chronic hypoxic wounds are usually administered daily but may be administered more frequently depending on wound severity and patient condition.

5. A therapeutic rise in PtcO2 values during treatment must be demonstrated. These values should be routinely measured in all patients as early in the course of adjunctive HBOT as possible. While some controversy exists as to the optimal PtcO2 values that must be achieved during treatment to predict successful wound healing, 200 mmHg is usually considered to be the minimum value necessary. In all cases, the clinical response of the wound to HBOT determines whether HBOT should be continued, with the PtcO2 value serving only as a general guide to exclude non-responders earlier to avoid futile treatment.

6. The response to treatment and/or evidence of continued requirement for treatment is frequently reassessed. This involves examination of the wound for evidence of resolution of infection and accelerated tissue growth or stability of the treated tissue graft or flap. The decision to discontinue HBOT can be as complicated as the one to initiate it. Is the patient intolerant of treatment or have other medical conditions occurred that limit the application of an effective treatment protocol? Is the wound failing to respond to adjunctive HBOT after a reasonable trial of treatment? Is the original indication for which adjunctive HBOT was initiated no longer present? Have PtcO2 values in the skin reasonably adjacent to the wound been raised to a level above the selection criteria for the particular patient? Has the wound healing response reached a plateau? The answers to these questions should help to determine when to discontinue treatment.

Adverse Events Occurring During HBOT

Although HBOT has been safely and successfully provided to thousands of patients representing a wide range of ischemic/hypoxic wound healing problems, complications associated with the hyperbaric environment can occur and require careful ongoing medical assessment and sometimes emergency intervention. ***Untreated pneumothorax and pregnancy*** (when not associated with carbon monoxide poisoning or life-threatening necrotizing soft tissue infection) are the only absolute contraindications. Relative contraindications should be considered from a risk-benefit perspective and optimized if the decision is made to initiate HBOT. A full discussion of these complications is beyond the scope of this chapter. However, adverse events from a large case series were recently reported.[34] The series included 17,394 patients with 453,749 HBOT sessions in monoplace chambers (average of 26 treatments per patient) provided primarily in outpatient settings. The authors noted the relative safety of HBOT, especially when patients received standardized medical evaluations prior to initiating treatment, standardized pretreatment education, and standardized assessments prior to each treatment. In 2010, 956 adverse events were reported for 252,599 treatments in 9,638 patients for an overall adverse event rate of 0.38%. In order of decreasing rate of occurrence were ***ear pain*** (of any description), ***confinement anxiety***, ***hypoglycemic events***, ***shortness of breath***, and ***seizure*** (35 events, 0.02%, in 2009 and 53 events, 0.02%, in 2010).

The Team in Hyperbaric Medicine: The Hyperbaric Physician, Nurse, and Technologist

The ***physician trained in hyperbaric medicine*** plays a valuable role as the leader of the HBOT team. A specific body of knowledge defines the scope of hyperbaric medicine practice in these patients. The Undersea and Hyperbaric Medical Society has defined minimum training requirements for physicians, nurses, and technicians. This organization also has defined facility operational standards to enhance the appropriateness and safety of HBOT administration in the United States. HBOT should never be administered in isolation from other aspects of care of the wound or the patient. Therefore, the most successful applications of HBOT occur when the treatment and the hyperbaric physician are fully integrated into an interprofessional wound care approach.

Once the physician decides that the patient is a candidate for HBOT, the hyperbaric therapy nurse performs much of the preparatory work. The varied clinical applications for hyperbarics

have led to the development of a unique, highly skilled nursing specialty. Hyperbaric nurses are responsible for the practical implementation of patient care during hyperbaric treatments. The Baromedical Nurses Association (BNA) established standards for practice and published a textbook, *Hyperbaric Nursing*,[35] which was revised in 2010. The BNA also made a copy of their Nursing Standards of Care available on their website (www.hyperbaricnurses.org). These standards of care provide hyperbaric nurses with exact criteria against which patient care can be evaluated for effectiveness and appropriateness.

Hyperbaric nurses start with a comprehensive nursing history and physical assessment, which always includes the assistance of potential hyperbaric patients and their significant others, if possible. The data collected is documented and communicated to all health team members involved in the care of the patient. This information is used to develop a nursing diagnosis, which is expressed as the sum of 3 parts: problem, etiology, and signs/symptoms. The nursing diagnosis must be continuously prioritized, reviewed, and revised as appropriate throughout the continuum of care. The nursing care plan is continuously evaluated for its impact on patient response to goal achievement. Nursing action should be designed to accomplish established goals, which are initiated based on the nursing plan of care.

The third member of the HBOT team is the ***qualified hyperbaric chamber operator***, often referred to as the hyperbaric technologist. The technologist is trained in hyperbaric medicine, safety, and technical aspects and plays a valuable role as a member of the wound care team. Training in hyperbaric medicine is not entry-level training but rather an added qualification for someone who has previously received formal training in an allied healthcare profession. Common examples are individuals certified or licensed as respiratory therapists, military corpsmen, EMTs/paramedics, registered nurses or LPNs/LVNs, nurse practitioners, certified nurse aides, and certified medical assistants.

Technologists can obtain certification through the National Board of Diving & Hyperbaric Medical Technology (NBDHMT) by demonstrating competency in specific areas; by documenting clinical practice experience; by possessing a qualifying allied healthcare profession; and by passing an examination, leading to designation as a Certified Hyperbaric Technologist (CHT).[35] The NBDHMT has defined minimum training requirements for hyperbaric nurses and technologists.[36]

The Undersea and Hyperbaric Medical Society and the National Fire Protection Association (NFPA) have defined facility operational guidelines to enhance the appropriateness and safety of HBOT administration in the United States.[37,38] Additionally, NFPA code standards call for a hyperbaric safety director to be designated at every hyperbaric facility. It is common practice for the lead hyperbaric technologist to be the designee. Further training in safety is recommended for the hyperbaric safety director.

The technologist focuses on patient orientation to the HBOT experience. Emphasis is placed upon the purpose of the treatment, the treatment schedule, special precautions to be taken for the patient's comfort and safety, and teaching the patient middle ear pressure equalization (ear clearing) techniques. Patients should be able to explain their role in the treatment to the technologist. During a treatment, it is important to note that the technologist's main role is to monitor patients and equipment in order to respond quickly to possible adverse events.

Conclusion

Gaps in our knowledge remain, especially as it relates to optimal HBOT candidates. However, when integrated into a system of interprofessional wound care, HBOT has been shown in multiple clinical trials over an extended period of time and in extensive clinical experience in inpatient and outpatient clinical settings to be an effective adjunct to wound healing and diabetic limb salvage. Careful attention to initial patient selection and careful ongoing monitoring to minimize the risk of adverse events and to optimize the therapeutic benefit enhance the value of HBOT in these patients. The interprofessional wound care hyperbaric medicine team has contributed significantly to the effectiveness of this intervention. HBOT should be available to all centers providing limb salvage and complex diabetic foot ulcer treatment services.

Take-Home Messages for Practice
- Topical oxygen, while perhaps finding value in the future, has yet to be established on firm clinical grounds for wound healing.
- The optimal application of HBOT requires an understanding of the physiology and pharmacology of elevated tissue PO2 and a systematic approach to evaluation and management of patients with wounds.
- The interprofessional hyperbaric medicine care team plays an essential role in achieving safe, optimal outcomes in these patients.

Self-Assessment Questions

1. Local hypoxia in the tissue surrounding a chronic wound has been shown to cause all of the following EXCEPT:
   A. Impaired local response of leukocytes to bacterial infection
   B. Improved rate and amount of collagen synthesis by fibroblasts
   C. Decreased effectiveness of certain antibiotics
   D. Decreased angiogenesis into the wound margin

2. HBOT has been shown to do all of the following EXCEPT:
   A. Stimulate angiogenesis
   B. Improve leukocyte response to bacterial infection
   C. Ameliorate post-ischemic reperfusion injury
   D. Restore normal tissue oxygen values in the absence of any local blood flow

3. HBOT provides the greatest benefit in the treatment of chronic wounds when all of the following conditions are met EXCEPT:
   A. It is administered in an interprofessional setting
   B. Prospective patients are evaluated by a physician specifically trained in the use of HBOT
   C. It is used to replace peripheral arterial angioplasty or surgical revascularization

D. PtcO2 measurements are used along with frequent examination of the wound to determine the course and duration of treatment

Answers: 1-B, 2-D, 3-C

References

1. Gesell LB. The Hyperbaric Oxygen Therapy Committee Report. *Hyperbaric Oxygen Therapy Indications.* 12th ed. Durham, NC: Undersea and Hyperbaric Medical Society; 2009.

2. Sen CK. Wound healing essentials: let there be oxygen. *Wound Repair Regen.* 2009;17(1):1–18.

3. Fife CE, Smart DR, Sheffield PJ, Hopf HW, Hawkins G, Clarke D. Transcutaneous oximetry in clinical practice: Consensus statements from an expert panel based on evidence. *Undersea Hyperb Med.* 2009;36(1):43–53.

4. Meyhoff CS, Wetterslev J, Jorgensen LN, et al; PROXI Trial Group. Effect of high perioperative oxygen fraction on surgical site infection and pulmonary complications after abdominal surgery: the PROXI randomized clinical trial. *JAMA.* 2009;302(14):1543–1550.

5. Whitney JD. Enhancing wound oxygen levels: effectiveness of hydration and transdermal oxygen therapies. In: Sen CK, ed. *Advances in Wound Care, Volume 2.* New Rochelle, NY: Mary Ann Liebert, Inc., Publishers; 2011:128–133.

6. Gordillo GM, Sen CK. Evidence-based recommendations for the use of topical oxygen therapy in the treatment of lower extremity wounds. *Int J Low Extrem Wounds.* 2009;8(2):105–111.

7. Said HK, Hijjawi J, Roy N, Mogford J, Mustoe T. Transdermal sustained-delivery oxygen improves epithelial healing in a rabbit ear wound model. *Arch Surg.* 2005;140(10):998–1004.

8. Kalliainen LK, Gordillo GM, Schlanger R, Sen CK. Topical oxygen as an adjunct to wound healing: a clinical case series. *Pathophysiology.* 2003;9(2):81–87.

9. Blackman E, Moore C, Hyatt J, Railton R, Frye C. Topical wound oxygen therapy in the treatment of severe diabetic foot ulcers: a prospective controlled study. *Ostomy Wound Manage.* 2010;56(6):24–31.

10. Bakri MH, Nagem H, Sessler DI, et al. Transdermal oxygen does not improve sternal wound oxygenation in patients recovering from cardiac surgery. *Anesth Analg.* 2008;106(6):1619–1626.

11. Mosteller JA, Sembrst MM, McGarveuy ST, Quinn JL, Klausner EG, Sloat GB. A comparison of transcutaneous oxygen pressures between hyperbaric oxygen and topical oxygen. Presented at the 1999 UHMS Annual Scientific Meeting in Boston, MA.

12. Leslie CA, Sapico FL, Ginunas VJ, Adkins RH. Randomized controlled trial of topical hyperbaric oxygen for treatment of diabetic foot ulcers. *Diabetes Care.* 1998;11(2):111–115.

13. Feldmeier JJ, Hopf HW, Warriner RA 3rd, Fife CE, Gesell LB, Bennett M. UHMS position statement: topical oxygen for chronic wounds. *Undersea Hyperb Med.* 2005;32(3):157–168.

14. Warriner RA. Physiology of hyperbaric oxygen treatment. In: Larson-Lohr V, Josefsen L, Wilcox J, eds. *Hyperbaric Nursing.* 2nd ed. Palm Beach Gardens, FL: Best Publishing Company; 2011:13–31.

15. Thom SR. Hyperbaric oxygen: its mechanisms and efficacy. *Plast Reconstr Surg.* 2011;127(Suppl 1):131S–141S.

16. Thom SR. The impact of hyperbaric oxygen on cutaneous wound repair. In: Sen CK, ed. *Advances in Wound Care, Volume 1.* New Rochelle, NY: Mary Ann Liebert, Inc., Publishers; 2010:321.

17. Thom SR, Bhopale VM, Velazquez OC, Goldstein LJ, Thom LH, Buerk DG. Stem cell mobilization by hyperbaric oxygen. *Am J Physiol Heart Circ Physiol.* 2006;290(4):H1378–H1386.

18. Gallagher KA, Liu ZJ, Xiao M, et al. Diabetic impairments in NO-mediated endothelial progenitor cell mobilization and homing are reversed by hyperoxia and SDF-1 alpha. *J Clin Invest.* 2007;117(5):1249–1259.

19. Liu ZJ, Velazquez OC. Hyperoxia, endothelial progenitor cell mobilization, and diabetic wound healing. *Antioxid Redox Signal.* 2008;10(11):1869–1882.

20. Milovanova TN, Bhopale VM, Sorokina EM, et al. Hyperbaric oxygen stimulates vasculogenic stem cell growth and differentiation *in vivo. J Appl Physiol.* 2009;106(2):711–728.

21. Faglia E, Favales F, Aldeghi A, et al. Adjunctive systemic hyperbaric oxygen therapy in treatment of severe prevalently ischemic diabetic foot ulcer. A randomized study. *Diabetes Care.* 1996;19(12):1338–1343.

22. Kranke P, Bennett M, Roeckl-Wiedmann I, Debus S. Hyperbaric oxygen therapy for chronic wounds. *Cochrane Database Syst Rev.* 2004;(2):CD004123.

23. Guo S, Counte MA, Gillespie KN, Schmitz H. Cost-effectiveness of adjunctive hyperbaric oxygen in the treatment of diabetic ulcers. *Int J Technol Assess Health Care.* 2003;19(4):731–737.

24. Rakel A, Huot C, Ekoe JM. Canadian Diabetes Association Technical Review: the diabetic foot and hyperbaric oxygen therapy. *Canadian J Diabetes.* 2006;30(4):411–421.

25. Goldman RJ. Hyperbaric oxygen therapy for wound healing and limb salvage: a systematic review. *PM R.* 2009;1(5):471–489.

26. Löndahl M, Katzman P, Nilsson A, Hammarlund C. Hyperbaric oxygen therapy facilitates healing of chronic foot ulcers in patients with diabetes. *Diabetes Care.* 2010;33(5):998–1003.

27. Steed DL, Attinger C, Colaizzi T, et al. Guidelines for the treatment of diabetic ulcers. *Wound Repair Regen.* 2006;14(6):680–692.

28. Hopf HW, Ueno C, Aslam R, et al. Guidelines for the treatment of arterial insufficiency ulcers. *Wound Repair Regen.* 2008;14(6):693–710.

29. Fife CE, Buyukcakir C, Otto G, Sheffield P, Love T, Warriner R 3rd. Factors influencing the outcome of lower-extremity diabetic ulcers treated with hyperbaric oxygen therapy. *Wound Repair Regen.* 2007;15(3):322–331.

30. Apelqvist J, Elgzyri T, Larsson J, Londahl M, Nyberg P, Thorne J. Factors related to outcome of neuroischemic/ischemic foot ulcer in diabetic patients. *J Vasc Surg.* 2001;53(6):1582–1588.

31. Guo S, Counte MA, Gillespie KN, Schmitz H. Cost-

effectiveness of adjunctive hyperbaric oxygen in the treatment of diabetic ulcers. *Int J Health Technology Assess Health Care*. 2003;19(4):731–737.

32. Hailey D, Jacobs P, Perry DC, Chuck A, Morrison A, Boudreau R. *Adjunctive Hyperbaric Oxygen Therapy for Diabetic Foot Ulcer: An Economic Analysis* [Technology report no 75]. Ottawa: Canadian Agency for Drugs and Technologies in Health; 2007.

33. Löndahl M, Landin-Olsson M, Katzman P. Hyperbaric oxygen therapy improves health-related quality of life in patients with diabetes and chronic foot ulcer. *Diabet Med*. 2011;28(2):186–190.

34. Beard T, Watson B, Barry R, Stewart D, Warriner R.

Analysis of adverse events occurring in patients undergoing adjunctive HBOT: 2009–2010. Presented at the 2011 UHMS Annual Scientific Meeting in Fort Worth, TX.

35. Larson-Lohr V, Norvell HC, eds. *Hyperbaric Nursing*. Flagstaff, AZ: Best Publishing Company; 2002.

36. Clarke D, ed. *Certified Hyperbaric Technologist Resource Manual*. Columbia, SC: National Board of Diving and Hyperbaric Medical Technology; 2011.

37. Workman WT, ed. *UHMS Guidelines for Hyperbaric Facility Operations*. Kensington, MD: UHMS; 2004.

38. Bielen R, ed. NFPA 99: Health Care Facilities Code. Quincy, MA: National Fire Protection Association; 2005.

*Authors' Note**

This chapter is dedicated to a pioneer in chronic wound healing, **Dr. Robert A. Warriner III†, MD, ABPM/UHM, FACA, FCCP, FCCWS.**

Dr. Warriner educated physicians and clinicians about hyperbaric oxygen therapy and developed the clinical practice guidelines necessary to heal chronic wounds. Dr. Warriner authored over 50 publications related to wound care and hyperbaric medicine. In 2008, he received the Lifetime Achievement Award from the World Union of Wound Healing Societies. The following year, Dr. Warriner was awarded the Sharon Branoski Founder's Award, which recognized him as an expert in wound care treatment and disease management. Dr. Warriner was the recipient of many awards from the Undersea and Hyperbaric Medical Society for contributions to advancing the field of clinical hyperbaric medicine. Our friend, mentor, and co-author of this chapter will be missed and long remembered.

CHAPTER 23

SCALE
Skin Changes At Life's End©

Final Consensus Statement

October 1, 2009

The content of this document is based on the results of a two-day round table discussion held on April 4-6, 2008 in Chicago, IL, and was made possible by an unrestricted educational grant from Gaymar Industries, Inc. Additional input was received from international panels of 49 and 52 distinguished reviewers using a modified Delphi Method process. The information contained herein does not necessarily represent the opinions of all panel members, distinguished reviewers, or Gaymar Industries, Inc.

Disclaimer: The content of this document is intended for general information purposes and is not intended to be a substitute for medical or legal advice. Do not rely on information in this article in place of medical or legal advice.

Abstract

An expert panel was established to formulate a consensus statement on Skin Changes At Life's End (SCALE). The panel consists of 18 internationally recognized key opinion leaders including clinicians, caregivers, medical researchers, legal experts, academicians, a medical writer and leaders of professional organizations. The inaugural forum was held on April 4-6, 2008 in Chicago, IL, and was made possible by an unrestricted educational grant from Gaymar Industries, Inc. The panel discussed the nature of SCALE, including the proposed concepts of the Kennedy Terminal Ulcer (KTU) and skin failure along with other end of life skin changes. The final consensus document and statements were edited and reviewed by the panel after the meeting. The document and statements were initially externally reviewed by 49 international distinguished reviewers. A modified Delphi process was used to determine the final statements and 52 international distinguished reviewers reached consensus on the final statements.

The skin is the body's largest organ and like any other organ is subject to a loss of integrity. It has an increased risk for injury due to both internal and external insults. The panel concluded that: our current comprehension of skin changes that can occur at life's end is limited; that SCALE process is insidious and difficult to prospectively determine; additional research and expert consensus is necessary; and contrary to popular myth, not all pressure ulcers are avoidable.

Originally published as: Sibbald RG, Krasner DL, Lutz JB, et al. The SCALE Expert Panel: Skin Changes At Life's End. Final Consensus Document. October 1, 2009. Used with permission.

Specific areas requiring research and consensus include: 1) the identification of critical etiological and pathophysiological factors involved in SCALE, 2) clinical and diagnostic criteria for describing conditions identified with SCALE, and 3) recommendations for evidence-informed pathways of care.

The statements from this consensus document are designed to facilitate the implementation of knowledge-transfer-into-practice techniques for quality patient outcomes. This implementation process should include interprofessional teams (clinicians, lay people and policy makers) concerned with the care of individuals at life's end to adequately address the medical, social, legal, and financial ramifications of SCALE.

SCALE Expert Panel Members

Co-Chairpersons:

R. Gary Sibbald, BSc, MD, FRCPC (Med, Derm),MACP, FAAD, MEd, FAPWCA University of Toronto, Toronto, Canada, gary. sibbald@utoronto.ca

Diane L. Krasner, PhD, RN, CWCN, CWS, MAPWCA, FAAN, Wound & Skin Care Consultant, York, PA, USA, dlkrasner@aol.com Corresponding Author: 212 East Market Street, York, PA 17403 USA

Medical Writer:

James Lutz, MS, CCRA, Lutz Consulting, LLC, Medical Writing Services, Buellton, CA, USA, jlutzmail@aol.com

Panel Facilitator:

Cynthia Sylvia, MSc, MA, RN, CWOCN, Gaymar Industries, Inc., Orchard Park, NY, USA, cindy.sylvia@stryker.com

Additional Panel Members:

Oscar Alvarez, PhD, CCT, FAPWCA, Center for Curative and Palliative Wound Care, Calvary Hospital, Bronx, NY, USA, oalvarez@calvaryhospital.org

Elizabeth A. Ayello, PhD, RN, ACNS-BC, ETN, FAPWCA, FAAN, Excelsior College School of Nursing, USA, elizabeth @ayello. com

Sharon Baranoski, MSN, RN, CWOCN, APN, DAPWCA, FAAN, Wound Care Dynamics, Inc., Shorewood, IL, USA, nrsebear@aol.com

William J. Ennis, DO, MBA, FACOS, University of Illinois, Palos Heights, IL, USA, w.ennis@comcast.net

Nancy Ann Faller, RN, MSN, PhD, ETN, CS, Carlisle, PA, USA, nafaller@aol.com

Jane Hall, Medical Malpractice Defense Attorney, Huie, Fernambucq & Stewart, LLP, Birmingham, AL, USA, jgh@hfsllp.com

Rick E. Hall, BA, RN, CWCN, Helping Hands Wound Care, Wichita, KS, USA, mnurse66@yahoo.com

Karen Lou Kennedy-Evans, RN, CS, FNP, KL Kennedy, LLC, Tucson, AZ, USA, ktulcer@me.com

Diane Langemo, PhD, RN, FAAN, Langemo & Assoc, Grand Forks, ND, USA, dianelangemo@aol.com

Joy Schank, RN, MSN, ANP, CWOCN, Schank Companies, Himrod, NY, USA, joyschank@yahoo.com

Thomas P. Stewart, PhD, Gaymar Industries, Inc., Orchard Park, NY & S.U.N.Y. at Buffalo, USA, drtomstew@roadrunner.com

Nancy A. Stotts, RN, CNS, EdD, FAAN, University of California, San Francisco, San Francisco, CA, USA, nancy.stotts@nursing.ucsf.edu

David R. Thomas, MD, FACP, AGSF, GSAF, CMD, St. Louis University, St. Louis, MO, USA, thomasdr@slu.edu

Dot Weir, RN, CWON, CWS, Osceola Regional Medical Center, Kissimmee, FL, USA, dorothy.weir@hcahealthcare.com

Background for Skin Changes At Life's End (SCALE)

Organ dysfunction is a familiar concept in the health sciences, and can occur at any time but most often occurs at life's end, during an acute critical illness or with severe trauma. Body organs particularly the heart and kidneys undergo progressive limitation of function as a normal process related to aging and the end of life. *End of life is defined as a phase of life when a person is living with an illness that will often worsen and eventually cause death. This time period is not limited to the short period of time when the person is moribund.*[1] It is well accepted that during the end stages of life, any of a number of vital body systems (eg, the renal, hepatic, cardiac, pulmonary, or nervous systems) can be compromised to varying degrees and will eventually totally cease functioning. The process of organ compromise can have devastating effects, resulting in injury or interference with functioning of other organ systems that may contribute to further deterioration and eventual death.

We propose that the skin, the largest organ of the body, is no different, and also can become dysfunctional with varying degrees of resultant compromise. *The skin is essentially a window into the health of the body, and if read correctly, can provide a great deal of insight into what is happening inside the body.* Skin compromise, including changes related to decreased cutaneous perfusion and localized hypoxia (blood supply and local tissue factors) can occur at the tissue, cellular, or molecular level. The end result is a reduced availability of oxygen and the body's ability to utilize vital nutrients and other factors required to sustain normal skin function. When this compromised state occurs, the manifestations are termed, Skin Changes At Life's End (SCALE). It should be noted that the acronym SCALE is a mnemonic used to describe a group of clinical phenomena, and should not be confused with a risk assessment tool. The term applies to all individuals across the continuum of care settings.

Skin organ compromise at life's end is not a new concept in the literature. The first clinical description in modern medical literature appeared in 1989 with the Kennedy Terminal Ulcer (KTU).[2] Kennedy described the KTU as a specific subgroup of pressure ulcers that some individuals develop as they are dying. They are usually shaped like a pear, butterfly, or horseshoe, and are located predominantly on the coccyx or sacrum (but have been reported in other anatomical areas). The ulcers are a variety of colors including red, yellow or black, are sudden in onset, typically deteriorate rapidly, and usually indicate that death is imminent.[2] This initial report was based on retrospective chart reviews of individuals with pressure ulcers. It sparked further inquiry into how long these individuals within the facility lived after occurrence of a pressure ulcer. Just over half (55.7%) died within six weeks of discovery of their pressure ulcer(s). The observations were further supported by Hanson and colleagues (1991), who reported that 62.5% of pressure ulcers in hospice patients occurred in the 2 weeks prior to death.[3] Further evidence for the existence of the KTU is mostly observational in nature, but is consistent with the premise that skin function can become compromised at life's end.

It is noteworthy that while Kennedy independently described the KTU in 1989, a similar condition was actually first described much earlier in the French medical literature by Jean-Martin Charcot (1825-1893).[4,5] In a medical textbook written in 1877, Charcot described a specific type of ulcer that is butterfly in shape and occurring over the sacrum. Patients that developed these ulcers usually died shortly thereafter, hence he termed the ulcer *Decubitus Ominosus*. However, Charcot attributed the ulcers to being neuropathic rather than pressure in origin. Charcot's writings of *Decubitus Ominosus* were all but forgotten in the medical literature until recently with renewed interest in skin organ compromise.[4] The fact that two experts in the field of chronic wounds independently reported the same clinical phenomenon, with very similar descriptions, 112 years apart, lends credence to the possible existence of terminal pressure ulcers as a result of end-of-life skin organ compromise.

Also of historical interest is the original work of Dr. Alois Alzheimer in Germany. He was on call in 1901 when a 51-year-old woman, Frau August D, was admitted to his asylum for the insane in Frankfort. Dr. Alzheimer followed this patient, studied her symptoms and presented her case to his colleagues as what came to be known as Alzheimer's Disease. When Frau Auguste D.

died on April 8, 1906, her medical record listed the cause of death as "septicemia due to decubitus."[6] Alzheimer noted, "at the end, she was confined to bed in a fetal position, was incontinent and in spite of all the care and attention given to her, she suffered from decubitus". So, here we have the first identified patient with Alzheimer's Disease having developed immobility and two pressure ulcers with end stage Alzheimer's. In our modern times, end stage Alzheimer's Disease has become an all-too-frequent scenario with multiple complications including SCALE.

In 2003, Langemo proposed a working definition of skin failure; that it is a result of hypoperfusion, creating an extreme inflammatory reaction concomitant with severe dysfunction or failure of multiple organ systems.[7] Three years later, Langemo and Brown (2006) conducted a comprehensive review of the literature on the concept of skin failure that focused largely on pressure ulcer development.[8] They presented a discussion of changes in the skin that can occur with aging, the development of pressure ulcers, multiorgan failure, and "skin failure" (both acute and chronic as well as end of life).[9-15] In the early 1990's two publications by Parish & Witkowski had presented logical arguments about the mechanism of pressure ulcer occurrence at the end of life, suggesting that they may not be preventable in those individuals with multiple organ failure.[11,16] Although the term skin failure has been introduced, it is not currently a widely accepted term in the dermatological or the wound literature.

Despite the limited scientific literature, there is consensus from the narrative literature that some pressure ulcers may be unavoidable including those that are manifestations of SCALE. We propose that at the end of life, failure of the homeostatic mechanisms that support the skin can occur, resulting in a diminished reserve to handle insults such as minimal pressure. Therefore, contrary to popular myth, not all pressure ulcers are avoidable.[17,18] Many members of the SCALE Panel acknowledge the need for systematic study of the phenomenon.

Goals and Objectives of the SCALE Panel

The overall goal of the SCALE Expert Panel was to initiate stakeholder discussion of skin changes at the end of life, a phenomenon that we have termed SCALE. An objective was to examine the concept of unavoidable pressure ulcers that can occur as a result of SCALE. While reaching consensus on the various aspects of this topic is an important outcome, this endeavor will require a more rigorous scientific investigative approach that was beyond the scope of this groundbreaking meeting. The purpose of this initial meeting was to generate a series of statements that will serve as a platform for future consensus discussions. The objective of this document is to present these panel statements, disseminate them for public discussion, and to further the development of the body of scientific knowledge on this important topic.

Methodology

A modified three phase *Delphi Method* approach was used to reach consensus on the 10 statements reported in this document. The Delphi Method relies on expert panel input to reach consensus on a topic of interest.[19] Our approach consisted of three separate phases of consensus building involving an international group of 69 noted experts in the field of wound care.

Phase 1: A panel of 18 experts in the field of wound care with expertise in wound and skin care convened in a round table format on April 4-6, 2008 in Chicago, IL, USA. Audio proceedings and written notes from this round table discussion were used to generate a *Preliminary Consensus Document (PCD)*. This PCD was returned to the original panel for review and was modified as necessary to reach panel consensus.

Phase 2: The PCD was presented and distributed at numerous international conferences seeking public comment from September 2008 through June 2009. The document was published,[20] and also available for public download from the web site of the panel sponsor (Gaymar Industries, Inc.).[21] The PCD was further reviewed by a selected international panel of 49 Distinguished Reviewers with noted expertise in wound care and palliative medicine.

Phase 3: Written input received from the panel of Distinguished Reviewers and from the various public presentations was used to generate A *Final Consensus Document (FCD)*. This FCD was then returned to the original 18-member Expert

Panel and a 52-member Distinguished Reviewer Panel for voting on each of the 10 statements for consensus. A quorum of 80% that *strongly agree* or *somewhat agree* with each statement was used as a pre-determined threshold for having achieved consensus on each of the statements. Fifty two individuals voted on the final consensus process.

In addition to the PCD and FCD documents, an annotated bibliography of literature pertinent to SCALE was generated and is available upon request from Dr. Diane L. Krasner (dlkrasner@ aol.com).[21]

Panel Statements

As a result of the two-day panel discussion and subsequent panel revisions, and with input from 69 noted wound care experts in a modified Delphi Method approach, the following 10 statements are proposed by the SCALE Expert Panel:

Statement 1
Physiologic changes that occur as a result of the dying process may affect the skin and soft tissues and may manifest as observable (objective) changes in skin color, turgor, or integrity, or as subjective symptoms such as localized pain. These changes can be unavoidable and may occur with the application of appropriate interventions that meet or exceed the standard of care.

When the dying process compromises the homeostatic mechanisms of the body, a number of vital organs may become compromised. The body may react by shunting blood away from the skin to these vital organs, resulting in decreased skin and soft tissue perfusion and a reduction of the normal cutaneous metabolic processes. Minor insults can lead to major complications such as skin hemorrhage, gangrene, infection, skin tears and pressure ulcers that may be markers of SCALE. See Statement 6 for further discussion.

Statement 2
The plan of care and patient response should be clearly documented and reflected in the entire medical record. Charting by exception is an appropriate method of documentation.

The record should document the patient's clinical condition including co-morbidities, pressure ulcer risk factors, significant changes, and clinical interventions that are consistent with the patient's wishes and recognized guidelines for care.[22] Facility policies and guidelines for record keeping should be followed and facilities should update these policies and guidelines as appropriate. The impact of the interventions should be assessed and revised as appropriate. This documentation may take many forms. Specific approaches to documentation of care should be consistent with professional, legal, and regulatory guidelines, and may involve narrative documentation, the use of flow sheets, or other documentation systems/ tools.

If a patient is to be treated as palliative, it should be stated in the medical record, ideally with a reference to a family/caregiver meeting, and that consensus was reached. If specific palliative scales such as the Palliative Performance Scale,[23] or other palliative tools were utilized,[24] they should be included in the medical record. Palliative care must be patient-centered, with skin and wound care being only a part of the total plan of care.

It is not reasonable to expect that the medical record will be an all-inclusive account of the individual's care. Charting by exception is an appropriate method of documentation. This form of documentation should allow the recording of unusual findings and pertinent patient risk factors. Some methods of clinical documentation are antiquated in light of today's complexity of patient care and rapidly changing interprofessional healthcare environment; many current documentation systems need to be revised and streamlined.

Statement 3
Patient centered concerns should be addressed including pain and activities of daily living.

A comprehensive, individualized plan of care should not only address the patient's skin changes and co-morbidities, but any patient concerns that impact quality of life including psychological and emotional issues. Research suggests that for wound patients, health-related quality of life is especially impacted by pain, change in body image, odors and mobility issues. It is not uncommon for these factors to have an effect on aspects of daily living, nutrition, mobility, psychological factors, sleep patterns and socialization.[25,26] Addressing these patient-centered concerns optimizes activities of daily living and enhances a patient's dignity.

Statement 4

Skin changes at life's end are a reflection of compromised skin (reduced soft tissue perfusion, decreased tolerance to external insults, and impaired removal of metabolic wastes).

When a patient experiences SCALE, tolerance to external insults (such as pressure) decreases to such an extent that it may become clinically and logistically impossible to prevent skin breakdown and the possible invasion of the skin by microorganisms. Compromised immune response may also play an important role, especially with advanced cancer patients and with the administration of corticosteroids and other immunosuppressant agents.

Skin changes may develop at life's end despite optimal care, as it may be impossible to protect the skin from environmental insults in its compromised state. These changes are often related to other cofactors including aging, co-existing diseases and drug adverse events. SCALE, by definition occurs at life's end, but skin compromise may not be limited to end of life situations; it may also occur with acute or chronic illnesses, and in the context of multiple organ failure that is not limited to the end of life.[8,27] However, these situations are beyond the scope of this panel's goals and objectives.

Statement 5

Expectations around the patient's end of life goals and concerns should be communicated among the members of the interprofessional team and the patient's circle of care. The discussion should include the potential for SCALE including other skin changes, skin breakdown and pressure ulcers.

It is important that the provider(s) communicate and document goals of care, interventions, and outcomes related to specific interventions (See Statement 2). The patient's circle of care includes the members of the patient unit including family, significant others, caregivers, and other healthcare professionals that may be external to the current interprofessional team. Communication with the interprofessional team and the patient's circle of care should be documented. The education plan should include realistic expectations surrounding end of life issues with input from the patient if possible. Communication of what to expect during end of life is important and this should include changes in skin integrity.

Being mindful of local protected health information disclosure regulations (eg, USA: HIPAA, 1996),[28] the patient's circle of care needs to be aware that an individual at the end of life may develop skin breakdown, even when care is appropriate. They need to understand that skin function may be compromised to a point where there is diminished reserve to tolerate even minimal pressure or external insult. Educating the patient's circle of care up front may help reduce the chances of shock and emotional reactions if end of life skin conditions occur.

This education includes information that as one nears end of life, mobility decreases. The individual frequently has a "position of comfort" that the patient may choose to maintain, resulting in a greater potential for skin breakdown. Some patients elect to continue to lie on the pressure ulcer, stating it is the most comfortable position for them. Respecting the coherent patient's wishes is important.

With the recognition that these skin conditions are sometimes a normal part of the dying process, there is less potential for assigning blame, and a greater understanding that skin organ compromise may be an unavoidable part of the dying process.

Discussions regarding specific trade-offs in skin care should be documented in the medical record. For example, patients may develop pressure ulcers when they cannot be (or do not want to be) turned due to pain or the existence of other medical conditions. Pressure ulcers may also occur in states of critical hypoperfusion due to underlying physical factors such as severe anemia, hypoxia, hypotension, peripheral arterial disease, or severe malnutrition. Care decisions must be made with the total goals of the patient in mind, and may be dependent on the setting of care, trajectory of the illness, and priorities for the patient and family. *Comfort may be the overriding and acceptable goal, even though it may be in conflict with best skin care practice.* In summary, the patient and family should have a greater understanding that skin organ compromise may be an unavoidable part of the dying process.

Statement 6

Risk factors symptoms and signs associated with SCALE have not been fully elucidated, but may include:

- *Weakness and progressive limitation of mobility.*
- *Suboptimal nutrition including loss of appetite, weight loss, cachexia and wasting, low serum albumin/pre-albumin, and low hemoglobin as well as dehydration.*
- *Diminished tissue perfusion, impaired skin oxygenation, decreased local skin temperature, mottled discoloration, and skin necrosis.*
- *Loss of skin integrity from any of a number of factors including equipment or devices, incontinence, chemical irritants, chronic exposure to*
- *body fluids, skin tears, pressure, shear, friction, and infections.*
- *Impaired immune function.*

Diminished tissue perfusion is the most significant risk factors for SCALE and generally occurs in areas of the body with end arteries, such as the fingers, toes, ears, and nose. These areas may exhibit early signs of vascular compromise and ultimate collapse, such as dusky erythema, mottled discoloration, local cooling, and eventually infarcts and gangrene.

As the body faces a critical illness or disease state, a normal protective function may be to shunt a larger percentage of cardiac output from the skin to more vital internal organs, thus averting immediate death. Chronic shunting of blood to the vital organs may also occur as a result of

Table 1. Useful dermatologic terms for describing areas of concern. Additional terms can be found in the Glossary included at end of this document.

Term	Description
Bruise	An injury producing a hematoma or diffuse extravasation of blood without rupture of the skin.[29] Often presents as a reddish, purple, black discoloration of the skin.
Crust	A hard outer layer or covering; cutaneous crusts are often formed by dried serum, pus or blood on the surface of a ruptured blister or pustule.[29]
Erosion (denudation)	A loss of surface skin with an epidermal base.
Eschar	Thick adherent, necrotic tissue that is typically dry and brown, black or gray in color.
Fissure	A thin linear loss of skin with a dermal or deeper base.
Hematoma	A collection of blood in the soft tissues.
Lesion	Any change in the skin that may be a normal or abnormal variant including a wound or injury[29]. It encompasses everything from macular lesions (color changes without elevation or depression of the skin) through total skin breakdown.
Mottling of skin due to vascular stasis	An area of skin composed of macular lesions of varying shades or colors over the smaller or medium sized blood vessels.[29]
Scale	Surface keratin that may be thick or thin, resembling a fish scale, cast off (desquamating) from the skin.[29]
Skin Tear	A traumatic wound occurring principally on the extremities of older adults as a result of friction alone or with shearing and frictional forces, that separate the epidermis from the dermis (partial-thickness wound) or which separate both the epidermis and the dermis from the underlying structures (full-thickness wound).[30]
Slough	Yellow, green, tan, or white putrefied debris often partly separated from the surface of the wound bed.[29]
Ulcer	A loss of surface skin with a dermal or deeper base.

Table 2. Dermatological descriptions of lesions based on characteristics and size.

Lesion Characteristic	Lesion Size	
	<1 cm	>1 cm
Flat	Macule	Patch
Elevated	Papule	Plaque
Blister	Vesicle	Bulla

limited fluid intake over a long period of time. Most of the skin has collateral vascular supply but distal locations such as the fingers, toes, ears and nose have a single vascular route and are more susceptible to a critical decrease in tissue oxygenation due to vasoconstriction. Furthermore, the ability to tolerate pressure is limited in poorly perfused body areas.

Additional literature reviews and clinical research are needed to more thoroughly comprehend and document all of the potential risk factors associated with SCALE and their clinical manifestations.

Statement 7
A total skin assessment should be performed regularly and document all areas of concern consistent with the wishes and condition of the patient. Pay special attention to bony prominences and skin areas with underlying cartilage. Areas of special concern include the sacrum, coccyx, ischial tuberosities, trochanters, scapulae, occiput, heels, digits, nose and ears. Describe the skin or wound abnormality exactly as assessed.

It is important to assess the whole body because there may be signs that relate to skin compromise. Table 1 provides a limited list of dermatologic terms that may be useful when describing areas of concern. Table 2 provides descriptive terms for lesions based on characteristics and size.

Statement 8
Consultation with a qualified health care professional is recommended for any skin changes associated with increased pain, signs of infection, skin breakdown (when the goal may be healing), and whenever the patient's circle of care expresses a significant concern.

There are very definite descriptive terms for

skin changes that can be used to facilitate communication between health care professionals (see Statement 7). Until more is known about SCALE, subjective symptoms need to be reported and objective skin changes described. This will allow for identification and characterization of potential end of life skin changes.

An accurate diagnosis can lead to decisions about the area of concern and whether it is related to end of life care and/or other factors. The diagnosis will help determine appropriate treatment and establish realistic outcomes for skin changes. For pressure ulcers, it is important to determine if the ulcer may be (i) healable within an individual's life expectancy, (ii) maintained, or (iii) non-healable or palliative.[17] The treatment plan will depend on an accurate diagnosis, the individual's life expectancy and wishes, family members' expectations, institutional policies, and the availability of an interprofessional team to optimize care.[31] Remember that patient status can change and appropriate reassessments with determination of likely outcomes may be necessary.

It is important to remember that a maintenance or non-healable wound classification does not necessarily equate with withholding treatment. For example, the patient may benefit with improved quality of life from surgical debridement and/or the use of advanced support surfaces.

Statement 9
The probable skin change etiology and goals of care should be determined. Consider the 5 Ps for determining appropriate intervention strategies:
- *Prevention*
- *Prescription (may heal with appropriate treatment)*
- *Preservation (maintenance without deterioration)*
- *Palliation (provide comfort and care)*
- *Preference (patient desires)*

Prevention is important for well being, enhanced quality of life, potential reimbursement, and to avoid unplanned medical consequences for end of life care. The skin becomes fragile when stressed with decreased oxygen availability associated with the end of life. The plan of care needs to address excessive pressure, friction, shear, moisture,

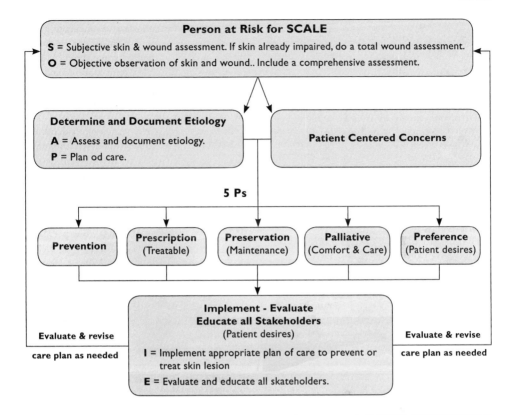

S = *Subjective skin & wound assessment:* The person at the end of life needs to be assessed by history, including an assessment of the risk for developing a skin change or pressure ulcer (Braden Scale or other valid and reliable risk assessment scale).[36]

O = *Objective observation of skin & wound:* A physical exam should identify and document skin changes that may be associated with the end of life or other etiologies including any existing pressure ulcers.

A = *Assess and document etiology:* An assessment should then be made of the general condition of the patient and a care plan.

P = *Plan of care:* A care plan should be developed that includes a decision on skin care considering the 5P's as outlined in the Figure 1. This plan of care should also consider input and wishes from the patient and the patient's circle of care.

I = *Implement appropriate plan of care:* For successful implementation, the plan of care must be matched with the healthcare system resources (availability of equipment and personnel) along with appropriate education and feedback from the patient's circle of care and as consistent with the patient's goals and wishes.

E = *Evaluate and educate all stakeholders:* The interprofessional team also needs to facilitate appropriate education, management, and periodic reevaluation of the care plan as the patient's health status changes.

Figure 3. The SOAPIE mnemonic with the 5P enabler.

suboptimal nutrition, and immobilization.

Prescription refers to the interventions for a treatable lesion. Even with the stress of dying, some lesions are healable after appropriate treatment. Interventions must be aimed at treating the cause and at patient centered concerns (pain, quality of life), before addressing the components of local wound care as consistent with the patient's goals and wishes.

Preservation refers to situations where the opportunity for wound healing or improvement is limited, so maintenance of the wound in its present clinical state is the desired outcome. A maintenance wound may have the potential to heal, but there may be other overriding medical factors that could direct the interprofessional team to maintain the status quo. For example there may be limited access to care, or the patient may simply refuse treatment.

Palliation refers to those situations in which the goal of treatment is comfort and care, not healing. A palliative or non-healable wound may deteriorate due to a general decline in the health of the patient as part of the dying process, or due to hypoperfusion associated with non-correctable critical ischemia.[32, 33] In some situations, palliative wounds may also benefit from some treatment interventions such as surgical debridement or support surfaces, even when the goal is not to heal the wound.[34]

Preference includes taking into account the preferences of the patient and the patient's circle of care.

The 5P enabler can be used in combination with the SOAPIE mnemonic to help explain the process of translating this recommendation into practice (Figure 1).[35] Realistic outcomes can be derived from appropriate SOAPIE processes with the 5 skin Ps becoming the guide to the realistic outcomes for each individual.

Statement 10
Patients and concerned individuals should be educated regarding SCALE and the plan of care.

Education needs to be directed not only to the patient but also the patient's circle of care. Within the confines allowed by local protected health information regulations (eg, HIPAA, 1996, USA),[28] the patient's circle of care needs to be included in decision making processes regarding goals of care and the communication of the meaning and method of accomplishing those decisions. Collaboration and communication should be ongoing with designated representatives from the patient's circle of care and the clinical team connecting at regular intervals. Documentation of decision making, educational efforts, and the patient's circle of care perspective is recommended. If adherence to the plan of care cannot be achieved, this should be documented in the medical record (including the reasons), and alternative plans proposed if available and feasible.

Education also extends beyond the patient's circle of care, to other involved healthcare professionals, healthcare administrators, policy makers, and to the payers. Healthcare professionals need to facilitate communication and collaboration across care settings and disciplines; organizations need to prepare staff to identify and manage SCALE. Ongoing discussions with key stakeholders will additionally provide a stimulus for additional evidence based research and education regarding all aspects of SCALE.

Recommendations for Future Research
Conduct and disseminate through publications and presentations:
- A thorough review of the literature concerning all aspects of SCALE.
- Research to identify the mechanisms for the proposed decreased hypoperfusion and oxygenation of the skin and soft tissues involved with SCALE and resulting outcomes.
- Research to determine the mechanisms for the proposed, tissue, cellular, and molecular dysfunctions that occur during SCALE.
- Research that helps to clarify and distinguish skin and soft tissue damage associated with SCALE from pressure ulcers and other skin disorders not associated with skin organ compromise or the end of life.
- Research into predictive tools for the onset and measurement of SCALE and the timing of life's end (possibly adaptive use of the Palliative Performance Scale (http://palliative.info/resource_material/PPSv2.pdf)
- Qualitative research to explore the impact of SCALE on the patient, the patient's circle of

care, and professional caregivers with regard to healthcare-related quality of life.

- Development of a database of patients (with histories) suspected of exhibiting SCALE to analyze them retrospectively for skin and soft tissue changes and risk factors that occurred just prior to death. Isolate the skin changes and risk factors involved and determine how important each individual variable is to the occurrence of SCALE.
- Research cataloging patients who do not exhibit SCALE to identify factors that may help prevent the occurrence of SCALE.
- Develop a registry of Kennedy Terminal Ulcers to better categorize this phenomenon, including location, clinical description, patient and ulcer outcomes, and the presence of other end of life skin changes including lesions in other locations.
- Both prospective and retrospective prevalence research of individuals suspected of exhibiting SCALE, particularly among hospice patients.
- Research on specific medical and physiologic conditions that may contribute to SCALE. These include but may not be limited to malignancy, hypotension and hemodynamic instability, administration of potent vasoconstrictors, peripheral arterial and vascular disease, hypoxia, malnutrition, and severe anemia.

Conclusions

SCALE Panel members are in agreement that there are observable changes in the skin at the end of life. Our current understanding of this complex phenomenon is limited and the panel concludes that additional research is necessary to assess the etiology of SCALE, to clinically describe and diagnose the related skin changes, and to recommend appropriate pathways of care. The panel recommends that clinicians, laypeople, and policy makers need to be better educated in the medical, social, legal and financial ramifications of SCALE. Health care organizations need to ensure the provision of resources that enable health care professionals to identify and care for SCALE while maintaining the dignity of the patient, family and circle of care to the end of life.

Glossary of Terms

Arterial Ulcer: An ulcer that occurs almost exclusively in the distal lower extremity due to inadequate perfusion/ischemia.[37]

Avoidable (pressure ulcer): The resident (individual) developed a pressure ulcer and the facility did not do one or more of the following: evaluate the resident's clinical condition and pressure ulcer risk factors; define and implement interventions that are consistent with resident needs, resident goals, and recognized standards of practice; monitor and evaluate the impact of the interventions; or revise the interventions as appropriate (CMS definition).[38]

Charting by Exception (CBE): Charting by exception is premised on an assumption that the patient has manifested a normal response to all interventions unless an abnormal response is charted.[39] This type of charting is often performed with flow sheets that are based on pre-established guidelines, protocols, and procedures that identify and document the standard patient management and care delivery. Clinicians need to make additional documentation when the patient's condition deviates from the standard or what's expected.[40]

Crust: A hard outer layer or covering; cutaneous crusts are often formed by dried serum, pus or blood (one or more components may co-exist) on the surface of a ruptured blister or pustule.[29]

Decubitus Ominosus: Medical term first used by Jean-Martin Charcot in the 19th century to signify a sacral ulcer that presages death.[5]

Delphi Method: A systematic, interactive forecasting method which relies on a panel of independent experts. The carefully selected experts answer questionnaires in two or more rounds. After each round, a facilitator provides an anonymous summary of the experts' forecasts from the previous round as well as the reasons they provided for their judgments. Thus, experts are encouraged to revise their earlier answers in light of the replies of other members of their panel. It is believed that during this process the range of the answers will decrease and the group will converge towards the "correct" answer. Finally, the process is stopped after a pre-defined stop criterion (e.g. number of rounds, achievement of consensus, stability of results) and the mean or median scores of the final rounds determine the results.[19]

Denudation: See erosion.

Diabetic Ulcer: A wound occurring most often in the feet of people with diabetes due most commonly to neuropathy and/or peripheral vascular disease.[41]

End of Life: End of life is defined as a phase of life when a person is living with an illness that will worsen and eventually cause death. It is not limited to the short period of time when the person is moribund.[1]

Erosion: A loss of surface skin with an epidermal base.

Fissure: A thin linear loss of skin with a dermal or deeper base.

Healable (wound): A wound occurring on an individual whose body can support the phases of wound healing within the individuals expected lifetime.

Healed (wound): A wound that has attained closure of the epidermal surface. A recently closed wound may only have 20% tensile strength of skin that has never been wounded and may be susceptible to recurrent ulceration.

Kennedy Terminal Ulcer: A pressure ulcer that some individuals develop as they are dying. It is usually shaped like a pear, butterfly, or horseshoe, usually on the coccyx or sacrum (but has been reported on other anatomical areas), has colors of red, yellow or black, is sudden in onset, and usually is associated with imminent death.[2, 42-49]

Lesion: Any change in the skin that may be a normal or abnormal variant including a wound or injury[29]. It encompasses everything from macular lesions (color changes without elevation or depression of the skin) through total skin breakdown.

Maintenance (wound): An attempt to keep an ulcer from deteriorating by providing good wound care. The wound may not heal due to patient choice or a lack of the health care system to provide optimal resources to promote healing.

Non-healable (wound): A wound that often deteriorates and occurs on an individual whose body cannot support the phases of wound healing within the individuals expected lifetime. There may be inadequate vascular supply to support healing or the cause of the wound cannot be corrected.

Palliative skin care: Providing comfort and support for the bodies cutaneous surface (part of the practice of palliative medicine) is not a time-confined but rather a goal-oriented and patient-centered care delivery model.[50] Palliative wound care is the evolving body of knowledge and skills that take a holistic approach to relieving suffering and improving quality of life for patients (individuals) and families living with chronic wounds, whether the wound is healable, can be maintained or may deteriorate.[32]

Patient circle of care: This is not a legal term, but rather a social term that includes all of the stakeholders in the patient's health and well being. The term includes, but is not limited to, the patient, a legal guardian or responsible party, a spouse or significant other, interested friends or family members, caregivers, and any other individual(s) who may have an interest in the patient's care and well being.

Pressure Ulcer: A pressure ulcer is localized injury to the skin and/or underlying tissue usually over a bony prominence, as a result of pressure, or pressure in combination with shear and/or friction. A number of contributing or confounding factors are also associated with pressure ulcers; the significance of these factors is yet to be elucidated.[51]

Scale (skin): Surface keratin that may be thick or thin, resembling a fish scale, cast off (desquamating) from the skin.[29]

SCALE: The acronym for Skin Changes At Life's End.

Skin breakdown: An interruption in the integrity of the skin surface leading to defect in the epidermal covering with an epidermal, dermal or deeper base.

Skin compromise: A state in which skin's protective function is at risk of breaking down.

Skin failure: An acute episode where the skin and subcutaneous tissues die (become necrotic) due to hypoperfusion that occurs concurrent with severe dysfunction or failure of other organ systems.[8]

Skin tear: A traumatic wound occurring principally on the extremities of older adults as a result of friction alone or with shearing and frictional forces that separate the epidermis from the dermis (partial-thickness wound) or a deeper split that separates both the epidermis and the dermis from the underlying structures (full-thickness wound).[30]

Stakeholders: An individual, facility, or organization with an interest in Skin Changes At Life's End (SCALE).

Stage I Pressure Ulcer: Intact skin with non-blanchable redness of a localized area usually over a bony prominence. Darkly pigmented skin may not have visible blanching; its color may differ from the surrounding area.[51]

Stage II Pressure Ulcer: Partial thickness loss of dermis presenting as a shallow open ulcer with a red pink wound bed, without slough. May also present as an intact or open/ruptured serum-filled blister.[51]

Stage III Pressure Ulcer: Full thickness tissue loss. Subcutaneous fat may be visible but bone, tendon or muscle are not exposed. Slough may be present but does not obscure the depth of tissue loss. May include undermining and tunneling.[51]

Stage IV Pressure Ulcer: Full thickness tissue loss with exposed bone, tendon or muscle. Slough or eschar may be present on some parts of the wound bed. Often include undermining and tunneling.[51]

Suspected Deep Tissue Injury: Purple or maroon localized area of discolored intact skin or blood-filled blister due to damage of underlying soft tissue from pressure and/or shear. The area may be preceded by tissue that is painful, firm, mushy, boggy, warmer or cooler as compared to adjacent tissue.[51]

Terminal tissue trauma: Damage to the integumentary system that has occurred at the end of life.

Ulcer: A loss of surface skin with a dermal or deeper base.

Unavoidable (pressure ulcer): The resident developed a pressure ulcer even though the facility had evaluated the resident's clinical condition and pressure ulcer risk factors; defined and implemented interventions that are consistent with resident needs, goals, and recognized standards of practice; monitored and evaluated the impact of the interventions; and revised the approaches as appropriate (CMS definition).[38]

Unstageable Pressure Ulcer: Full thickness tissue loss in which the base of the ulcer is covered by slough (yellow, tan, gray, green or brown) and/or eschar (tan, brown or black) in the wound bed.[51]

Venous Ulcer: A ulceration that occurs on the lower limb secondary to underlying venous disease; formerly called stasis ulcers.[52]

References

1. Qaseem A, Snow V, Shekelle P, et al. Evidence-based interventions to improve the palliative care of pain, dyspnea, and depression at the end of life: a clinical practice guideline from the American College of Physicians. *Ann Intern Med.* 2008;148(2):141-146.

2. Kennedy KL. The prevalence of pressure ulcers in an intermediate care facility. *Decubitus.* 1989;2(2):44-45.

3. Hanson D, Langemo DK, Olson B, et al. The prevalence and incidence of pressure ulcers in the hospice setting: analysis of two methodologies. *Am J Hosp Palliat Care.* 1991;8(5):18-22.

4. Levine JM. Historical perspective on pressure ulcers: the decubitus ominosus of Jean-Martin Charcot. *J Am Geriatr Soc.* 2005;53(7):1248-51.

5. Charcot JM. *Lectures on the Diseases of the Nervous System.* Translated by G. Sigerson. London: The New Sydenham Society; 1877.

6. Shenk D. The Forgetting: Alzheimer's: Portrait of an Epidemic. In: *I Have Lost Myself.* Anchor; 2003.

7. Langemo DK. The hot seat: the reality of skin failure. 18th Annual Clinical Symposium on Advances in Skin & Wound Care. Chicago, IL 2003.

8. Langemo DK, Brown G. Skin fails too: acute, chronic, and end-stage skin failure. *Adv Skin Wound Care.* 2006;19(4):206-211.

9. Goode PS, Allman RM. The prevention and management of pressure ulcers. *Med Clin North Am.* 1989;73(6):1511-1524.

10. La Puma J. The ethics of pressure ulcers. *Decubitus.* 1991;4(2):43-44.

11. Witkowski JA, Parish LC. Skin failure and the pressure ulcer. *Decubitus.* 1993;6(5):4.

12. Leijten FS, De Weerd AW, Poortvliet DC, De Ridder VA, Ulrich C, Harink-De Weerd JE. Critical illness polyneuropathy in multiple organ dysfunction syndrome and weaning from the ventilator. *Intensive Care Med.* 1996;22(9):856-861.

13. Hobbs L, Spahn JG, Duncan C. Skin failure: what happens when this organ system fails. Poster presented at the 32nd Annual Wound, Ostomy, and Continence Nurses Society, Toronto, Canada June 2000.

14. Witkowski JA, Parish LC. The decubitus ulcer: skin failure and destructive behavior. *Int J Dermatol.* 2000;39(12):894-896.

15. Brown G. Long-term outcomes of full-thickness pressure ulcers: healing and mortality. *Ostomy Wound Manage.* 2003;49(10):42-50.

16. Parish LC, Witkowski JA. Chronic wounds: myths about decubitus ulcers. *Int J Dermatol.* 1994;33(9):623-624.

17. Alvarez OM, Kalinski C, Nusbaum J, et al. Incorporating wound healing strategies to improve palliation (symptom management) in patients with chronic wounds. *J Palliat Med.* 2007;10(5):1161-1189.

18. Thomas DR. Are all pressure ulcers avoidable? *J Am Med Dir Assoc.* 2003;4(2 Suppl):S43-48.

19. Wikipedia The Free Encyclopedia: Delphi Method. Available at URL: http://en.wikipedia.org/wiki/Delphi_method. Last Accessed July 20,2009.

20. Sibbald RG, Krasner DL, Lutz JB, et al. Skin changes at life's end (SCALE): a preliminary consensus statement. *World Council of Enterostomal Therapists Journal.* 2008;28(4):15-22.

21. Sibbald RG, Krasner DL, Lutz JB, et al. Skin Changes At life's End (SCALE) Preliminary Consensus Statement. Available at URL: www.Gaymar.com >Medical Research and Education>SCALE Consensus Documents. 2008;Last accessed July 20, 2009.

22. Ayello EA, Capitulo KL, Fife CE, et al. Legal Issues in the Care of Pressure Ulcer Patients: Key Concepts for Healthcare Providers.White Paper Available from URL: WWW.Medline.com 2009.

23. Victoria Hospice Society, Palliative Performance Scale version 2 (PPSv2). Available at URL: http://palliative.info/resource_material/PPSv2.pdf 2001.

24. International Association for Hospice & Palliative Care: Assessment and Research Tools: Assessment and Research Tools. 2009;Available at URL: http://www.hospicecare.com/resources/pain-research.htm.

25. Price P. Health-Related Quality of Life. In: Krasner D, Rodeheaver GT, Sibbald RG, es. *Chronic Wound Care: A Clinical Source Book for Healthcare Professionals.* 4th ed. Malvern, Pa: HMP Communications; 2007:79-83.

26. Krasner DL, Papen J, Sibbald RG. Helping Patients Out of the SWAMP©: Skin and Wound Assessment and Management of Pain. In: Krasner D, Rodeheaver GT, Sibbald RG, eds. *Chronic Wound Care: A Clinical Source Book for Healthcare Professionals.* 4th ed. Malvern, Pa: HMP Communications; 2007:85-97.

27. Langemo DK. When the goal is palliative care. *Adv Skin Wound Care.* 2006;19(3):148-154.

28. U.S. Department of Health and Human Services. Standards for Privacy of Individually Identifiable Health Information; Final Rule, 45 C.F.R. Parts 160, and 164. Code of Federal Regulations Available at: http://wedi.org/snip/public/articles/45CFR160&164.pdf. Accessed May 13, 2009.

29. Stedman's Medical Dictionary, 27th Edition. Lippincott Williams & Wilkins. 2008 Available from URL: http://www.stedmans.com.

30. Payne RL, Martin ML. Defining and classifying skin tears: need for a common language. *Ostomy Wound Manage.* 1993;39(5):16-20, 22-4, 26.

31. Krasner D, Rodeheaver GT, Sibbald RG. Interprofessional Wound Caring. In: Krasner D, Rodeheaver GT, Sibbald RG, eds. *Chronic Wound Care: A Clinical Source Book for Healthcare Professionals.* 4th ed. Malvern, Pa: HMP Communications; 2007:3-9.

32. Ferris FD, Al Khateib AA, Fromantin I, et al. Palliative wound care: managing chronic wounds across life's continuum: a consensus statement from the International Palliative Wound Care Initiative. *J Palliat Med.* 2007;10(1):37-39.

33. Romanelli M, Dini V, Williamson D, Paterson D, Pope M, Sibbald R. Measurement: Lower Leg Ulcer Vascular and Wound Assessment. In: Krasner D, Rodeheaver GT, Sibbald RG, eds. *Chronic Wound Care: A Clinical Source Book for Healthcare Professionals.* 4th ed. Malvern, Pa: HMP Communications; 2007:463-480.

34. Lee KF, Ennis WJ, Dunn GP. Surgical palliative care of advanced wounds. *Am J Hosp Palliat Care.* 2007;24(2):154-160.

35. Weed LJ. The problem oriented record as a basic tool in medical education, patient care and clinical research. *Ann Clin Res.* 1971;3(3):131-134.

36. Bergstrom N, Braden BJ, Laguzza A, Holman V. The Braden Scale for Predicting Pressure Sore Risk. *Nurs Res.* 1987;36(4):205-210.

37. Holloway GA. Arterial Ulcers: Assessment, Classification, and Management. In: Krasner D, Rodeheaver GT, Sibbald RG, eds. *Chronic Wound Care: A Clinical Source Book for Healthcare Professionals.* 4th ed. Malvern, Pa: HMP Communications; 2007:443-449.

38. CMS Manual System Department of Health & Human Services (DHHS). Pub. 100-07 State Operations. Provider Certification. Centers for Medicare & Medicaid Services (CMS).Transmittal 4. Date: November 12, 2004.

39. Murphy EK. Charting by exception - OR Nursing Law. *AORN J.* 2003 (NOV).

CHRONIC WOUND CARE: The Essentials,

40. Smith LM. How to chart by exception. *Nursing.* 2002 (SEPT).

41. Steed DL. Wounds in People with Diabetes: Assessment, Classification, and Management. In: Krasner D, Rodeheaver GT, Sibbald RG, eds. *Chronic Wound Care: A Clinical Source Book for Healthcare Professionals.* 4th ed. Malvern, Pa: HMP Communications; 2007:537-542.

42. Kozier B, Erb G, Olivieri R. *Fundamentals of nursing: concepts, process and practice.* 4th ed. Redwood City, Calif.: Addison-Wesley Nursing; 1991.

43. Milne CT, Corbett LQ. The Kennedy Terminal Ulcer. In: *Wound, Ostomy, and Continence Secrets.* Philadelphia, Pa: Hanley & Belfus; 2003:198-199.

44. Kennedy KL. *Gaymar Pictoral Guide to Pressure Ulcer Assessment.* Second ed. Orchard Park, NY: Gaymar Industries, Inc.; 2006.

45. Weir D. Pressure ulcers: assessment, classification, and management. In: Krasner DL, Rodeheaver GT, Sibbald RG, eds. *Chronic Wound Care: A Clinical Source Book for Healthcare Professionals.* 4th ed. Malvern, Pennsylvania: HMP Communications; 2007:577-578.

46. The different types of wounds. In: *The Wound Care Handbook.* Mundelein, IL: Medline Industries, Inc.; 2007:110-111.

47. Ayello EA, Shank JE. Ulcerative lesions. In: Kuebler KK, Heidrich DE, Esper P, eds. *Palliative & end-of-life care: clinical practice guidelines.* 2nd ed. Philadelphia, Pa: Edinburgh: Elsevier Saunders; 2007:523.

48. Turnbull GB. Year's end notables. *Ostomy Wound Manage.* 2001;47(12):10.

49. Hogue EE. Key legal issues for wound care practitioners in 2005. *The Remmington Report.* May/June 2005;13(3):14-16.

50. Davis MP, Walsh D, LeGrand SB, Lagman R. End-of-Life care: the death of palliative medicine? *J Palliat Med.* 2002;5(6):813-814.

51. National Pressure Ulcer advisory Panel: Updated Staging System. Available at URL: http://www.npuap.org/pr2.htm. 2007.

52. Sibbald RG, Williamson D, Contreras-Ruiz J, et al. Venous Leg Ulcers. In: Krasner D, Rodeheaver GT, Sibbald RG, eds. *Chronic Wound Care: A Clinical Source Book for Healthcare Professionals.* 4th ed. Malvern, Pa: HMP Communications; 2007:429-442.

Distinguished Reviewers

Sadanori Akai	Japan	Kathleen Lawrence	USA
Mona Baharestani	USA	Michele Lee	Hong Kong
Jane Ellen Barr	USA	Jeffrey Levine	USA
Scott Bolhack	USA	Larry Liebrach	Canada
Barbara Braden	USA	Christina Lindholm	Sweden
Barbara Bates-Jensen	USA	Maartin Lubbers	Netherlands
Janice Beitz	USA	Vera Lucia de Gouevia Santos	Brazil
Pauline Beldon	UK	JoAnn Maklebust	USA
Nancy Bergstrom	USA	Marge Meehan	USA
Dan Berlowitz	USA	Gerit Mulder	USA
Joyce Black	USA	Linda Norton	Canada
Keryln Carville	Australia	Jeanne Nusbaum	USA
Pat Coutts	Canada	Nancy Parslow	Canada
Carol Dealey	UK	Christine Pearson	Canada
Tom Defloor	Belgium	Ben Peirce	USA
Dorothy Doughty	USA	Patricia Price	UK
Caroline Fife	USA	Madhuri Reddy	USA
Chris Glynn	UK	George Rodeheaver	USA
Laurie Goodman	Canada	Marco Romanelli	Italy
Robert Gunther	USA	James Spahn	USA
Terese Henn	USA	Aletha Tippett	USA
Heather Hettrick	USA	Charles Von Gunten	USA
Cathy Kalinski	USA	Robert Warriner	USA
David Keast	Canada	Kevin Woo	Canada
Kathryn Kozell	Canada	Gail Woodbury	Canada
Steven Kravitz	USA		

Best Practice Guidelines, Algorithms, and Standards: Tools to Make the Right Thing Easier to Do

Heather L. Orsted, RN, BN, ET, MSc; **David Keast**, BSc(Hon), MSc, DipEd, MD, CCFP, FCFP; **Heather McConnell**, RN, BScN, MA(Ed); **Catherine R. Ratliff**, PhD, APRN-BC, CWOCN, CFCN

Objectives

The reader will be challenged to:

- Differentiate between the terms best practice guideline, algorithm, and standard
- Describe the relationship between best practice guidelines, algorithms, and standards
- Identify the stages in the development of best practice guidelines
- Summarize a process to evaluate the quality of existing best practice guidelines
- Analyze barriers to the implementation of best practice guidelines and describe methods to overcome them
- Propose effective interventions aimed at adoption and translation of best practice guidelines into practice.

Introduction

As evidence accumulates regarding healthcare practices, doing things "the way we have always done them" is no longer acceptable. In the past, part of the art and necessity of the practice in healthcare was making decisions on the basis of tradition and, in many cases, inadequate evidence. This often led to variations in practice, inappropriate care, and uncontrolled costs.[1,2] Rapid advances in healthcare make it almost impossible to keep up to date on what is "known." Inadequate care is now a result of inadequate production, evaluation, dissemination, and use of information. The provision of care based on evidence is required to support the creation of best practice cultures that require standards of quality, performance measures, and review criteria.

Comparative effectiveness research helps determine healthcare decisions by providing evidence on the effectiveness, benefits, and harms of different treatment options. Comparative effectiveness research requires the use of a variety of data sources and methods to conduct research and disseminate the results in a form that is quickly usable by clinicians, patients, policymakers, and health plans and other payers.[3]

In the United States, the Effective Health Care Program funds researchers to work together with the *Agency for Healthcare Research and Quality (AHRQ)* to produce effectiveness and comparative effectiveness research for clinicians, consumers, and policymakers. The AHRQ is the federal agency in the United States charged with improving the quality, safety, efficiency, and effectiveness of healthcare for all Americans. The Effective Health Care Program:

Orsted HL, Keast D, McConnell H, Ratliff CR. Best practice guidelines, algorithms, and standards: tools to make the right thing easier to do. In: Krasner DL, ed. *Chronic Wound Care: The Essentials.* Malvern, PA: HMP Communications; 2014:319–330.

- Reviews and synthesizes published and unpublished scientific evidence
- Facilitates the generation of new scientific evidence and analytic tools
- Compiles research findings that are synthesized and/or generated and translates them into useful formats for various audiences.

The AHRQ summary guides are reviews of research findings pertaining to the benefits and harms of different treatment options, and various versions are tailored to clinicians, consumers, or policy makers. Consumer guides provide useful background information on health conditions.

The *National Guideline Clearinghouse*™ *(NGC)* is a publicly available database of evidence-based clinical practice guidelines available at http://www.guideline.gov. It provides Internet users with weekly updates highlighting new content. The NGC is produced by the AHRQ in partnership with the American Medical Association (AMA) and the American Association of Health Plans (AAHP) Foundation. Key components of the NGC include:

- Structured, standardized abstracts (summaries) about each guideline
- Side-by-side comparisons of two or more guidelines
- Syntheses of guidelines covering similar topics, highlighting similarities and differences in the guidelines
- Links to full-text guidelines, where available, and/or ordering information for print copies
- Annotated bibliographies on guideline development methodology, structure, implementation, and evaluation.

In Canada, the Canadian Medical Association (CMA) maintains a database of clinical practice guidelines along with resources for development, evaluation, and implementation. To be included in the *CMA Infobase*, each guideline must:

1. Include information to help patients and physicians make decisions about appropriate healthcare for specific clinical circumstances. Ethics guidelines are included only if they help in decision-making concerning appropriate care. Guidelines on facilities, management, training, or professional qualifications are not included unless they also contain guidelines on clinical practice.
2. Be produced in Canada by a medical or

health organization, professional society, government agency, or expert panel at the national, provincial/territorial, or regional level (clinical practice guidelines produced by individuals are excluded) or be produced outside Canada by one of the foregoing types of groups and officially endorsed by an authoritative Canadian organization.
3. Have been developed or reviewed in the last 5 years (rolling date).
4. Have evidence that a literature search was performed during guideline development.

The CMA Infobase is available at http://www.cma.ca/cpgs.

The *Centre for Evidence-based Medicine (CEBM)* in Oxford, England, promotes evidence-based healthcare and provides resources for clinicians interested in learning more about evidence-based practice. Their goal is to develop, teach, and promote evidence-based healthcare and provide support and resources to doctors and healthcare professionals to help maintain the highest standards of medicine. The CEBM is available at http://www.cebm.net/index.aspx.

Best Practice Approach to Care

Evidence alone is not enough to ensure best practice. *In 2000, Sackett et al[4] defined evidence-based medicine (EBM) as follows: "Evidence-based medicine is the integration of best research evidence with clinical expertise and patient values."* Kitson, Harvey, and McCormack[5] suggest that a synergy of actions is required to enable successful implementation of the evidence to support best practice. The evidence is required to be scientifically robust, the environment or context has to be ready for change, and the change process has to be appropriately facilitated. Evidence-based medicine is not restricted to randomized trials and meta-analyses but involves finding the best evidence with which to answer clinical questions.[6]

Best practice needs to be more than a theory. In clinical practice settings, multiple modalities are required to provide and transform the evidence into usable frameworks that enable appropriate facilitation and adoption of best practice by healthcare providers and the agencies in which they work.

Best practice guidelines (BPGs), also sometimes called clinical practice guidelines (CPGs), are systematically developed statements to assist practitioner decisions about appropriate healthcare for specific clinical circumstances.[7] They combine research evidence, experience, and expert opinion to improve patient care through reducing inappropriate variations in practice and promoting the delivery of high-quality, evidence-based healthcare.[8] Guidelines form the framework for practice in supporting policy and procedure recommendations. *Algorithms* or *pathways*, by contrast, are graphic maps that visualize the major cognitive components required to resolve a problem. They can act as clinical decision-making frameworks to guide the implementation of BPGs.[9–11] *Standards* differ in that they are rules or models of care established by professional organizations or regulatory bodies. Standards often set the minimal acceptable level of performance. Some standards may be specific to each discipline and may be enshrined in legislation in certain jurisdictions. Other standards may be flexible and responsive. For example, a common legal standard of care is to compare the care provided to that of a reasonable clinician in similar circumstances.

In practice, BPGs help healthcare clinicians define effective and appropriate practices based on current and extensive scientific research and available evidence; algorithms represent tools or enablers that aid in the implementation of BPGs; and standards set minimal levels of performance. The three, though different, are intimately related.[12]

The BPG, Assessment and Management of Foot Ulcers for People with Diabetes, from the *Registered Nurses' Association of Ontario (RNAO)* illustrates this relationship in many sections. For example, the BPG rationale is presented under the heading "Background Context" and then accompanied by an algorithm (Pathway to Diabetic Foot Ulcers) to enable further understanding of the concepts discussed. The same document contains a discussion relating to sharp debridement that asks the clinician to consider if the task is within his or her standard of practice.[13]

How are BPGs Developed?

In the years that have passed since BPGs or CPGs were introduced into the healthcare system, they have permeated into every area of clinical practice. Originally, healthcare chief executive officers regarded BPGs as "the answer" to reduce inappropriate or unnecessary variation in clinical practice.[8] Between 1990 and 1996, the Agency for Health Care Policy and Research (AHCPR), now the AHRQ, introduced 19 practice guidelines in an effort to support evidence-based methods to assess medical treatments and to set high standards for the development of guidelines.

In Canada, the International Affairs and Best Practice Guidelines Program, a signature program of the RNAO, is being funded by the Ministry of Health and Long-Term Care in Ontario to develop, implement, evaluate, disseminate, and support the uptake of both clinical and healthy work environment BPGs.[14] Though the RNAO is a professional nursing association, its guidelines are developed with interprofessional support as well as patient guidance and advice. Since 1999, the RNAO has developed and maintained (through regularly scheduled revisions) 44 clinical and healthy work environment BPGs. Translation into a range of languages including French, Italian, Spanish, Japanese, and Chinese has made these resources accessible to a range of practitioners provincially, nationally, and internationally. Additionally, the RNAO utilizes the *Appraisal of Guidelines for Research and Evaluation (AGREE II instrument)* to support a best practice approach to guideline development.[15]

The International Affairs and Best Practice Guidelines Program's goals are to:
- Improve patient care
- Reduce variation in care
- Transfer research evidence into practice
- Promote nursing knowledge base
- Assist with clinical decision-making
- Identify gaps in research
- Stop interventions that have little effect or cause harm
- Reduce cost.

Guidelines are designed to be used as recommendations to inform care decisions rather than rules for care to enable the practitioner to provide the best possible care by adopting new information and changing practice.[16] Guidelines must provide healthcare professionals with adequate notice of the boundaries of acceptable and prescribed behaviors yet not be so narrow or rigid that they create a detrimental effect on innovative and individualized patient care.[15]

Quality guideline development requires that rel-

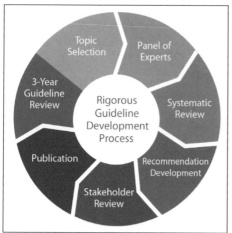

Figure 1. RNAO guideline development methodology process. Reprinted with permission from the Registered Nurses' Association of Ontario. Transforming Nursing Though Knowledge. Available at: http://www.rnao.org/Page.asp?PageID=122&ContentID=1557&SiteNodeID=158&BL_ExpandID=.

evant literature and practice patterns are reviewed and the data appraised for weight of evidence. The results are then distilled and collated into a succinct, user-friendly format. In the final stage, these guidelines are reviewed widely and modified based on feedback by experts in the field before being endorsed by a credible sponsoring body or association. At this point, the guideline is ready for dissemination to appropriate bodies leading to knowledge transfer or implementation into practice.

The final important stage in the cycle of BPGs is a feedback loop of ongoing reevaluation and refinement through gathering of new evidence as the cycle continues. Regularly scheduled reviews should include changing practice patterns, new evidence, and barriers and enablers to implementation. For example, the RNAO guidelines are revised every 3–5 years (Figure 1).[17]

According to Roberts, *attributes of a good practice guideline are validity, reliability, reproducibility, clinical applicability, clinical flexibility, clarity, interdisciplinary process, scheduled review and documentation, and simplicity*.[8]

Selecting a Best Practice Guideline for Implementation

Developing BPGs is an expensive and time-

consuming process. If one wishes to adopt an existing guideline into practice, how does one select the most rigorous yet practical one? The AGREE II instrument is the new international tool for the assessment of guidelines. The AGREE II is both valid and reliable and comprises 23 items organized into the original 6 quality domains. It helps guideline developers and users assess the methodological quality of CPGs.[18] The AGREE II instrument has 3 goals: 1) to assess the quality of CPGs, 2) to provide a methodological strategy for guideline development, and 3) to recommend what information should be reported in guidelines.

Assessment of a guideline involves evaluation of its quality (using the AGREE II tool), how up-to-date it is, and the consistency of the recommendation with the underlying evidence. Assessment also consists of the feasibility of applying recommendations. This process can result in different alternatives ranging from adopting a guideline unchanged, to adapting the format, modifying single recommendations, and producing a customized guideline based on various guidelines used as sources.[19]

The AGREE II instrument is a tool designed primarily to help guideline developers and users assess the methodological quality of CPGs.[15] The 6 quality domains include:

1. Scope and purpose: overall aim of the guideline, clinical question, and target population
2. Stakeholder involvement: extent to which the guideline represents the views of the intended users
3. Rigor of development: process used to gather and synthesize the evidence and methods to formulate the recommendations and to update them
4. Clarity and presentation: the language and format of the guideline
5. Applicability: organizational, behavioral, and cost implications of application
6. Editorial independence: independence of the recommendations and acknowledgement of possible conflict of interest from the development group.

Once the review is complete, a quality score is calculated for each of the 6 AGREE II domains. The 6 domain scores are independent and should not be aggregated into a single quality score. Reviewers are provided with the opportunity to comment on the overall quality of the guideline and whether the guideline would be recommended for use in practice.

Wimpenny and van Zelm compared 4 national pressure ulcer guidelines from Australia, Canada, the Netherlands, and the United Kingdom to identify similarities and differences in their quality and content.[20] The domain scores for each guideline show some but not total agreement among reviewers. One guideline was identified as scoring highest in a majority of AGREE II domains.

While the AGREE II tool identifies the quality of the guideline development process, it still requires practitioners to determine which guideline would be most appropriate to implement in their clinical settings. The potential for evidence overload also suggests that brevity might be best, even in algorithm or decision-tree format.

National and international bodies have made major efforts to improve the quality of guidelines, but less time has been spent understanding how guidelines can be implemented. Developing BPGs is an expensive and time-consuming process. If one wishes to adopt or modify an existing guideline, how does one select the most rigorous yet practical one? Adaptation of existing guidelines for individual facility use enhances applicability. National guidelines often lack specific details on what changes in the organization are required to apply the recommendations. Adaptation of evidence may promote a sense of ownership by those who are engaged in this process.[19]

The **ADAPTE collaboration** (www.adapte. org) is a group whose purpose is to increase the use of evidence-based guidelines. The ADAPTE process consists of 3 phases, including planning, adaptation, and development of the guideline. The planning phase outlines the tasks to be completed before adapting the guideline, including identifying necessary skills and resources and determining who should be on the panel. The panel should include end users of the guideline, such as clinicians and patients.[19]

Since 2000, the **Canadian Association of Wound Care (CAWC)** has authored best practice recommendations relating to wound bed preparation and the prevention and management of pressure ulcers, diabetic foot ulcers, and venous leg ulcers. These were not intended to be BPGs but rather a distillation of existing guidelines into a succinct practice article and bedside enabler (the **Quick Reference Guide** or **QRG**) backed by the existing articles, research, and guidelines for more in-depth information.

When it came time to update and revise the CAWC recommendations, the CAWC board recognized the quality of the RNAO guidelines and decided to create regional teams to revise the recommendations utilizing the RNAO wound-related guidelines. The updated articles and **QRGs serve as practice enablers** that help to interpret these guidelines for the multiple healthcare professionals involved in the management of chronic wounds. Each article takes the practice enabling statements and discusses their relationship to the corresponding RNAO guideline as well as additional resources from the literature to enhance and support an interprofessional approach. To further enable practice, each QRG is related to a Pathway to Assessment and Treatment, which provides an algorithm to guide clinical decision-making.

A Health Canada initiative to encourage adaptation of the RNAO guidelines stimulated the development of regional wound care guidelines in Saskatchewan. In January 2004, the Health Quality Council (HQC) and the Saskatchewan Association of Health Organizations (SAHO) convened a provincial Skin and Wound Care Action Committee to develop a strategy to ensure that patients receive consistent, high-quality skin and wound care. The results of their initiative involved a partnership between the HQC and the RNAO to adapt the RNAO guidelines to produce a regionally specific pressure ulcer guideline.[21]

The **Wound, Ostomy, and Continence Nurses Society (WOCN)** developed evidence-based guidelines using a clinically diverse panel of WOCN nurses, a topical outline with specific questions to guide the literature search for evidence, and studies reporting primary data relevant to the topic with specific diagnostic modalities and treatment therapies included in the review. The search targeted meta-analyses, randomized controlled trials, prospective and retrospective clinical trials, and systemic reviews.

In early 2003, the **Wound Healing Foundation** put out a request for proposal (RFP) for a project to formulate and publish chronic wound care guidelines. Multidisciplinary committees were set up to complete the project with the majority of the group members in agreement with the recommendations. Publically held forums on the National Institutes of Health (NIH) campus solicited input from other interested parties, societies, and industry.

The American **National Pressure Ulcer Advisory Panel (NPUAP)** and the **European Pressure Ulcer Advisory Panel (EPUAP)** collaborated to develop guidelines on the prevention and treatment of pressure ulcers. The guidelines were produced by a guideline development group along with several small working groups. The entire process of the guideline development could be followed on a designated website by stakeholders of this process.

The first step in any guideline development process is identifying the evidence. Generally, electronic databases are searched with specific predetermined inclusion criteria, such as dates of the searches, subject titles, such as pressure ulcers, pressure sores, and decubitus ulcers, and type of studies to be included, such as randomized controlled trials, meta-analyses, systematic reviews, etc. All retrieved references are then sorted by topic and placed in evidence tables. The level of evidence is then noted for each study based on a predetermined classification system set up by the guideline group. Recommendations about the body of available evidence are then identified based on the level of evidence found in the tables.

Implementing Best Practice Guidelines and Algorithms

Many BPGs have been developed and disseminated; however, their implementation across all disciplines and delivery sites remains a major challenge.

In a Minnesota study, approximately two-thirds of family physicians were unaware of the existence of the AHCPR guidelines for pressure ulcers (#3 and #15). Ninety percent of the physicians who had browsed the prevention guidelines had found them helpful, and all who read them in entirety said they were helpful.[22] A survey of Ontario family physicians showed that 78% indicated that they complied with lipid-lowering guidelines, but further questioning revealed that only 5% actually followed them.[23] Davis and Taylor-Vaisey[14] reviewed the literature on adop-

tion of CPGs by healthcare professionals. They found that the variables affecting adoption include the qualities of the guidelines, the characteristics of the healthcare professional, the characteristics of the practice setting, incentives, regulation, and patient factors.

Davis and Taylor-Vaisey[14] also reviewed interventions aimed at the adoption of guidelines and classified them as weak (didactic, traditional continuing medical education, and mailings), moderately effective (audit and feedback, especially concurrent, targeted to specific providers and delivery by peers or opinion leaders), and relatively strong (reminder systems, academic detailing, and multiple interventions).

The first hurdle is promoting a culture or environment that supports the adoption and application of evidence-based practice. Guidelines involve change, and any change must be based on a need. Therefore, any system's change should be based on a needs assessment that identifies care gaps. The needs assessment should involve the users, recipients, educators, and appropriate administrators who may be involved in ultimate implementation. Toward this end (system change), the RNAO clinical guidelines not only identify clinical practice recommendations but also contain a recommendation section directed toward **organization and policy** (identifying the structures and resources that need to be in place to support evidence-based practice) as well as a section dedicated to the educational requirements (the knowledge and skills) required to successfully implement the guideline recommendations.[21] This approach to guideline development recognizes that the nature of nursing practice falls on a continuum from being a solo practitioner to being interdependent team members, which requires organizational structures and resources to ensure consistency in practice.

An often overlooked element in creating evidence-based practice cultures is sustainability. The **Knowledge-to-Action Cycle** identifies attention to sustaining knowledge use as a critical element of moving knowledge to action[22] (Figure 2). A study by Higuchi et al reported on a 3-year follow-up evaluation of nursing care indicators following the implementation of 2 RNAO BPGs.[23] They found that clinical guidelines provide credible resources for evaluating and improving prac-

Table I. Barriers and bridges to best practice

Category	Barrier	Bridge
Financial Issues	• Support for programs and interdisciplinary teams • Technology • Infrastructure to support guidelines	• Clear identification of outcomes will support a cost-effective delivery of best practices • Efficiencies regarding supply/equipment acquisition and purchase
Educational Issues	• Location of existing guidelines • Dissemination of guideline-specific education and knowledge • Changing the attitudes and expectations of healthcare providers • Understanding the tools for documentation • Lack of leadership • Educational resources and time • Patients refusing evidence-based practice	• Websites specific to needs • Program leader to integrate guidelines into policies, procedures, and protocols • Regular communication to provide ongoing information (newsletter, emails, alerts) • Regularly scheduled staff and team meetings to educate, learn, provide a forum for discussion, and support change • Easy-to-read, healthcare provider-specific, and client-specific evidence-based educational material (current, simple, holistic, and easy to adapt based on client need and clinical judgment)
Practice Issues	• Clinical integration of evidence-based practice among healthcare providers • Staff skill level • Staff stress level and staff shortages	• Clinical integration of evidence-based practice among healthcare providers • Clinical pathway • User-friendly format for protocols and procedures • Interdisciplinary team (opinion leaders) to provide ongoing support to staff regarding clinical issues and change • Agency support and effective resource management • Alternative, cost-effective methods of service delivery (clinics) • Continuity of care and care providers

tice, but the changes required at the individual and system levels are frequently significant and require considerable time. Two significant contributors to guideline sustainability they identified were documentation and reminder systems, which support change at the systems level.

Challenges to implementing wound care BPGs occur across all service delivery sites (hospital, outpatient clinics, home, and long-term care). These challenges include information transfer, integration of payment sources into the dialogue to realize potential savings in overall program costs, consistency of wound management approaches among all service delivery sites, and development and maintenance of interdisciplinary care teams. Successful implementation strategies:

• Provide educational offerings that teach concepts of the BPG
• Provide an educational offering for each new BPG
• Include a pathophysiology review during each educational offering
• Provide routine, ongoing educational offerings on BPG information.[6]

The literature is replete with barriers to guideline implementation, which can be condensed into 3 main categories.[17–20,24] No listing of barriers would be complete, however, without dis-

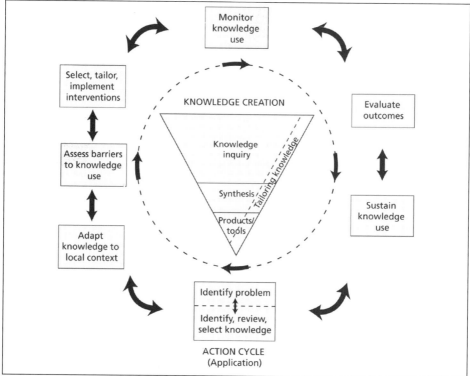

Figure 2. Knowledge-to-Action Cycle. Reprinted with permission from Graham ID, Logan J, Harrison MB, et al. Lost in knowledge translation: time for a map? *J Contin Educ Health Prof.* 2006;26(1):13–24.

cussing recommended solutions (bridges). Table 1 reviews "bridges for barriers," discussing solutions from the literature and from clinical experience.[25]

Best practice guideline implementation requires strong leadership from clinicians who understand concepts of planned change, program planning and evaluation, and research utilization. This knowledge will support the development of a program plan that enables the transformation of organizations toward best practice. In 2002, the RNAO developed a toolkit to assist organizations through a planned change process for successful implementation.[26]

Graham et al indicated that in order for guidelines to be implemented successfully, a critical initial step must be the *formal adoption of the guideline recommendations into the policy and procedure structure.*[27] This key step provides direction regarding the expectations of the organization and facilitates integration of the guideline into systems, such as the quality management process.[27]

Shiffman and colleagues developed the *Guideline Implementability Appraisal (GLIA)* to facilitate guideline implementation. The instrument is designed to systematically highlight barriers to implementation including executability, decidability, validity, flexibility, effect on process of care, measurability, novelty/innovation, and computability. The GLIA is intended to provide feedback about a guideline's ability to be implemented to the authors of the guideline and to those individuals who choose to apply the guideline within a healthcare system. The GLIA consists of 31 items, arranged into 10 dimensions, and is applied individually to each recommendation of the guideline. Evidence of content validity and preliminary support for construct validity was obtained by the authors.[28]

It is understood that if healthcare professionals are to provide best practices, they must seek valid, reproducible, useful, and relevant studies and support material that enable the growth of their practice into a best practice standard.[29] However, how does that information get into practice? Healthcare professionals also need to participate in recognized, accredited continuing educational opportunities that allow them to participate with skill and confidence as members of interprofessional wound care teams. Agencies need to provide a full scope of support for nurses seeking professional education.[30,31]

The question remains: How can we be assured that knowledge is developed, delivered, evaluated, and sustained by an educational event or program, such as described in the Knowledge-to-Action Cycle?[22]

The CAWC and the Canadian Association for Enterostomal Therapy (CAET) collaborated toward the development, evaluation, and publication of a standard for wound management education and programming that can be used by healthcare professionals and their employers to appraise existing and future investments in wound care education.[32] The *Wound CARE Instrument* contains standards obtained from literature focused on knowledge mobilization that support a collaborative and evidence-informed approach to the appraisal and recommendation process of wound management education and programming. This instrument supports decision-makers in their efforts to improve wound care knowledge, skills, and attitude and to improve the health of patients at risk for or suffering from wounds.

The Wound CARE Instrument:

1. Provides a foundation to identify the components required to plan, develop, implement, evaluate, and sustain evidence-informed wound management education and programming
2. Provides a benchmark to appraise the quality of wound management education and programming
3. Supports collaboration in the development and implementation of wound management education and programming
4. Informs decisions related to the endorsement, adoption, adaptation, purchase, or rejection of wound management education and programming
5. Improves patient care and health outcomes relating to the prevention and management of wounds.

The Wound CARE Instrument has dem-onstrated that it is a valuable tool to aid in the appraisal and evaluation of wound management education and programming within a clinical setting. The Wound CARE Instrument is now available online and downloadable for no cost at http://www.cawc.net or http://www.caet.ca.

Are Algorithms and Best Practice Guidelines Effective?

Algorithms. Beitz and van Rijswijk published a study in which they attempted to establish content validation data for a set of wound care algorithms.[33] They tried to identify strengths and weaknesses of the algorithms in order to gain further insight into the wound care decision-making process. With this set of wound care algorithms, they identified 11 themes of difficulty in 5 areas. These 5 areas included the length of the algorithm, wound care terminology, wound assessment, wound context (patient issues), and clinical decision-making. The algorithms provided 3 positive aspects to care: a focus on goals, an ability to improve consistency, and a high content validity index of the wound assessment and care concepts. They concluded that the wound care algorithm studies were valid; however, the algorithms lacked valid and reliable wound assessment and care definitions.

Best practice guidelines. In a study of 5 client care settings, including a home care agency, the prevalence rates of pressure ulcers showed a decrease from 19% to 7.4% 4 months after the introduction of guidelines. The decrease continued to 6.7% after 8 months and 6.1% after 1 year.[34]

The response to BPGs varies. Many practitioners, especially physicians, worry that CPGs will lead to "cookbook medicine" with little room for clinical decision-making, consideration of patient and local condition variations, or innovation. Many practitioners fear that even the slightest variation from the guidelines will make them more liable to be successfully sued. Legal concerns relating to guidelines have been addressed by Goebel and Goebel who reviewed legal databases for malpractice awards for pressure ulcers.[16] The authors found that substantial savings in malpractice costs would have occurred and only 4 of 14 findings in favor of the defendant would have been reversed had guidelines been followed.

It is important to remember that in the com-

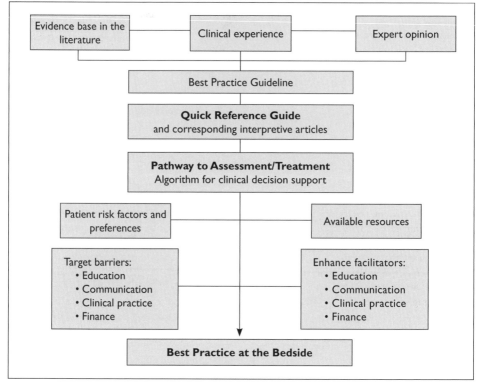

Figure 3. The pathway to best practice.[38] Reprinted with permission from Keast D, Orsted H. The pathway to best practice. *Wound Care Canada.* 2006;4(1):10.

plex wound-healing environment, interventions — even those based on guidelines — need to be regularly assessed by skilled professionals to ensure that outcomes of care are achieved. Care delivery must be based on lifestyle and client choice as well as best evidence.

Conclusion

A Health Policy Forum convened an interprofessional summit in Toronto, Canada, including patient representatives, practicing physicians (both generalists and specialists), nurses, researchers, and healthcare administrators.[35] The following 3 questions were asked:

• What goals should underlie CPG development?
• How can we improve CPGs?
• Who should participate in CPG development, use, and evaluation?

The results from the various working groups were remarkably consistent. They agreed that

CPGs should serve one central goal: providing better care for patients.

The forum made a number of recommendations regarding the production and role of CPGs that include the following:

1. Education: CPGs are an educational tool and must not be used to regulate medical practice
2. Flexibility: CPGs must be flexible enough to meet the needs of individual patients while incorporating all aspects of care
3. Multidisciplinary: The CPG process must be truly interprofessional with a focus on frontline caregivers rather than academics — the process must include all parties involved in care
4. Patient input: Patient representatives must have meaningful input at all stages of CPG development, including outcome measures used
5. Quality assurance: A standardized process for developing and evaluating CPGs should be employed with periodic or continuous re-

view processes incorporated to keep CPGs up to date

6. Accountability: The CPG process must be visible and accountable to healthcare professional and patient groups; the level of evidence used to formulate a CPG must be explicitly stated, as must potential bias

7. Outcomes orientation: CPGs should facilitate treatment choices by providing clear information about what works and what does not work — the outcomes examined should reflect patient priorities

8. Accessible: Successful strategies to encourage adoption of CPGs must be shared and materials and technologies developed to make them immediately available for consultation

9. National clearinghouse: Many participants identified the need for a central body to oversee CPG development, funding, and use. This central body would ensure that existing CPGs are regularly updated and reviewed and that implementation strategies are shared.

Marketing experts have suggested that organizations *focus on the exchange rather than on the change about to be encountered*.[36] The adoption and implementation of new tools can provide the implementers and the users support for knowledge exchange. Through expert opinion and current extensive scientific research and available evidence, guidelines define best practices that in turn support the attainment of competency and skill level. Basing a wound care program on tools that enable evidence-based practice will promote excellence in skin care, foster collegial relationships, and permit replication with other clinical populations.[37]

Guidelines and algorithms integrated into the continuum of care can provide:

• Cost-effective care delivery

• Documentation that is consistent, complete, standardized, comparable, outcome generated, and shared

• Care that will be evidence based, holistic, and patient specific.

To support the implementation of best practice at the bedside, clinicians and facilities must integrate BPGs that endorse recommendations related not only to practice but also to educational, organizational, and policy changes. Re-

gional differences related to population and resources need to be considered when program development is considered. To accomplish this, the clinician must be supported in an environment that breaks down barriers related to communication, education, practice, and resources. Barriers to best practice must be identified and modified, and bridges to best practice must be identified and enhanced. This is an active process that requires a receptive environment supported by administrators, the allocation of appropriate resources, and the cooperation of interprofessional team members. Figure 3 summarizes the entire process.

Most importantly, when it comes to best practice, you may know best practice, but are you providing it?

Take-Home Messages for Practice

• Not all guidelines are created equal.

• Awareness of the best evidence does not ensure a change in practice.

• The strength of the evidence must be combined with a willingness of the environment to change practice and appropriate facilitation of the new information.

• Practice change needs to be system-wide and supported by policy.

Self-Assessment Questions

1. A guideline is a document that outlines the best available evidence for a health-related problem.
   A. True
   B. False

2. The AGREE II instrument allows the clinician to evaluate if the recommendations outlined in the guideline will work at the bedside.
   A. True
   B. False

3. Guideline recommendations are more effective if supported by agency policy and procedure.
   A. True
   B. False

Answers: 1-A, 2-B, 3-A

References

1. Leape LL. Practice guidelines and standards: an overview. *QRB Qual Rev Bull.* 1990;16(2):42–49.

2. Atkins D, Kamerow D, Eisenberg JM. Evidence-based medicine at the Agency for Health Care Policy and Research. *ACP J Club.* 1998;128(2):A12–A14.

3. US Department of Health & Human Services. Agency for Healthcare Research and Quality. What is comparative effectiveness research? Available at: http://www.effectivehealthcare.ahrq.gov/index.cfm/what-is-comparative-effectiveness-research1/. Accessed February 2010.

4. Sackett DL, Straus SE, Richardson WS, Rosenberg W, Haynes RB. *Evidence-Based Medicine: How to Practice and Teach EBM.* 2nd ed. New York, NY: Churchill Livingstone; 2000:1.

5. Kitson A, Harvey G, McCormack B. Enabling the implementation of evidence based practice: a conceptual framework. *Qual Health Care.* 1998;7(3):149–158.

6. Centre for Evidence Based Medicine. What is EBM? Available at: http://www.cebm.net/index.aspx?o=1914. Accessed February 2010.

7. Field MJ, Lohr KN. *Clinical Practice Guidelines: Directions for a New Program.* Washington, DC: National Academy Press; 1990.

8. Roberts KA. Best practices in the development of clinical practice guidelines. *J Healthc Qual.* 1998;20(6):16–32.

9. Gaines C. Concept mapping and synthesizers: instructional strategies for encoding and recalling. *J N Y State Nurses Assoc.* 1996;27(1):14–18.

10. Hadorn DC, McCormick K, Diokno A. An annotated algorithm approach to clinical guideline development. *JAMA.* 1992;267(24):3311–3314.

11. Tallon R. Critical paths for wound care. *Adv Wound Care.* 1995;8(1):26–34.

12. Tellez RD. Wound care 2000: challenges to integration across the continuum. *Home Care Provid.* 1997;2(4):192–196.

13. Registered Nurses' Association of Ontario. Assessment and management of foot ulcers for people with diabetes. Available at: http://www.rnao.org/Page.asp?PageID=924&ContentID=719. Accessed September 2010.

14. Davis DA, Taylor-Vaisey A. Translating guidelines into practice. A systematic review of theoretic concepts, practical experience and research evidence in the adoption of clinical practice guidelines. *CMAJ.* 1997;157(4):408–416.

15. Registered Nurses' Association of Ontario. Nursing best practice guidelines. Available at: http://www.rnao.org/Page.asp?PageID=861&SiteNodeID=133. Accessed September 2010.

16. Goebel RH, Goebel MR. Clinical practice guidelines for pressure ulcer prevention can prevent malpractice lawsuits in older patients. *J Wound Ostomy Continence Nurs.* 1999;26(4):175–184.

17. The AGREE Collaboration. Appraisal of guidelines research and evaluation. Available at: http://www.agreetrust.org/. Accessed September 2010.

18. Dans AL, Dans LF. Appraising a tool for guideline appraisal (the AGREE II instrument). *J Clin Epidemiol.* 2010;63(12):1281–1282.

19. Harrison MB, Légaré F, Graham ID, Fervers B. Adapting clinical practice guidelines to local context and assessing barriers to their use. *CMAJ.* 2010;182(2):E78–E84.

20. Wimpenny P, van Zelm R. Appraising and comparing pressure ulcer guidelines. *Worldviews Evid Based Nurs.* 2007;4(1):40–50.

21. Edwards N, Davies B, Ploeg J, et al. Evaluating best practice guidelines. *Can Nurse.* 2005;101(2):18–23.

22. Graham ID, Logan J, Harrison MB, et al. Lost in knowledge translation: time for a map? *J Contin Educ Health Prof.* 2006;26(1):13–24.

23. Higuchi KS, Davies BL, Edwards N, Ploeg J, Virani T. Implementation of clinical guidelines for adults with asthma and diabetes: a three-year follow-up evaluation of nursing care. *J Clin Nurs.* 2011;20(9-10):1329–1338.

24. Gander L, Delaney C. Saskatchewan Health Quality Council test drives new pressure-ulcer guidelines. *Wound Care Canada.* 2006;4(2):26–27.

25. Kimura S, Pacala JT. Pressure ulcers in adults: family physicians' knowledge, attitudes, practice preferences, and awareness of AHCPR guidelines. *J Fam Pract.* 1997;44(4):361–368.

26. Registered Nurses' Association of Ontario. Toolkit: implementation of clinical practice guidelines. Available at: http://www.rnao.org/Page.asp?PageID=924&ContentID=823. Accessed September 2010.

27. Graham ID, Harrison MB, Brouwers M, Davies BL, Dunn S. Facilitating the use of evidence in practice: evaluating and adapting clinical practice guidelines for local use by health care organizations. *J Obstet Gynecol Neonatal Nurs.* 2002;31(5):599–611.

28. Shiffman RN, Dixon J, Brandt C, et al. The Guideline Implementability Appraisal (GLIA): development of an instrument to identify obstacles to guideline implementation. *BMC Med Inform Decis Mak.* 2005;5:23.

29. Ryan S, Perrier L, Sibbald RG. Searching for evidence-based medicine in wound care: an introduction. *Ostomy Wound Manage.* 2003;49(11):67–75.

30. Best MF, Thurston NE. Measuring nurse job satisfaction. *J Nurs Adm.* 2004;34(6):283–290.

31. Gottrup F. Optimizing wound treatment through health care structuring and professional education. *Wound Repair Regen.* 2004;12(2):129–133.

32. Orsted HL, Woodbury G, Stevenson K. The Wound CARE Instrument. *International Wound Journal.* In press.

33. Beitz JM, van Rijswijk L. Using wound care algorithms: a content validation study. *J Wound Ostomy Continence Nurs.* 1999;26(5):238–249.

34. Hanson DS, Langemo D, Olson B, Hunter S, Burd C. Decreasing the prevalence of pressure ulcers using agency standards. *Home Healthc Nurse.* 1996;14(7):525–531.

35. Usher S, ed. *Health Policy Forum.* Montreal, Canada: June, 1999.

36. Landrum BJ. Marketing innovations to nurses, Part 2: marketing's role in the adoption of innovations. *J Wound Ostomy Continence Nurs.* 1998;25(5):227–232.

37. Suntken G, Starr B, Ermer-Seltun J, Hopkins L, Preftakes D. Implementation of a comprehensive skin care program across care settings using the AHCPR pressure ulcer prevention and treatment guidelines. *Ostomy Wound Manage.* 1996;42(2):20–32.

38. Keast D, Orsted H. The pathway to best practice. *Wound Care Canada.* 2006;4(1):10.

CHAPTER 25

The Outpatient Wound Clinic

Laurel A. Wiersema-Bryant, APRN-BC, CWS;
Linda A. Stamm[†], APRN-BC, CWS[*];
Jennifer A. Berry, FNP-BC;
John P. Kirby, MD, MS, FCCWS, FACS

Objectives

The reader will be challenged to:

- Appraise the need for a dedicated outpatient facility for the coordination and care of patients with wounds
- Assess a wound clinic's ability to coordinate care across medical specialties and to concentrate the use of available resources, both personnel and supplies, to optimally heal wounds
- Fulfill the increased patient demand for wound care excellence as the field develops as an interprofessional specialty.

Introduction

This chapter presents the development of an outpatient wound clinic for the care and management of nonhealing and chronic wounds. The coordinated management of patients with wounds is the focus of an outpatient wound clinic. The concept of an interprofessional team approach to the care of patients with wounds is not new. Utilization of the team approach in the care and management of wounds has been encouraged in acute care and long-term care for some time. Data exist to support the influence of the team approach in achieving cost-effective outcomes.[1] Patients with wounds increasingly are being cared for in the outpatient arena. Reimbursement by third-party payers is largely for wound care given in the outpatient setting. A quick look at the practices in which these patients are being managed traditionally reveals home care, general practitioner offices, general surgery offices, dermatology, rheumatology, hematology/oncology, internal medicine, plastic surgery, orthopedic surgery, cardiology, and vascular surgery. Management of these patients is as varied as the practice settings, so coordination of care can be difficult.

In response to the increasing number of patients with nonhealing and chronic wounds, more wound clinics are being developed. A recent Internet search with the key word "wound clinic" was answered with 4,800,000 results in 0.17 seconds. The key word "wound center" was answered with 25,000,000 results in 0.13 seconds. While there were certainly duplicates in the responses, clearly the concept of moving the challenging wound care patient to a focused

Wiersema-Bryant LA, Stamm LA, Berry JA, Kirby JP. The outpatient wound clinic. In: Krasner DL, ed. *Chronic Wound Care: The Essentials*. Malvern, PA: HMP Communications; 2014:331–340.

Attribute	Facility/Room Design	Equipment Needs
Ambulatory	• Routine • Easy access to parking helpful	• Standard
Wheelchair dependent	• ADA compatible • May need lift assist or ceiling-mounted lift • Evaluate width of doorways and ability to turn into rooms/hallways • Restrooms accessible	• Valet parking helpful • Wheelchairs near entrance • Lift equipment or lift orderlies/techs; check facility for lift policy • Consider ceiling lift in new construction
Stretcher/ambulance	• Easy access for ambulance to deliver • May require more time or additional space for wait for return trip	• Stretcher or bed
Weight challenged	• Exam rooms to accommodate bariatric furniture • Waiting room furniture to accommodate bariatric patients • Doorway/hallway access accommodates bariatric wheelchair/bed/stretcher • Bariatric restroom	• Bed or standing scale that weighs to 1,000 lb • Assorted sizes of blood pressure cuffs • Patient gowns in size 5X to 8X
Cultural diversity	• Exam room furniture to accommodate language interpreter, privacy curtain, etc.	• Mobile video phone if interpreter cannot be physically present

Table 1. Client attributes for consideration

care center is widely accepted. A well planned, well coordinated wound care clinic provides comprehensive assessment, medical and surgical management, state-of-the-art treatment, and follow-up care. The clinic should not be conceived as a place of last resort for treatment failures but as a central place for the management of wounds and patient/caregiver education. This chapter will discuss the process of establishing a wound clinic, ongoing management of the clinic, and areas for further support for the practice of wound care and caring.

Establish the Need

The hospital and/or individuals planning for a wound healing center have several options when developing a model for the practice.[2] A hospital planning for a wound healing center may have the staff and financial support to develop the practice with little or no outside or commercial support. It is estimated that *opening a new practice may cost approximately $350,000 US to $500,000 US* in equipment, space construction/remodeling, and furnishings. The hospital planning committee will also need to develop procedure man-

uals, documentation tools, training costs for staff, recruitment and hiring of staff to supplement current employees, and a plan for ongoing salary needs. The hospital planning group will also want to plan for monitoring of outcomes and collection of data to monitor cost data and to identify persons skilled in maximizing reimbursement and insurance authorization.

Alternatively, *the planning group may elect to work with a commercial company to develop and manage the wound healing center.* The commercial entity then provides the staff, training, and practice policies and assumes the burden of the start-up costs and, in many cases, the salary expenses. This option transfers the cost of start-up and equipment needs to the industry sponsor. In return, the wound care company enters into a fee sharing or monthly management fee to operate the center.

A hybrid of the aforementioned options exists when a planning group retains a consultant to set up the wound healing center. This option allows the facility to maintain ownership of the practice while utilizing procedure manuals, quality assurance programs, documentation systems, and access to established treatment algorithms. The hospital retains ownership of the facility, equipment, billing, and staff hiring and salaries.

The business plan should incorporate the data obtained during the market research phase of the project. Key elements of the business plan include the introduction, vision and mission of the clinic, description of the business, market and competition analysis, product development, marketing and distribution plan, organizational plan, development schedule, financial plan, and executive summary. In determining the direction and focus of the wound clinic, it is important to write a mission statement. The *mission statement* should be global in scope and provide a shared sense of purpose, direction, and achievement both in terms of focusing the clinic and for team building among the clinic staff. Once written, the mission statement will help to define and focus the remainder of the plan. The plan should include both short-term (1 year) and long-term (3 to 5 years) goals. The *goals* should include, but not be limited to, patient visit volume projections, growth in the type of services provided, continued professional development of the clinic staff, research opportunities, monitors for success of the clinic, and cost savings to the institution (if hospital-based). Assuming the market research phase has supported the need for the wound clinic, there are a few additional operational issues that need to be assessed. These issues include the size and type of space needed by the expected population to be served, any special equipment that will be needed, and staffing needs.

A careful and critical look at the business side of the wound healing center is necessary early in the planning process. The selection of a strategy for the formation of the practice and business aspects of the center (or clinic) may prevent struggles in the future.

Needs Assessment

The initial step in the development of a wound clinic is the identification of the need for such a service. Market research must provide clear, concise information about the need for the clinic. *Utilize a marketing department, if available, to assist in the needs assessment process.* In gathering demographic information, a variety of sources may be used:

- Hospital/facility/health authority demographics of patient types
  o Determine the geographic area of the population to be targeted for care
  o Drill down to understand clinical needs of the population to be served (Table 1)
  o Where are patients currently receiving care?
  o Is there sufficient physician/provider commitment for appropriate patient referrals to maintain a stable patient volume?
- Demographic studies by the Centers for Disease Control and Prevention (CDC)/consensus data
- Prevalence data on people with diabetes that may be included in the American Diabetes Association (ADA) database
- State and county health department databases
- American Association of Retired Persons (AARP) database

In essence, the marketing research refines the clinical needs of the patients the center will serve, how many patients the center will serve, and how they will reach the center.

The formation of a center for wound management and healing is a must for most hospitals, as the challenge of chronic wounds is complex and involves multifactorial problems and interprofessional solutions.

Services Offered

The identified needs of the population to be served must be carefully evaluated. The characteristics of the population to whom services will be offered will help to define the professional staff, support/clerical staff, physical design, and location of the wound healing center.

The wound healing center should have available the equipment and staff needed to perform the majority of diagnostic evaluations and treatment modalities within or in close proximity to the clinic. *Universal precautions should be employed for the entire patient population as indicated by the individual facility's policy and procedures.* Diagnostics needed may include radiologic evaluation, vascular laboratory testing, laboratory testing including analysis of blood chemistry and hematology, wound culture (quantitative), and

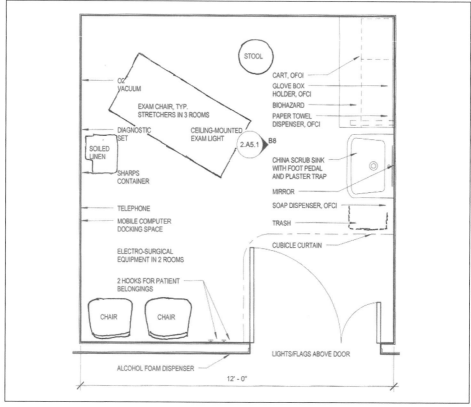

Figure 1. Basic room design.

pathology. Treatment modalities may include surgical intervention and debridement, hyperbaric oxygen, ultrasound therapy, offloading of the neuropathic foot/limb, application of tissue substitutes and grafts, and compression therapy. Planning should include a view to the future with respect to diagnostics and treatment modalities not yet available in clinical practice.

A survey monitoring *the evolving wound care clinic identified 6 basic themes with respect to practice expansion.*[3] The 6 themes are summarized as:

1. Increasing clinic volume
2. Addition of services not currently provided
3. Development of new clinic sites linked to the parent clinic
4. Addition of physician specialists to the clinic staff
5. Increased education
6. A contract with a management company.

Physical Space

The space needed requires a careful, thorough evaluation of the expected patient population. Figure 1 represents a standard exam room that will accommodate a standard exam table, a stretcher, a podiatric chair, or a bariatric exam table/chair. Other configurations exist for multiplace hyperbaric chambers and room configurations from a variety of online resources.

The current obesity epidemic highlights the need for logistical forethought to accommodate patients with special needs or handicaps. This information should be available as a result of the market research data. The following questions must be explored:

- Is existing space available for the clinic?
- Where is the space located?
- If the space is a multifunctional area, is the time needed to efficiently run the clinic available?
- If the clinic is open for patients on a part-

time basis, how will emergency calls/visits be handled?

- How and by whom is the staff to be trained? How will ongoing education be provided?
- How accessible is the location to patients?
- Do you anticipate patients arriving by ambulance, by wheelchair, or ambulatory?
- If the patients are wheelchair- or bed-bound, are stretcher-beds available for them in the facility?
- Is space available to accommodate stretcher- or bed-bound patients?
- If a patient requires lift or transfer assistance, is the clinic able to properly provide this?
- Is public transit available?
- Is accessible parking available?

Portable cautery that can be moved to exam rooms as needed for potential bleeding problems should be made available and staff should be trained on this equipment. Again, universal precautions should be employed for every patient and rooms stocked with protective equipment. Patients of high acuity will most likely need access to parenteral fluids, suction, and oxygen. If every patient exam room does not have these capabilities, patient scheduling is further complicated. If the room space available does not accommodate patients on stretchers, the type of patient seen may need to be restricted to those who are ambulatory or wheelchair-bound. Likewise, *if the appropriate lift equipment is not available, this equipment will need to be added to the start-up costs*. The time to turn a room around will be impacted negatively when patients must be held waiting for lift assistance or ambulance transport.

Staffing and Personnel

Methods of staffing the wound clinic and developing the organizational structure may take on a variety of forms. Generally, staffing requires a medical director and clinic manager, providers representing a variety of specialties, nurses skilled in performing wound care, and a secretary and/or receptionist. Larger clinics may include additional staff (eg, additional physicians specializing in areas not represented by a medical director, physical therapists, a dietitian, an orthoprosthetist, a social worker, home-health nurses, or a combination of these). Providers may be a combination of physicians, nurse practitioners, physician assis-

tants, and others as determined by practice rules as defined by state/country rules. The wound patient population tends to require more nursing time in care and teaching.[4] It may be beneficial to staff the clinic with technical persons who are trained to perform the basics, such as vital signs, dressing removal, and basic wound care. Ancillary staff includes laboratory technicians and financial, legal, supply, and housekeeping personnel. If hyperbaric oxygen therapy is to be offered, trained hyperbaric technicians will need to be added to the treatment team.

The organizational structure establishes the chain of command, and the authority ascribed to the members of the structure can be delineated in the job descriptions. The job descriptions should provide the minimum preparation steps for the position as well as detailed responsibilities for each member of the team. Expectations should be clear and accepted by both the employer and employee. Intervals for performance appraisal should also be identified.

Staffing and Scheduling

The actual daily operations of the wound clinic will depend on a number of factors. If the clinic is set up as a part-time service in a multifunctional area, the time of actual patient visits will be confined to designated hours and day(s) of the week. The opportunity afforded by initially opening as a part-time service takes advantage of existing space and, to some degree, existing staff. This scenario provides low start-up cost relative to hiring staff and renting space for a full-time service. A part-time service also allows for patient volume to build gradually, which is especially important if the volume data gathered during the assessment phase was largely theoretical. One difficulty with a part-time service is providing patients with access to the staff in order to have questions or problems managed after clinic hours. This problem can be easily handled with appropriate telephone triage but needs to be planned prior to the first patient visit (problems or concerns rarely seem to occur during operating clinic hours).

The number of patients scheduled during a given time will depend on the type of visit and the level of acuity. Scheduling is a challenge, as patient visits generally require a disproportionate amount of nursing to physician time. This difficulty can result in lack of efficiency, especially for the physicians/providers. The amount of time needed for direct care, for teaching and support, and for assessment needs to be taken carefully into account. It may be helpful to have a schedule that allows for patient support and teaching after evaluation by the provider(s) and after physician hours in the clinic. Optimally, the reception staff can organize the schedule as it occurs with initial patient evaluations, patients with known time-consuming dressings, or therapies accorded sufficient time. It is helpful to be generous when initially scheduling patients, as well as allowing a greater amount of time for initial visits than for follow-up visits.

The patient visit will be further expedited if additional information is available prior to the visit. If testing is required, it is beneficial to schedule the test to allow time for the results to be obtained by the clinic staff prior to the patient's next appointment. Ideally, noninvasive testing can be performed at the time of the initial visit. Patients referred to the wound clinic may arrive with test results from their referral source, which further facilitates the visit. When testing is required, the patient may require an appointment of several hours in duration; this needs to be considered in the schedule.

Another opportunity for scheduling is managing time for patients participating in clinical trials. In general, the visits for participation in clinical trials are longer and require separate documentation and additional procedures from what may be routine in the clinic. This needs to be communicated to the person scheduling patient visits.

Patients with special needs must have these details communicated to the scheduler. For example, when a patient arrives on a stretcher, requiring a specific exam room, this information should be communicated and the appropriate room reserved. Perhaps a patient is bed-bound and needs to be weighed. With appropriate planning, an appropriate bed scale can be available, as well as the staff to perform the weighing procedure. Patients requiring special assistance may be coded on the schedule to allow for further efficiency in, for example, lift assistance, a specific exam room, testing, and procedures. Other special needs of the patient may also be obtained prior to the visit, including, but not limited to:

- An interpreter for non-English-speaking patients

- An interpreter for the hearing impaired
- Family members if the patient is cognitively impaired
- Coordination with appointments in the facility.

Optimal scheduling requires good communication between the office staff and the clinical staff.

Management of Referrals

The management of patient referrals to the wound clinic depends on timely communication with the referring source. The referral source may be a self-referral, but more likely, it is from a physician or other healthcare provider. *One common complaint about specialty-type clinics is that of inadequate communication with referral sources.* A plan to provide such communication should be in place before the first patient is seen. Another method of minimizing "referral anxiety" is to establish the wound clinic as a "consult" service by stressing that it does not intend to take over primary care of the patient but assists with the management of the patient only with respect to wound care. In fact, in a busy wound clinic, many chronically ill patients can overload the clinic with non-direct wound care activities. Having the primary care physician manage these problems improves wound clinic flow and patient outcome. Rapid communication of the wound care plan and progress to the primary care physician leads to optimal care and future referrals. Unless the wound clinic plans to provide primary care, it is important that all patients seen have a primary care physician.

A wound clinic evaluation plan should be in place from the inception and planning phases. The goal of the evaluation process is to measure progress, monitor outcomes, and evaluate established goals and objectives. Program evaluation may include such issues as infection rate, time to wound closure, recidivism rate, rehospitalization rate, and others. Another aspect of the program to monitor is in the area of demographics. How closely does the actual patient population match the projected statistic? This information is useful for concurrent planning and for the marketing department that may have facilitated the research during the planning phase. Conflicts are minimized if the original mission statement is adhered to and alternative agendas are rejected. Finally, it is helpful to have *periodic team meetings* to discuss the evaluation of findings. Staff meetings provide the opportunity to hear the data, comment on the results, and formulate ideas for future research.

Clinical Management

Assessment. Patient assessment and, specifically, wound assessment can take many forms. As previously described, the first portion of the assessment begins with the receptionist scheduling the patient. *Upon presentation to the clinic, the intake evaluation forms should include an assessment of the history of the wound, any associated pain, and the patient's expectations for the visit.* A wound clinic operating as an outpatient clinic of a hospital will likely have required assessments and forms already in place. A careful medical history and physical exam should be performed. Laboratory studies, including routine hematology, chemistries, nutritional indices, as well as wound culture and possibly tissue for pathology, may be ordered. A nutritional history is also helpful, as is assessment for familial medical history. During the initial interview, it is helpful to obtain social information with respect to smoking, alcohol consumption, exercise regimen, and the availability of support persons. Finally, it is suggested to take an inventory of past and current wound care. When eliciting this information, it is most helpful to identify actual wound care being performed, as this may differ considerably from the current order. The wound profile should be carefully documented. Both quantitative and qualitative information should be gathered.

Quantitative information includes wound size and depth, surface area, a photograph of the wound and surrounding skin, and wound perimeter tracing. If the wound is venous in nature, additional information regarding leg volume with ankle and calf circumference measurements is appropriate. The patient with a diabetic foot ulcer may need neurosensory testing, pressure mapping of the foot, and assessment of the non-involved foot. Tools to assist in quantitative assessment continue to be developed and may be integrated into practice as they become available for bedside use.

Qualitative information includes wound description, description of the peri-wound skin, odor, exudate, edema, anatomic location, pain, type of tissue exposed, and color. (Pain should be quantified with a self-report using a pain scale if possible; we include this assessment as the "5th" vital sign when recording vital signs.)

Depending on the differentiation of wound by type, other testing may be required. Wounds with a potential vascular origin may require vascular testing. Vascular testing generally involves noninvasive testing of pulses, Doppler waveform analysis, ankle brachial Doppler pressure, and transcutaneous oxygen analysis. Invasive vascular testing may involve arteriography. Other vascular testing may be indicated based on clinical assessment. Diagnostic radiography may be indicated to rule out the presence of osteomyelitis. This testing may require plain films, bone scan, or magnetic resonance imaging (MRI). If infection is suspected, a wound bone biopsy may be indicated with operative debridement of the wound.

Many documentation systems exist, including utilization of one of the commercially available computerized tools. A facility may opt to purchase an existing computer-based documentation system or develop a computer database internally. Whichever system is chosen, it should facilitate data management for the tracking of clinical outcomes, cost of care, and other facility needs.

Guidelines. Applicable institutional guidelines may be utilized to the extent to which they fit the needs of the clinic. Applicable general policies may include patient scheduling, staffing, medical authority, documentation, and infection control. The wound clinic team will want to develop guidelines specific to the service. These guidelines may include wound cleansing and debridement, use of sedation, wound culturing, topical wound care, and use of adjuvant management, such as sequential compression therapy, orthotic devices, and pressure relief.

Financial considerations. The responsible provider needs to consider the reimbursement pattern for the expected patient volume. The probable mix of private pay, private insurance, Medicare, Medicaid, and healthcare contracts is important to assess. If an outpatient facility depends heavily on negotiated contracts, it is critical that those in the position of negotiating the contracts be aware of the proposed service. Recommended treatments may not be covered, resulting in potentially suboptimal clinical outcomes and frustrated clients who are unable to obtain supplies and adjuvants for care. Furthermore, these payer mixes and reimbursement contracts are not static and need to be reviewed regularly to align them. Assumptions need to be made from the geographic and demographic information regarding the anticipated volume of patients to be seen during years 1 to 5. The projected volume of service should be described by visit type, procedures, and diagnostic codes so that the capabilities of the clinic can meet (or exceed) the anticipated patient population needs. Another aspect of volume projection is the opportunity for secondary inpatient admissions, surgical procedures, and referrals to other ancillary services as a result of the clinic volume. For example, there should be an anticipated increase in the volume of outpatient vascular studies documenting a wound patient's blood flow. *Cost justification will be apparent to the parent institution through a reduction of inpatient days and hospital re-admission.* Does the proposed patient population require expanded services, such as lymphedema care or hyperbaric oxygen therapy? The field of wound care is an evolving interprofessional specialty and as such needs continued administrative support, physician leadership, and nursing expertise.

When appropriate, individuals may be referred to home care services to provide the wound care needed. Home care then responds by assisting the patient and the family with caring for the wound and assisting with obtaining necessary supplies. If home care is not available, the family and/or significant other is instructed on wound care, and supplies can be ordered through an outside durable medical equipment company.

Additional potential influences on the success of the clinic require one to take a critical look at future trends in healthcare that may impact the clinic. These trends may include but are not limited to political, legal, economical, and social arenas. The economics of a clinic are complex and require the clinician and financial analyst to be clear on financial targets. As clinicians, we advocate that a comprehensive wound clinic is cost effective in managing the patient with a chronic wound. However, from a financial perspective, concentrating this population in one area looks expensive. When the costs of caring for this population are dispersed throughout the healthcare setting, the actual cost of care is offset by those patients whose care is not

as expensive in terms of both dollars and resource utilization. Therefore, this concept, which concentrates the care of the wound patient, now exposes these costs, and the clinician may be faced with developing a strategy to "lose less money" rather than to break even or potentially show a profit.

Billing issues can be a concern for the facility and the practitioner. How the billing will be managed needs to be addressed at this stage of development. Will there be one bill to the patient, which includes professional services as well as facility procedure and dressing charges, or will there be separate professional and facility charges? Standard office reimbursements may not cover the cost of the dressings, which redirects the need for careful discussion with the insurance providers before the clinic opens.

Summary

Running an outpatient wound clinic can be an exciting process. The concept is continuing to evolve. The vitality that can be brought to such a setting will make a difference for the staff, patients, and caregivers. A center focused on the care and management of people with nonhealing and chronic wounds brings together interested professionals who are willing to learn, to teach, and to share with the patient a coordinated approach to an often difficult to manage problem. It is an area where clinical research can be accomplished with a coordinated team effort.

This chapter has focused on the process of formalizing an idea and bringing it to reality with careful research and planning. It is our hope that the concepts presented in this chapter will facilitate the process of opening a wound clinic for those individuals contemplating such a service. Certainly, additional areas could be covered, including the development and use of guidelines for both diagnosis and topical wound care. For additional information on these aspects of operating a wound clinic, we recommend other chapters of this book and other articles on selecting treatment modalities and wound healing and repair (Table 2).

Conclusion

It should be stressed that there are many methods for achieving organized treatment of nonhealing and chronic wounds. Establishing an outpatient wound clinic is simply one of these ways. Even

Table 2. Resources for the clinician		
Publications:	*Advances in Skin and Wound Care*	*Podiatry Today*
	Journal of Wound Care	*Today's Wound Clinic*
	Journal of Wound Ostomy & Continence Nursing	*WoundSource*
	Ostomy Wound Management	*Wound Care Canada*
Guidelines:	AHRQ Clinical Practice Guidelines	
	AMDA Clinical Practice Guideline: Pressure Ulcers	
	Association for the Advancement of Wound Care (AAWC) Guidelines	
	EPUAP NPUAP Pressure Ulcer Guidelines	
	International Pressure Ulcer Prevention Guidelines	
	International Pressure Ulcer Treatment Guidelines	
	Medical Algorithms Project	
	Wound Healing Society Guidelines	
	Wound Ostomy Continence Nursing Society Guidelines	
	World Union of Wound Healing Societies Best Practice Consensus Statements	
Organizations:	American Professional Wound Care Association	
	Association for the Advancement of Wound Care	
	Canadian Association of Wound Care	
	European Pressure Ulcer Advisory Panel	
	National Pressure Ulcer Advisory Panel	
	National Alliance of Wound Care	
	World Union of Wound Healing Societies	
	Wound Healing Society	
	Wound Ostomy Continence Nursing Society	

with respect to the wound clinic, the structure may take many different forms from the model presented here or from any of a number of variations including a "virtual" clinic. The clinic, if it is to be successful, must meet the needs of the population to be served. Therefore, careful analysis of that population cannot be underestimated. Likewise, a careful, realistic appraisal of potential referral sources and competitors needs to be completed. The best designed, best planned clinic will not survive without patients. However, a properly positioned clinic offering a comprehensive approach for patients and their wounds is an opportunity for clinical excellence with cost savings for the institution, improved

outcomes for the patients, and continued professional development for the involved clinicians.

While the primary goal for most wound clinics is achieving wound healing, that goal is not realistic for some of our patients. The team needs to acknowledge that not all patients have wounds that will heal or remain healed. The team should have a plan for those patients who are not following a "healing" trajectory. These patients may require a palliative approach or even referral to other centers. In all instances, qualitative management of wound-related symptoms and wound pain should be recognized as a component of care in the wound clinic.[5]

Self-Assessment Questions

1. What are the key elements in identification of the need for an outpatient wound clinic?
   A. Physician commitment to support and referral is lacking
   B. Market analysis identifies an existing wound center in a nearby facility
   C. The demographics of the population to be served match the proposed service plan
   D. All of the above

2. What are the necessary components of the mission statement?
   A. It is based on one person's ideas
   B. The mission statement is global in scope with a shared sense of purpose, direction, and achievement
   C. The mission statement contains only short-term goals
   D. Team building of staff is not essential in planning for the clinic

3. The business plan should include the following:
   A. Concern regarding costs of operation is not considered in the business plan
   B. Billing issues are not a concern for the facility or practitioner
   C. The marketing plan does not influence the business plan
   D. The economics of a wound clinic are complex and require the clinician and financial analyst to be clear on financial targets

Answers: 1–C, 2–B, 3–D

References

1. Seaman S. Outpatient wound care in a capitated environment: quality care for the patient and an ideal practice for the wound specialist. *Today's Wound Clinic.* 2011;July/August:12–15.
2. Pruneda RC. Development of a wound healing center. In: Sheffield PJ, Smith APS, Fife CE, eds. *Wound Care Practice.* Flagstaff, Ariz: Best Publishing Company; 2004:731–746.
3. Fife C. Reader survey: monitoring the changing wound care clinic. *Today's Wound Clinic.* 2011;July/August:16–18.
4. Sheehan DD, Zeigler MH. Developing an outpatient wound care clinic in an acute rehabilitation setting. *Rehabil Nurs.* 2010;35(3):91–98.
5. Woo K, Sibbald G, Fogh K, et al. Assessment and management of persistent (chronic) and total wound pain. *Int Wound J.* 2008;5(2):205–213.

Authors' Note*
This chapter is dedicated to a pioneer in chronic wound healing, **Linda A. Stamm†, APRN, BC, CWS.**

Since the last edition of Chronic Wound Care, our friend, colleague, and chapter co-author, Linda Stamm, passed away. She was a dedicated nurse who cared for her patients with passionate excellence and ensured that they received the best in care. She helped shape many of the principles covered in this chapter and we dedicate it to the memory of a true wound and ostomy professional.

In conclusion, make a commitment to these **SKILLS** and **PRINCIPLES:**

Seven Chronic Wound Care Skills

1. Respect for patients and caregivers

2. Respect for patient preferences

3. Tenacity

4. Perseverance

5. Creativity

6. Compassion

7. Sharing & Caring

Five Chronic Wound Care Principles

1. Focus on prevention

2. Use gentle techniques

3. Provide timely interventions that meet or exceed the standard of care

4. Be respectful of patient preferences

5. Maintain a holistic perspective

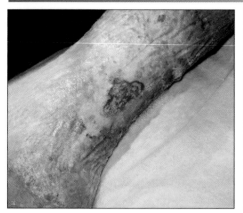

Plate 1. Venous leg ulcer. Chapter 1, p1.

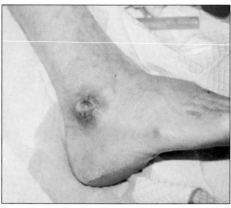

Plate 2. Exquisitely painful pressure ulcer of the lateral malleolus. Chapter 1, p1.

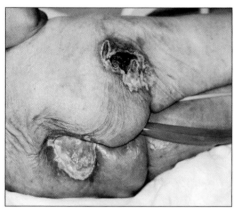

Plate 3. Sacral and trochanteric pressure ulcers with slough and eschar. Chapter 1, p1.

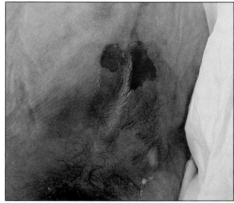

Plate 4. Deep tissue injury. Chapter 1, p1.

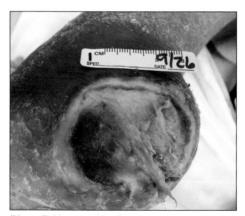

Plate 5. Unstageable. Chapter 1, p1.

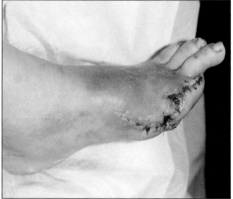

Plate 6. Nonhealing surgical wound with infection in a person with a diabetic neuropathic foot. Chapter 1, p1.

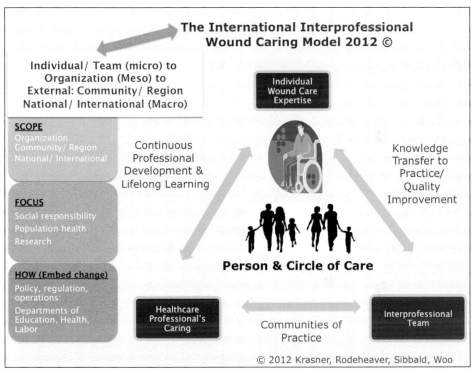

Plate 7. The International Interprofessional Wound Caring Model 2012. Chapter 2, p7.

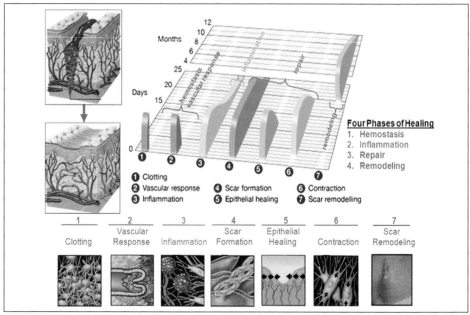

Plate 8. Sequence of wound healing. Normal skin wound healing proceeds through the 4 phases of hemostasis, inflammation, repair, and remodeling. Most chronic wounds get "stuck" in a prolonged inflammatory phase that prevents the wound from moving into an effective repair phase. Adapted from Schultz GS, Ladwig G, Wysocki A. Extracellular matrix: review of its roles in acute and chronic wounds. Available at: http://www.worldwidewounds.com/2005/august/Schultz/Extrace-Matric-Acute-Chronic-Wounds.html. Chapter 3, p17.

Respiratory burst in activated neutrophils and macrophages generates reactive oxygen species (ROS) that chemically kill engulfed bacteria

Activated neutrophils and macrophages secrete proteases that remove damaged extracellular matrix (ECM) components so new scar can form

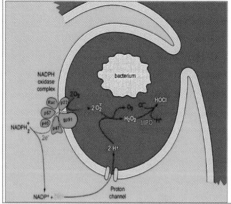

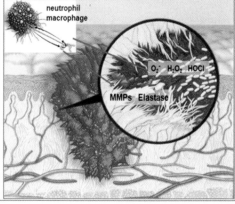

Plate 9. Neutrophils and macrophages perform critical functions in acute wounds by engulfing and killing bacteria and fungi by generation of ROS in endosomes and by releasing proteases that debride the acute wound bed. Chapter 3, p18.

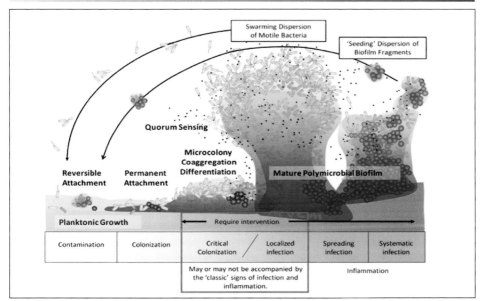

Plate 10. Biofilms in chronic wounds. Planktonic bacteria typically convert into biofilm communities when the levels of quorum molecules reach a threshold and change the pattern of bacterial gene expression. In the spectrum of bacterial bioburden, the concept of critical colonization probably reflects the presence of biofilms, which are not detected by standard clinical microbiology laboratory measurements. Reprinted from Phillips P, Sampson E, Yang Q, et al. Bacterial biofilms in wounds. *Wound Healing S Africa*. Available at: http://www.woundhealingsa.co.za/index.php/WHSA/article/view/17. Chapter 3, p20.

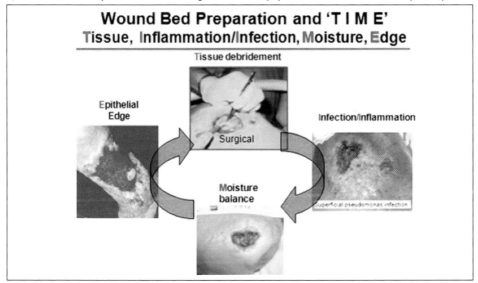

Plate 11. Imbalanced molecular and cellular environments of healing and chronic wounds. The molecular and cellular environment of acute healing wounds is dramatically different than that of chronic wounds and must be "rebalanced" to approximate the environment of healing wounds before healing can progress. Adapted with permission from Mast BA, Schultz GS. Interactions of cytokines, growth factors, and proteases in acute and chronic wounds. *Wound Repair Regen*. 1996;4(4):411. Chapter 3, p23.

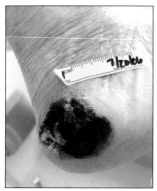

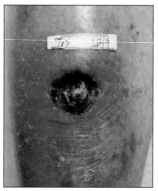

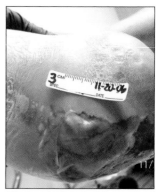

Plate 12. Intact heel eschar on ischemic foot. Chapter 6, p64.

Plate 13. Infected LE wound. Note eschar liquefying in center. Chapter 6, p64.

Plate 14. Acutely infected heel ulcer requiring debridement. Chapter 35, p64.

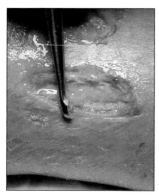

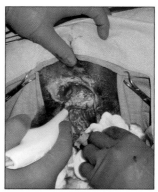

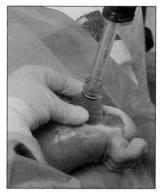

Plate 15. Use of currette to debride ulcer. Chapter 6, p65.

Plate 16. Use of high powered waterjet. Chapter 6, p67.

Plate 17. Pulsed lavage with suction. Chapter 6, p67.

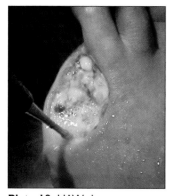

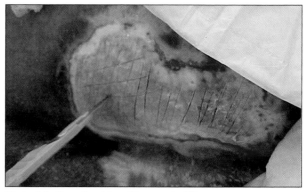

Plate 18. UAW therapy. Chapter 6, p70.

Plate 19. Crosshatching. Chapter 6, p73.

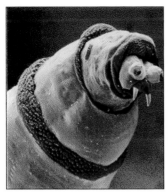

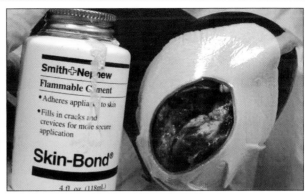

Plate 20. Electron scan of a maggot. Chapter 36 p74.

Plate 21. Hydrocolloid border with skin cement. Chapter 6, p75.

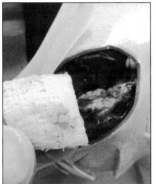

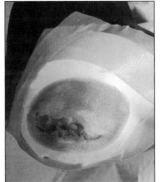

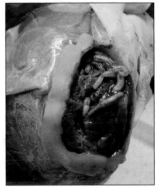

Plate 22. Application of maggots. Chapter 6, p75.

Plate 23. Sealing wound area with veil dressing and taping edges. Chapter 6, p75.

Plate 24. Removal of dressing after 72 hours. Chapter 6, p75.

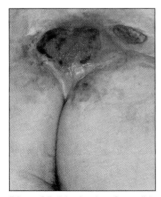

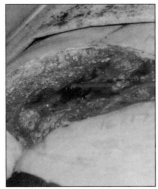

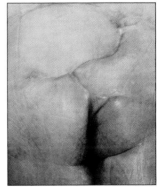

Plate 25. Nonhealing Stage IV sacral pressure ulcer, cleared of candidasis and ready for reconstruction. Chapter 21, p285.

Plate 26. Acute wound following ulcer excision and ostectomy. Chapter 21, p285.

Plate 27. Left gluteal rotation and right gluteal V-Y myocutaneous flap reconstruction. Chapter 21, p285.

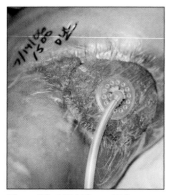

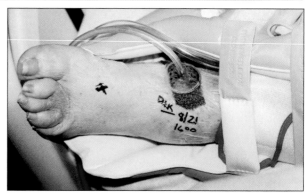

Plate 28. NPWT on thigh wound of IV drug abuser. Chapter 16, p200.

Plate 29. NPWT on debrided heel ulcer bridged to dorsum of foot. Chapter 16, p200.

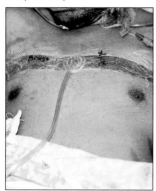

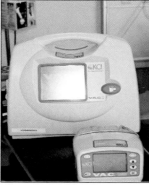

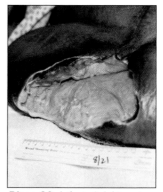

Plate 30. NPWT bridged axilla to axilla s/p excision for hidradenitis suppurativa. Chapter 16, p200.

Plate 31. VAC® ATS pump and VAC® Freedom pump (KCI®). Chapter 16, p200.

Plate 32. Infected dehisced surgical wound s/p bowel resection. Chapter 16, p200.

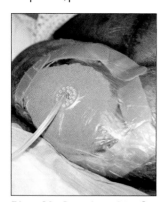

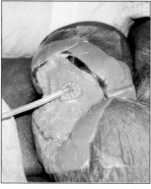

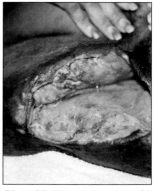

Plate 33. Granufoam Silver® (KCI®) dressing applied to wound from Plate 32. Chapter 16, p200.

Plate 34. Granufoam Silver® (KCI®) at 120 mmHg pressure. Chapter 16, p200.

Plate 35. Wound from Plate 32 with infection clear and wound granulating. Chapter 16, p200.

INDEX

A

AAWC *see Association for the Advancement of Wound Care*

ABPI (Ankle Brachial Pressure Index) 176, 261-2, 266, 268

abrasion 1-2, 32, 34, 151, 153-154, 157, 252

acetaminophen 117-19, 121

acute healing wounds 20-1, 345

acute procedure-related wound pain 122

acute wounds 1-2, 5, 18-19, 21, 24-6, 32, 75, 79, 85, 90, 177-8, 210, 213, 344, 347

ADA *see American Diabetes Association, American Dietetic Association*

adherence 5, 9, 15, 149-50, 153-4, 172, 177, 202-4, 207, 216, 234, 262, 267-8, 274, 286

dressing 155, 170, 200

advanced moist wound therapy (AMWT) 208, 221

Agency for Health Care Policy and Research (AHCPR) *see AHCPR (Agency for Health Care Policy and Research)*

Agency for Healthcare Research and Quality *see AHRQ*

AGREE II instrument 321-2, 329-30

AHCPR (Agency for Health Care Policy and Research) 76, 241, 256-7, 291, 321, 330

AHRQ (Agency for Healthcare Research and Quality) 131, 227, 319-21, 339

albumin 89, 135, 138, 226, 256, 266, 283, 309

alginates 156-7, 159, 162, 169, 187, 208

calcium 157, 169

algorithm 208, 221, 254, 319, 321, 323-5, 327-9

wound classification 32

AMDA (American Medical Directors Association) 144, 339

American Diabetes Association (ADA) 333

American Dietetic Association (ADA) 137, 140, 143-4, 332-3

American Medical Directors Association (AMDA) 144, 339

American Professional Wound Care Association (APWCA) 172, 339

amino acids 81, 134

amputation 2, 126-7, 208, 280, 283-4, 290-1

AMWT *see advanced moist wound therapy*

anaerobes 20, 88-90, 92-3, 96, 99

anemia 80, 85, 107, 140, 144, 179

angiogenesis 64, 69, 73, 80-81, 84, 90, 133, 160-161, 177, 215, 217, 294-295

ankle brachial pressure index *see ABPI*

anti-inflammatory 18, 84, 98, 100, 103, 118-120, 199, 218, 290

anti-inflammatory drugs, nonsteroidal 118-20, 284

antibiotics 21, 24, 52, 54, 58, 72, 74, 87, 97, 100, 103, 106-8, 286, 289, 295

antimicrobial dressings 120, 186, 200, 202, 205

antimicrobial gauze dressings 202

antimicrobials 21, 47, 49, 58, 98, 105, 107, 177, 190, 204, 217

systemic 177

topical 21, 58, 107

antioxidant 135, 157, 160, 280, 289-290

antiseptics 47-8, 54-8, 60-1, 97-8, 161, 169, 190, 282

anxiety 2, 65-6, 72, 113, 116, 118, 121-2, 127

APWCA (American Professional Wound Care Association) 172, 339

arginine 81, 134, 141-2

arterial disease 84, 176, 259, 261, 268

arterial ulcers 5, 100, 283, 313, 316

ascorbic acid 134-5, 141, 143

assessment 29-31, 33-6, 42-5, 116-17, 127-9, 135-7, 191-2, 240, 256-7, 268-9, 288, 311, 316-17, 321-4, 336-7

needs 192, 235, 324, 333

nutrition 136-138, 140

risk *see risk assessment*

vascular 261, 267, 294

wound *see wound assessment*

Association for the Advancement of Wound Care (AAWC) 43-4, 339

ATA 177, 294, 296-7

autolytic debridement 71-2, 74, 100, 156, 168-9

B

bacteria 18-21, 50, 52-7, 65, 69-70, 72, 82, 88-9, 92, 94, 104-5, 109, 150, 152, 168
 planktonic 19, 345
bandages 83, 148, 168, 190, 260, 262-6
Baromedical Nurses Association (BNA) 298
Bates-Jensen Wound Assessment Tool 38
bed, specialty 137, 173, 234-235, 250
bedsores *see pressure ulcers*
best practice guidelines 319-21, 323, 325, 327-30
bioburden 20-1, 23-4, 82, 345
biofilm 17-22, 26, 65, 218, 345
blood supply, adequate 177
BMI (body mass indices) 134, 136-7, 179, 252
BNA (Baromedical Nurses Association) 298
body mass indices *see BMI*
BPGs (Best practice guidelines) 319-25, 327, 329-30
Braden scale 133, 225-242, 254, 311
burn wounds 32-3, 56, 77, 94, 101
burns 34, 61, 101, 103, 110, 143, 150-1, 153-4, 157, 178, 212, 215, 222, 242, 251

C

CAET (Canadian Association for Enterostomal Therapy) 327
calcium 157, 169
calories 135, 139-41, 283
Canada 120, 122, 183, 198, 220, 268, 304, 316-17, 320-1, 323, 328, 330
Canadian Association for Enterostomal Therapy (CAET) 327
Canadian Association of Wound Care *see CAWC*
Cardiff Wound Impact Schedule 126
caregiver education 175, 332
case studies 13, 74, 201, 203
CAWC (Canadian Association of Wound Care) 323, 327, 339
CE (continuing education) 12, 15, 327
CEBM (Centre for Evidence-based Medicine) 320
cellulitis 41, 70, 91-2, 103, 177, 288
Centers for Disease Control and Prevention (CDC) 20, 108, 333

Centers for Medicare & Medicaid Services (CMS) 44, 123, 132, 142, 172, 174, 295, 316
Centre for Evidence-based Medicine (CEBM) *see CEBM (Centre for Evidence-based Medicine)*
chemotherapy 84-5
chlorhexidine 54, 98, 108, 151, 167, 204
chronic inflammation 19, 41
chronic leg ulcers 21-2, 26-7, 45, 60, 76, 158, 210, 222
chronic venous insufficiency *see venous insufficiency*
chronic wound pain experience (CWPE) 112, 121
circle of care 7-9, 11-2, 14-5, 115, 120, 123-4, 129, 171, 308, 310-4
cleansers 48-9, 186
cleansing 38, 40-1, 47-61, 65, 67, 70, 72, 74, 108, 121, 133, 149
clinic *see wound clinic*
clinical practice guidelines *see guidelines*
clinical trials 125, 128, 161, 191, 242, 293-6, 336
 controlled 293, 295
codeine 118-19
cofactors 79-80, 82-5, 135, 308
collagen 18, 27, 72-3, 80-2, 85, 102, 133-5, 152, 161, 187, 197, 217-18, 280, 283, 285-6
collagenase 73-4
colonization 47, 87-9, 106, 288
color 23, 37-8, 40, 102, 284-5, 305, 309, 314-15, 337
communication 12, 33, 43, 141, 204, 308, 310, 312, 328-9, 336
 physician-patient 12, 126, 312
communities 13, 15, 20-1, 140, 157, 345
community of practice (CoP) 13-15
comorbidities 91, 126, 138, 240, 280
compliance 9, 25, 42, 203, 218, 240, 274, 277
compression 10, 100, 103, 175-6, 178, 183, 218, 257, 259-69, 283
 stockings 83, 182, 266-8
compression therapy 103, 176, 259-268, 334
 devices 173
 pneumatic 218, 267
contact layers, intervening 197, 199, 201-3
contamination 43, 51, 54, 68, 82, 88, 94, 158, 198, 210, 288
contraindications 70, 174, 182, 205, 207, 260
controlled trial 27, 53, 57, 75, 110, 114, 178, 208-11, 242, 259, 266

CoP *see community of practice*

cost   9-11, 132, 142, 166-7, 191-2, 211, 225-6, 236, 248-51, 253-4, 256-7, 263-4, 332, 337-8, 340

creams   98, 165, 187, 190

critical colonization   20, 53, 54, 58, 64, 87-8, 92, 100, 103, 120, 167, 345

culture   21-2, 42, 57, 60, 72, 91, 95-7, 109, 140, 156, 324

CWPE *see chronic wound pain experience*

cytokines   20, 22-3, 25-7, 90, 146-7, 160, 163, 217-18, 280, 290, 345

   inflammatory   17-8, 20-3, 26, 64, 177

D

Dakin's   56, 58, 165

debridement   21, 23, 54-5, 58, 63-77, 83, 86, 112, 114, 277, 280, 282-4, 334, 337

   autolytic   71-2

   biotherapy   74-5

   collagenase   73-4

   enzymatic   72, 77

   maggot therapy   74-5

   mechanical   31, 67

decubitus ulcers *see pressure ulcers*

dehisced wounds   70, 196, 202, 205, 213, 218-19

dehydration   135, 138-9, 143, 153, 155, 199, 215, 309

dementia   2, 116

depression   2, 9, 88, 113, 118, 127-8, 130, 178, 309, 314-15

depth   31-5, 38-9, 52, 66, 104, 168, 205, 208-9, 218, 236, 246, 255, 278, 315, 337

dermis   34-5, 281, 309, 315

devices   35, 37, 50-1, 56, 65-6, 70-1, 173-184, 185, 196-201, 219, 230-1, 272-7, 294

DFUs *see diabetic foot ulcers*

diabetes   2, 4, 80-1, 84, 103, 105, 109-10, 126-7, 129-30, 271, 275, 277-8, 281-4, 300-1, 330

diabetic foot ulcers (DFUs)   27, 33-5, 38, 40-1, 44-5, 61, 70-1, 76-7, 126-7, 130, 177-8, 183, 208, 271-278, 300-1

   pain   113, 130

diagnosis   7, 13, 32, 34, 44-5, 60, 81-2, 90-1, 93, 108-9, 183, 281, 283-4, 310, 313

   accurate wound   168

diet   134, 137, 140-4

Dietary Reference Intake (DRI)   135, 143

dietitian   8, 136, 139, 335

   registered   137-8, 238

disability   7, 9

documentation   2, 29, 31, 33, 35, 37-9, 41-3, 45, 55, 307, 312, 322, 325, 329, 336-7

donor sites   156, 159, 211, 282-3, 285

   skin graft   32, 153, 161

doxycycline   24, 27, 107

drainage   25, 64, 70, 72, 82, 91, 168, 170, 180, 190, 195, 218, 264, 280, 282-4, 290

draining wounds   134-5, 139

dressing adherence   155, 170, 200

dressing change   31, 111-12, 114, 116, 120-2, 125, 149-50, 153-4, 159, 162, 167, 171-2, 202, 206-7, 212-13

dressing formulary   171-2

dressing selection   167, 171, 208

dressings, occlusive   88, 202

DRI (Dietary Reference Intake)   135, 143

E

ECM   18, 22, 177, 214-15, 217-18

ECM proteins   18, 22, 25

economics   338

edema   39-41, 90, 92, 105, 113-14, 176-7, 179-80, 212, 215, 218-19, 229, 231, 266-7, 290, 294

edge   18, 23, 36, 64-5, 83, 181

education   16, 89, 112, 117, 120-1, 128, 182-3, 308, 312, 316, 325, 328-9

   caregiver   175, 332

   family   72

   healthcare   15

   patient   117, 208, 268

educational programs   240

effects

   antimicrobial   89, 98, 161, 169

   bactericidal   56, 152, 161

EGF (epidermal growth factor)   22, 160

electrical stimulation (ES)   173, 188

energy source   133-4

enteral nutrition   136, 138, 143

enzyme *see debridement, enzymatic*

INDEX

H

hair follicles 18, 34, 285

hardware, exposed orthopedic 212-13

HBOT 173-4, 177-8, 293-9

    adjunctive 293, 296-7, 301

healability 89

healable wounds 31, 98, 168, 178

healing 17-20, 22-7, 42-4, 53, 55-7, 59-61, 63-4, 74-7, 79-85, 123-5, 127-31, 140-2, 159-63, 276-8, 282-5

    phases of 17, 84

healing process 1, 30, 34, 53, 74, 76, 80, 137, 145-7, 150, 167, 215, 282, 290

healing rates 9, 24, 79-80, 159-60, 196, 211, 260, 275, 278

healing wounds 5, 17, 19-20, 22-3, 61, 74, 82, 85, 133, 345

    cellular environment of acute 20, 345

    environment of 20, 345

Health-related quality of life 123-130

health-related quality of life *see HRQoL*

healthcare 9, 12, 124, 129, 132, 188, 254, 319, 324-5, 329, 338

    evidence-based 320-1

    evidence-informed 13

heel 179-80, 200, 230-2, 240, 247, 253, 257, 273, 282, 310

hemoglobin 66, 80, 140, 309

hemostasis 17, 149, 153, 169, 205, 2007, 288, 344

herbal 118, 140, 218

HIF (hypoxia-inducing factor) 217

high-risk patients 213

holistic 124, 165, 171-3, 191, 325, 329

home care 4, 68, 107, 112, 171, 191-2, 209, 229, 246, 252-4, 327, 331, 338

honey 87, 151, 188-9

hospitals 51, 107, 109, 132, 142, 146-7, 157, 161, 204, 212, 238, 240-2, 325, 332-3, 337

HRQoL (health-related quality of life) 123-30, 301, 307

HRQoL data 125, 129

HRQoL measures 126-9

hyaluronic acid 159, 215, 218

hydrocolloids 75, 93, 102, 152, 157-8, 161-3, 169-71, 189, 207

hydrogels 75, 152, 155-8, 160-3, 169, 171, 188-9, 203, 208

hydrogen peroxide 56, 73, 98, 157, 159-60, 294

hydromorphone 118-19

hydrophobic 154, 169, 200-1

hyperbaric medicine 293-301

hyperbaric oxygen 130, 167, 173, 177, 183, 207, 293-301, 335, 338

hypovolemia 80-1

    subclinical 81

hypoxia, periwound 294, 296

hypoxia-inducing factor (HIF) 217

hypoxic wounds 80, 293, 295

I

immobility 113, 235, 252, 281-2, 284, 286, 290

immune function 134-5, 309

immunocompromise 53, 65, 82, 84, 95, 288

impaired healing 54, 79-85

in-growth 202-4, 207, 216

incidence 2, 3, 50, 101, 104, 151, 178, 208, 210, 225, 253, 268, 283-4

incontinence 1, 113, 132, 149, 158, 178, 186, 208, 226, 237-8, 245, 247, 255, 282, 288, 309

induration 39-40, 82, 288, 290

infected wounds 19, 59-60, 66, 70, 72, 74, 76-7, 90, 106, 150, 152-3, 155, 206, 264, 273

    chronic 90

infection 40-2, 48, 64-5, 80-2, 84-92, 94-6, 98, 103-10, 113-14, 126-7, 140, 177, 205-7, 282-4, 288-90

    acute wound 90

    bacterial 92-6, 299

    chronic wound 88, 90-2, 97, 99, 108, 215

    deep 32, 87, 92, 98, 108, 167

    diagnose 40-1, 90-2

    exotoxin-producing wound 293

    fungal 21, 96, 290

    postoperative wound 59, 294

    risk of 31, 41-2, 67, 84, 89

    signs of 31, 41, 64, 92, 106-7, 121, 310

    treatment 97-109

inflammation 10, 16-19, 23, 39, 41, 83-4, 91-2, 105, 109, 113-14, 140, 143, 161, 163, 290

V

vacuum-assisted closure *see also NPWT* 183, 219-23, 348

vascular ulcers 178

venous insufficiency 2, 67, 92

venous leg ulcers (VLUs) 9, 15, 19, 27, 43, 45, 109, 111, 176, 182-3, 259, 262, 268-9, 317, 323

venous ulcer pain 113

venous ulcers 22, 27, 39, 53, 70, 74, 83, 86, 152, 154, 157-8, 161, 259, 263, 266-9

  chronic 2, 22, 60, 268

vitamins 81-2, 84, 134-5, 139-43, 238, 284, 288, 290

VLUs see venous leg ulcers

W

warmth 39, 41, 82, 92, 168, 288

water 48, 53, 55, 58, 66-7, 74, 94, 100, 134, 143, 149, 151, 153-6, 246, 248

WBP see wound bed preparation

weight 54, 101, 136-7, 139, 157, 178, 233, 236, 246, 248, 252, 322, 332

weight loss 137, 139, 143, 309

  unintentional 137, 143

wet-to-dry dressings 68-9

wheelchair 232-6, 252, 276-7, 332, 335

World Union of Wound Healing Societies (WUWHS) 15, 171, 175-6, 183, 301, 339

World Wide Wounds 171-2, 175

wound assessment 5, 29-45, 85, 106, 166, 183, 311, 316, 327, 337

  comprehensive 112

  daily 31

wound-associated pain 111-14, 118, 121

wound base 40, 70, 168-9, 195, 197, 208, 216-17

wound bed preparation (WBP) 16, 23, 25-7, 76, 86, 97, 109, 122, 166, 183, 215, 223, 323

  assessment tool 23

  paradigm 10, 175, 181

  principles of 25-6

wound cleansing 33, 47-51, 53, 55, 57-9, 61, 113-14, 120, 337

wound clinic 4, 11, 36, 100, 109, 264-5, 325, 331-340

  outpatient 331, 333, 335, 337-40

wound closure 44, 92, 106, 111, 181, 208-10, 280, 284, 288, 336

  accelerated 135

  complete 24, 112

wound contamination 87, 197

wound contraction 200-1, 216, 223

wound culture 82, 106, 333, 337

wound depth 31-3, 35, 39, 43, 102, 209

wound dimensions 35, 201

wound disinfection 47, 49, 51, 53, 55, 57, 59, 61

wound dressings 53, 112, 145-163, 165-172, 185-193, 221, 291

wound edges 16, 31, 36-40, 43, 65, 91, 177, 183, 214, 288

  rolled 39

wound fluids 22, 24, 26-7, 30, 69, 72, 77, 114, 168-9

wound healing 17-19, 21-3, 25-7, 43-5, 69-72, 74-6, 79-81, 83-5, 88-9, 133-5, 160-1, 195-6, 280, 290-1, 293-5

  aid 157, 162

  cascade 63, 90, 146-7, 157, 159-61, 217

  center 332-3, 340

  chronic diabetic foot 23

  complete 30, 282, 296

  cutaneous 2, 81, 83

  delaying 87, 112, 140

  diabetes-related 295

  factors impacting 218

  inflammatory phase of 18, 90, 284, 344

  influence 168

  moist 25, 60, 160, 167, 185

  normal 17-18, 61, 293

  phases of 18, 314

  poor 134

  process 9, 20, 29, 131, 133, 135, 280, 287

Wound Healing Society (WHS) 1, 296, 339

wound infection 2, 40-1, 50-1, 58-9, 61, 74, 80, 82, 88-9, 107-9, 114, 141, 207

  clinical signs of 40

  diagnosing 82

  identifying 45, 110, 122

  local 45

  localized 168

  localized chronic 110, 122

Z